Golden Notes for
Community Health Nursing-I

Golden Notes for Community Health Nursing-I

As per the Revised Syllabus

Parimal Patel
MD (Gold Medalist) DNB (Gold Medalist) PGDMRCH
Faculty
Department of Community Medicine
BJ Medical College
Ahmedabad, Gujarat, India

Khushbu Makadia
MD PGDMRCH
Faculty
Department of Community Medicine
GMERS Medical College
Himmatnagar, Gujarat, India

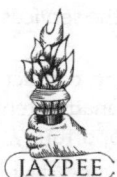

JAYPEE BROTHERS MEDICAL PUBLISHERS
The Health Sciences Publisher
New Delhi | London

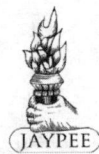 **Jaypee Brothers Medical Publishers (P) Ltd**

Headquarter
Jaypee Brothers Medical Publishers (P) Ltd
EMCA House, 23/23-B
Ansari Road, Daryaganj
New Delhi 110 002, India
Landline: +91-11-23272143, +91-11-23272703
+91-11-23282021, +91-11-23245672
Email: jaypee@jaypeebrothers.com

Corporate Office
Jaypee Brothers Medical Publishers (P) Ltd
4838/24, Ansari Road, Daryaganj
New Delhi 110 002, India
Phone: +91-11-43574357
Fax: +91-11-43574314
Email: jaypee@jaypeebrothers.com

Overseas Office
J.P. Medical Ltd
83 Victoria Street, London
SW1H 0HW (UK)
Phone: +44 20 3170 8910
Fax: +44 (0)20 3008 6180
Email: info@jpmedpub.com

Website: www.jaypeebrothers.com
Website: www.jaypeedigital.com

© 2023, Jaypee Brothers Medical Publishers

The views and opinions expressed in this book are solely those of the original contributor(s)/author(s) and do not necessarily represent those of editor(s) and publisher of the book.

All rights reserved. No part of this publication may be reproduced, stored or transmitted in any form or by any means, electronic, mechanical, photocopying, recording or otherwise, without the prior permission in writing of the publishers.

All brand names and product names used in this book are trade names, service marks, trademarks or registered trademarks of their respective owners. The publisher is not associated with any product or vendor mentioned in this book.

Medical knowledge and practice change constantly. This book is designed to provide accurate, authoritative information about the subject matter in question. However, readers are advised to check the most current information available on procedures included and check information from the manufacturer of each product to be administered, to verify the recommended dose, formula, method and duration of administration, adverse effects and contraindications. It is the responsibility of the practitioner to take all appropriate safety precautions. Neither the publisher nor the author(s)/editor(s) assume any liability for any injury and/or damage to persons or property arising from or related to use of material in this book.

This book is sold on the understanding that the publisher is not engaged in providing professional medical services. If such advice or services are required, the services of a competent medical professional should be sought.

Every effort has been made where necessary to contact holders of copyright to obtain permission to reproduce copyright material. If any have been inadvertently overlooked, the publisher will be pleased to make the necessary arrangements at the first opportunity.

Inquiries for bulk sales may be solicited at: jaypee@jaypeebrothers.com

Golden Notes for Community Health Nursing-I

First Edition: **2023**
ISBN: 978-93-5696-237-8

Printed at: Sterling Graphics Pvt. Ltd. India.

Dedicated to

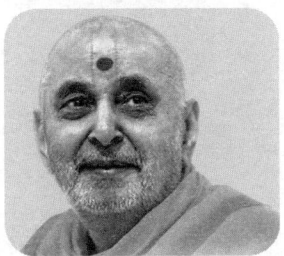

"In the joy of others, lies our own"
Brahmaswarup Shri Pramukh Swami Maharaj

All students S.t.S. are blessed by Pramukh Swami Maharaj

Pragat Brahmaswarup Shri Mahant Swami Maharaj

and
Our Parents

Preface

विद्या नाम नरस्य कीर्तिरतुला भाग्यक्षये चाश्रयो
धेनुः कामदुधा रतिश्च विरहे नेत्रं तृतीयं च सा।।
सत्कारायतनं कुलस्य महिमा रत्नैर्विना भूषणम्
तस्मादन्यमुपेक्ष्य सर्वविषयं विद्याधिकारं कुरू।।

Community Health Nursing is a vital subject for all frontline healthcare workers. It encompasses all the competencies needed to perform the activities of the healthcare delivery system, particularly, National Health Programs. So, this book; **Golden Notes for Community Health Nursing** is our genuine attempt to provide competency-based knowledge of the subject.

This book is designed as per the revised nursing syllabus. This will eliminate the need to refer to any other supplementary books to learn the subject.

Each chapter contains updated information. This book would be the first of its kind as it is written by subject matter experts who have vast experience in academics as well as fieldwork. All the chapters are written in bullet point format along with flowcharts and tables to make it easy for students to learn.

The major extent of *Community Health Nursing-I* is communicable diseases which have been covered extensively in this book. This book is not only for theory purposes but also covers practical aspects of the subject. All chapters of this book is prepared based on the latest information from the Ministry of Health and Family Welfare (MOHFW) guidelines, advisories, and program modules.

Community Health Nursing is a pertinent subject not only from an academic point of view but also from a career point of view, especially for those interested in joining the government sector. We can assure you that this book will help all the students not only to secure good marks in exams but also excel in professional life also.

We are confident that our book **"Golden Notes for Community Health Nursing"** will enable students to function in a variety of settings in either public/government or private healthcare settings.

We always welcome constructive criticism!

Parimal Patel (drparimalpsm3787@gmail.com)
Khushbu Makadia (khushbu20makadia@gmail.com)

Acknowledgments

First of all, we would like to thank Almighty God and our parents for giving us an opportunity to serve society and for placing us where we are today.

We would also like to thank all the nursing college faculties and all nursing students who have helped us in understanding the need of such book and also helping us by reviewing the chapters that helped in improving the content of the book.

Last but not the least; we would like to thank and appreciate Shri Jitendar P Vij (Group Chairman), Mr Ankit Vij (Managing Director), Mr MS Mani (Group President), Dr Madhu Choudhary (Director–Educational Publishing), Ms Pooja Bhandari [Director–Production (Books and Journals)], Ms Sunita Katla (Executive Assistant to Group Chairman and Publishing Manager), Ms Samina Khan (Executive Assistant to Director–Educational Publishing), Ms Alisha Talwar (Content Strategist), Mr Rajesh Sharma (Production Coordinator), Ms Seema Dogra (Cover Visualizer), Mr Deep Dogra (Typesetter), Mr Anil Singh (Proofreader), Mr Pappu Yadav (Graphic Designer), and all the staff of the M/s Jaypee Brothers Medical Publishers (P) Ltd, New Delhi, India, for doing appreciable work in their respective field of printing and publishing.

I also thank Manager and staff of Ahmedabad branch of M/s Jaypee Brothers Medical Publishers (P) Ltd.

Contents

CHAPTER 1: Concepts of Community Health and Community Health Nursing 1

1.1 Definition of Public Health, Community Health and Community Health Nursing 1
1.2 Public Health in India and its Evolution 5
1.3 Scope of Community Health Nursing 10
1.4 Concept, Definition, Dimensions and Determinants of Health and Disease 13
1.5 Health Problems (Profile) of India 23

CHAPTER 2: Healthcare Planning and Organization of Healthcare at Various Levels 26

2.1 Basics of Health Planning 26
2.2 Brief note on Health Planning in India (Various Committees, Commissions on Health and Five-Year Plans) 32
2.3 Community Participation in Health Planning 41
2.4 Overview of Healthcare Delivery System in India 45
2.5 Primary Healthcare and Comprehensive Primary Healthcare 50
2.6 Role of MLHP in CPHC at SC/Health Wellness Center (HWC) 53
2.7 Sustainable Development Goals (2015–2030) 55
2.8 National Health Policy (1983, 2002, 2017) 61
2.9 National Health Mission (NHM) 66
2.10 PM Ayushman Bharat Health Infrastructure Mission (PM-ABHIM) 70
2.11 National Digital Health Mission (Ayushman Bharat Digital Mission) 71
2.12 Ayushman Bharat PMJAY 74
2.13 Universal Health Coverage 77

CHAPTER 3: Environmental Science, Environmental Health, and Sanitation 82

3.1 Brief Note Natural Resources, Ecosystem and Biodiversity 82
3.2 Concept of Environment and Health (House, Water, Air, Noise, Light) 85
3.3 Basics of Different Kinds of Pollution 98
3.4 Climate Change and National Program on Climate Change and Human Health (NPCCHH) 101
3.5 Waste Management 106
3.6 Acts Related to Environment 111
3.7 National Clean Air Program 118

CHAPTER 4: Nutrition Assessment and Nutrition Education 121

4.1 Basics of Nutrition 121
4.2 Nutrition Assessment Methods for Individuals, Families and Community 129
4.3 Concept of Meal and Diet Planning 132
4.4 Purpose, Principles and Methods of Nutrition Education 136
4.5 Overview of Common Nutritional Disorders in India 139
4.6 National Nutrition Policy 1993 142
4.7 Different National Health Programs Related to Nutrition 144
    4.7.1 Poshan Abhiyaan and Mission Poshan 2.0 144
    4.7.2 Pradhan Mantri Matru Vandana Yojana (PMMVY) 146
    4.7.3 Integrated Child Development Services (ICDS) Scheme 147
    4.7.4 Infant and Young Child Feeding (IYCF) 150
    4.7.5 Anemia Mukt Bharat (I-NIPI) 152
    4.7.6 Basics of Vitamin A and Nutritional Blindness 157
    4.7.7 Intensified Mission Indradhanush 4.0 158

Contents

    4.7.8   Intensified Diarrhea Control Fortnight   160
    4.7.9   Nutrition Rehabilitation Center   163
    4.7.10 Home Based Newborn Care and Home Based Care for Young Child   166
    4.7.11 Pradhan Mantri Poshan Shakti Nirman (PM Poshan)   168
4.8   Brief Note on Food-related diseases and Food Safety   169
4.9   Food Safety and Standards Act (FSSA), 2006 and Food Safety and Standards Rules, 2011   178
4.10 Consumer Protection Act (CPA), 1986 and Amended in 2019   181

CHAPTER 5: Concepts of Communication in Health Education   183

5.1   Behavior Change: Concept, Steps, Techniques and Models   183
5.2   Basic Methods of Communication   189
5.3   Barriers to Effective Communication   192
5.4   Social and Behavior Change Communication   194
5.5   Basics of Health Education and Health Promotion   198

CHAPTER 6: Roles, Responsibilities and Approaches of Community Health Nurse   206

6.1   Community Health Nursing Approaches   206
6.2   Role and Responsibilities of Community Health Nurse in Family Health Services (MCH)   208
6.3   Role and Responsibilities of Community Health Nurse during Home Visit
      (Including Bag Technique)   212
6.4   Basics of Counseling   215
6.5   Role and Responsibilities of Community Health Nurse in Supportive
      Supervision and Training   218

CHAPTER 7: Community Health Nurse's Role in Health Promotion and Maintenance   220

7.1   Assessment of Health Status (Anthropometry, BP and Temperature Measurement,
      Breast Self-examination and Lab Tests Like Hb, Urine Sugar and Albumin)   220
7.2   Provision of Primary Health Care   223
      (Routine Health Check-up, Immunization, Counseling, Management of
      Common Health Problems)   223
7.3   Record Keeping   228
7.4   Social Issues Affecting Health and Development of the Family (Women Empowerment, Child
      Abuse, Abuse of Elders, Female Feticide, Commercial Sex Workers, Substance Abuse)   232
7.5   Brief Introduction of Community Resources
      (Old Age homes, Orphanages, Palliative Care Centers, Hospice Care Centers)   236

CHAPTER 8: Epidemiology Made Easy   241

8.1   Epidemiology: Concept and Definition   241
8.2   Basic Tools of Epidemiology   245
8.3   Uses of Epidemiology   246
8.4   Theories of Disease Causation   247
8.5   Modes of Disease Transmission   254
8.6   Glimpse about Important Concepts of Epidemiology   259
8.7   Classification of Different Epidemiological Study Designs   265
8.8   Cross-sectional Study: Design, Steps, Analysis and Interpretation   265
8.9   Case Control Study: Design, Steps, Analysis and Interpretation   267
8.10 Cohort Study: Design, Steps, Analysis and Interpretation   269

8.11	Randomized Control Trial (RCT) Study: Design, Steps, Analysis and Interpretation	271
8.12	Levels of Prevention: Primordial, Primary, Secondary and Tertiary	273
8.13	Outbreak Investigation	275
8.14	Evidence-based Public Health	283
8.15	Screening	285

CHAPTER 9: Communicable Diseases and Relevant National Health Programs — 287

- 9.1 Respiratory Infections 287
  Smallpox 287; Chickenpox 288; Measles 289; Mumps 290; Rubella 291; Influenza 292; Diphtheria 293; Pertussis 294; Tuberculosis 295; Meningitis 295; COVID-19 296; Monkeypox 297
- 9.2 Intestinal Infections 298
  Cholera 298; Typhoid 299; Food Poisoning 300; Poliomyelitis 301; Viral Hepatitis 302; Amebiasis 304; Soil transmitted Helminths 305
- 9.3 Arthropod Infection 309
  Malaria 309; Dengue 312; Chikungunya 314; Filariasis 314; Leishmaniasis 316; Japanese Encephalitis 318
- 9.4 Zoonotic Infections/Diseases 319
  Rabies 321; Plague 323; Anthrax 324; Leptospirosis 325; Brucellosis 326; Kyasanur Foreset Disease 327; Rickettsial 329; Taeniasis 330; Hydatid Disease 331; Hanta Virus 332; Nipah Virus 332; Ebola Virus Disease 334; Crimean Congo Hemorrhagic Fever 334
- 9.5 Other Important Diseases 335
  HIV/AIDS 335; Sexually Transmitted Diseases 336; Trachoma 338; Tetanus 339; Leprosy 340; Yaws 340; Scabies 341; Pediculosis 342
- 9.6 Universal Immunization Program (UIP) 343
- 9.7 National Leprosy Eradication Program (NLEP) 354
- 9.8 The National Tuberculosis Elimination Program (NTEP) 358
- 9.9 Integrated Disease Surveillance Program (IDSP) 372
- 9.10 National AIDS Control Program (NACP) 376
- 9.11 National Vector Borne Disease Control Program (NVBDCP) 380
- 9.12 National Action Plan for Dog Mediated Rabies Elimination from India by 2030 386
- 9.13 National Viral Hepatitis Control Program (NVHCP) 389

CHAPTER 10: Non-communicable Diseases and Relevant National Health Programs — 393

- 10.1 Basics of Non-Communicable Diseases (NCDs) 393
- 10.2 Common Non-Communicable Diseases 400
- 10.3 Common Cancers (Breast, Cervical and Oral) 418
- 10.4 National Program for Prevention and Control of Cancer, Diabetes, Cardiovascular Diseases and Stroke (NPCDCS) and National Program for Healthcare of the Elderly (NPHCE) 424
- 10.5 National Cancer Control Program 428
- 10.6 National Program for Palliative Care 429
- 10.7 National Program for Control of Blindness and Visual Impairment (NPCBVI) 431
- 10.8 National Program for Prevention and Control of Deafness (NPPCD) 432
- 10.9 National Iodine Deficiency Disorders Control Program (NIDDCP) 434
- 10.10 National Tobacco Control Program 435

CHAPTER 11: School Health Program — 439

- 11.1 History of School Health 439
- 11.2 Objectives of School Health 441
- 11.3 Health Problems of School Children 442
- 11.4 Components of School Health Services 443
- 11.5 Initiation and planning of School Health Services 443
- 11.6 Role of a School Health Nurse 445
- 11.7 RBSK/School Health Program 445

Annexures 451
Index 465

Syllabus (BSc Nursing)

COMMUNITY HEALTH NURSING—I

Including Environmental Science and Epidemiology

Theory: 5 Credits (100 hours) includes Lab hours also

Practicum: Clinical: 2 Credits (160 hours)

Description: This course is designed to help students develop broad perspectives of health, its determinants, about community health nursing and understanding about the healthcare delivery services, healthcare policies and regulations in India. It helps the students to develop knowledge and understanding of environmental science. It further helps them to apply the principles and concepts of BCC and health education for health promotion and maintenance of health within the community in wellness and illness continuum. It helps students to practice Community Health Nursing for the individuals, family and groups at rural, urban and tribal settings by applying principles of community health nursing and epidemiological approach. It also helps the students to develop knowledge and competencies required to screen, assess, diagnose, manage and refer clients appropriately in various healthcare settings. It prepares the students to provide primary healthcare to clients of all ages in the community, DH, PHC, CHC, SC/HWC and develop beginning skills in participating in all the National Health Programs.

Competencies: On completion of the course, the students will be able to:
- Explore the evolution of public health in India and community health nursing.
- Explain the concepts and determinants of health.
- Identify the levels of prevention and health problems of India.
- Develop basic understanding about the healthcare planning and the present healthcare delivery system in India at various levels.
- Locate the significance of primary healthcare and comprehensive primary healthcare as part of current healthcare delivery system focus.
- Discuss health care policies and regulations in India.
- Demonstrate understanding about an overview of environmental science, environmental health and sanitation.
- Demonstrate skill in nutritional assessment for different age groups in the community and provide appropriate nutritional counseling.
- Provide health education to individuals and families applying the principles and techniques of behavior change appropriate to community settings.
- Describe community health nursing approaches and concepts.
- Describe the role and responsibilities of community health nursing personnel.
- Utilize the knowledge and skills in providing comprehensive primary health care across the life span at various settings.
- Make effective home visits applying principles and methods used for home visiting.
- Use epidemiological approach in community diagnosis.
- Utilize the knowledge of epidemiology, epidemiological approaches in caring for people with communicable and non-communicable diseases.
- Investigate an epidemic of communicable diseases.

Syllabus (BSc Nursing)

- Assess, diagnose, manage and refer clients for various communicable and non-communicable diseases appropriately at the primary health care level.
- Identify and perform the roles and responsibilities of nurses in implementing various national health programs in the community for the prevention, control and management of communicable and non-communicable diseases particularly in screening, identification, primary management and referral to a health facility/First Referral Unit (FRU).

COURSE OUTLINE

T–Theory

Unit	Time (Hrs)	Learning outcomes	Content	Teaching/learning activities	Assessment methods
I	4 (T)	Define public health, community health and community health nursing Explain the evolution of public health in India and scope of community health nursing Explain various concepts of health and disease, dimensions and determinants of health Explain the natural history of disease and levels of prevention Discuss the health problems of India	**Concepts of Community Health and Community Health Nursing** • Definition of public health, community health and community health nursing • Public health in India and its evolution and scope of community health nursing • *Review:* Concepts of Health and Illness/disease: Definition, dimensions and determinants of health and disease • Natural history of disease • Levels of prevention: Primary, secondary and tertiary prevention–Review • Health problems (Profile) of India	• Lecture • Discussion • Explain using chart, graphs • Community needs assessment (Field survey on identification of demographic characteristics, health determinants and resources of a rural and an urban community) • Explain using examples	• Short answer • Essay • Objective type • Survey report
II	8 (T)	Describe health planning and its steps, and various health plans, and committees Discuss health care delivery system in India at various levels	**Health Care Planning and Organization of Health Care at Various Levels** • Health planning steps • Health planning in India: various committees and commissions on health and family welfare and Five Year plans • Participation of community and stakeholders in health planning • Healthcare delivery system in India: Infrastructure and Health sectors, Delivery of health services at sub-centre (SC), PHC, CHC, District level, state level and national level	• Lecture • Discussion • Field visits to CHC, PHC, SC/ Health Wellness Centers (HWC)	• Short answer • Essay • Evaluation of Field visit reports and presentation

Syllabus (BSc Nursing)

Unit	Time (Hrs)	Learning outcomes	Content	Teaching/learning activities	Assessment methods

		Describe SDGs, primary health care and comprehensive primary health care (CPHC)
		
		Explain health care policies and regulations in India
			• Sustainable development goals (SDGs), Primary Health Care and Comprehensive Primary Health Care (CPHC): elements, principles
			• CPHC through SC/Health Wellness Center (HWC)
			• Role of MLHP/CHP
			• National Health Care Policies and Regulations
			  ▪ National Health Policy (1983, 2002, 2017)
			  ▪ National Health Mission (NHM): National Rural Health Mission (NRHM), National Urban Health Mission (NUHM), NHM
			  ▪ National Health Protection Mission (NHPM)
			  ▪ Ayushman Bharat
			  ▪ Universal Health Coverage
				• Directed reading	

III	15 (T)	Identify the role of an individual in the conservation of natural resources Describe ecosystem, its structure, types and functions Explain the classification, value and threats to biodiversity Enumerate the causes, effects and control measures of environmental pollution Discuss about climate change, global warming, acid rain, and ozone layer depletion	**Environmental Science, Environmental Health, and Sanitation** • *Natural resources:* Renewable and non-renewable resources, natural resources and associated problems: Forest resources, water resources, mineral resources, food resources, energy resources and land resources • Role of individuals in conservation of natural resources, and equitable use of resources for sustainable lifestyles • *Ecosystem:* Concept, structure and functions of ecosystems, types and characteristics—forest ecosystem, grassland ecosystem, desert ecosystem, Aquatic ecosystem, energy flow in ecosystem	• Lecture • Discussion • Debates on environmental protection and preservation • Explain using charts, graphs, models, films, slides	• Short answer • Essay • Field visit reports

Syllabus (BSc Nursing)

Unit	Time (Hrs)	Learning outcomes	Content	Teaching/learning activities	Assessment methods
		Enumerate the role of an individual in creating awareness about the social issues related to environment	• *Biodiversity:* Classification, value of biodiversity, threats to biodiversity, conservation of biodiversity • *Environmental pollution:* Introduction, causes, effects and control measures of air pollution, water pollution, soil pollution, marine pollution, noise pollution, thermal pollution, nuclear hazards and their impact on health • *Climate change, global warming:* e.g., heat wave, acid rain, ozone layer depletion, waste land reclamation and its impact on health • *Social issues and environment:* Sustainable development, urban problems related to energy, water and environmental ethics • Acts related to environmental protection and preservation	• Directed reading • Visits to water supply and purification sites	
		List the Acts related to environmental protection and preservation	**Environmental Health and Sanitation** • Concept of environment health and sanitation • Concept of safe water, sources of water, waterborne diseases, water purification processes, household purification of water	• Observe rain water harvesting plants • Visit to sewage disposal and treatment sites, and waste disposal sites	
		Describe the concept of environmental health and sanitation	• Physical and chemical standards of drinking water quality and tests for assessing bacteriological quality of water • Concepts of water conservation: rain water harvesting and water shed management		
		Describe water conservation, rain water harvesting and water shed management	• Concept of Pollution prevention • Air and noise pollution • Role of nurse in prevention of pollution		

Syllabus (BSc Nursing)

Unit	Time (Hrs)	Learning outcomes	Content	Teaching/learning activities	Assessment methods
		Explain waste management	• Solid waste management, human excreta disposal and management, and sewage disposal and management • Commonly used insecticides and pesticides		

IV	7 (T)	Describe the various nutrition assessment methods at the community level
		
		Plan and provide diet plans for all age groups including therapeutic diet
		
		Provide nutrition counseling and education to all age groups and describe the national nutrition programs
		
		Identify early the food borne diseases, and perform initial management and referral appropriately
			Nutrition Assessment and Nutrition Education
			• Review of Nutrition
			  ▪ Concepts, types
			  ▪ Meal planning: Aims, steps and diet plan for different age groups
			  ▪ Nutrition assessment of individuals, families and community by using appropriate methods
			• Planning suitable diet for individuals and families according to local availability of foods, dietary habits and economic status
			• General nutritional advice
			• Nutrition education: Purpose, principles and methods and rehabilitation
			
			• *Review:* Nutritional deficiency disorders
			• National nutritional policy and programs in India
			Food Borne Diseases and Food Safety
			Food borne diseases
			• Definition, and burden, causes and classification
			• Signs and symptoms
			• Transmission of food borne pathogens and toxins
			• Early identification, initial management and referral
			Food poisoning and food intoxication
			• Epidemiological features/clinical characteristics, types of food poisoning
			• Food intoxication-features, preventive and control measures
			• Public health response to food borne diseases
				• Lecture
				• Discussion
				• Demonstration
				• Role play
				• Market visit
				• Nutritional assessment for different age groups
				
				• Lecture
				• Discussion
				
				• Field visits to milk purification plants, slaughterhouse
				• Refer Nutrition module-BPCCHN Block 2-unit I and UNIT 5
					• Performance assessment of nutrition assessment for different age groups
					• Evaluation on nutritional assessment reports
					
					• Short answer
					• Essay
					
					• Field visit reports

Syllabus (BSc Nursing)

Unit	Time (Hrs)	Learning outcomes	Content	Teaching/learning activities	Assessment methods

V	6 (T)	Describe behavior change communication skills
		
		Counsel and provide health education to individuals, families and community for promotion of healthy life style practices using appropriate methods and media
			Communication management and Health Education
			• Behaviour change communication skills
			  ▪ Communication
			  ▪ Human behaviour
			  ▪ Health belief model: concepts and definition, ways to influence behaviour
			  ▪ Steps of behaviour change
			  ▪ Techniques of behaviour change: Guiding principles in planning BCC activity
			  ▪ Steps of BCC
			  ▪ Social and Behaviour Change Communication strategies (SBCC): techniques to collect social history from clients
			  ▪ Barriers to effective
			• communication, and methods to overcome them
			• Health promotion and Health education: methods/techniques, and audio-visual aids
				• Lecture
				• Discussion
				• Role play
				• Demonstration: BCC skills
				• Supervised field practice
				• Refer: BCC/SBCC module (MoHFW and USAID)
					• Short answer
					• Essay
					• Performance evaluation of health education sessions to individuals and families

VI	7 (T)	Describe community health nursing approaches and concepts	**Community Health Nursing Approaches, Concepts, Roles and Responsibilities of Community Health Nursing Personnel**
			• *Approaches:*
			  ▪ Nursing process
			  ▪ Epidemiological approach
			  ▪ Problem solving approach
			  ▪ Evidence based approach
			  ▪ Empowering people to care for themselves
			• *Review:* Primary health care and Comprehensive Primary Health Care (CPHC)
			Home Visits:
			• Concept, principles, process, and techniques: Bag technique
			• Qualities of community healthnurse
				• Lecture
				• Discussion
				• Demonstration
				• Role plays
					• Short answer
					• Essays

Syllabus (BSc Nursing)

Unit	Time (Hrs)	Learning outcomes	Content	Teaching/learning activities	Assessment methods
		Describe and identify the activities of community health nurse to promote and maintain family health through home visits	• Roles and responsibilities of community health nursing personnel in family health services • *Review:* Principles and techniques of counseling	• Supervised field practice	• Assessment of supervised field practice

VII	10 (T)	Explain the specific activities of community health nurse in assisting individuals and groups to promote and maintain their health	**Assisting Individuals and Families to Promote and Maintain their Health**
			A. *Assessment of individuals and families* (Review from Child health nursing, Medical surgical nursing and OBG nursing)
			• Assessment of children, women, adolescents, elderly, etc.
			• Children: Monitoring growth and development, milestones
			• Anthropometric measurements, BMI
			• Social development
			• Temperature and blood pressure monitoring
			• Menstrual cycle
			• Breast self-examination (BSE) and testicles self-examination (TSE)
			• Warning signs of various diseases
			• Tests: Urine for sugar and albumin, blood sugar, hemoglobin
			B. *Provision of health services/primary health care:*
			• Routine check-up, immunization, counseling, and diagnosis
			• Management of common diseases at home and health centre level
			  ▪ Care based on standing orders/protocols approved by MoHandFW
			  ▪ Drugs dispensing and injections at health centre
			C. *Continue medical care and follow up* in community for various diseases/disabilities
				• Lecture
				• Discussion
				• Demonstration
				• Role plays
					• Short answer
					• Essay
					• Assessment of clinical performance in the field practice area
					
					• Assessment of procedural skills in lab procedures

Syllabus (BSc Nursing)

Unit	Time (Hrs)	Learning outcomes	Content	Teaching/learning activities	Assessment methods
		Provide primary care at home/health centers (HWC) using standing orders/protocols as per public health standards/approved by MoHandFW and INC regulation Develop skill in maintenance of records and reports Develop beginning skills in handling social issues affecting the health and development of the family Identify and assist the families to utilize the community resources appropriately	D. Carry out therapeutic procedures as prescribed/required for client and family E. Maintenance of health records and reports • Maintenance of client records • Maintenance of health records at the facility level • Report writing and documentation of activities carried out during home visits, in the clinics/centers and field visits F. Sensitize and handle social issues affecting health and development of the family • Women empowerment • Women and child abuse • Abuse of elders • Female foeticide • Commercial sex workers • Substance abuse G. Utilize community resources for client and family • Trauma services • Old age homes • Orphanages • Homes for physically challenged individuals • Homes for destitute • Palliative care centres • Hospice care centres • Assisted living facility	• Document and maintain: • Individual records • Family records • Health center records • Field visits	• Evaluation of records and reports • Evaluation of field visit reports
VIII	10 (T)	Describe the concepts, approaches and methods of epidemiology	**Introduction to Epidemiology – Epidemiological Approaches and Processes** • Epidemiology: Concept and definition • Distribution and frequency of disease • Aims and uses of epidemiology • Epidemiological models of causation of disease • Concepts of disease transmission • Modes of transmission: Direct, indirect and chain of infection	• Lecture • Discussion • Demonstration • Role play • Field visits: communicable disease hospital and Entomology office	• Short answer • Essay • Report on visit to communicable disease hospital • Report on visit to entomology office

Syllabus (BSc Nursing)

Unit	Time (Hrs)	Learning outcomes	Content	Teaching/learning activities	Assessment methods
		Investigate an epidemic of communicable disease	• Time trends or fluctuations in disease occurrence • Epidemiological approaches: Descriptive, analytical and experimental • Principles of control measures/levels of prevention of disease • Investigation of an epidemic of communicable disease • Use of basic epidemiological tools to make community diagnosis for effective planning and intervention	Investigation of an epidemic of communicable disease	• Report and presentation on investigating an epidemic of communicable disease

IX	15 (T)	Explain the epidemiology of specific communicable diseases
		
		Describe the various methods of prevention, control and management of communicable diseases and the role of nurses in screening, diagnosing, primary management and referral to a health facility
			Communicable Diseases and National Health Programs
			1. Communicable Diseases – Vector borne diseases (Every disease will be dealt under the following headlines)
			• Epidemiology of the following vector born diseases
			• Prevention and control measures
			• Screening, and diagnosing the following conditions, primary management, referral and follow up
			  ▪ Malaria
			  ▪ Filaria
			  ▪ Kala-azar
			  ▪ Japanese encephalitis
			  ▪ Dengue
			  ▪ Chikungunya
			2. Communicable diseases: Infectious diseases (Every disease will be dealt under the following headlines)
			• Epidemiology of the following infectious diseases
			• Prevention and control measures
			• Screening, diagnosing the following conditions, primary management, referral and follow-up
				• Lecture
				• Discussion
				• Demonstration
				• Role play
				• Suggested field visits
				• Field practice
				• Assessment of clients with communicable diseases
					• Field visit reports
					• Assessment of family case study
					• OSCE assessment
					• Short answer
					• Essay

Syllabus (BSc Nursing)

Unit	Time (Hrs)	Learning outcomes	Content	Teaching/learning activities	Assessment methods
			<ul><li>Leprosy</li><li>Tuberculosis</li><li>Vaccine preventable diseases—diphtheria, whooping cough, tetanus, poliomyelitis and measles</li><li>Enteric fever</li><li>Viral hepatitis</li><li>HIV/AIDS/RTI</li><li>infections</li><li>HIV/AIDS, and Sexually Transmitted Diseases/ Reproductive tract infections (STIs/RTIs)</li><li>Diarrhoea</li><li>Respiratory tract infections</li><li>COVID-19</li><li>Helminthic – soil and food transmitted and parasitic infections – scabies and pediculosis</li></ul>3. Communicable diseases: Zoonotic diseases<ul><li>Epidemiology of zoonotic diseases</li><li>Prevention and control measures</li><li>Screening and diagnosing the following conditions, primary management, referral and follow up<ul><li>Rabies: Identify, suspect, primary management and referral to a health facility</li></ul></li><li>Role of a nurses in control of communicable diseases</li></ul>**National Health Programs** 1. UIP: Universal Immunization Program (Diphtheria, Whooping cough, Tetanus, Poliomyelitis, Measles and Hepatitis B) 2. National Leprosy Eradication Program (NLEP) 3. Revised National Tuberculosis Control Program (RNTCP) 4. Integrated Disease Surveillance Program (IDSP): Enteric fever,		
		Identify the national health programs relevant to communicable diseases and explain the role of nurses in implementation of these programs			

Syllabus (BSc Nursing)

Unit	Time (Hrs)	Learning outcomes	Content	Teaching/learning activities	Assessment methods
			5. Diarrhea, Respiratory infections and Scabies 6. National Aids Control Organization (NACO) 7. National Vector Borne Disease Control Program 8. National Air Quality Monitoring Program 9. Any other newly added program		
X	15 (T)	Describe the national health program for the control of non-communicable diseases and the role of nurses in screening, identification, primary management and referral to a health facility	**Non-Communicable Diseases and National Health Program (NCD)** • National response to NCDs (Every disease will be dealt under the following headlines • Epidemiology of specific diseases • Prevention and control measures • Screening, diagnosing/ identification and primary management, referral and follow up care **NCD-1** • Diabetes mellitus • Hypertension • Cardiovascular diseases • Stroke and obesity • **Blindness:** Categories of visual impairment and national program for control of blindness • **Deafness:** National program for prevention and control of deafness • **Thyroid diseases** • **Injury and accidents:** Risk factors for road traffic injuries and operational guidelines for trauma care facility on highways **NCD-2 Cancers** • Cervical Cancer • Breast Cancer • Oral cancer • Epidemiology of specific cancers, risk factors/ causes, prevention, screening, diagnosis – signs, signs and symptoms, and early management and referral	• Lecture • Discussion • Demonstration • Role play • Suggested field visits • Field practice • Assessment of clients with non-communicable diseases Participation in national health programs	• Field visit reports • Assessment of family case study • OSCE assessment • Short answer • Essay

Syllabus (BSc Nursing)

Unit	Time (Hrs)	Learning outcomes	Content	Teaching/learning activities	Assessment methods
			• Palliative care • Role of a nurse in non-communicable disease control program **National Health Programs** • National Program for Prevention and Control of Cancer, Diabetes, Cardiovascular Diseases and Stroke (NPCDCS) • National Program for Control of Blindness • National Program for Prevention and Control of Deafness • National Tobacco Control Program • **Standard treatment protocols used in National Health Programs**		
XI	3 (T)	Enumerate the school health activities and the role functions of a school health nurse	**School Health Services** • Objectives • Health problems of school children • Components of school health services • Maintenance of school health records • Initiation and planning of school health services • Role of a school health nurse	• Lecture • Discussion • Demonstration • Role play • Suggested field visits • Field practice	• Short answer • Essay • Evaluation of health counseling to school children • Screen, diagnose, manage and refer school children • OSCE assessment

Note: Lab hours less than 1 credit is not specified separately.

Syllabus (GNM)

COMMUNITY HEALTH NURSING-I

Placement- First Year **Time- 180 hours**

CHN-I – 80 hours Environmental Hygiene- 30 hours
Health Education and Communication skills- 40 hours
Nutrition- 30 hours

Course Description

This course is designed to help students gain an understanding of the concept of community health in order to introduce them to the wider horizons of rendering nursing services in a community set-up, both in urban and rural areas.

General Objectives

Upon completion of this course, the students shall be able to:
- Describe the concept of health, community health and community health nursing.
- State the principles of epidemiology and epidemiological methods in community health nursing practice.
- Explain the various services provided to the community and role of the nurse.
- Demonstrate skills to practice effective nursing care of the individuals and families in the clinics as well as in their homes, using scientific principles.

Total Hours – 80

Unit No.	Learning objectives	Content	Hrs	Teaching/learning activities	Method of assessment
I	Describe the concept of health and disease and community health	**Introduction to Community Health** • Definitions: Community, community health, community health nursing • Concept of health and disease, dimensions and indicators of health, health determinants • History and development of community health in India and its present concept • Primary health care, Millennium Development Goals • Promotion and maintenance of Health	10	Lecture-cum-discussions	Short answers
II	Explain various aspects of Community Health Nursing. Demonstrate skills in applying nursing process in Community Health Nursing settings	**Community Health Nursing** • Philosophy, goals, objectives and principles, concept and importance of Community Health Nursing, • Qualities and functions of Community Health Nurse	14	Lecture-cum-discussions	• Short answers • Essay type

Syllabus (GNM)

Unit No.	Learning objectives	Content	Hrs	Teaching/learning activities	Method of assessment
		• Steps of nursing process; community identification, population composition, health and allied resources, community assessment, planning and conducting community nursing care services.			
III	Demonstrate skill in assessing the health status and identify deviations from normal parameters in different age groups.	**Health Assessment** • Characteristics of a healthy individual • Health assessment of infant, preschool, school going, adolescent, adult, antenatal woman, postnatal woman, and elderly.	10	Lecture-cum-discussions Demonstration Role play Videos	• Short answers Objective type Essay type • Return demonstration
IV	Describe the principles of epidemiology and epidemiological methods in community health nursing practice.	**Principles of Epidemiology and Epidemiological methods** • Definition and aims of epidemiology, communicable and non-communicable diseases. • Basic tools of measurement in epidemiology • Uses of epidemiology • Disease cycle • Spectrum of disease • Levels of prevention of disease. • Disease transmission—direct and indirect. • Immunizing agents, immunization and national immunization schedule. • Control of infectious diseases. • Disinfection.	10	Lecture cum discussions Non-communicable disease module of government of India. Field visit	• Short answers Objective type Essay type
V	Demonstrate skill in providing comprehensive nursing care to the family.	**Family Health Nursing Care** • Family as a unit of health • Concept, goals, objectives • Family health care services • Family health care plan and nursing process. • Family health services—maternal, child care and family welfare services. • Roles and function of a community health nurse in family health service. • Family health records.	12	• Lecture-cum-discussions • Role play • Family visit	• Short answers • Essay type
VI	Describe the principles and techniques of family health care services at home and in clinics	**Family Health Care Settings Home Visit:** • Purposes, principles • Planning and evaluation • Bag technique • Clinic: Purposes, type of clinics and their functions • Function of health personnel in clinics	10	• Lecture-cum-discussions • Demonstration • Visits – Home, health center	• Short answer • Return demonstration

Syllabus (GNM)

Unit No.	Learning objectives	Content	Hrs	Teaching/learning activities	Method of assessment
VII	Describe the referral system and community resources for referral	**Referral System** • Levels of health care and health care settings. • Referral services available • Steps in referral. • Role of a nurse in referral	6	• Lecture-cum-discussions • Mock drill	• Short answer • Objective type
VIII	List the records and reports used in community health nursing practice	**Records and Reports** • Types and uses • Essential requirements of records and reports • Preparation and Maintenance	3	• Lecture-cum-discussions • Exhibit the records	• Short answer • Objective type
IX	Explain the management of minor ailments	**Minor Ailments** • Principles of management • Management as per standing instructions/orders.	5	• Lecture-cum-discussions	• Short answer • Objective type

CHAPTER 1

Concepts of Community Health and Community Health Nursing

CHAPTER OUTLINE
- 1.1 Definition of public health, community health and community health nursing
- 1.2 Public health in india and its evolution
- 1.3 Scope of community health nursing
- 1.4 Concept, definition, dimensions and determinants of health and disease
- 1.5 Health problems (profile) of India

1.1 DEFINITION OF PUBLIC HEALTH, COMMUNITY HEALTH AND COMMUNITY HEALTH NURSING

PUBLIC HEALTH
- Public health: "The science and art of preventing disease, prolonging life and promoting health and efficiency through organized community effort" (Winslow).
- Henry Siegerist: He stated that there is a system of medicine in every culture.
- Dubos: He believed that ancient medicine is the mother of all sciences and human development has organic relationship with the medicine.

Primitive Medicine
During this phase people used to believe that diseases occur due to wrath of gods or due to invasion of evil spirits or due to influence of stars and planets (this is collectively called as **supernatural theory of disease**).

Ayurveda
- Ayurveda means knowledge of life.
- It is derived from Atharveda.

- It is practiced throughout the India.
- It is based on **Tridosha (humors)** theory:
  - Vata (Wind)
  - Pitta (Gall)
  - Kapha (Mucus)
- Disease occurs as result of disequilibrium between these three doshos (humors).
- Dhanvantri is God of Ayurveda.
- Atreya is known as great Indian physician and teacher.
- Charak is father of Indian Medicine.
- Susruta is father of Indian Surgery.

Chinese Medicine

- It is the world's first organized system of medicine.
- It is based on **Yang and Yin principle**.
- Good health depends on balance between Yin (negative, dark, and feminine) and Yang (positive, bright, and masculine).
- Chinese medicine is known for acupuncture and barefoot doctors.
- They are the pioneer for the immunization.

Egyptian Medicine

- No anatomy practice allowed during this phase as they believed in preservation of human body as "mummies".
- They were known for the civilization, sanitation, etc.
- Famous manuscripts of these periods are:
  - Edwin Smith Papyrus: for surgery
  - Ebers Papyrus: for medicine

Mesopotamian Medicine

- Mesopotamia is the region between two rivers namely Eupharates and Tigris.
- This area also known as "Cradle of Civilization".
- There were the group of doctors during this period:
  - Herb doctors: Just like internists
  - Knife doctors: Like surgeons
  - Spell doctors: Like psychiatrists

Greek Medicine (Unani System of Medicine)

- Aesculapius (Greek medicine leader) had two daughters:
  1. Hygiea (Goddess of Health)—gaves rise to Primitive Medicine
  2. Panacea (Goddess of Medicine)—It formed Curative Medicine
- Greek medicine is based on four humors:
  1. Phlegm
  2. Yellow Bile
  3. Black Bile
  4. Blood
- Disease occurs as result of disequilibrium between these four humors.

Homeopathic Medicine

- **Samuel Hahneman** was German physician and known as **Father of Homeopathy**.
- There are 4 principles of homeopathy:
  1. **Similia Similbus Curentur:** A homeopathic drug produces same set of signs and symptoms that normally disease does.
  2. **Single Remedy:** Only one homeopathic drug is given at one point of time.
  3. **The Minimum Dose:** Minimum possible dose of drug is used.
  4. **The Potentized Remedy:** Drug is diluted many times.

Siddha System of Medicine

- Siddha system of medicine is used by Tamil people in India and abroad as well.
- This system is based on three physiological component as below:
  1. Air (Vaadham)
  2. Fire (Pitham)
  3. Earth and water (Kabam)
- It is believed that success of the treatment depends on environment, age, sex and other factors.

COMMUNITY HEALTH: AN INTRODUCTION

- **Community:** It is a social group determined by geographical boundaries and/common values and interests. Its members know and interact with each other. It functions within a particular social structure and exhibits and creates certain norms, values and social institutions. Example of Community can be like rural community and urban community, etc.
- **Community Health:** It refers to the health status of the members of the community, to the problems affecting the health and to the totality of healthcare provided for the community. The major determinants of community health are the health status, disease patterns and health expectations of the people. Community health postulates a unified and balanced integration of promotive, preventive, curative and rehabilitative services.
- Rapid social and economic growth it has resulted in an increase both in the number of elderly people who are prone to degenerative and chronic diseases, and new patterns of illnesses that are brought on by social and economic factors, such as occupational hazards, accidents, and environmental poisonings caused by air pollution, noise and contaminated water.
- Communities are struggling as they receive minimal or no healthcare because they cannot afford or access services.
- Nurses have always cared for individuals, families and communities in their practice, primarily in community-based settings that focus on individuals and families.
- There is also increasing emphasis on community focused nursing care with the community as the client.
- Evidence suggests that increasing attention to healthy lifestyles and healthy behaviors prevents health problems and reduces health risk and threats. Strengthening the community healthcare system based on primary healthcare is thus the focus of healthcare reform.
- Practically and preferably, professional nursing services focusing on providing health care and services to the entire community is an ideal solution to meeting the demands of community healthcare.
- Students must be prepared to meet the needs of populations rather than institutions.

COMMUNITY HEALTH NURSING: CONCEPT, SCOPE, EVOLUTION AND PRINCIPLES

- **Definition of Community Health Nursing by WHO:** A special field of nursing that combines the skills of nursing, public health and some phases of social assistance and functions as part of the total public health program for the promotion of health, the improvement of the conditions in the social and physical environment, rehabilitation of illness and disability.
- **Definition of Community Health Nursing/Public Health Nursing by American Nursing Association (ANA):** Public health nursing is the practice of promoting and protecting the health of populations using knowledge from nursing, social and public health sciences (Waldorf, 1999).
- Community Health Nursing combines nursing and public health. It synthesizes the body of knowledge from the public health sciences and professional nursing theories. The purpose of this synthesis is to improve the health of the entire community. Thus, community health nursing can be defined as a field of practice that synthesizes, knowledge and skills in nursing, public health and applies them toward the promotion of optimal health for the total community.
- The primary goal of community health nursing is to help a community protect and preserve the health of its members, while the secondary goal is to promote self-care among individuals and families.
- Many factors have influenced the growth of community health nursing like advanced technology, progress in casual thinking, changes in education, the changing role of the nurse and the consumer movement.
- **Characteristics of Community Health Nursing:** Six characteristics of community health nursing are:
  1. Basically a field of nursing as basic knowledge and skills are of professional nursing practice are applied here also. Basic Nursing skills with addition of concepts, knowledge and skills from other disciplines makes community health nursing a distinctive discipline.
  2. Combination of two disciplines like public health and nursing.
  3. Population oriented with mission to improve the health of the population groups.
  4. Emphasizes on positive health or wellness. Community health nursing aims to prevent health problems and to promote a higher level of health.
  5. Involves interdisciplinary collaboration as health always requires support from different sectors. Community health nurses working as dedicated team member and at the same time contributing by thinking and acting independently can make great contribution to the team effort and over organizational goals.
  6. Encourages community participation by promoting their sense of responsibility for their own health.

The Four Major Goals of Community Health Nursing

1. Helping the individual, family, groups and community to reach the optimum level of well being
2. Providing comprehensive care
3. Preserving the autonomy
4. Improving nursing and community health practice

The Four Core Functions of Community Health Nursing Practice

1. Community social capital, including community culture, and identification of resources as key actors in the community healthcare system
2. Assessment of community health conditions, health risks and problems to identify the healthcare demands of the people
3. Design and implementation of comprehensive community health interventions, care, services and programs, and
4. Health policies/agreements developed at the local community level to drive policies/agreements at the state and national levels for collaborative endeavors and actions.

BIBLIOGRAPHY

1. https://www.nursingworld.org/
2. https://apps.who.int/iris/bitstream/handle/10665/204726/B4816.pdf
3. https://www.egyankosh.ac.in/bitstream/123456789/34331/1/Unit-1.pdf

1.2 PUBLIC HEALTH IN INDIA AND ITS EVOLUTION

DEVELOPMENT OF PUBLIC HEALTH IN INDIA BEFORE INDEPENDENCE

- **Vedic Period (3000 BC to 1400 BC):** It was period of ancient civilization existed in Indus valley. During this time there were planned cities and practice of good environmental sanitation. Ayurveda and Siddha systems of medicine were also in practice.
- **Post Vedic Period (600 BC to 600 AD):** Jainism and Buddhism were most accepted religions during this time period. Ancient universities of Nalanda and Taxila were the main hub for medical education. Expansion of Hospital system was done by King Ashoka.
- **Mughals Period (650 AD to 1750 AD):** Under the rule of Muslim emperor, Unani system of medicine was introduced for the first time in India and gradually it became part of Indian System of Medicine.
- **British Period (19th Century to Mid 20th Century):** During this phase many good initiatives were taken for better community health and examples are:
  - Quarantine Act, 1825
  - Birth and Death Registration Act, 1873
  - Vaccination Act, 1880
  - First Census and First Indian Factories Act, 1881
  - Epidemic Disease Act, 1897
  - Establishment of Lady Reading Health School in 1918 for training of Lady Health Visitors for rural and urban health centers
  - Workmen Compensation Act, 1923
  - Child Marriage Restraint Act (SARDA) 1929–1930, age of marriage is 14 years for girls and 18 years for boys
  - All India Institute of Hygiene and Public Health was established in 1930 in Calcutta
  - Maternal and Child Welfare Bureau was established in 1931 by Red Cross Society

Concepts of Community Health and Community Health Nursing

- Pre-Independence Period (1943–1946): During this period in 1943, Bhore Committee was set up to survey the existing health conditions of the people in India and final report submitted in 1946 with recommendations for improvement of health of people in India.
- In 1947, MOH-Established with creation of post of DGHS.

Development of Public Health in India after Independence

Year	Act/Program/Plan/Other
1948	ESI Act
1951	• First Five Year Plan • National Family Planning Program • BCG Vaccination Started
1952	• Community Development Program • Central Council of Health Formed
1953	National Malaria Control Program
1954	• National Water Supply and Sanitation Program • PFA Act
1955	• National Filaria Control Program • National Leprosy Control Program
1956	• Second Five Year Plan (1956–1961) • The Immoral Traffic Act
1958	• The National Malaria Eradication Programme • Panchayati Raj (Balwantrai committee)
1959	• Mudaliar Committee (Report In 1961) • Panchayati Raj Adopted For The First Time By Rajasthan State
1961	• 3rd FYP (1961–1966) • Dowry Prohibition Act • Maternity Benefit Act
1962	• National Smallpox Eradication Program • School Health Program • National TB Control Program • National Goiter Control Program
1963	• National Trachoma Control Program • Chadha Committee
1966	• Mukherjee Committee • Department of Family Planning Constituted
1969	• 4th FYP (1969–1974) • The Central Birth And Death Registration Act (1969)
1970	• The Drugs (Price Control) Order • All India Hospital (Postpartum) Family Planning Program
1971	• The Medical Termination of Pregnancy • Urban Malaria Scheme
1973	• Kartar Singh Committee (Multipurpose Health Worker)
1974	• 5th FYP • Water (Prevention and Control of Pollution) Act, 1974

Concepts of Community Health and Community Health Nursing

Year	Act/Program/Plan/Other
1975	ICDS
1976	NPCB
1977	• ROME Scheme • Kalaazar Control Program • Modified Plan of Operation
1980	• On 8th May, Smallpox was Eradicated • 6th FYP
1981	• The Air (Prevention and Control of Pollution) Act • 20 Point Program
1982	National Mental Health Program
1983	• NLEP • National Health Policy • Guinea Worm Eradication Program • National Plan of Action Against Available Disablement Known As "Impact India"
1984	Bhopal Gas Tragedy
1985	• 7th FYP (1985–1990) • Universal Immunization Program • Narcotics Drugs and Psychotropic Substance Act
1986	• Juvenile Justice Act • Consumer Protection Act (CPA)
1987	• NACP • Mental Health Act
1989	Blood Safety Program
1991	Baby Friendly Hospital Initiative
1992	• 8th FYP (1992–1997) • National Iodine Deficiency Disorder Control Program (It has replaced National Goiter Control Program) • CSSM • The Infant Milk Substitute, Feeding Bottles and Infant Foods (Regulation of Production, Supply and Distribution Act) • NACP-1 (1992–1997) • NFHS-1 (1992–1993)
1993	• RNTCP as pilot project • Protection of Human Rights
1994	• PNDT (Came into Force in 1996) • Transplantation of Human Organ Act
1995	Pulse Polio Immunization (First Round: 9th Dec-1995, 20th Jan 1996)
1996	Yaws Eradication Program Launched
1997	• RCH-I Launched • 9th FYP Launched
1998–2004	Modified Leprosy Elimination Campaign

Year	Act/Program/Plan/Other
1998–99	• NFHS-II • NMEP Renamed As National Anti Malaria Program • NACP-II (1992-2004) • Biomedical Waste (Management and Handling-1998)
2000	• National Population Policy • Information Technology Act
2001	National Policy for Empowerment of Women
2002	• National Health Policy • National AIDS Prevention and Control Policy
2003	• 10th FYP • COTPA Act • NVBDCP
2004	• IDSP Launched • Launching of Vandemataram Scheme • Low Dose Osmolarity ORS
2005	• RCH-II • JSY • NRHM • IPHS for CHC • Disaster Management Act • NAREGA • RTI
2006	• New Growth Chart (WHO) • RNTCP-Implementation in whole Country • NFHS-III (2005-2006) • IMNCI • Food Standard and Safety Act
2007	• 11th FYP • NACP-III (2007-2012) • IPHS for PHC and SC
2008	NPCDCS
2009	Pandemic Swine (H1N1) Flu
2011	NPHCE
2012	• 12th FYP • Protection of Children of POCSO Act • NACP-IV (2012-17)
2013	• RMNCH+A • NHM
2014	• Indian Newborn Action Plan (27th March) • Mission Indradhanush (25th December)
2015	• NITI Aayog replaced Yojana Aayog • Introduction of IPV • Swachh Bharat Abhiyan
2016	• SDG • Malaria Eradication Plan (2016-2030) • Introduction of bOPV(Switch)

Concepts of Community Health and Community Health Nursing

Year	Act/Program/Plan/Other
2017	- National Strategic Plan for HIV/AIDS and STI 2017–2024 - National Action Plan to combat Antimicrobial Resistance (2017–2021) - National Nutrition Mission - National Health Policy, 2017 - National Mental Health Care Act, 2017
2018	- Ayushman Bharat (PM-JAY) - Allied and Healthcare Professions Bill, 2018 - Nikshay Poshan Yojna (April 2018) - National Viral Hepatitis Control Program (28th July, 2018)
2019	- National Medical Commission Bill, 2019 - IDCF (28th May–8th June, 2019) - E-Cigarettes Prohibition Act (18th September, 2019) - TB Harega, Desh Jitega Campaign (25th September, 2019) - RNTCP renamed as NTEP - SUMAN (October, 2019) - SAANS (November, 2019) - IMI 2.0 (1st Round)-December, 2019
2020	- COVID-19 declared as Public Health Emergency of International Concern (30th January) - COVID-19 nomenclature declared on 11th February, 2020 - COVID-19 Declared as Pandemic by WHO (11th March, 2020) - IMI 2.0 (4th Round)-March, 2020
2021	- Nationwide COVID-19 vaccination started on 16th January, 2021 - National Policy for Rare Diseases on 30th March, 2021 - Polio Eradication Strategy 2022–2026: Delivering on a Promise launched on 10th June, 2021 - Ministry of Health and family Welfare (MoHFW) approved the vaccination of pregnant women against COVID-19 on 2nd July, 2021 - Global Youth Tobacco Survey (GYTS-4), India, 2019 National Fact Sheet released on 10th August, 2021 - Ayushman Bharat Digital Mission launched on 27th September, 2021 - National Action Plan for dog Mediated Rabies Elimination by 2030 launched on 28th September, 2021 - WHO approved use of the RTS,S/AS01 (RTS,S) malaria vaccine among children in sub-Saharan Africa and in other regions with moderate to high P. falciparum malaria transmission on 6th October, 2021 - PM Ayushman Bharat Health Infrastructure Mission on 25th October, 2021 - Nationwide expansion of Pneumococcal Conjugate Vaccine (PCV) under the Universal Immunization Program (UIP) on 29th October, 2021 - IMI 3.0 (November, 2021)
2022	- IMI 4.0 (Feb-April 2022) - NACP-5 (2021-2026)-approved on 21st March, 2022 - IDCF-2022 launched on 13th June, 2022 - Pradhan Mantri TB Mukt Bharat Abhiyan launched on 9th September, 2022 - National list of Essential Medicines (13th September)
2023	- Introduction of third dose of fIPV to be given at 9 months of age - International Year of Millets

1.3 SCOPE OF COMMUNITY HEALTH NURSING

AREAS OF CONCERN FOR COMMUNITY HEALTH NURSING

Areas of Concern for Community Health Nursing
- Chronic diseases and prolonged hospitalization
- Problems of the geriatric population
- Population explosion and sociocultural factors affecting family planning
- Pollution including air, water, soil, noise, and radiation
- Industrialization and urbanization
- Addiction to tobacco, alcohol, and drugs
- Adulteration of drugs and food
- Home care, nursing home, school health, mental health, and rehabilitation centers.

Objectives of Community Health Nursing
- Provide antenatal, intranatal, and postnatal care to ensure safe pregnancy and delivery
- Immunization
- Provide under five children care
- Health education
- Community empowerment to improve their ability to deal with their own health problems
- To strengthen the community resources
- To prevent and control communicable and noncommunicable diseases
- To provide specialized services
- To conduct research

Principles of Community Health Nursing
- Community health nurse must know the community thoroughly.
- Community health nurse must have ability to work effectively as team.
- Community health nurse is answerable to the appointing authority.
- Community health nurse must maintain professional relationship with authority from health and other related department. She must also maintain etiquette with every member of the community.
- Community health nurse should provide services to all the members of the community irrespective of age, gender, religion, caste, or socioeconomic condition.
- Community health nurse should not indulge in any nonprofessional activity.
- Community health nurse should never accept any bribes in any form including cash or gifts.
- Community health nurse should give priority to felt needs of the people.
- The expectations of services from community health nurse must be realistic in manner with taking into consideration the availability of manpower and other facilities.
- Community health nurse must impart health education at every opportunity.
- Community health nurse must provide continuum of care and continuous care by strengthening follow-up.
- Services provided by community health nurse to be assessed periodically.
- Community health nurse must be maintaining all the records of services provided.
- Career progression options for community health nurse must be clearly defined.

- Community health nurse must practice first before teaching to the community members or even colleagues.
- Integration of health education, guidance, and supervision with community health nursing services.
- Community participation is the integral part of the community health services.
- Individual and family member's participation in decision making.
- Proper evaluation of health services.

Competencies for Community Health Nurse

- Basically, there are two sets of competencies: (1) core competencies and (2) the complementary competencies.
- While in core competencies, there are two competencies like one for clinical care, and another for implementing the four functions of community healthcare.
- Competencies for clinical care range from health assessment, disease management, case finding, case management, observation, and treatment according to delegated responsibility, etc.
- Competencies for the four functions rely heavily on the means and methods employed to implement each function.
- Another set of complementary competencies may include cultural sensitivity, participatory research, leadership, development of tools and guidelines for data collection and analysis, and experiential learning through action.
- Competency mapping is crucial for designing both the theory and the practice aspects of community health nursing courses.

Aspects of Community Heath Nurse can be easily depicted by the each alphabet of the word itself: **COMMUNITY HEALTH NURSE.**

- **C:** Consultant (care provider), Counselor, Collaborator
- **O:** Organizer
- **M:** Motivator
- **M:** Manager
- **U:** Utilizer of manpower
- **N:** Nurse practitioner
- **I:** Independent
- **T:** Teacher, Trainer
- **Y:** Youth at Heart
- **H:** Helper
- **E:** Educator, Encouraging
- **A:** Advocate, Accessible, Adequate provision of services
- **L:** Leader
- **T:** Team member
- **H:** Honest
- **N:** Neutral, Nobility
- **U:** Unbiased
- **R:** Responsible
- **S:** Sympathetic
- **E:** Efficient

Six major roles of community health nurse have been identified:
1. Care provider
2. Educator
3. Advocate
4. Manager
5. Collaborator
6. Leader

Qualities of community health nurse are shown in **Figure 1.1**.

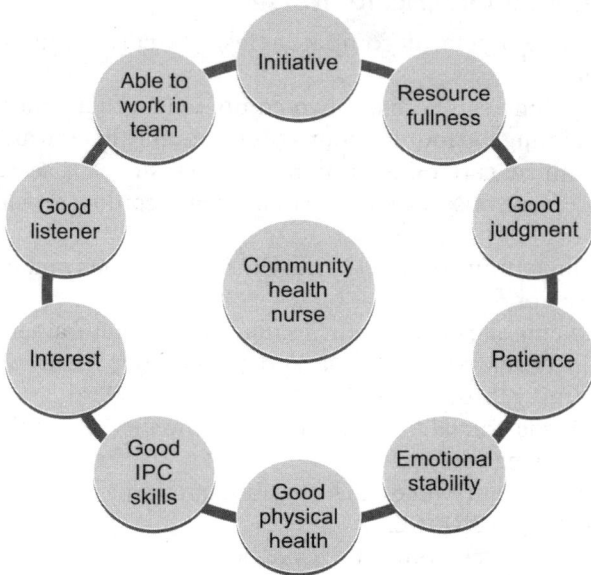

Fig. 1.1: Qualities of community health nurse.

The community healthcare system represents at least five layers of care that respond to the comprehensive healthcare demands of its people. The five layers include:
1. Individual self-care,
2. Family care,
3. Care and support among neighbors and groups in the community,
4. Care and support given by healthcare providers and healers, and
5. Welfare and support provided by community allies such as the local administrative government, community organizations such as community health funds, community funds, and cremation fund, social welfare office, etc.

BIBLIOGRAPHY

1. eGyanKosh—a National Digital Repository. (2017). Community health nursing: Concepts and principles. [online] Available from https://www.egyankosh.ac.in/bitstream/123456789/34331/1/Unit-1.pdf. [Accessed December, 2022]
2. eGyanKosh—a National Digital Repository. (2017). Roles and responsibilities of community health nursing personnel. [online] Available from http://egyankosh.ac.in/bitstream/123456789/33204/5/Unit-2.pdf. [Accessed December, 2022]

1.4 CONCEPT, DEFINITION, DIMENSIONS AND DETERMINANTS OF HEALTH AND DISEASE

CONCEPT OF HEALTH

Biomedical Concept:
The biomedical concept based on the "germ theory of disease".
The biomedical concept of health has been considered unsatisfactory as it ignores the role of environmental, social, cultural and psychological determinants of health.
The Biomedical concept of health has been proven inadequate to explain some of the major problems like malnutrition, chronic diseases, drug abuse, mental illness, etc.

↓

Ecological Concept:
As per the ecological concept, health is a state of harmonious equilibrium between human beings and their environment, and disease a state of mal-adjustment of the human being to the environment.
For example, deforestation on a large scale has changed the climate which in turn leading to famine, floods and starvation with consequent disease problems.
It is argued that better adaptation of human beings to natural environments leads to a longer life expectancy and a better quality of life.

↓

Psychosocial Concept:
This concept is based on the fact that health is not only a biological phenomenon, but also a social one.
Factors such as psychological, socio-cultural and economic also affect health. Social customs and practices relating to diet of a pregnant or lactating woman, feeding an infant, and marriage between relatives have major impact on the health status of the individuals, such as those.

↓

Holistic Concept:
The holistic concept of Health is the synthesis of all above mentioed concepts of health and thus it is the most acceptable concept of health.
The holistic concept implies a sound mind, in a sound body, in a congenial family, in a good environment. The holistic concept thus recognizes that all sectors of society have an effect on health, and emphasizes the protection and promotion of health.

Definition of Health

- World Health Organization's definition of health: "Health is a state of complete physical, mental and social well-being and not merely an absence of disease or infirmity." In recent time, this definition has been expanded to include the ability to lead a "socially and economically productive life".
- This concept of health by WHO is broad and positive in its implications.
- It sets out the standard; the standard of "positive health", towards which all of us should strive.

Positive Health

- The Positive Health implies "perfect functioning of the body and mind in the social environment".
- It means
  - Biologically: Every cell and organ of the body is functioning at optimum capacity and in perfect harmony.
  - Psychologically: The individual feels a sense of well-being.
  - Socially: Individual's capacities for participation in the social system are optimal.
- In short, a person enjoys health at all physical, mental and social levels.

Quality of Life

- It is defined by WHO as "the product of the interplay between social, health, economic, and environmental conditions which affect human and social development".
- It is a broad-ranging concept, incorporating a person's physical health, psychological state, level of independence, social relationships, personal belief and relationship to salient features in the environment.
- It is consisting of individual's own subjective evaluation like feelings of happiness.

HUMAN DEVELOPMENT INDEX (HDI) VS. PHYSICAL QUALITY OF LIFE INDEX (PQLI)

	HDI (developed by Indian economist Amartya Sen and Pakistani economist Mahbub ul Haq)	PQLI (developed by Morris David Morris)
Components	1. Longevity – Life expectancy at birth (LEB/ LE0) 2. Income (Real GDP per capita in PPP US$) 3. Knowledge (Mean years of schooling – Gross enrolment ratio & Literacy rate)	1. Life expectancy at 1 year age (LE1) 2. Infant mortality rate (IMR) 3. Literacy rate
Range	0 to +1	0 to 100
Value of India	0.633	65
Rank of India	132	–

Dimensions of Health

Physical Dimension

- Physical well-being implies a "state in which every cell and organ is functioning at optimum capacity and in harmony with the rest of the body".
- It is a very important dimension of health.
- Physical dimension of health is easy to identify as signs of physical well-being of a person are:
  - Lustrous hair, healthy scalp and good complexion
  - Clean skin and firm flesh
  - Bright, clear eyes
  - No skeleton malformation
  - Normal weight and height for age
  - Well-developed and firm muscles
  - Smooth, easy, coordinated body movements
  - Bowels and bladder function are intact and regular
  - Good appetite and sound sleep
- In such a state, the organs of the body are of normal size and function normally, and all the senses (such as sight and hearing) are intact.
- Physical health can be assessed by measures such as clinical examination, dietary and nutritional assessment and laboratory investigations.

Mental Dimension
- Mental health is a vital component of total health.
- It is basic for dealing effectively with reality, with oneself and with others.
- Only a mentally healthy person is able to handle life problems in such a way as to provide a feeling of personal satisfaction and to contribute satisfactorily to the welfare of the society.
- **A person who is mentally healthy is one who is:**
  - Free from unsolvable internal conflicts and is able to arrive at decisions
  - Is confident about own abilities but also recognizes own faults
  - Has high self-esteem
  - Assumes responsibilities according to own capacity and finds satisfaction in their accomplishment
  - Is not in the habit of condemning or pitying all the time
  - Is able to handle any situation without getting too upset or tense
  - Has good control over own emotions and does not give in frequently to strong Feelings of fear, jealousy, anger or guilt
  - Adapts to situations and people
  - Is sensitive to the emotional needs of others
  - Deals with others with consideration
  - Is well adjusted and gets along well with others
- Poor mental health affects physical health and vice-versa.
- Psychological factors play a major role in physical disorders like stomach ulcer, bronchial asthma and high blood pressure just like that congenital heart condition is likely to influence mental health.

Social Dimension
- Along with taking care of physical and mental well-being we need to take care of social dimension of health as well.
- As per social dimension a healthy person should be able to adjust in the community to function for the betterment of the community. It is possible when person sees him or herself as member of a larger community, the quantity and quality of interpersonal relationships and the extent of involvement with the community.
- Person should fulfil own social obligations to the family as well as the community.
- The three dimensions of health, physical, mental and social well-being are closely interrelated and change in any one of them is normally accompanied by changes in the other aspects too.
- For example, if we are suffering from any mental issue then due to that we may lose our appetite and gradually our physical well-being may get affected. The same is true vice versa as if we are having any chronic physical problem then it definitely affects out mental health.

Spiritual Dimension
- With widely acceptance of holistic concept of health, spiritual dimension getting its due consideration.
- Spiritual dimension talks about the meaning and purpose of life.
- Spiritual health includes integrity, ethics, belief in concepts that may not have a scientific explanation, commitment to some higher being.
- A person has to be at peace with oneself before can be at peace with the world.

Emotional Dimension

- Normally it seems that emotional dimension is closely related to mental dimension.
- However, with advancement of research it has been found there is definite difference between these two dimensions.
- Mental health which something related to knowing or cognitive while emotional dimension talks about feeling.

Vocational Dimension

- The vocational aspect of life is part of human existence.
- When work is fully adapted to human goals, capacities and limitations, it often plays a role in promoting both physical and mental health.
- Completion of work is usually associated with an improvement in physical capacity (physical health) and satisfaction and enhanced self-esteem (mental health).
- The vocational aspect influences and is influenced by the other dimensions of health.
- For example: Unsatisfied person with own job is likely to feel frustrated all the time, with accompanying feelings of anxiety, anger and/or low self-esteem. These affect both physical and social health.
- And Person is not likely to be at peace either with oneself or with the world. This affects spiritual well-being.

Other Dimensions

Other dimensions include: Philosophical dimension, cultural dimension, socio-economic, environmental dimension, educational dimension, nutritional dimension, curative dimension and preventive dimension.

Determinants of Health (Fig. 1.2)

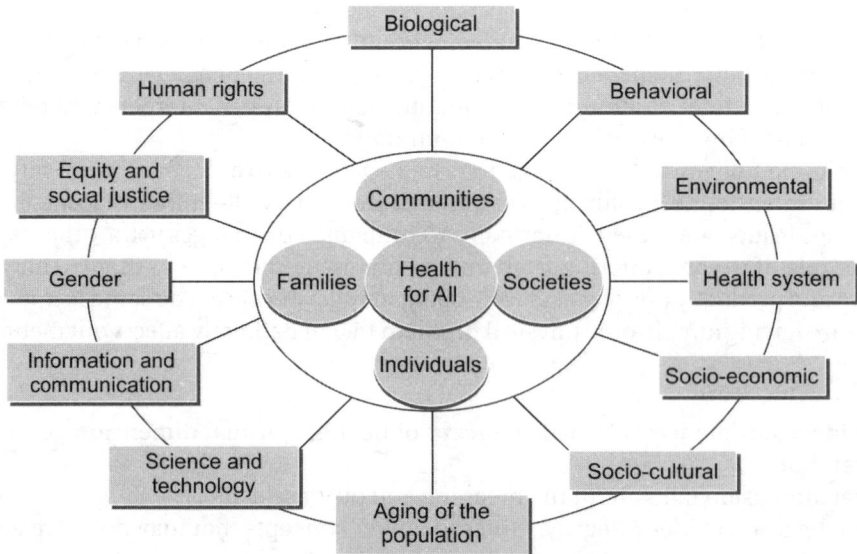

Fig. 1.2: Determinants of health.

The Determinants of Health

- **Biological determinants of health**
  - Biological determinants, also referred to as "inborn" factors influencing health, are mainly genetic. Diseases due to genetic origin are, e.g., chromosomal anomalies, mental retardation, errors of metabolism, etc.
- **Behavioral and sociocultural determinants of health**
  - Evidence suggests that there is an association between health and lifestyle of individuals.
  - Health problems like coronary heart disease, obesity, addiction, etc. are associated with lifestyle changes. Healthy lifestyle promotes the health through physical activity, proper nutrition, adequate sleep, good habits and better cultural patterns, etc.
- **The environmental determinants of health**
  - Initially Hippocrates and later on Pettenkofer revived the concept of disease environment association.
  - Environment is classified as "internal" and "external". The **internal** environment includes "each and every component part, every tissue, organ and organ system and their harmonious functioning within the system".
  - The **external** is also known as macro-environment. It is defined as all that which is external to the individual human host. It can be divided into physical, biological and psychosocial components, any or all of which can affect the health of man and his susceptibility to illness. It also includes eating habits, addiction, occupation, etc.
- **Health services**
  - It includes immunization, maternal and child health services, provision of safe water, etc. All the health services must be accessible, acceptable, affordable and equitably distributed.
- **Socio-economic conditions**
  - **Economic status:** The per capita GNP is the measure of general economic performance. The economic status determines the purchasing power, standard of living, quality of life, health seeking behavior and the pattern of disease and deviant. Currently disease like obesity, coronary heart disease are more found in higher socio-economic population.
  - **Education:** Education plays most important role in better health. It indirectly affects the higher infant mortality, malnutrition, poor health, etc. Kerala having higher female literacy and lower infant mortality.
  - **Occupation:** Individual having productive work promotes the health. In reverse scenario like loss of employment leads to loss of income, psychological and social damage.
  - **Political system:** The percentage of GNP spent on health is a quantitative indicator of political commitment. The WHO has set the target of at least 5% expenditure of each country's GNP on healthcare. Political commitment and leadership can be helpful to eliminate health hazard and diseases.
- **Aging of the population**
  - More than two-thirds of people aged 60 and over, are of living in developing countries. Aging process require special attention.
- **Gender**
  - Men and women suffer from different types of diseases at different ages.
  - Gender discrimination might affect the health.
- **Other factors**
  - Health related systems, e.g., education, food and agriculture, industry, etc., are also helpful.

- In recent era, information and technology department plays important role to dissemination of health information worldwide.

Indicators of Health

Characteristics of indicators: Reliable, valid, sensitive, specific, feasible, relevant.

Classifications

- Morbidity indicators
- Mortality indicators
- Disability rates
- Nutritional status indicators
- Healthcare delivery indicators
- Utilization rates
- Indicators of social and mental health
- Environmental indicators
- Socio-economic indicators
- Health policy indicators
- Indicators of quality of life, and
- Other indicators

Morbidity Indicators

Morbidity is generally measured by following indicators:
- Incidence and prevalence
- Notification rates
- Admission, readmission and discharge rate
- Duration of hospital stay
- Spells of sickness

Incidence

- We usually measure incidence of any disease through conducting longitudinal studies like cohort study.
- It is calculation of occurrence of new cases of specified disease in a given area during specified period of time in population at risk for developing disease.
- For meaningful calculation of incidence every individual included in the denominator must have the potential to be part of the numerator.
- For example: To calculate incidence of uterine cancer the denominator should include only women because men are not at risk of developing uterine cancer.

Formula: (number of new cases of a disease in the population during specified period of time/ number of persons who are at risk of developing disease during that period of time) × 1000
- Multiplier can be anything from 1000....to 1 million or any other figure.

Prevalence

- **Definition of prevalence:** 'The total number of all individuals who have an attribute or disease at a particular time (or during a particular period) divided by the population at risk of having the attribute or disease at this point in time or midway through the period'.
- It is total cases (new plus old) in a given population over a point or period of time.

Concepts of Community Health and Community Health Nursing

- It measures through cross sectional study.
- Prevalence = incidence * duration of disease. (it must be steady situation in which rates are not changing and in-migration equals out-migration)
- Prevalence measures burden of disease in the community that's why it is valuable for planning health services.
- **There are two types:**
  1. **Point prevalence.**
  2. **Period prevalence.**

Point Prevalence
- Number of all current new cases plus old cases of a specified disease in the population existed at given point in time/total estimated population at the same point in time* 100
- If we ask do you currently have the disease? Then this will get us point prevalence of that disease at that point of time.

Period Prevalence
- Number of new cases plus old cases of a disease for given time period/total population at risk* 100
- If we ask have you had the disease during the last ten years? Then this will get us period prevalence for that period.
- Period prevalence is less commonly used measure of morbidity.

Mortality Indicators
- Crude death rate
- Specific death rate
- Age specific death rate
- Case fatality rate
- Disease specific proportional mortality rate
- Infant mortality rate
- Under-5 proportionate mortality rate
- Child mortality rate
- Maternal mortality rate
- Proportional mortality rate
- Years of potential life lost
- Survival rate

Crude Death Rate
Crude death rates have major limitation like lack of comparability between population or community that differ by age, gender, etc.

$$= \frac{\text{Total number of deaths during the year}}{\text{Mid-year population}} \times 1000$$

Specific Death Rate
- It helps to know the etiology.
- There are broadly classified as cause or disease specific (e.g., cancer, tuberculosis, accident) and age or gender specific

Age Specific Death Rate

$$= \frac{\text{Total number of deaths in specific age group during the year}}{\text{Mid-year population of same age group}} \times 1000$$

Case Fatality Rate (Ratio)

$$= \frac{\text{Number of deaths due to a particular disease}}{\text{Total number of cases due to the same disease}} \times 100$$

- It denotes the killing power of a disease and virulence of an organism.
- It is more useful for the acute infectious diseases (e.g., food poisoning, cholera, measles).
- It has limited role in chronic disease.

Proportional Mortality Rate (Ratio)

- It is generally used to measure the burden of the disease.
- It helps to calculate proportion of total deaths due to particular cause (e.g., tuberculosis) or proportion of total deaths in a particular age group (e.g., above the age of 60 years).

Proportional Mortality from a Specific Disease

$$= \frac{\text{Number of deaths from the specific disease in a year}}{\text{Total deaths (including all causes) in that year}} \times 100$$

Infant Mortality Rate (IMR)

$$= \frac{\text{Number of deaths of children less than 1 year of age in a year}}{\text{Number of live births in the same year}} \times 1000$$

Under-5 Proportionate Mortality Rate

$$= \frac{\text{Number of deaths less than 5 years of age in the given year}}{\text{Total number of deaths during that year}} \times 100$$

Maternal Mortality Ratio

$$\text{MMR} = \frac{\text{Total no. of female deaths due to complications of pregnancy, childbirth or within 42 days of delivery from ``puerperal causes'' in an area in a given year}}{\text{Total no. of live births in the same area and year}} \times 100{,}000$$

Years of Potential Life Lost (YPLL)

- It is defined as one that occurs before the age to which a dying person could have expected to survive.
- It is calculated based on the years of life lost through premature death.

Survival Rate

- It is useful to know prognosis of disease and assessment of outcome of standard of therapy.

$$\text{Survival rate} = \frac{\text{Total number of patients alive after 5 years}}{\text{Total number of patients diagnose or treated}}$$

Disability Rates
Types

Event-type indicators	• Number of days of restricted activity • Bed disability days • Work-loss days (or school-loss days) within a specified period
Person-type indicators	• Limitation of mobility (ex like confined to bed or house) • Limitation of activity (it includes eating, moving, work etc)

Health-adjusted Life Expectancy (HALE)

HALE is based on life expectancy at birth but includes an adjustment for time spent in poor health. It is most easily understood as the equivalent number of years in full health that a newborn can expect to live based on current rates of ill-health and mortality.

Quality-adjusted Life Years (QALY)

QALY is a measure of disease burden including both the quality and quantity of life lived. It is used in assessing the value for money of a medical intervention. The QALY is based on the number of years of life that would be added by intervention

Disability-free Life Expectancy (Syn: Active Life Expectancy)

Disability-free life expectancy (DFLE) is the average number of years an individual is expected to live free of disability if current pattern of mortality and disability continue to apply.

Disability-adjusted Life Years (DALY)

DALY is a measure of overall disease burden, expressed as a number of years lost due to ill-health, disability or early death.
It is calculated by formula: DALY = YLL + YLD

Years of lost life (YLL) calculated from the number of deaths at each age multiplied by the expected remaining years of life according to a global standard life expectancy.

Years lost to disability (YLD) where the number of incident cases due to injury and illness is multiplied by the average duration of the disease and a weighting factor reflecting the severity of the disease on a scale from 0 (perfect health) to 1 (dead).

Health Care Delivery Indicators

- Doctor-population ratio
- Doctor-nurse ratio
- Population-bed ratio
- Population per health/subcentre, and
- Population per trained birth attendant

Nutritional Status Indicators

- Anthropometric measurements
- Prevalence of low birth weight (less than 2.5 kg)

Utilization Rates
- Proportion of infants who are "fully immunized'"
- Proportion of pregnant women who receive antenatal care, or have their deliveries supervised by a trained birth attendant.
- Percentage of the population using the various methods of family planning.
- Bed-occupancy rate: $\dfrac{\text{Number of inpatient days in a given month}}{\text{Number of available bed days in that month}} \times 100$
- Average length of stay: $\dfrac{\text{Number of inpatient days in a given month}}{\text{Number of discharge and deaths in that month}}$
- Bed turnover ratio (i.e., discharges/average beds).

Environmental Indicators
They include indicators relating to pollution of air and water, radiation, solid wastes, noise, exposure to toxic substances in food or drink.

Socio-economic Indicators
These indicators do not directly measure health.
- Population growth rate
- Per capita GNP
- Level of unemployment
- Dependency ratio
- Literacy rates, especially female literacy rates
- Family size
- Housing: the number of persons per room, and
- Per capita "calorie" availability.

Health Policy Indicators
- Proportion of GNP spent on health services
- Proportion of GNP spent on health related activities (including water supply and sanitation, housing and nutrition, community development), and
- Proportion of total health resources devoted to primary healthcare.

Indicators of Quality of Life
The physical quality of life index consolidates three indicators, viz. infant mortality, life expectancy at age one, and literacy.

Social Indicators
There are 12 categories including population; family formation, families and households; learning and educational services; earning activities; distribution of income, consumption, and accumulation; social security and welfare services; health services and nutrition; housing and its environment; public order and safety; time use; leisure and culture; social stratification and mobility.

Basic Needs Indicators

It is used by ILO. It includes calorie consumption; access to water; life expectancy; deaths due to disease; illiteracy, doctors and nurses per population; rooms per person; GNP per capita.

BIBLIOGRAPHY

1. https://apps.who.int/iris/bitstream/handle/10665/63933/IDHL_1998_49_p1-296_Special_issue_eng.pdf?sequence=1
2. https://www.nabh.co/Images/PDF/10MandatoryQI.pdf
3. https://www.undp.org/india/press-releases/india-ranks-132-human-development-index-global-development-stalls
4. Park K. Park's Textbook of Preventive and Social Medicine, 25th edition. Jabalpur: Bhanot Publishers; 2019

1.5 HEALTH PROBLEMS (PROFILE) OF INDIA

Table 1.1: Health problems (profile) of India.

Parameter	India's contribution globally
Population	17%
Total deaths	17%
Child deaths	16%
Childhood vaccine preventable disease	26%
Maternal deaths	15 %
Leprosy new cases	60%
Tuberculosis cases	26%
HIV infected persons	6%

Table 1.2: Status of health facilities as per rural health statistics (RHS) 2021–22.

Health facility type	Numbers
Subcenters (SCs)	1,61,829
Primary Health Centers (PHCs)	31,053
Community Health Centers (CHCs)	6,064
Subdivisional/Subdistrict Hospital	1,275
District Hospitals (DHs)	767

Table 1.3: Status of key vital statistics (SRS 2022 report).

Birth rate	19.5/1000 live birth
Death rate	6/1000 live birth
Infant mortality rate	28/1000 live birth
Maternal mortality ratio	97/1,00,000 live birth

Concepts of Community Health and Community Health Nursing

Table 1.4: Comparison of key RCH and nutrition related indicators as per NFHS-4 and NFHS-5.

Indicators	NFHS-4	NFHS-5
Total fertility rate (TFR)	2.2	2.0
Contraceptive prevalence rate (CPR)	53.5%	66.7%
Unmet needs of family planning	12.9%	9.4%
Proportion of ANC visit in the first trimester	58.6%	70%
Mother who had at least 4 ANC visits (%)	51.2%	58.1%
Institutional births	78.9%	88.6%
Children age 12–23 months fully immunized	62%	76.4%
Sex ratio at birth (female per 1000 male)	919	929
Anemia prevalence (%)		
All women (15–49 years)	53.1	57
Pregnant women (15–49 years)	50.4	52.2
Adolescent girls (15–19 years)	54.1	59.1
Children (6–59 months)	58.6	67.1
Adolescent boys (15–19 years)	29.2	31.1
Nutritional status of children under 5 years of age (%)		
Stunting	38.4	35.5
Wasting	21.0	19.3
Severely wasted	7.5	7.7
Overweight	2.1	3.4
Infant and child mortality rate		
Neonatal mortality rate per 1000 live birth	29.5	24.9
Infant mortality rate per 1000 live birth	40.7	35.2
Under 5 mortality rate per 1000 live birth	49.7	41.9

Table 1.5: Disease specific profile.

Malaria

Malaria (as per 2021)	
ABER	8.25
API	0.12
SPR	0.14
% Falciparum cases	63.09

HIV and Tuberculosis

NACO HIV Estimation report 2020	
Adult prevalence	0.22%
GLOBAL TB Report 2022 India	**Rate per 1,00,000 population**
Total TB incidence	210
HIV positive TB incidence	3.9
HIV negative TB mortality	35
HIV positive TB mortality	0.81

Leprosy

Indicators	
Annual case detection rate	5.52 per 1,00,000 population
Prevalence rate	0.45 per 10,000 population
Child proportion	6.87%
Grade 2 disability proportion	2.41%
Grade 2 disability rate	1.96 per million population

Cancer Statistics (GLOBOCAN 2020)

Number of new cases of common cancer					
Both genders		**Male**		**Female**	
Type	% of total cases	Type	% of total cases	Type	% of total cases
Breast	13.5	Lip, oral cavity	16.2	Breast	26
Lip, oral cavity	10.3	Lung	8	Cervix uteri	18.3
Cervix uteri	9.4	Stomach	6.3	Ovary	6.7
Lung	5.5	Colorectal	6.3	Lip, oral cavity	4.6
Colorectal	4.9	Esophagus	6.2	Colorectal	3.7
Other	56.5	Other	57	Other	40.4

BIBLIOGRAPHY

1. https://pib.gov.in/PressReleseDetailm.aspx?PRID=1843842
2. http://rchiips.org/nfhs/NFHS-5_FCTS/India.pdf
3. https://main.mohfw.gov.in/sites/default/files/rhs20-21.pdf
4. https://gco.iarc.fr/today/data/factsheets/populations/356-india-fact-sheets.pdf
5. https://censusindia.gov.in/census.website/data/SRSB
6. https://censusindia.gov.in/census.website/data/SRSMMB

CHAPTER 2

Healthcare Planning and Organization of Healthcare at Various Levels

CHAPTER OUTLINE

2.1 Basics of health planning
2.2 Brief note on health planning in India (various committees, commissions on health and five-year plans)
2.3 Community participation in health planning
2.4 Overview of healthcare delivery system in India
2.5 Primary healthcare and comprehensive primary healthcare
2.6 Role of MLHP in CPHC at SC/Health Wellness Center (HWC)
2.7 Sustainable Development Goals (SDGs—2015–2030)
2.8 National Health Policy (1983, 2002, 2017)
2.9 National Health Mission (NHM) including National Rural Health Mission (NRHM), National Urban Health Mission (NUHM)
2.10 PM Ayushman Bharat Health Infrastructure Mission (PM-ABHIM)
2.11 National Digital Health Mission (Ayushman Bharat Digital Mission)
2.12 Ayushman Bharat PMJAY
2.13 Universal Health Coverage

2.1 BASICS OF HEALTH PLANNING

SOME IMPORTANT CONCEPTS OF PLANNING

Vision
- It is an inspirational statement of what an organization would like to achieve or accomplish in the mid-term or long-term future.
- It is intended to serve as a clear guide for choosing current and future courses of action.
- Simply vision refers to where an organization wants to be in the future.

Mission

- It is a statement of the purpose of an organization, i.e., what it wants to do to accomplish its vision.
- The mission of an organization is the base or foundation and on that all the strategies are built upon.
- The mission statement guides the actions of the organization, spell out its overall goal, provide a path, and helps in decision-making.

Policies: They are guiding principle stated as per an expectation, not as a commandment, i.e. they are directive not bindings.

Program is a sequence of activities designed to implement policies and accomplish objectives.

Goal: The ultimate desired state towards which all resources and objectives are directed. Goals are broad in nature and focus on long-term achievements in same specific area, i.e. population stabilization, halting HIV epidemic, etc. They are long-term outcome or Health impact.

An objective is precise, time bound, measurable and action oriented desired result. Objectives must be **SMART** (Specific, Measurable, Achievable, Realistic, Time Bound). Objectives are short-term outcomes or output.

Target: It often refers to a discrete activity such as the number of blood films collected or vasectomies done; it permits the concept of degree of achievement. Targets are thus concerned with the factors involved in a problem.

Schedule is a time sequence for the work to be done.

Procedures: It is a set of rules for carrying out the work.

Resources: Manpower, Money, Material, Minutes (Time), Methods (Skills-Strategies)

Difference between GDP and GNP

Parameters	GDP (by Indians and other foreign nationals in India)	GNP (by Indians in India or in any other country)
Definition	• The value of goods and services produced within the geographical limits of the particular country is known as Gross Domestic Product (GDP) • It is decided on the basis of location of production.	• The worth of goods and services produced by the country's citizens irrespective of the geographical location is known as Gross National Product (GNP). • It is decided on the basis of citizenship of producers.
Location of production	Production of products within the country's boundary (within India only)	Production of products by the companies owned by the residents of the country. (It means Indian company production in India and its other plant in other country production also taken into consideration.)
Conclusion	It reflects the strength of the country's domestic economy.	It reflects the contribution of countrymen towards the country's economy.

NDP (net domestic product): GDP minus value of depreciation on fixed assets.

NNP (net national product): GNP minus capital we consume.

Purchasing Power Parity (PPP)

- It is used worldwide to compare the income levels in different countries and thus it makes easy to understand the data of each country.
- **Definition:** It is an economic concept which states citizen of one country should be able to buy the goods and services at the same price as inhabitants of any other country over time.
- **Example:** No. of units of INDIA's currency required to buy the same amount of goods and services in own domestic market as 1 dollar would buy in USA.

TYPES OF ECONOMIC EVALUATION

Cost Minimization Analysis

- It is comparison between two or more interventions whose outcomes are assumed to be exactly the same.
- It means choosing least costly intervention among available interventions with similar outcomes.
- **Example:** Choosing generic drug against costly branded drug
- And we assume that all consequences of the alternative interventions will be same.
- If therapeutic equivalence cannot be proved then cost-minimization analysis is inappropriate.
- Generally it is not recommended tool for economic evaluation.

Cost Effectiveness Analysis

- In this type of evaluation benefits are measured in the form of natural units like life years gained or stroke attacks avoided.
- It measures degree of attainment of predetermined targets of the program.
- Most common type of economic evaluation in healthcare.
- It measures lives saved by a health program.
- CEA = cost per number of lives saved.

Cost Utility Analysis

- When alternative interventions produce different levels of effect in terms of both quantity and quality of life the cost utility analysis will be better method to use.
- It measures both length of life and subjective levels of well-being.
- Cost effective analysis measures only the numbers of lives saved while cost utility analysis measures both quantity and quality of life.
- The best known utility measure is the quality-adjusted life year (QALY).
- Other utility measures include DALY and HALE.
- CUA = cost per QALY gained or DALY averted.
- When after doing cost effective and cost utility analysis it is found that intervention A is equal to intervention B then do the cost minimization analysis to decide which intervention to be replicated.
- Cost-utility analysis is used to compare two different drugs whose benefits may be different.

Cost Benefit Analysis

- Measures all outcomes in monetary terms.
- Commonly expressed as cost-benefit ratio: it is used to assess overall value of money for program.
- Useful for comparing interventions with many diverse outcomes—most appropriate for economic evaluation of inter-sectoral interventions.
- It measures cost saved by health program.
- CBA = cost in monetary terms per benefits in monetary terms

Definition of Health Planning: The orderly process of defining community health problems, identifying unmet needs and surveying the resources to meet them, establishing priority goals that are realistic and feasible and projecting administrative action to accomplish the purpose of the proposed program.

Health Planning Cycle

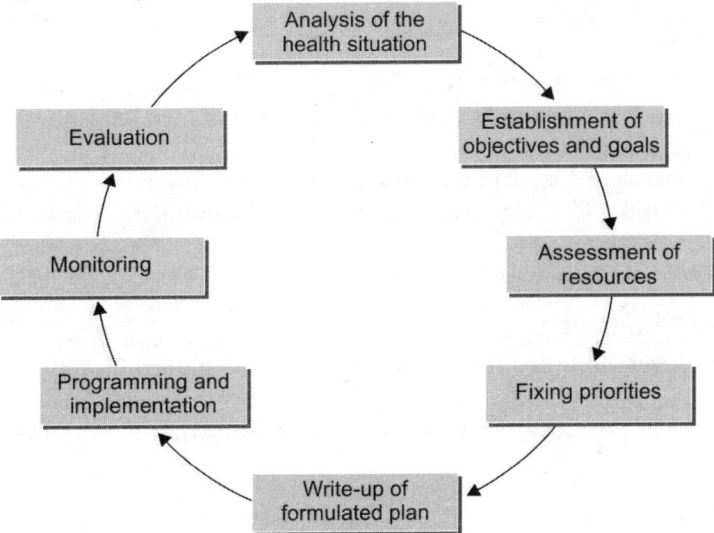

Fig. 2.1: Stages of health planning cycle.

Stages of Health Planning (Fig. 2.1)

- Analysis of the health situation
- Establishment of objectives and goals
- Assessment of resources
- Fixing priorities
- Write-up of formulated plan
- Programming and implementation
- Monitoring
- Evaluation

1. Analysis of the Health Situation

- It involves the collection, assessment and interpretation of information to get the clear picture of the health situation.
- The following information is very essential for health planning:
  - The population, its age and sex structure
  - Morbidity and mortality indicators
  - The epidemiology and geographical distribution of different diseases
  - Medical care facilities such as hospitals, health centers, and other health agencies—both public and private
  - The technical manpower of various categories
  - Availability of training facilities
  - Attitudes and beliefs of the population towards disease, its cure and prevention
- The analysis and interpretation of the these data brings out the:
  - Health problems
  - Health needs
  - Health demands

2. Establishment of Objectives and Goals

- Objectives and goals are needed to guide efforts which in turn helps for better economical use of funds and overall better performance of the program.
- Objectives are also a yard-stick to measure work after it is done.
- Objectives are at upper levels, general in nature but becoming more specific at successively lower levels.
- The objectives could be short-term or long-term.

3. Assessment of Resources

- The term resources includes the manpower, money, materials, skills, knowledge and techniques.
- These resources are assessed as what is required and what is available, or likely to be available.

4. Fixing Priorities

Once the problems, resources and objectives have been determined, the next most important step in planning is establishment of priorities in order of importance or magnitude, since the resources always fall short of the total requirement.

Decision of priorities based on:

- Financial constraints
- Mortality and morbidity data
- Diseases prevention cost
- Lives of younger people
- Political and community interests and pressures
- Once priorities have been established, alternate plans for achieving them are also formulated and assessed in order to determine whether they are practicable and feasible. Alternate plans with greater effectiveness are chosen.

5. Write-up of Formulated Plan
- The plan must be complete in all respects for the execution of a project.
- Expected cost and time for each stage of the plan is defined.
- It must be having working guidance to all those responsible for execution.
- It must be having a "built-in" system of evaluation.
- Central planning authority of the government considers modifications of the plan relating to allocation of resources.

6. Programming and Implementation
- Plan execution depends upon the existence of effective organization.
- The main considerations at the implementation stage include:
  - Definition of roles and tasks
  - The selection, training, motivation and supervision of the manpower
  - Organization and communication, and
  - The efficiency of individual institutions such as hospitals or health centers.

7. Monitoring
- Monitoring is the day-to-day follow-up of activities during their implementation to ensure that they are proceeding as planned and are on schedule.
- It is a continuous process of observing, recording, and reporting on the activities of the organization or project.
- Monitoring, thus, consists of keeping track of the course of activities and identifying deviations and taking corrective action if excessive deviations occur.

8. Evaluation
- The purpose of evaluation is to assess the achievement of the stated objectives of a program, its adequacy, its efficiency and its acceptance by all parties involved.
- While monitoring is confined to day-to-day or on-going operations, evaluation is mostly concerned with the final outcome and with factors associated with it.
- As per WHO Expert Committee on National Health Planning in Developing Countries, evaluation "measures the degree to which objectives and targets are fulfilled and the quality of the results obtained.
- It measures the productivity of available resources in achieving clearly-defined objectives.
- It measures how much output or cost-effectiveness is achieved.
- It makes possible the reallocation of priorities and of resources on the basis of changing health needs".

BIBLIOGRAPHY

1. Introduction to drug utilization research, available at; http://apps.who.int/medicinedocs/en/d/Js4876e/5.5.html, accessed on 20 December 2016.
2. Joseph B. Babigumira, Types of Economic Evaluation in Healthcare, center for AIDS research, Washington. Available at; http://depts.washington.edu/cfar/sites/default/files/uploads/coreprogram/user164/Session%201%20CFAR%20Methods%20of%20EE%20(2).pdf

2.2 BRIEF NOTE ON HEALTH PLANNING IN INDIA (VARIOUS COMMITTEES, COMMISSIONS ON HEALTH AND FIVE-YEAR PLANS)

BHORE COMMITTEE

- **Chairman:** Sir Joseph Bhore
- **Launching year:** 1943
- **Reporting year:** 1946
- **Committee name:** "Health Survey and Development Committee"
- **Recommendations:** It is the most comprehensive health policy and plan document ever prepared in India.
  - Preventive and curative services should be integrated at all the administrative levels.
  - Primary health centers (PHC) to be developed in two stages as follows:
    1. **Short-term:**
       - One PHC per 40,000 populations.
       - In every PHC:

Staff name	Number
Doctors	2
Nurse	1
Public Health Nurse	4
Midwives	4
Trained Dais	4
Sanitary Inspectors	2
Health Assistants	2
Pharmacist	1
Class IV	15

   2. **Long-term (also known as the 3 million plan):**
      - Primary health units with 75 beds for 10,000–20,000 population
      - Secondary health units with 650 beds
      - District hospitals with 2,500 beds.
  - **Significant changes in medical education:** 3 months training in preventive and social medicine to prepare **"social physicians"**.

MUDALIAR COMMITTEE

- **Chairman:** Dr AL Mudaliar
- **Launching year:** 1959
- **Reporting year:** 1962
- **Committee name:** **"Health Survey and Planning Committee"**
- **Recommendations:**
  - Consolidation of gains of previous two FYP.
  - Provision of specialist services for strengthening of district hospital.
  - A PHC should serve less than 40,000 population.
  - Formation of All India Health services as Indian Administrative Services.
  - Integration of medical and health services.

Healthcare Planning and Organization of Healthcare at Various Levels

CHADAH COMMITTEE

- **Chairman:** Dr MS Chadah (DGHS)
- **Launching year:** 1963
- **Reporting year:** 1963
- Committee name: **"Basic Health Worker (BHW) Committee"**
- **Recommendations:** Committee was appointed to advise about the necessary arrangements for the maintenance phase of National Malaria Eradication Program:
  - Main recommendation was for the integration of health and family planning services.
  - Vigilance Operations regarding malaria program should be carried out by general health services.
  - This vigilance work can be done through monthly home visit by "Basic Health Worker (BHW)" (1 BHW per 10,000 population). "Basic Health Worker (BHW)" in addition to malaria work, used to perform the duties of family planning and vital statistics related data collection.

MUKERJI-1 COMMITTEE

- **Chairman:** Shri Mukerji (Secretary)
- **Launching year:** 1965
- **Reporting year:** 1965
- **Committee Name: Committee to Review (Delink Committee)**
- **Recommendations:** Delink was necessary as basic health workers, with their multiple tasks, were not able to do either malaria work or family planning work properly.
  - Separate staff for family planning activities
  - Delinking of malaria activities from family planning
  - Basic Health Worker to be involved in the activities other than family planning.

MUKERJI-2 COMMITTEE

- **Chairman:** Shri Mukerji (Secretary)
- **Launching year:** 1966
- **Reporting year:** 1966
- **Committee name: Committees on basic Health Services.**
- **Recommendations:** Provision of "Basic Health Services" at block level.

JUNGALWALA COMMITTEE

- **Chairman:** Dr N Jungalwala (Director, NIHAE)
- **Launching year:** 1964
- **Reporting year:** 1967
- **Committee name: Committee on Integration of Health Services**
- **Recommendations:** Main areas of integration are:
  - Cadre must be unified
  - Common seniority
  - Extra qualifications must be recognized
  - Equal work-equal pay

- Specialized work-specialized pay
- Private practice not allowed.

KARTAR SINGH COMMITTEE

- **Chairman:** Kartar Singh (Add. Secretary, MOH and Family Planning)
- **Launching year:** 1972
- **Reporting year:** 1973
- **Committee name:** The Committee on Multipurpose Workers under Health and Family Planning
- **Recommendations:**
  - ANMs to become Female Health Workers and all others (present basic health workers, malaria surveillance workers, vaccinators, health education assistance of trachoma) to be replaced Male Health worker.
  - PHC for 50,000 population
  - Each PHC should be divided into 16 subcenters each having population 3000-3500 and should be staffed by 1 male and 1 female health worker.
  - Male and Female Health supervisors for every 3-4 health workers

SHRIVASTAV COMMITTEE, 1975

- **Chairman:** Shrivastav
- **Launching year:** 1974
- **Reporting year:** 1975
- **Committee name:** Group on Medical Education and Support Manpower
- **Recommendations:**
  - Development of "Referral services Complex" by establishing proper linkage between PHC and higher referral services.
  - Creation of bands of para-professional and semi-professional health workers from within the community itself.
  - Creation of two cadres of health workers namely multipurpose health worker and health assistant.
  - Establishment of Medical and Health Education Commission.
  - Rural health scheme (primary healthcare should be provided within the community itself through specially trained workers so that the health of the people is placed in people's hand).
  - ROME scheme.

BAJAJ COMMITTEE, 1986

- **Chairman:** Dr JS Bajaj, Professor at AIIMS
- **Launching year:** 1985
- **Reporting year:** 1986
- **Committee name:** Expert Committee for Health Manpower Planning, Production and Management

Healthcare Planning and Organization of Healthcare at Various Levels

❏ **Recommendations:**
- Formulation of Essential Policies like National Medical and Health Education Policy and National Health Manpower Policy.
- Like UGC, it was recommended to establish an educational commission for health sciences (ECHS).
- Establishment of Health Science Universities and Health Manpower Cells at center and in the states.
- Curriculum of education at 10+2 levels should incorporate the concepts of health-related fields with appropriate incentives, so that good quality paramedical personnel may be available in adequate numbers.
- Carrying out a realistic health manpower survey.

Some other important committees include **Krishnan Committee** "Urban Revamping (renewing) Scheme", **High Level Expert Group Committee** (Universal Health Coverage), etc.

FIRST FIVE-YEAR PLAN: LAUNCHED ON 8TH DECEMBER (1951–1956)

Mainly focused on agrarian sector.
Main objectives for health sector of First Five-Year Plan were:
❏ Provision of water-supply and sanitation.
❏ Control of malaria.
❏ Preventive healthcare of the rural population through health units and mobile units.
❏ Health services for mothers and children.
❏ Education and training, and health education.
❏ Self-sufficiency in drugs and equipment.
❏ Family planning and population control.

SECOND FIVE-YEAR PLAN: 1956–1961

Mainly focused on industrial sector. This plan based on Mahalanobis model.
Main objectives for health sector of Second Five-Year Plan were:
❏ Establishment of institutional facilities to serve as bases from which services can be rendered to the people both locally and in surrounding territories;
❏ Development of technical manpower through appropriate training programs and employment of persons trained;
❏ As the first step in the improvement of public health, institution of measures to control communicable diseases which may be widely prevalent in a community;
❏ An active campaign for environmental hygiene; and
❏ Family planning and other supporting programs for raising the standard of health of the people.

THIRD FIVE-YEAR PLAN: 1961–1966

Main objectives for Health Sector of Third Five-Year Plan were:
❏ To expand health services.
❏ To bring about progressive improvement in the health of the people by ensuring a certain minimum of physical well-being and to create conditions favourable to greater efficiency and productivity.

- To improve environmental sanitation, especially rural and urban water supply.
- Control of communicable diseases.
- Organization of institutional facilities for providing health services and for the training of medical and health personnel.
- Provision of services such as maternal and child welfare, health education, nutrition and family planning.

Note: Due to Indo-China war, the scarcity of fund led to postponed the fourth five-year plan and during 1966 to 1969, annual plans were formed.

FOURTH FIVE-YEAR PLAN: 1969–1974

It was formulated based on the report of Mudaliar "Health Survey and Planning Committee"-1961 Committee.

This was the first five-year plan formulated under the leadership of Prime Minister Indira Gandhi.

Main objectives for health sector of Third Five-Year Plan were:
- To control and eradicate communicable diseases
- To provide curative and preventive health services in rural areas through the establishment of a primary health center in each community development block and
- To expand medical and nursing education and training of paramedical personnel to meet the minimum technical manpower requirements.
- Subdivisional and district hospitals will be strengthened to serve as referral centers.

FIFTH FIVE-YEAR PLAN: 1974–1979

Main focus: Poverty Alleviation and Achievement of Self-Reliance
Main achievements:
- Minimum Needs Program
- 20 Point Program
- The concept of family planning was changed into family welfare
- The country was declared free from smallpox in April, 1977
- The Water (Prevention and Control of Pollution) Act 1974
- The Integrated Child Development scheme, 1975.
- Child Marriage Restraint (Amendment) Bill fixing the minimum age of marriage of 21 years for boys and 18 years for girls in 1978.

Note: Newly Elected Government of Morarji Desai Rejected fifth five-year plan in 1978 so during 1978-1980 again annual health plans were formed.

SIXTH FIVE-YEAR PLAN: 1980–1985

Also Known as Janata Government Plan

The objectives were:
- Increasing the accessibility of health services to rural areas.
- Correcting regional imbalances.
- Further development of referral services by removal of deficiencies in district/subdivisional hospitals and by providing specialist attention to common diseases in rural areas.

Healthcare Planning and Organization of Healthcare at Various Levels

- Intensification of the control/eradication of communicable diseases especially Malaria and smallpox.
- Qualitative improvement in the education and training of health personnel.
- National programs for immunization and nutrition of mothers and children have also been initiated.
- Adoption of the National Health Policy.

SEVENTH FIVE-YEAR PLAN: 1985–1989

This plan was formulated under the leadership of Rajiv Gandhi as Prime minister. Major thrusts were given in the following areas:
- The Minimum Needs Program would continue with back up by adequately strengthened infrastructural facilities.
- Strengthening of inter-sectoral coordination and cooperation will be made as part of the package for achieving the goal of Health for All by 2000 AD.
- Community participation and people's involvement in the program
- Qualitative improvements along with management of supplies and logistics to ensure adequate provision of essential drugs, vaccines and sera need special attention for ensuring production, pricing and distribution and universal accessibility, availability and affordability.
- Urban health services, school health services, mental and dental health services.
- For the control and eradication of communicable diseases.
- Cancer, coronary heart diseases, hypertension, diabetes, and traffic and other accidents are emerging as major health problems and required to initiate appropriate action for their control and containment.
- Training and education of doctors and paramedical personnel to be need-based, problem-centred and community-oriented.
- Medical research of special relevance to the common health problems of the people, would be pursued.
- Integration of the Indian systems of medicine.

Note: During 1990–1992 again annual health plans were formed.

EIGHTH FIVE-YEAR PLAN: 1992–1997

This was the beginning of liberalization, privatization and globalization (LPG) in India.
- Population control
- Provision of safe drinking water and
- Primary healthcare facilities, including immunization
- The transplantation of human organs bill 1994.

NINTH FIVE-YEAR PLAN: 1997–2002

New Initiatives in the Ninth Plan:
- Horizontal integration of vertical programs
- Develop Disease Surveillance and Response mechanism with focus on rapid recognition, report and response at district level
- Develop and implement integrated Non-Communicable Disease Control Program

- Health Impact Assessment as a part of environmental impact assessment in developmental projects.
- Implement appropriate management systems for emergency, disaster, accident and trauma care at all levels of healthcare.
- Improve HMIS and logistics of supplies.

Ninth Plan Priorities for Rural Primary Healthcare Institutions
- Ensure existing SC, PHC are fully operational
- Fill the gaps in CHCs through re-structuring existing block level PHC, Taluk, Subdivisional hospital
- Establish functional referral linkages
- Provide need based manpower on the basis of distances, difficulties and work load.

Strategies to Improve Healthcare in Tribal Areas
- Ensuring availability of adequate infrastructure and personnel.
- Area specific RCH programs.
- 100% central plan funds for NMEP.
- Effective implementation of the health and FW programs.
- Close monitoring, early detection of problems in implementation and midcourse correction.

Ninth Plan Strategies for Improving Urban Primary Healthcare
Create and strengthen primary healthcare infrastructure through:
- Reorganization and restructuring of existing institutions
- Redeploy existing manpower to operationalize these institutions
- Link primary healthcare infrastructure with existing secondary and tertiary care institutions in the same geographically delineated areas
- Establish effective referral services
- Involve Nagar Palikas in effective inter-sectoral coordination and improving community participation.

TENTH FIVE-YEAR PLAN: 2002–2007
- Reorganization and restructuring the existing government healthcare system including the ISM and H infrastructure at the primary, secondary and tertiary care levels with appropriate referral linkages.
- Development of appropriate two-way referral systems utilizing information technology (IT) tools to improve communication, consultation and referral right from primary care to tertiary care level.
- Building up an efficient and effective logistics system for the supply of drugs, vaccines and consumables based on need and utilization.
- Horizontal integration of all aspects of the current vertical programs with progressive convergence of funding, implementation and monitoring of all health and family welfare programs under a single field of administration beginning at and below district level
- Improvement in the quality of care at all levels and settings.
- Exploring alternative systems of healthcare financing including health insurance so that essential, need based and affordable healthcare is available to all.

Healthcare Planning and Organization of Healthcare at Various Levels

- Improving content and quality of education of health professionals and para-professionals and skill upgradation of all healthcare providers through CME and reorientation.
- Research and development to solve major health problems confronting the country including basic and clinical research on drugs needed for the management of emerging diseases and operational research to improve efficiency of service delivery.
- Building up a fully functional, accurate health management information system (HMIS) utilizing currently available IT tools.
- Building up an effective system of disease surveillance and response at the district, state and national level as a part of existing health services.
- Strengthening and sustaining Civil Registration, Sample Registration System; improving medical certification of death so that information on specific causes of death throughout the country are available;
- Increasing the involvement of voluntary and private organizations, self-help groups and social marketing organization in improving access to healthcare.
- Improving inter-sectoral coordination; devolution of responsibilities and funds to Panchayati Raj Institutions (PRIs).
- Strengthening programs for the prevention, detection and management of health consequences of the continuing deterioration of the ecosystems.
- Improving the safety of the work environment in organized and unorganized industrial and agricultural sectors especially among vulnerable groups of the population.
- Developing capabilities at all levels, for emergency and disaster prevention and management; evolving appropriate management systems for emergency, disaster, accident and trauma care at all levels of healthcare.
- Effective implementation of the provisions for food and drug safety; strengthening the food and drug administration both at the center and in the states.
- Screening for common nutritional deficiencies especially in vulnerable groups and initiating appropriate remedial measures; evolving and effectively implementing programs for improving nutritional status, including micronutrient nutritional status of the population.

ELEVENTH FIVE-YEAR PLAN: 2007–2012

This Plan was formulated under the leadership of Prime Minister Dr Manmohan Singh.

Objectives of Eleventh Five-Year Plan
- Rapid and Inclusive growth especially the poor and the underprivileged
- To give special attention to the health of marginalized groups like adolescent girls, women of all ages, children below the age of three, older persons, disabled, and primitive tribal groups
- Increasing survival through responsive healthcare by convergence and development of public health systems and services
- Reduction of gender inequality
- System-centric approach
- Prevention of catastrophic health expenditure
- Decentralizing governance
- Increasing role of telemedicine
- Quality healthcare
- Increasing focus on health human resources.

Time-Bound Goals for the Eleventh Five-Year Plan
- Reducing Maternal Mortality Ratio (MMR) to 1 per 1,000 live births.
- Reducing Infant Mortality Rate (IMR) to 28 per 1000 live births.
- Reducing Total Fertility Rate (TFR) to 2.1.
- Providing clean drinking water for all by 2009 and ensuring no slip-backs.
- Reducing malnutrition among children of age group 0–3 to half its present level.
- Reducing anemia among women and girls by 50%.
- Raising the sex ratio for age group 0–6 to 935 by 2011–12 and 950 by 2016–17.

TWELFTH FIVE-YEAR PLAN: 2012–2017

Outcome Indicators for Twelfth Plan:
- Reduction of Infant Mortality Rate (IMR) to 25 per 1000 live births
- Reduction of Maternal Mortality Ratio (MMR) to 100 per 1,00,000 live births
- Reduction of Total Fertility Rate (TFR) to 2.1
- Prevention, and reduction of undernutrition in children under 3 years to half of NFHS-3 (2005–06) levels
- Prevention and reduction of anemia among women aged 15–49 years to 28 percent
- Raising child sex ratio in the 0–6 year age group from 914 to 950
- Prevention and reduction of burden of communicable and non-communicable diseases (including mental illnesses) and injuries
- Reduction of poor households' out-of-pocket expenditure.

NITI (National Institution for Transforming India) AYOG
- It was formed on 1st January, 2015 as replacement of Planning Commission.
- NITI Aayog is itself as a state-of-the-art resource center.
- NITI Aayog is the premier policy think tank of the Government of India, providing directional and policy inputs. Apart from designing strategic and long-term policies and programs for the Government of India, NITI Aayog also provides relevant technical advice to the center, States, and Union Territories.
- Prime minister used to be chairperson of NITI Ayog.
- The Governing Council of NITI Aayog is chaired by the Hon'ble Prime Minister and comprises Chief Ministers of all the States and Union Territories with legislatures and Lt Governors of other Union Territories.
- NITI Aayog's activities divided into four main areas:
  - Policy and Program Framework
  - Cooperative Federalism
  - Monitoring and Evaluation
  - Think Tank, and Knowledge and Innovation Hub.

OBJECTIVES
- To evolve a shared vision of national development priorities, sectors and strategies with the active involvement of States.
- To foster cooperative federalism through structured support initiatives and mechanisms with the States on a continuous basis, recognizing that strong States make a strong nation.

Healthcare Planning and Organization of Healthcare at Various Levels

- To develop mechanisms to formulate credible plans at the village level and aggregate these progressively at higher levels of government.
- To ensure, on areas that are specifically referred to it, that the interests of national security are incorporated in economic strategy and policy.
- To pay special attention to the sections of our society that may be at risk of not benefiting adequately from economic progress.
- To design strategic and long-term policy and program frameworks and initiatives, and monitor their progress and their efficacy. The lessons learned through monitoring and feedback will be used for making innovative improvements, including necessary mid-course corrections.
- To provide advice and encourage partnerships between key stakeholders and national and international like-minded think tanks, as well as educational and policy research institutions.
- To create a knowledge, innovation and entrepreneurial support system through a collaborative community of national and international experts, practitioners and other partners.
- To offer a platform for the resolution of inter-sectoral and inter-departmental issues in order to accelerate the implementation of the development agenda.
- To maintain a state-of-the-art resource center, be a repository of research on good governance and best practices in sustainable and equitable development as well as help their dissemination to stake-holders.
- To actively monitor and evaluate the implementation of programs and initiatives, including the identification of the needed resources so as to strengthen the probability of success and scope of delivery.
- To focus on technology upgradation and capacity building for implementation of programs and initiatives.

BIBLIOGRAPHY

1. Committees and Commission, available at; http://www.nihfw.org/ReportsOfNCC.aspx, accessed on 21-1-18.
2. http://niu.edu.in/son/online-classes/committee..pdf
3. http://www.gmch.gov.in/sites/default/files/documents/Health%20Planning%20in%20India.pdf
4. https://www.niti.gov.in/content/overview
5. https://www.niti.gov.in/planningcommission.gov.in/docs/sectors/health.php?sectors=hea
6. Suthanthiraveeran, Sathia. (2011). The five year plans in India: Overview of Public Health Policies.

2.3 COMMUNITY PARTICIPATION IN HEALTH PLANNING

- Community participation means the ability to make informed health decisions and be an active participant in improving one's own health. It also means active participation in the health sector at the community and national level to create, influence and mobilize public opinion for improved public policy on health.
- Community participation is one of the four main principles of primary healthcare.

ADVANTAGES OF A COMMUNITY PARTICIPATION

- It is a cost-effective way of extending a healthcare system to the geographical and social periphery of a country.
- Communities that begin to understand their health status objectively rather than fatalistically may be moved to take a series of preventive measures.
- Communities that invest labor, time, money and materials in health-promoting activities are more committed to the use and maintenance of the things they produce, such as water supplies.
- Health education is most effective as part and parcel of village activities.
- Community health workers, if they are well chosen, have the people's confidence. They may know the most effective techniques for achieving commitment from their neighbors and, at the very least, are not likely to exploit them. They come under strong social pressure to help the community carry out its health-promoting activities.

Initiatives for Community Participation in Indian Health System

- **Village Health Sanitation and Nutrition Committee**
- **ASHA**
- **Village Health Nutrition Day (VHND)**
- **Rogi Kalyan Samiti**

Village Health Sanitation and Nutrition Committee

- The committee takes collective actions on issues related to health and its social determinants at the village level.
- It is example of Decentralized Health Planning.
- This committee is envisaged to take leadership in improving health awareness, access of community for health services and address specific local needs.
- It serves as a mechanism for community-based planning and monitoring.
- The committee is formed at the revenue village level and it should act as a subcommittee of the Gram Panchayat.
- It should have a minimum of 15 members.
- Members include elected member of the Panchayat, all those working for health and health related services, community members/beneficiaries and representation from all community sub-groups especially the vulnerable sections and hamlets/habitations.
- ASHA residing in the village shall be the member secretary and convener of the committee.

Roles and responsibilities

- Create awareness about nutritional issues and significance of nutrition as an important determinant of health.
- Carry out survey on nutritional status and nutritional deficiencies in the village especially among women and children.
- Identify locally available foodstuffs of high nutrient value as well as disseminate and promote best practices (traditional wisdom) congruent with local culture, capabilities and physical environment through a process of community consultation.
- Inclusion of Nutritional needs in the Village Health Plan—The committee will do an in-depth analysis of causes of malnutrition at the community and household levels, by involving the ANM, AWW, ASHA and ICDS Supervisors.

- Monitoring and Supervision of Village Health and Nutrition Day to ensure that it is organized every month in the village with the active participation of the whole village.
- Facilitate early detection of malnourished children in the community; tie up referral to the nearest Nutritional Rehabilitation Center (NRC) as well as follow-up for sustained outcome.
- Supervise the functioning of Anganwadi Center (AWC) in the village and facilitate its working in improving nutritional status of women and children.
- Act as a grievances redressal forum on health and nutrition issues.

Accredited Social Health Activist (ASHA)

- ASHA is one of the key components of the National Rural Health Mission.
- ASHA Selected from the village itself and accountable to it.
- ASHA is trained to work as an interface between the community and the public health system.
- ASHA is supported by Women's committees (like self-help groups or women's health committees), village Health and Sanitation Committee, ANMs and Anganwadi workers, and the trainers of ASHA and in-service periodic training.
- **Following are the key components of ASHA:**
  - ASHA must primarily be a woman resident of the village married/ widowed/ divorced, preferably in the age group of 25 to 45 years.
  - She should be a literate woman with due preference in selection to those who are qualified up to 8th standard wherever they are interested and available in good numbers. This may be relaxed only if no suitable person with this qualification is available.
  - ASHA is chosen through a rigorous process of selection involving various community groups, self-help groups, Anganwadi Institutions, the Block Nodal officer, District Nodal officer, the village Health Committee and the Gram Sabha.
  - ASHA undergoes series of training episodes to acquire the necessary knowledge, skills and confidence for performing her spelled out roles.
  - The ASHA receives performance-based incentives for promoting universal immunization, referral and escort services for Reproductive and Child Health (RCH) and other healthcare programs, and construction of household toilets.
  - Empowered with knowledge and a drug-kit to deliver first-contact healthcare.
  - ASHA is the first port of call for any health related demands of deprived sections of the population, especially women and children, who find it difficult to access health services.
  - ASHA is a health activist in the community who will create awareness on health and its social determinants and mobilise the community towards local health planning and increased utilization and accountability of the existing health services.
  - She is a promoter of good health practices and will also provide a minimum package of curative care as appropriate and feasible for that level and make timely referrals.
  - ASHA provides information to the community on determinants of health such as nutrition, basic sanitation and hygienic practices, healthy living and working conditions, information on existing health services and the need for timely utilisation of health and family welfare services.
  - She counsels women on birth preparedness, importance of safe delivery, breastfeeding and complementary feeding, immunization, contraception and prevention of common infections including Reproductive Tract Infection/Sexually Transmitted Infections (RTIs/STIs) and care of the young child.

- ASHA mobilizes the community and facilitate them in accessing health and health related services available at the Anganwadi/sub-center/primary health centers, such as immunization, Antenatal Check-up (ANC), Postnatal Check-up supplementary nutrition, sanitation and other services being provided by the government.
- She acts as a depot older for essential provisions being made available to all habitations like Oral Rehydration Therapy (ORS), Iron Folic Acid Tablet (IFA), chloroquine, Disposable Delivery Kits (DDK), Oral Pills and Condoms, etc.

Village Health Nutrition Day

- The VHND is organized once every month (preferably on Wednesdays) mostly at the AWC in the village. It ensures uniformity in organizing the VHND.
- The AWC is identified as the hub for service provision and also as a platform for inter-sectoral convergence.
- As VHND being held at a site very close to the people, they don't need to spend money or time on travel. Through VHND Health services are being provided at the villagers' doorstep.
- VHND provides platform for interfacing between the community and the health system.
- ASHAs, AWWs, and other will mobilize the villagers, especially women and children to assemble at the nearest AWC.
- On the VHND, the villagers can obtain basic services and information and also learn about the preventive and promotive aspects of healthcare.
- The VHSC is fully involved in organizing the event, can bring about dramatic changes in the way that people perceive health and healthcare practices.

Rogi Kalyan Samiti

- Rogi Kalyan Samiti (Patient Welfare Committee)/Hospital Management Committee is registered society, acts as a group of trustees for the hospitals to manage the affairs of the hospital.
- It consists of members from local Panchayati Raj Institutions (PRIs), NGOs, local elected representatives and officials from Government sector who are responsible for proper functioning and management of the hospital/Community Health Center/FRUs.
- RKS/HMS is free to prescribe, generate and use the funds with it as per its best judgement for smooth functioning and maintaining the quality of services.

OBJECTIVES THE RKS/HMS

- Ensure compliance to minimal standard for facility and hospital care and protocols of treatment as issued by the government
- Ensure accountability of the public health providers to the community
- Introduce transparency with regard to management of funds
- Upgrade and modernize the health services provided by the hospital and any associated outreach services
- Supervise the implementation of National Health Programs at the hospital and other health institutions that may be placed under its administrative jurisdiction
- Organize outreach services/health camps at facilities under the jurisdiction of the hospital
- Display a Citizens Charter in the Health facility and ensure its compliance through operationalization of a grievance redress mechanism (GRM)
- Generate resources locally through donations, user fees and other means

- Establish affiliations with private institutions to upgrade services
- Undertake construction and expansion in the hospital building
- Ensure optimal use of hospital land as per government guidelines
- Improve participation of the Society in the running of the hospital
- Ensure scientific disposal of hospital waste
- Ensure proper training for doctors and staff
- Ensure subsidized food, medicines and drinking water and cleanliness to the patients and their attendants
- Ensure proper use, timely maintenance and repair of hospital building equipment and machinery.

COMPOSITION OF RKS/HMS

- People's representatives MLA/MP
- Health officials (including an Ayush doctor)
- Local district officials
- Leading members of the community
- Local CHC/ FRU in-charge
- Representatives of the Indian Medical Association
- Members of the local bodies and Panchayati Raj representative
- Leading donors.

Note: Concept of Jan Arogya Samiti is being evolved and detail of the same is given in the relevant chapter.

BIBLIOGRAPHY

1. CP MacCormack. Community participation in primary Healthcare. Tropical doctor, 13 (2). 51-54 (1983).
2. https://vikaspedia.in/health/nrhm/national-health-mission/initiatives-for-community-participation-under-nhm/rogi-kalyan-samiti-rks

2.4 OVERVIEW OF HEALTHCARE DELIVERY SYSTEM IN INDIA

HEALTHCARE IS PROVIDED BY FIVE MAJOR SECTORS IN INDIA

- Public Health Sector
  - Primary Healthcare: PHCs and Sub-centers (Health and Wellness Centers)
  - Secondary Healthcare: District Hospitals and Community Health Centers including first referral unit
  - Tertiary Healthcare: Medical College Hospitals, All India Institutes, Regional Hospitals, Specialized Hospitals and other Apex Institutions
  - Health Insurance Schemes Providing Healthcare: ESI, CGHS
  - Other agencies: Defence services, Railways, Public Sector Units

- Private sector
  - Private Hospitals, Nursing Homes, Polyclinics, etc.
  - General Practitioners
- Indigenous Systems of Medicine
  - Ayurveda, Yoga, Unani, Siddha and Homeopathy: AYUSH
- Voluntary Health Agencies
- National Health Programs

Institutional Framework of Healthcare Delivery System (Fig. 2.2)

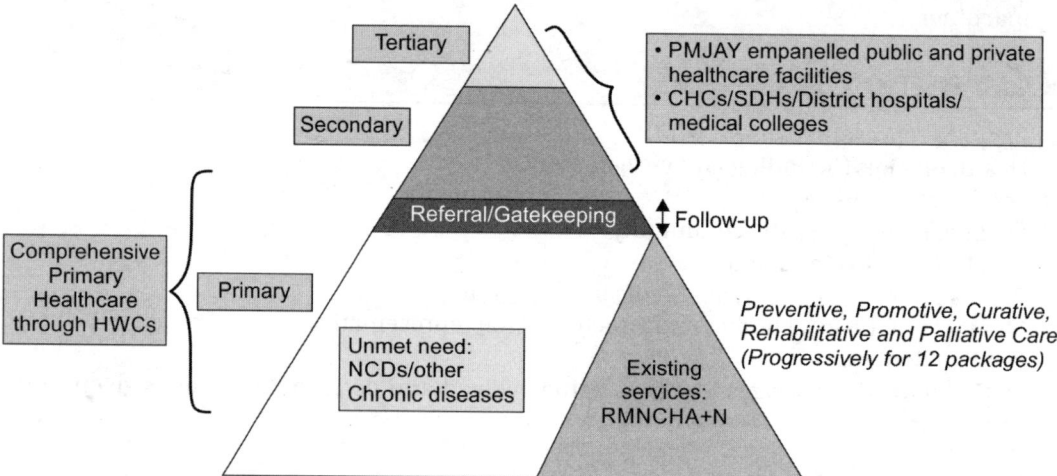

Fig. 2.2: Continuum of care—comprehensive primary health care and Pradhan Mantri Jan Arogya Yojana (PMJAY).

Health System at Different Levels

At National Level
- Union Ministry of Health and Family Welfare (MOHFW)
- Directorate General of Health Services (DGHS)
- Central Council of Health

Union Ministry of Health and Family Welfare (MOHFW)
- Headed by Cabinet Minister, a Minister of State and Deputy Health Minister
- Two Departments: Department of Health and Department of Family Welfare (Since 1966)
- Department of Health Headed by Secretary to GOI and Assisted by Joint secretaries and Dy. Secretaries.
- Department of Family Welfare Assisted by Additional Secretary and Commissioner (FW) and joint secretary

The division of powers between Union and State is notified through three kinds of the list mentioned in the seventh schedule of the Indian Constitution:
- Union List – List I
- State List – List II
- Concurrent List – List III

Union list	Concurrent list
• International health relations and administration of port quarantine • Administration of central institutes like NICD (Delhi), AIIHPH (Kolkata), etc. • Promotion of research • Regulation of medical, pharmaceutical, dental and nursing professions • Establishment and maintenance of drug standards (CDSCO) • Census, collection and publication of other statistical data, IDSP • Immigration and emigration • Regulation of labor in the working of mines and oil fields • Coordination with states and other ministries for promotion of health	• Prevention of extension of communicable diseases from one unit to another • Prevention of adulteration of foodstuffs • Control of drugs and poisons • Vital statistics, IDSP • Labor welfare • Economic and Social planning • Population control and family planning

Directorate General of Health Services (DGHS)

- Principal adviser to the Union Govt. in both Medical and Public Health matters.
- Headed by the Director General (DG) and assisted by an additional DG and a team of deputies.
- Three main units
    1. **Medical Care and Hospitals**
    2. **Public Health**
    3. **General Administration**
- Surveys, planning, coordination, programming, appraisal of all health matters
- International health relations and quarantine at all the major ports and international airports
- Lay down and enforce standards for manufacturing and distribution of drugs through both central and state officers
- National Health Programs
    - Postgraduate training: Administration of National Institutes for like AIIHPH, NICD, NIHFW, NTI, etc.
    - Medical education: Through medical colleges like Maulana Azad, Lady Harding, JIPMER, etc.
    - Medical research: Organized through ICMR (since 1911), which runs many research institutes all over the country.
    - Central Govt. Health Scheme
    - National Medical Library
    - Central Health Education Bureau
    - Health Intelligence—CBHI

Central Council of Health

- Set up by the Presidential order in 1952
- For promoting coordinated and concerted action between the Center and States in implementing all the programs and measures pertaining to health
- Union Health Minister is the Chairman and the State Health Ministers are the members.
- Functions:
    - Consider and recommend broad outline of policy
    - Make proposals for legislation in health related matters

- Make recommendations for distribution of available grant-in-aid for health purposes to the States and to review periodically the work accomplished with the grant
- Establish any organization for promoting and maintaining cooperation between center and state health administrations.

At the State Level
- As per the state list, the responsibility of state includes provision of medical care and preventive health services.
- State Ministry of Health Headed by a Minister of Health and Family Welfare and Dy. Minister of H and FW.
- Health Secretariat is headed by a secretary who is assisted by Dy. Secretaries, Undersecretaries, joint secretaries, etc.
- For example in Gujarat following departments headed by Additional Directors: Public Health, Family Welfare, Medical Services and Medical Education
- Some other additional directors, joint directors, deputy directors and assistant directors are there for various national health programs
- Dy. and Assistant Directors of Health are of 2 types: Regional and Functional
- Regional Dy. Directors: Inspects all the branches of public health within their jurisdiction. There are 6 RDDs in Gujarat state.
- Functional Dy. Directors: Looks after a particular branch of public health, e.g. ,RCH, NVBDCP, Epidemic, Tuberculosis, Leprosy, etc.

At the District Level
- District is the principal unit of administration headed by Collector.
- Six types of administrative areas in each district: Subdivisions, Talukas, Blocks, Municipalities and Corporations, Villages, Panchayats
- The Urban areas
    - Town area committees (5,000 to 1,0000)
    - Municipal Boards (10,000 to 2 Lakhs)
    - Corporations (>2 Lakhs)
- Authorities related to health at district level includes Chief District Health Officer, ADHO, RCHO, EMO/DSO, DMO, etc.

Panchayati Raj
- The Panchayati Raj is a 3-tier structure of rural local self-government in India, linking village to the district.
    - Panchayat- at the village level
    - Panchayat samiti- at the block level
    - Zila parishad- at the district level

Healthcare Delivery System in Rural Area

Population norms	Plain area	Hilly/Tribal/Difficult Area
Subcenter/HWC	5,000	3,000
Primary Health Center	30,000	20000
Community Health Center	1,20,000	80,000

Subcenter/AB-HWCs

- **A subcenter** (SC) is the most peripheral and first contact point between the primary healthcare system and the community.
- SCs provide services in relation to maternal and child health, family welfare, nutrition, immunization, diarrhea control and control of communicable diseases programs.
- Type A Subcenter provides recommended services except that the facilities for conducting delivery. IPHS recommends two ANM (one essential and one desirable) and one Health Worker Male (essential).
- Type B Subcenter provides all recommended services including facilities for conducting deliveries at the Subcenter itself.
- For Type B Subcenters, IPHS recommends to provide two ANMs (essential) and one Health Worker Male (essential). One Staff Nurse or ANM (if Staff Nurse not available) is to be provided, if number of deliveries at the Subcentre is 20 or more in a month.
- Sanitation services should be provided through outsourcing on part time basis at Type A and full-time basis at Type B.
- AB-HWCs are being set up as an upgraded version of existing GPHCFs such as Health Sub-Centers (HSC); Primary Health Centers and Urban Primary Health Centers (UPHCs).
- The first HWCs was launched in Jangla village in Bhairamgarh tehsil of Bijapur district of Chhattisgarh state in India on 14 April 2018.

Primary Health Center (PHC)

- PHC is the first contact point between the village community and the medical officer.
- PHCs to provide integrated curative and preventive healthcare to the rural population with emphasis on the preventive and promotive aspects of healthcare.
- PHCs may be of two types depending upon the delivery case load – Type A and Type B. The PHCs with delivery case load of less than 20 deliveries in a month will be of Type A and those with delivery case load of 20 or more in a month will be of Type B.

Community Health Centers (CHCs)

- CHCs are established and maintained by the State Government under the MNP/BMS program in an area with a population of 120 000 people and in hilly/difficult to reach/tribal areas with a population of 80 000. It serves as a referral center for PHCs within the block and also provides facilities for obstetric care and specialist consultations.
- An existing facility (**district hospital, subdivisional hospital, CHC**) can be declared a fully operational **first referral unit (FRU)** only if it is equipped to provide round-the-clock services for emergency obstetric and newborn care, in addition to all emergencies that any hospital is required to provide.

Healthcare Delivery System in Urban Area

Set up	Population norms
Mahila Arogya Samiti (MAS)	50–100 HHs or 250–500 population
USHA/LW	200–500 HHs or 1,000–2,500 population
ANM	10,000 Population
Urban-Primary Health Center	50,000 Population
Urban-CHC	2.5 Lakh Population (5 lakh for metros)

BIBLIOGRAPHY

1. Chokshi M, Patil B, Khanna R, Neogi SB, Sharma J, Paul VK, Zodpey S. Health systems in India. J Perinatol. 2016 Dec;36(s3):S9-S12. doi: 10.1038/jp.2016.184. PMID: 27924110; PMCID: PMC5144115.
2. https://nhm.gov.in/images/pdf/guidelines/iphs/iphs-revised-guidlines-2012/sub-centers.pdf
3. https://www.brainkart.com/article/Health-Care-Delivery-System-in-India_35450/
4. http://www.ihatepsm.com/blog/health-care-delivery-india
5. https://nhm.gov.in/images/pdf/guidelines/iphs/iphs-revised-guidlines-2012/primay-health-centers.pdf

2.5 PRIMARY HEALTHCARE AND COMPREHENSIVE PRIMARY HEALTHCARE

PRIMARY HEALTHCARE

- **Definition:** Primary healthcare is essential healthcare based on practical, scientifically sound and socially acceptable methods and technology made universally accessible to individuals and families in the community through their full participation and at a cost that the community and country can afford to maintain at every stage of their development in the spirit of self-reliance and self-determination.
- **Elements of primary healthcare:**
  - Education concerning prevailing health problems and the methods of preventing and controlling them
  - Promotion of food supply and proper nutrition
  - Adequate supply of safe water and basic sanitation
  - Maternal and child healthcare including family planning
  - Immunization against major infectious diseases
  - Prevention and control of locally endemic diseases
  - Appropriate treatment of common diseases and injuries
  - Provision of essential drugs
- **Principles of primary healthcare:**
  - Equitable Distribution
  - Community Participation
  - Appropriate Technology
  - Intersectoral Coordination

Comprehensive Primary Healthcare (CPHC)

- Comprehensive Primary Healthcare reduces morbidity and mortality at much lower costs.
- It significantly reduces the need for secondary and tertiary care by gate keeping approach.
- Primary Healthcare could be called as comprehensive when its span includes preventive, promotive, curative, rehabilitative and palliative aspects of care.
- Comprehensive Primary Healthcare should be as close to the beneficiaries as possible, have the widest cooperation between the people, the service and the profession and is available to all irrespective of their ability to pay specifically the vulnerable and weaker sections of the community.
- As Primary Healthcare becomes comprehensive it goes beyond first contact care, and is expected to mediate a two-way referral support to higher-level facilities and ensure follow up support for individual and population health interventions.

Healthcare Planning and Organization of Healthcare at Various Levels

- Strengthening Primary Healthcare Emphasized in the various guiding documents like:
  - Bhore Committee Report 1946
  - Alma Ata declaration for Health for All 1978.
  - National Health Policy 1983 and 2002.
  - The Twelfth Five-Year Plan: Universal Health Coverage as a key goal and based on the recommendations of the High-Level Expert Group Report on UHC had called for 70% budgetary allocation to Primary Healthcare in pursuit of UHC for India.
  - The National Health Policy, 2017 recommended strengthening the delivery of Primary Healthcare, through establishment of "Health and Wellness Centers" as the platform to deliver Comprehensive Primary Healthcare and called for a commitment of two thirds of the health budget to primary Healthcare.
- In February 2018, the Government of India announced that 1,50,000 Health and Wellness Centers (HWCs) would be created by transforming existing Sub Health Centers and Primary Health Centers to deliver Comprehensive Primary Healthcare.
- This was the first step in the conversion of policy articulations to a budgetary commitment.
- The delivery of CPHC through HWCs rests substantially on the institutional mechanisms, governance structures, and systems created under the National Health Mission (NHM).

Key Principles

- Transform existing Sub-Health Centers and Primary Health Centers to Health and Wellness Centers to ensure universal access to an expanded range of Comprehensive Primary Healthcare services **(Fig. 2.3)**.

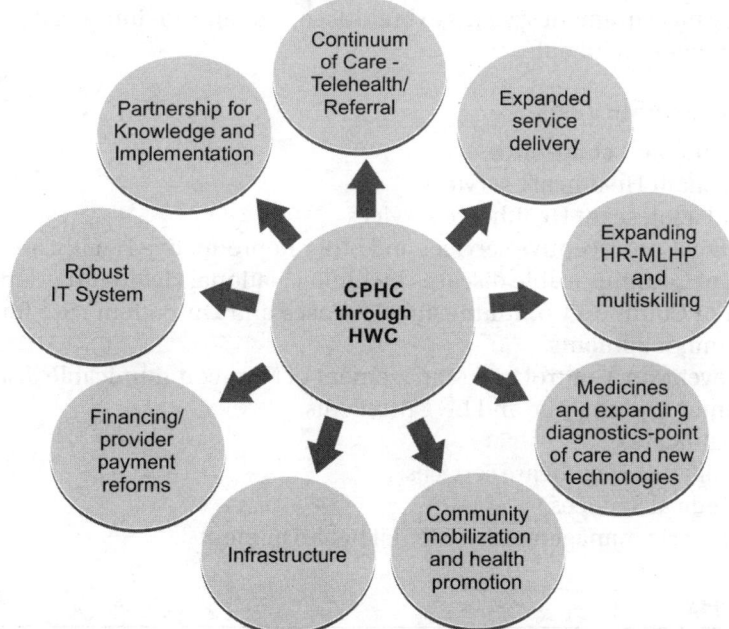

Fig. 2.3: Key elements of HWC.
(CPHC: Comprehensive Primary Health Care; HWC: Health and Wellness Center)

- Ensure a people centered, holistic, equity sensitive response to people's health needs through a process of population empanelment, regular home and community interactions and people's participation.
- Enable delivery of high quality care that spans health risks and disease conditions through a commensurate expansion in availability of medicines and diagnostics, use of standard treatment and referral protocols and advanced technologies including IT systems.
- Instill the culture of a team-based approach to delivery of quality Healthcare encompassing: preventive, promotive, curative, rehabilitative and palliative care.
- Ensure continuity of care with a two way referral system and follow up support.
- Emphasize health promotion (including through school education and individual centric awareness) and promote public health action through active engagement and capacity building of community platforms and individual volunteers.
- Implement appropriate mechanisms for flexible financing, including performance-based incentives and responsive resource allocations.
- Enable the integration of Yoga and AYUSH as appropriate to people's needs.
- Facilitate the use of appropriate technology for improving access to Healthcare advice and treatment initiation, enable reporting and recording, eventually progressing to electronic records for individuals and families.
- Institutionalize participation of civil society for social accountability.
- Partner with not for profit agencies and private sector for gap filling in a range of primary Healthcare functions.
- Facilitate systematic learning and sharing to enable feedback, and improvements and identify innovations for scale up.
- Develop strong measurement systems to build accountability for improved performance on measures that matter to people.

Expanded Range of Services

- Care in pregnancy and child-birth.
- Neonatal and infant Healthcare services.
- Childhood and adolescent Healthcare services.
- Family planning, Contraceptive services and other Reproductive Healthcare services.
- Management of Communicable diseases including National Health Programs.
- Management of Common Communicable Diseases and Outpatient care for acute simple illnesses and minor ailments.
- Screening, Prevention, Control and Management of Non-communicable diseases.
- Care for Common Ophthalmic and ENT problems.
- Basic Oral Healthcare.
- Elderly and Palliative Healthcare services.
- Emergency Medical Services.
- Screening and Basic management of Mental health ailments.

BIBLIOGRAPHY

1. https://www.nhm.gov.in/New_Updates_2018/NHM_Components/Health_System_Stregthening/Comprehensive_primary_health_care/letter/Operational_Guidelines_For_CPHC.pdf.

2.6 ROLE OF MLHP IN CPHC AT SC/HEALTH WELLNESS CENTER (HWC)

- Comprehensive Primary Healthcare (CPHC) services being delivered through converting the existing Sub-Health Centers covering a population of 3000-5000 to Health and Wellness Centers (HWC), with the principle being "time to care" to be no more than 30 minutes.
- Primary Health Centers in rural and urban areas would also be converted to HWCs.
- The HWC would be having appropriately trained Primary Healthcare team, comprising of multi-Purpose Workers (male and female) and ASHAs and Mid-Level Health Provider (MLHP)/Community Health Officer.

MID-LEVEL HEALTH PROVIDER (MLHP)

Rationale

- To Augment the capacity of the Health and Wellness Centre to offer expanded range of services closer to community, thus improving coverage with a reduction in OOPE.
- To Improve clinical management, care coordination and ensure continuity of care
- To Improve public health activities related to preventive and promotive health and the measurement of health outcomes
- To improve utilization of health services at primary care level, reduce fragmentation of care, and work load at secondary and tertiary care facilities.

Role of The Mid-Level Health Provider

- Listing of all the households in the service areas and this data to be maintained in digital format/paper format.
- Provide clinical care as specified in the standard treatment guidelines for the range of services expected of the HWC.
- Mid level Healthcare provider coordinate care or manage the cases of chronic illnesses who diagnosed and put on treatment by Medical Officer/specialists. MLHP can use telehealth for better coordination. In some cases they can provide medicines as well based on Schedule K.
- Screening for chronic conditions, enabling suspected cases confirmed and initiating treatment based on appropriate STGs. As a team, ensure adherence, along with counselling and support as needed for primary and secondary prevention efforts.
- Coordinate and lead local response to diseases outbreaks, emergencies and disaster situations and support the medical team or joint investigation teams for disease outbreaks.
- Support the team of MPWs and ASHAs on their tasks, including on the job mentoring, support and supervision and undertaking the monitoring, management, reporting and administrative functions of the HWC such as inventory management, upkeep and maintenance, and management of untied funds.
- Support and supervise the collection of population based data by frontline workers, collate and analyse data for planning and report the data to the next level in an accurate and timely fashion. Use HWC and population data to understand key causes of mortality, morbidity in the community and work with the team to develop a local action plan with measurable targets, including a particular focus on vulnerable communities.

- Coordinate with community platforms such as the VHSNC/MAS/SHGs and work closely with PRI/ULB, to address social determinants of health and promote behavior change for improved health outcomes.
- Address issues of social and environmental determinants of health with extension workers of other departments related to gender based violence, education, safe potable water, sanitation, safe collection of refuse, proper disposal of waste water, indoor air pollution, and on specific environmental hazards such as fluorosis, silicosis, arsenic contamination, etc.
- Guide and be actively engaged in community health promotion including behavior change communication.

Training and Mentorship

- The Mid Level Health providers would be trained in either Certificate Program in Community Health, managed and certified by IGNOU/state universities or have a B.Sc. degree in Community Health.
- The curriculum will enable the MLHP to attain a set of competencies related to public health and primary Healthcare.
- To improve training quality states shall also institutionalize District Level Committee of Observers to monitor the ongoing trainings. These committees can have representation from-Service providers of NGO run hospitals/Nurse Training Colleges/Faculty of MPW Training Centers/Medical Colleges and Counsellors from programme study centers and may submit feedback to State NHM/District Health Officers/CMHOs on improvement areas if any.
- In addition, states will need to create a strong mentorship program including through programs like ECHO (Extension for Community Healthcare Outcomes) for supporting the MLHPs through handholding, trouble shooting, problem solving, to enable building of technical competencies and sustaining motivation.
- The mentors could be drawn from schools of public health/medical colleges/district health teams/Technical support agencies and development partners.

Summary

- 6 months Certificate Program in Community Health
- 5–7 days Supplementary Training on new health programs new skills and refreshers every year.
- 3 days training on use of IT application and telehealth
- Regular monitoring/training through ECHO platform.

Skills

- Public Health Skills
- General Skills of Bio-Medical Waste management, medicine dispensation, medicine refills and injections, suturing of superficial wounds
- Laboratory Skills
- Skills for Management of common conditions fever, aches and pains
- First aid stabilization care for common emergencies
- Maternal Health Skills

- Reproductive and Adolescent Health Skills
- Newborn and Child Health Skills
- Skills to use digital applications wherever applicable for reporting, inventory management, record maintenance and use population based
- Maintaining Family Health Folders and Individual Health Records
- Supportive supervision of field level functionaries.

BIBLIOGRAPHY

1. https://www.nhm.gov.in/New_Updates_2018/NHM_Compo-nents/Health_System_Stregthening/Comprehensive_primary_health_care/letter/Operational_Guidelines_For_CPHC.pdf

2.7 SUSTAINABLE DEVELOPMENT GOALS (SDGS—2015–2030)

- Sustainable development is development that meets the need of the present without compromising the ability of future generations to meet their own needs.
- Sustainable development means meeting the diverse needs of all people in existing and future communities, promoting personal well-being, social cohesion, and inclusion, and creating equal opportunity.
- UN Sustainable Development summit entitled as **"transforming our world: the 2030 agenda for Sustainable development"** was accepted by the 193 Member States of the United Nations, and this document includes **17 Sustainable Development Goals and 169 targets.**
- **Three** interlinked elements of sustainable development namely **economic growth, social inclusion and environmental sustainability** have been addressed in SDGs. It means end all forms of poverty, fight inequalities and tackle climate change while ensuring that no one was left behind.
- Without addressing human rights and complex humanitarian issues at the same time, we can't build peaceful, inclusive and well-governed societies. SDGs have taken care of such issues.
- The SDGs are people-centered and planet-sensitive.
- They are universal, applying to all countries with considering realities and capabilities of different countries.
- The goals are need to be implemented in an integrated manner.
- The SDGs will guide us for the next 15 years in the following 5 aspects of development: **People, Planet, Prosperity, Peace and Partnership.**

SDGs Different from the MDGs

- SDGs are broader in scope than the MDGs and SDGs are framed to address the root causes of poverty.
- SDGs will cover some important and newer issues like inequalities, economic growth, employment, cities and human settlements, industrialization, energy, climate change, sustainable consumption and production, peace and justice.

- SDGs are universal and apply to all countries (both developed and developing) while MDGs were more focused on developing countries only.
- According to SDGs, climate change is key factor for sustainable development and poverty eradication.

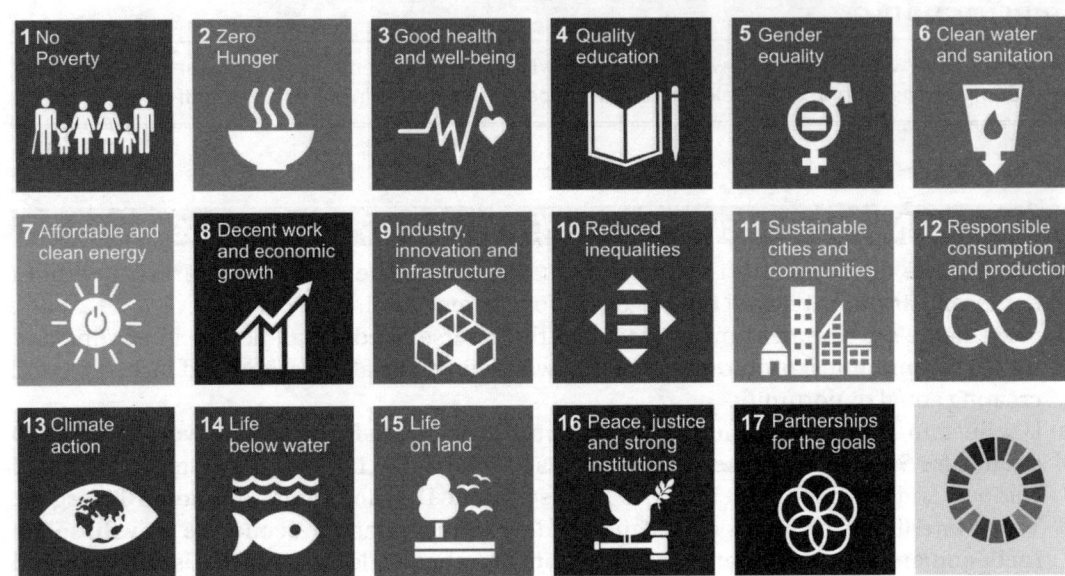

Fig. 2.4: Sustainable development goals (SDGs).

- **List of SDGs (Fig. 2.4):**
    - SDG 1 No Poverty
    - SDG 2 Zero Hunger
    - SDG 3 Good Health and Well-being
    - SDG 4 Quality Education
    - SDG 5 Gender Equality
    - SDG 6 Clean Water and Sanitation
    - SDG 7 Affordable and Clean Energy
    - SDG 8 Decent Work and Economic Growth
    - SDG 9 Industry, Innovation and Infrastructure
    - SDG 10 Reduce Inequalities
    - SDG 11 Sustainable Cities and Communities
    - SDG 12 Responsible Consumption and Production
    - SDG 13 Climate Action
    - SDG 14 Life Below Water
    - SDG 15 Life on Land
    - SDG 16 Peace, Justice and Strong Institutions
    - SDG 17 Partnerships for the Goals

Road Map of Different Ministries of India to Achieve the SDG

Goal no.	Goal	Nodal ministry	Related interventions
1.	End poverty in all its forms everywhere	Rural Development	• Pradhan Mantri Jan Dhan Yojana • Pradhan Mantri Jeevan Jyoti Bima Yojana • Atal Pension Yojana (APY) • Mahatma Gandhi National Rural Employment Guarantee Act (MGNREGA) • Deen Dayal Antyodaya Yojana (DAY)-National Rural Livelihood Mission (NRLM) • National Social Assistance Program (NSAP) • Ayushman Bharat (National Health Protection Mission)
2.	End hunger, achieve food security and improved nutrition and promote sustainable agriculture	Agriculture and Farmers Welfare	• Targeted Public Distribution System (TPDS) • National Nutrition Mission (NNM) • National Food Security Act (NFSA) • Mid-Day Meal Scheme • Pradhan Mantri Matru Vandana Yojana (PMMVY)
3.	Ensure healthy lives and promote well-being for all at all ages	It is explained in detail in the next table	
4.	Ensure inclusive and equitable quality education and promote lifelong learning opportunities for all	HRD	• Sarva Shiksha Abhiyan • National Program of Mid Day Meal in Schools (MDM) • Pradhan Mantri Kaushal Vikas Yojana
5.	Achieve gender equality and empower all women and girls	WCD	• Beti Bachao Beti Padhao • Sukanya Samridhi Yojana • Support to Training And Employment Program For Women (STEP) 2014 • Janani Suraksha Yojana (JSY) • SWADHAR 2011 (A scheme for women in difficult circumstances) • Pradhan Mantri Matru Vandana Yojana (PMMVY) • Pradhan Mantri Mahila Shakti Kendra (PMMSK) • Ujjawala • One Stop Centre, • Women Helpline, hostels
6.	Ensure availability and sustainable management of water and sanitation for all	Ministry of Water Resources, River Development and Ganga Rejuvenation	• National Rural Drinking Water Program (NRDWP) • Swachh Bharat Mission • Namami Gange • Inter-linking of rivers

Goal no.	Goal	Nodal ministry	Related interventions
7.	Ensure access to affordable, reliable, sustainable and modern energy for all	Power	• Deen Dayal Upadhyaya Gram Jyoti Yojana • National Solar Mission • Pradhan Mantri Ujjwala Yojana • Power (2015): grid Solar Power by 2020 • Five new Ultra Mega Power Projects • UJALA
8.	Promote sustained, inclusive and sustainable Economic growth, full and productive employment and decent work for all	Labor and Employment	• Deendayal Upadhyaya Antodaya Yojana. • National Urban Development Mission • STAND UP and STAR UP India • Pradhan Mantri Kaushal Vikas Yojana
9.	Build resilient infrastructure, promote inclusive and sustainable industrialization and foster innovation	Commerce and Industry	• Pt. Deendayal Upadhyaya Shramev Jayate Karyakram • Shyama Prasad Mukherjee Rurban Mission • Minimum Government Maximum Governance • Make in India • Start Up India • Ease of doing business initiative • FDI Policy
10.	Reduce inequality within and among countries	Social Justice and Empowerment	• Grants from Central Pool of Resources for North Eastern Region and Sikkim • Udaan Scheme for youth of Jammu and Kashmir • PAHAL-LPG (DBTL) consumers scheme • Give it Up Campaign (for LPG subsidy) • Mudra Yojana
11.	Make cities and human settlements inclusive, safe, resilient and sustainable	Urban Development	• Smart Cities Mission • Pradhan Mantri Awas Yojana (Housing for All-2022) • Atal Mission for Rejuvenation and Urban Transformation (AMRUT) • Heritage City Development and Augmentation Yojana (HRIDAY)
12.	Ensure sustainable consumption and production Patterns	MoEF and CC*	• National Policy on Biofuels • National Clean India Fund • National Clean Energy Fund (NCEF) • Soil Health Card Scheme
13.	Take urgent action to combat climate change and its impacts	MoEF and CC	• National Action Plan on Climate Change • National Mission for a Green India • National Solar Mission • National Mission for Enhanced Energy Efficiency • National Mission for Sustainable Habitat • National Water Mission • National Mission for Sustaining the Himalayan Ecosystem • National Mission for Sustainable Agriculture • National Mission on Strategic Knowledge for Climate Change.

Goal no.	Goal	Nodal ministry	Related interventions
14.	Conserve and sustainably use the oceans, seas and marine resources for sustainable development	Earth sciences	• National Plan for Conservation of Aquatic Ecosystem • Sagarmala Project (Blue Revolution)
15.	Protect, restore and promote sustainable use of terrestrial ecosystems, sustainably manage forests, combat desertification, and halt and reverse land degradation and halt biodiversity loss	MoEF and CC	• Project Elephant • National Environmental Policy 2006 • National Agroforestry Policy (2014) • National Action Program to Combat Desertification (2001)
16.	Promote peaceful and inclusive societies for sustainable development, provide access to justice for all and build effective, accountable and inclusive institutions at all levels	Home Affairs	• Digital India • Pragati Platform (Public Grievance Redressal System) • RTI (Right to Information Act)
17.	Strengthen the means of implementation and revitalize the global partnership for sustainable development	• Finance • Science and Technology • MEA • Commerce and Industry • Finance • MOEF and CC • MOSPI	• South-South Cooperation • India Africa Summit • SCO (Shanghai Cooperation Organization) • BRICS (Brazil, Russia, India, China, and South Africa) • NDB (New Development Bank–BRICS) • SAARC Satellite (South Asian Association for Regional Cooperation)

*Ministry of Environment, Forest and Climate Change.

Details of Goal Number 3

Goal No. 3	Nodal ministry	Targets	Means of implementation
Ensure healthy lives and promote well-being for all at all ages	Health and Family Welfare	**3.1** By 2030, reduce the global maternal mortality ratio to less than 70 per 100,000 live births **3.2** By 2030, end preventable deaths of newborns and children under 5 years of age **3.3** By 2030, end the epidemics of AIDS, tuberculosis, malaria and neglected tropical diseases and combat hepatitis, water-borne diseases and other communicable diseases **3.4** By 2030, reduce by one third premature mortality from non-communicable diseases through prevention and treatment and promote mental health and well being **3.5** Strengthen the prevention and treatment of substance abuse, including narcotic drug abuse and harmful use of alcohol **3.6** By 2020, halve the number of global deaths and injuries from road traffic accidents **3.7** By 2030, ensure universal access to sexual and reproductive healthcare services, including for family planning, information and education, and the integration of reproductive health into national strategies and programs **3.8** Achieve universal health coverage, including financial risk protection, access to quality essential healthcare services and access to safe, effective, quality and affordable essential medicines and vaccines for all **3.9** By 2030, substantially reduce the number of deaths and illnesses from hazardous chemicals and air, water and soil pollution and contamination	**3.a** Strengthen the implementation of the Framework Convention on Tobacco Control **3.b** *3.b.1* Support the research and development of vaccines and medicines for the communicable and non-communicable diseases that mainly affect developing countries, *3.b.2* Provide access to affordable essential medicines and vaccines (as per Doha Declaration on the TRIPS Agreement). **3.c** Substantially increase health financing and the recruitment, development, training and retention of the health workforce in developing countries **3.d** Strengthen the capacity for early warning, risk reduction and management of national and global health risks

SDG India Index
- NITI Aayog has developed SDG India Index to measure India and its States' progress towards the SDGs for 2030.
- The SDG India Index is intended to provide a holistic view of the social, economic and environmental status of the country and its States and UTs.
- The SDG India Index computes goal-wise scores on the 115 indicators incorporate 16 out of 17 SDGs, with a qualitative assessment on Goal 17, and cover 70 SDG targets.
- These scores range between 0–100, and if a State/UT achieves a score of 100, it signifies it has achieved the 2030 targets.
- States and Union Territories are classified in four categories based on their SDG India Index score: Aspirant (0–49), Performer (50–64), Front-Runner (65–99), Achiever (100).

BIBLIOGRAPHY
1. https://www.drishtiias.com/daily-news-analysis/sdg-india-index-2020-21-niti-aayog
2. https://www.niti.gov.in/sites/default/files/2019-01/SDGMapping-Document-NITI_0.pdf
3. Sustainable Development Goals (SDGs), Targets, CSS, Interventions, Nodal and other Ministries (As on 04.04.2016). Available at: http://niti.gov.in/content/SDGs.php
4. www.undp.org/content/undp/en/home/sustainable-development-goals.html

2.8 NATIONAL HEALTH POLICY (1983, 2002, 2017)

National Health Policy (NHP) 1983: The National Health Policy (NHP) was a response to the commitment to the Alma Ata Declaration to achieve "Health for All by 2000".

Initiatives Under NHP 1983
- A phased, time-bound program for setting up a well-dispersed network of comprehensive primary healthcare services.
- Intermediation through 'health volunteers' having appropriate knowledge, simple skills.
- Establishment of a well worked out referral system.
- An integrated network of evenly spread specialty and superspecialty services.

Indicators to be Achieved by the Year 2000
- Reduction of Infant Mortality Rate from 125 to below 60
- Reduction of Maternal Mortality Rate from 4.5 to below 2
- To raise life expectancy at birth from 52.6 to 64
- To reduce Crude Death Rate from 14 to 9
- To reduce Crude Birth Rate from 35 to 21
- To achieve a Net Reproductive Rate of 1
- To provide portable water to the entire rural population

National Health Policy 2002
Objectives
- To achieve and acceptable standard of good health among the general population of the country
- The approach would be increase access to decentralize public health system by establishing new infrastructure in the existing institutes
- Ensure equitable access to health services across the social and geographical expanse of the country
- Primacy will be given to preventive and first line curative initiatives at primary health level
- Focus on those diseases which are principally contributing to disease burden such as TB, HIV/AIDS, malaria, blindness, etc
- Emphasis will be laid on rational use of drugs within the allopathic system.

Note: Goals of NHP 2002 has been compared with NHP 2017 in the table given in the end of this chapter.

National Health Policy 2017
- The National Health Policy of 1983 and the National Health Policy of 2002 have served us well as guiding approach for the health.
- Since last health policy, the scenario has changed in four following ways:

First way: Health priorities have changed because
- Maternal and child mortality have been declined but still are at unacceptable level
- Infectious diseases are still major public health problems
- Drastic rise being seen in the prevalence of non communicable diseases.

Second Way: Emergence of a robust Healthcare industry growing at 15% compound annual growth rate (CAGR).

Third way: Catastrophic expenditure due to Healthcare costs is increasing which is an important contributor to poverty.

Fourth way: Fiscal capacity has increased due to economic growth.

Goal NHP-2017
The attainment of the highest possible level of good health and well-being, through a preventive and promotive Healthcare orientation in all developmental policies, and universal access to good quality Healthcare services without anyone having to face financial hardship as a consequence.

Objectives
- Improve population health status through concerted policy action in all sectors and expand preventive, promotive, curative, palliative and rehabilitative services provided by the public health sector.
- Achieve a significant reduction in out of pocket expenditure due to Healthcare costs and reduction in proportion of households experiencing catastrophic health expenditures and consequent impoverishment.

- Assure universal availability of free, comprehensive primary healthcare services, as an entitlement, for all aspects of reproductive, maternal, child and adolescent health and for the most prevalent communicable and non-communicable diseases in the population.
- Enable universal access to free essential drugs, diagnostics, emergency ambulance services, and emergency medical and surgical care services in public health facilities, so as to enhance the financial protection role of public facilities for all sections of the population.
- Ensure improved access and affordability of secondary and tertiary care services through a combination of public hospitals and strategic purchasing of services from the private health sector.
- Influence the growth of the private healthcare industry and medical technologies to ensure alignment with public health goals, and enable contribution to making healthcare systems more effective, efficient, rational, safe, affordable and ethical.

Key Policy Principles

- **Equity**:
  - By prioritizing the needs of the most vulnerable will give financial protection to the poor.
- **Universality**:
  - Systems and services are for the entire population and not only for targeted sub-group.
- **Patient Centered and Quality of Care**:
  - Effective, safe, and convenient Healthcare services would be provided with dignity and confidentiality at all health facilities across all sectors and they will be assessed, certified and incentivized to maintain quality of care.
- **Inclusive Partnerships**:
  - The task of providing Healthcare for all requires the participation of communities and community should take this participation as a means and a goal, as a right and as a duty.
  - Partnerships with medical institutions, NGOs and with the private sector are required to achieve these goals.
- **Pluralism (both allopathic and non-allopathic)**:
  - Patient would have access both allopathic **and** AYUSH care providers.
- **Subsidiarity:**
  - For ensuring responsiveness and greater participation, decentralization in decision making is required.
- **Accountability:**
  - Performance accountability, transparency in decision making, and elimination of corruption in both public and private Healthcare systems would be essential.
- **Professionalism, Integrity and Ethics**
- **Learning and Adaptive System:**
- **Affordability**:
  - When Healthcare cost of a family exceeding 10% of its total monthly consumption expenditures or 40% of its non-food consumption expenditure- is known as **catastrophic health expenditures**.
  - Poverty due to Healthcare costs is unacceptable.

Seven priority areas for improving the environment for health includes:
1. **The Swachh Bharat Abhiyan:** it will be measured by reduction in proportion of open air defecation.
2. **Balanced and Healthy Diets:** mainly at Anganwadi centers and schools and it will be measured by the reduction of malnutrition and improved food safety.
3. **Nasha Mukti Abhiyan:** achievement will be measured in terms of reduction in use of tobacco, alcohol and substance abuse.
4. **Yatri Suraksha:** Rail and road traffic accidents related deaths should decrease through a combination of response and prevention measures.
5. **Nirbhaya Nari:** Action must be taken against gender violence like sex determination sexual violence through a combination of legal measures, health sector responses.
6. **Reduce Stress and Safety at Workplace**
7. **Reducing Indoor and Outdoor air Pollution**

All these 7 approaches could be called together as **the SWASTH NAGRIK ABHIYAN**—a social movement for health.

Organization of Healthcare Services: The 7 Key Policy Shifts:
1. **In Primary Care:** From a Selective Care that is fragmented from secondary/tertiary care to Assured Comprehensive care that has continuity with higher levels.
2. **In Secondary and Tertiary Care:** From an input oriented, budget line financing to an output based strategic purchasing.
3. **In Public Hospitals:** From User Fees and Cost Recovery Based Public Hospitals to Assured Free Drugs, Diagnostic and Emergency Services to all in Public Health Facilities.
4. **In Infrastructure and Human Resource Development:** From normative approaches in their development to targeted approaches to reach under-serviced areas.
5. **In Urban Health:** From token under-financed interventions to on-scale assured interventions that reach the Urban Poor and establish linkages with national programmes: Scaling up of the interventions with focus on the urban poor and achieving convergence among the wider determinants of health.
6. **In National Health Programs:** Integration with health systems for effectiveness, and contributing to strengthening health systems for efficiency.
7. **In AYUSH Services:** From Stand-Alone AYUSH to a three dimensional mainstreaming.

Comparison of Targets of National Health Policy 2002 and 2017

Target	NHP 2002	NHP 2017	Current status 2022
Eradicate Polio	by 2005	—	Eliminated on 27th March 2014
Eradicate Yaws	by 2005	—	Eliminated on 14th July 2016
Eliminate Leprosy	by 2005	By 2018	Eliminated on 1st December 2005 (<1/10,000 criteria)
Establish an integrated system of surveillance, National Health Accounts and Health Statistics	By 2005	—	

Healthcare Planning and Organization of Healthcare at Various Levels

Target	NHP 2002	NHP 2017	Current status 2022
HIV/AIDS	Achieve zero level growth by 2007	90:90:90 by 2020 and 95:95:95 by 2024 • 90 percent of all people living with HIV know their HIV status, • 90 percent of all people diagnosed with HIV infection receive sustained antiretroviral therapy • 90 percent of all people receiving antiretroviral therapy will have viral suppression	
Eliminate Kala Azar	by 2010	by 2017	>70% of endemic blocks have achieved elimination
TB, Malaria and Other Vector and Water-borne diseases	Reduce Mortality by 50% by 2010	TB Elimination by 2025 and Malaria Elimination by 2030	
Blindness	Reduce prevalence to 0.5% by 2010	Reduce prevalence to 0.25/ 1000 by 2025	
Maternal Mortality Ratio (per 100,000 live births)	Reduce to 100 by 2010	Reduce to 100 by 2020	97
Infant Mortality Rate	Reduce to 30 by 2010	Reduce to 28 by 2019	28
Utilization of Public Health Facilities	Increase from current 20% to >75% by 2010	Increase by 50% of current levels by 2025	
Govt. health expenditure (as a % of GDP)	Increase from 0.9% to 2% by 2010	Increase to 2.5% by 2025	1.35% of country's total GDP
State Sector health spending	Increase from 5.5% to 7% by 2005 and 8% by 2010	Increase to >8% by 2020	

Target	NHP 2002	NHP 2017	Current status 2022
Eliminate Lymphatic Filariasis	by 2015	By 2017	Eliminated in 203 out of 255 endemic districts
Life expectancy	--	70 years by 2025	70.19 years
TFR	--	2.1 by 2025	2.0
Under-five Mortality Rate	--	23 per 1000 live births by 2025	32 per 1000 live births
Neonatal Mortality Rate	--	16 per 1000 live births by 2025	20 per 1000 live births
Stillbirth Rate	--	Single digit by 2025	3
Number of beds per 1000 population	--	2 beds per 1000 population by 2025	

BIBLIOGRAPHY

1. Dahiya, Heaven. (2018). National Health Policy of India. 9. 27842-27844. 10.24327/ijrsr.2018.0907.2343.
2. https://www.egyankosh.ac.in/bitstream/123456789/76672/1/Unit-11.pdf
3. https://www.nhp.gov.in/sites/default/files/pdf/nhp_1983.pdf
4. National Health Policy-2015 (draft), Ministry of Health and Family Welfare, New Delhi, (2014), available at; http://www.mohfw.nic.in/showfile.php?lid=3014, accessed on 10 July, 2016.

2.9 NATIONAL HEALTH MISSION (NHM)

- The National Health Mission encompasses its two Sub-Missions, the National Rural Health Mission (NRHM) and the National Urban Health Mission (NUHM).
- The NHM envisages achievement of universal access to equitable, affordable and quality healthcare services that are accountable and responsive to people's needs.

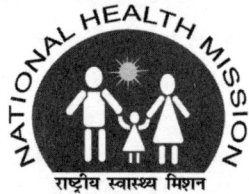

NATIONAL RURAL HEALTH MISSION (NRHM)

Objectives

- To provide quality healthcare to the rural population, especially the vulnerable groups.
- To establish a fully functional, community owned, decentralized health delivery system with inter-sectoral convergence at all levels
- To ensure simultaneous action on a wide range of determinants of health such as water, sanitation, education, nutrition, social and gender equality.

Goals of NRHM

- Reduce MMR to 1/1,000 live births
- Reduce IMR to 25/1,000 live births

Healthcare Planning and Organization of Healthcare at Various Levels

- Reduce TFR to 2.1
- Prevention and reduction of anemia in women aged 15–49 years
- Prevent and reduce mortality and morbidity from communicable, non-communicable; injuries and emerging diseases
- Reduce household out-of-pocket expenditure on total Healthcare expenditure
- Reduce annual incidence and mortality from Tuberculosis by half
- Reduce the prevalence of Leprosy to <1/10,000 population and incidence to zero in all districts
- Annual Malaria Incidence to be <1/1,000
- Less than 1 percent microfilaria prevalence in all districts
- Kala-azar Elimination by 2015, <1 case per 10,000 population in all blocks.

Major Initiatives Under NRHM/NHM

- ASHA
- Rogi Kalyan Samiti/Hospital Management Society
- The Untied Grants to Sub-Center (SCs)
- The Village Health Sanitation and Nutrition Committee (VHSNC)
- Janani Suraksha Yojana (JSY)
- Janani Shishu Suraksha Karyakram (JSSK)
- Facility Based Newborn Care
- National Mobile Medical Units (NMMUs)
- National Ambulance Services (NAS)
- Mainstreaming of AYUSH
- National Quality Assurance Framework for Health facilities
- Kayakalp—an initiative for Award to Public Health facilities
- Free Drugs Service Initiative
- Free Diagnostics Service Initiative
- Comprehensive Primary Healthcare
- Kilkari
- Mobile Academy

NATIONAL URBAN HEALTH MISSION (NUHM)

- The National Urban Health Mission (NUHM), launched on 1st May, 2013, is a sub-mission under the National Health Mission, which aims to cater to the unique and diverse needs of the urban poor and vulnerable population.
- Proportion of Urban population is 31.2% in 2011 and is expected to increase to 50% in next few decades.
- **Hashim Committee** has identified three main vulnerable categories as below:
  1. Residential or habitat-based vulnerability
  2. Social vulnerability
  3. Occupational vulnerability
- All people facing disproportionate burden of ill-health often linked with low-incomes, social exclusions, poor housing, risky occupational settings, gender, disability, singleness, age, debilitating ailments and others constitute vulnerability.

- Urban pull factors (like employment) and Rural push factors (like inadequate amenities and infrastructure) leads to migration and in turn increase the vulnerability of migrated people in urban area.
- Marginalization along with migration makes people more prone to have multiple health related issues.
- SDGs also have addressed urban health by defining SDG goal **"Sustainable Cities and Communities"**.
- MOHFW recommended establishment of 'Urban Health Posts' for 50,000 population, to be located in and around urban slums, with strong linkages with secondary and tertiary level facilities which were supported by World Bank through India Population Projects (IPPs).

Target Population
- 29.95 Crore urban population (Census 2011)
- 942 cities/towns with population above 50,000 (29.69 Crore)
- 64 District Headquarter towns with population between 30,000–50,000 (0.26 Crore)

Special focus on
- People living in listed, unlisted slums and other low income neighborhoods
- All other vulnerable population such as homeless, rag-pickers, street children, rickshaw pullers, and other temporary migrants.

Aim
To address unique and diverse needs of urban poor and vulnerable population.

Mission
To provide **essential primary health services** to the entire urban population, while urban poor and vulnerable sections remaining its prime concern

Urban issues and their solutions require:
- Inter-sectoral coordination
- Equity
- Community involvement
- Sustainability

Principles of Urban Primary Healthcare (Fig. 2.5)
- **Universal access:** No one shall be turned away or refused any health service.
- **Assured minimum package of services**: Delivered as close to home as possible to ensure universal access with quality.
- **Preventive and promotive care:** Enhanced focus on screening of NCDs, early identification of communicable diseases, early outbreak identification and management
- **Effective Gatekeeping:** Reduced patient load at higher facilities by strengthening primary health services
- **Outreach:** Special efforts to identify, reach out to and address health needs of marginalized
- **Reduction in out of pocket expenditure:** Provision of free drugs, diagnostics and consultation
- **Integration:** Collaboration with ULBs and other departments to tackle cross cutting issues
- **Continuity of Care:** Continued care through referral and follow ups.

Institutional Framework of NUHM

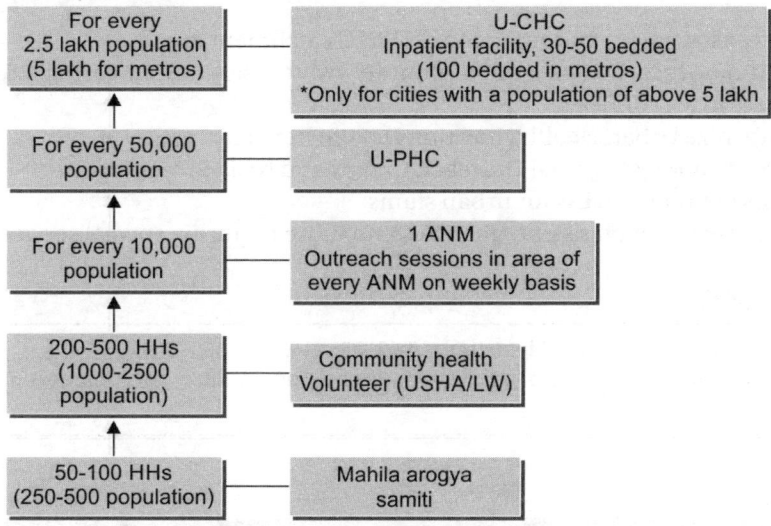

Fig. 2.5: Urban health care facilities.

URBAN ASHA (USHA: URBAN SOCIAL HEALTH ACTIVIST)

- Each Urban ASHA will cater area with 1,000–2,500 population. She preferably should be the Resident of the "slum clusters" and belong to a vulnerable group. Formal education of at least Tenth class is desired.
- She should undertake a vulnerability assessment of the households in her area.
- Her essential task to create awareness on social determinants and entitlements for health and other public services.
- She shall counsel women, families and adolescents on reproductive, maternal and child health, prevention of common infections, substance abuse, and prevention of domestic and sexual violence.
- Curative care for common ailments, first aid, other communicable diseases like malaria, Japanese encephalitis, chikungunya, leprosy, etc. also to be provided in her area.
- She facilitates UHND and outreach activities including home visits.
- She works as coordinator MAS formation and their functioning.

Mahila Arogya Samiti (MAS)

- One MAS is Group of 10-15 community women and it will be per 50-100 households.
- It is formed in slum and slum-like areas.
- MAS is coordinated by Urban ASHA.
- Groups will conduct monthly meetings to discuss issues faced by the community.
- Mobilize action for resolving them.
- Untied Funds of Rs. 5,000 per year transferred to their accounts.

ANM under NUHM

Functions and duties of ANM under NUHM are wider and expanded under NUHM, as compared to her traditional RCH centric role:

- Not just RCH services provision, but also services for communicable and non-communicable diseases
- Vulnerability assessment and mapping of UPHC catchment area
- Understand non-health issues of community (water, sanitation, garbage disposal) and communicate to MO or PHM
- Plan and organize Urban Health Nutrition Days in her areas
- Support organization of Special Outreach Camps and NCD Screening
- Supervisions of urban ASHAs for urban slums
- Make home visits for high risk pregnancies and those requiring special services.

BIBLIOGRAPHY

1. https://main.mohfw.gov.in/sites/default/files/56987532145632566578.pdf
2. https://www.nhm.gov.in/images/pdf/NUHM/Orientation_module_for_planners_implementers_and_partners.pdf

2.10 PM AYUSHMAN BHARAT HEALTH INFRASTRUCTURE MISSION (PM-ABHIM)

- The on-going COVID-19 pandemic has demonstrated that India's health systems need to be better equipped to address public health needs across primary, secondary, and tertiary care levels.
- India's current epidemiological and demographic status, with the rapid rise in non-communicable diseases, a double burden of chronic and infectious diseases, and unfinished agenda of reproductive, maternal new-born and child health services has created an increasing demand on Healthcare and public health services.
- So, answer to these issues resulted in launch of PM-ABHIM.
- **The PM Ayushman Bharat Health Infrastructure Mission** is one of the largest Pan-India health schemes for strengthening healthcare infrastructure and to accomplish the vision of comprehensive healthcare across the country.
- It was launched on 25 October 2021 with an outlay of ₹64,180 crore.

Objective: To fill the critical gaps in public health infrastructure, especially in critical care facilities and primary care in both the urban and rural areas.

There are 3 major aspects:
1. **The first**: to strengthen grass root public health institutions to deliver universal comprehensive primary healthcare and critical care services.
2. **The second**: to expand and build an IT enabled disease surveillance system by developing a network of surveillance laboratories for effectively detecting, investigating, preventing and combating Public Health Emergencies and Disease Outbreaks.
3. **The third**: the expansion of research on COVID-19 and other infectious diseases and to develop the core capacity to deliver the One Health Approach to prevent, detect, and respond to infectious disease outbreaks in animals and humans.

Components: It has Centrally Sponsored Scheme Components and Central Sector Components.

Centrally Sponsored Scheme (CSS) Components: (2021-22 to 2025-26)
- **Ayushman Bharat—Health and Wellness Center (AB-HWCs) in rural areas:** Support for infrastructure development for 17788 Sub-Health Center is proposed in 7 High Focus States (Bihar, Jharkhand, Odisha, Punjab, Rajasthan, Uttar Pradesh and West Bengal) and 3 North Eastern States (Assam, Manipur and Meghalaya).
- **Ayushman Bharat—Health and Wellness Centers (AB-HWCs) in Urban areas:** Support for 11044 Urban Health and Wellness Centers across the country is proposed under this component.
- **Block Public Health Units (BPHUs):** Support for 3382 BPHUs in 11 High Focus States/UTs (Assam, Bihar, Chhattisgarh, Himachal Pradesh, UT - Jammu and Kashmir, Jharkhand, Madhya Pradesh, Odisha, Rajasthan, Uttar Pradesh and Uttarakhand), is proposed under this component
- **Integrated District Public Health Laboratories** in all districts.
- **Critical Care Hospital Blocks** in all districts with a population more than 5 lakhs, in State Government Medical Colleges/District Hospitals.

Central Sector (CS) Components
- **Critical Care Hospital Blocks** in 12 Central Institutions.
- **Strengthening Surveillance of Infectious Diseases and Outbreak Response:** Support for 20 Metropolitan Surveillance Units, 5 new Regional NCDCs and implementation of Integrated Health Information Platform (IHIP) in all states.
- **Strengthening Surveillance Capacities at Points of Entry:** Support for 17 new Points of Entry Health Units and Strengthening of 33 existing Units.
- **Strengthening Disaster and Epidemic Preparedness:** Support for 15 Health Emergency Operation Centers and 2 Container based mobile hospitals.
- **Bio-security Preparedness and Strengthening Pandemic Research, National Institutions and Platforms for One Health:**
  - Support for setting up of a National Institution for One Health
  - A Regional Research Platform for WHO South-East Asia Region
  - 9 Bio-Safety Level III Laboratories and
  - 4 new Regional National Institutes of Virology (NIV).

BIBLIOGRAPHY

1. https://www.nhp.gov.in/pm-ayushman-bharat-health-infrastructure-mission_pg
2. https://nhsrcindia.org/sites/default/files/FINAL%20PM-ABHIM__15-12-21.pdf

2.11 NATIONAL DIGITAL HEALTH MISSION (AYUSHMAN BHARAT DIGITAL MISSION)

- The Ayushman Bharat Digital Mission (ABDM) aims to develop the backbone necessary to support the integrated digital health infrastructure of the country.
- Based on recommendation of committee of Shri J Satyanarayana.

- **National Digital Health Mission (NDHM)** has been launched on 27th September, 2021.
- **National Health Authority (NHA)** under the Ministry of Health and Family Welfare will be the core implementing agency for the **National Digital Health Mission** (NDHM).
- Jan Dhan, Aadhaar and Mobile (JAM) trinity and other digital initiatives of the government, Ayushman Bharat Digital Mission will create a seamless online platform through the provision of a wide-range of data, information and infrastructure services, duly leveraging open, interoperable, standards-based digital systems while ensuring the security, confidentiality and privacy of health-related personal information.

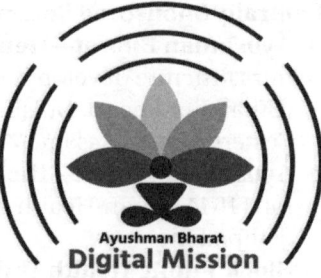

- The Mission will enable access and exchange of longitudinal health records of citizens with their consent.
- This Mission will create interoperability within the digital health ecosystem, Citizens will only be a click-away from accessing healthcare facilities.
- The NDHM is a complete **digital health ecosystem** comprising of five key features or components;
    1. **Health ID/ABHA Number**
    2. **Personal Health Records**
    3. **Digi Doctor**
    4. **Health Facility Registry**
    5. **Electronic Medical Record (EMR) web app**
- It is also going to include **e-pharmacy and telemedicine** services in near future.
- The platform is based on both **app** and **website.**

1. HEALTH ID/ABHA NUMBER

- It is important to standardize the process of identification of an individual across healthcare providers.
- The national health ID will be **a repository of all health-related information** of every Indian.
- The Health ID will be used for the purposes of uniquely identifying persons, authenticating them, and threading their health records (only with the informed consent of the patient) across multiple systems and stakeholders.
- **Various healthcare providers**—such as hospitals, laboratories, insurance companies, online pharmacies, telemedicine firms—will be expected to participate in the health ID system.
- Every patient who wishes to have their health records available digitally must create a **Unique Health ID,** using their basic details including demographic and location, family/relationship, and contact details and mobile or **Aadhaar** number.
- A Digital Health ID was proposed to "greatly reduce the risk of preventable medical errors and significantly increase quality of care".

2. PERSONAL HEALTH RECORDS (PHR)

- The most salient feature of the PHR, and the one that distinguishes it from the EMR and EHR, is that the information it contains is under the control of the individual.
- Each Health ID will be linked to a **health data consent manager,** which will be used to seek the patient's consent and allow for seamless **flow of health information from the Personal Health Records module.**
- The Health ID will be **voluntary** and **applicable across states,** hospitals, diagnostic laboratories and pharmacies.

3. DIGI DOCTOR (DOCTORS DIRECTORY)/HEALTHCARE PROFESSIONALS REGISTRY (HPR)

- A single, updated repository of all doctors enrolled in nation with all the relevant details of the doctors such as name, qualifications, name of the institutions of qualifications, specializations, registration number with State medical councils, years of experience, etc. would be an essential building block of the digital health infrastructure of the country.
- The directory must be designed to be kept up-to-date as doctors gain skills via fellowships and map them to the facilities they are associated with.
- The **Digi Doctor** option will allow doctors from all over the country to enroll and enter their details like their contact numbers, etc.
- These enrolled doctors will also be **assigned digital signatures for free** which can be used for **writing prescriptions.**
- It will be **voluntary for the hospitals and doctors** to provide details for the app.

4. HEALTH FACILITY REGISTRY

The Health Facility Registry is a single repository of all the health facilities in the country. The registry should be centrally maintained, store and facilitate the exchange of standardized data of both public and private health facilities in the country. The registry must allow health facilities to access their profile and update it periodically with specialties and services they offer, as well as provide a secure common platform to the facilities to maintain all essential information. Facilities should be able to e-sign documents such as patient records, apply for empanelment, have easier claims processing, as well as improve access to all healthcare ecosystem elements.

5. ELECTRONIC MEDICAL RECORD (EMR) WEB APP

- An EMR is a digital version of a patient's chart.
- It contains the patient's medical and treatment history from a SINGLE health facility.
- EMRs helps service providers to identify which patients are due for screening, monitoring of certain indicators like blood pressure or due for vaccinations, etc.
- The EMR envisages to be the comprehensive view of the patients Health Information at a given facility.

Expected Outcomes of NDHM

- It will improve the efficiency, effectiveness, and transparency of health service delivery.
- Patients will be able to securely store and access their medical records (such as prescriptions, diagnostic reports and discharge summaries), and share them with Healthcare providers to ensure appropriate treatment and follow-up.
- They will also have access to more accurate information on health facilities and service providers. NDHM will empower individuals with accurate information to enable informed decision making and increase accountability of healthcare providers.
- Patients will have the option to access health services remotely through tele-consultation and e-pharmacy.
- NDHM will provide choice to individuals to access both public and private health services, facilitate compliance with laid down guidelines and protocols, and ensure transparency in pricing of services and accountability for the health services being rendered.

BIBLIOGRAPHY

1. https://www.mygov.in/task/name-logo-and-tagline-contest-national-digital-health-mission-0/
2. https://www.drishtiias.com/daily-updates/daily-news-analysis/national-digital-health-mission
3. https://pib.gov.in/PressReleseDetail.aspx?PRID=1758248
4. https://ndhm.gov.in/abdm

2.12 AYUSHMAN BHARAT PMJAY

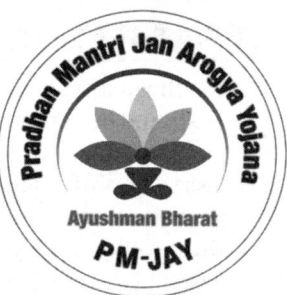

- India's economy has been one of the top three fastest growing economies in the world. However, more than 20 percent of India's population still lives under USD 1.9 per day (2011 PPP).
- As India's demographic dividend enables us to be highly optimistic about a sustained economic growth for few more decades before a higher dependency ratio sets in.
- However, the perceived benefits of the higher demographic dividend are threatened by the epidemiological transition in India.
- India is currently facing the unique situation of a 'triple burden of disease'. As the mission of eradication of major communicable diseases remained unfinished, the population is also bearing the high burden of non-communicable diseases (NCDs) and injuries.
- Nearly 50 percent of beds in India are in the private sector and nearly 70 percent of visits for Healthcare needs are served by the private sector.
- Public sector hospitals in India are overburdened, underfunded and their utilization varies widely. They face shortage of workers, physicians and other medical staff and also the issue of deficient supply of drugs and equipment which adversely impacts their functioning.
- One of the major causes of this situation is the persistent underfunding of the country's public Healthcare system. India's general Government expenditure on health has remained stagnant over the last two decades at close to 1.35% of its GDP (Source: National Health Accounts, 2019–2020).

Healthcare Planning and Organization of Healthcare at Various Levels

- India spends only 21 percent of its total health expenditure from the general Government revenue and as high as 47.1 per cent of total health expenditure is out-of-pocket (Source: National Health Accounts, 2019–2020).
- Increasing healthcare needs coupled with high out-of-pocket expenditure is a leading cause of poverty in India. It is not only keeping people poor but also pulling back those people who have moved out of poverty.
- Ayushman Bharat, a flagship scheme of Government of India, was launched as recommended by the National Health Policy 2017, to achieve the vision of Universal Health Coverage (UHC). This initiative has been designed to meet Sustainable Development Goals (SDGs) and its underlining commitment, which is to "leave no one behind."
- Ayushman Bharat is an attempt to move from sectoral and segmented approach of health service delivery to a comprehensive need-based Healthcare service. This scheme aims to undertake path breaking interventions to holistically address the healthcare system (covering prevention, promotion and ambulatory care) at the primary, secondary and tertiary level.
- Ayushman Bharat adopts a continuum of care approach, comprising of two inter-related components, which are:
  1. **Health and Wellness Centers (HWCs)**
  2. **Pradhan Mantri Jan Arogya Yojana (PM-JAY)**

1. HEALTH AND WELLNESS CENTERS (HWCS)

- In February 2018, the Government of India announced the creation of 1,50,000 Health and Wellness Centers (HWCs) by transforming the existing Sub Centers and Primary Health Centers.
- These centers are to deliver **Comprehensive Primary Healthcare (CPHC)** bringing healthcare closer to the homes of people.
- Health and Wellness Centers are envisaged to deliver an expanded range of services to address the primary Healthcare needs of the entire population in their area, expanding access, universality and equity close to the community.
- The emphasis of health promotion and prevention is designed to bring focus on keeping people healthy by engaging and empowering individuals and communities to choose healthy behaviours and make changes that reduce the risk of developing chronic diseases and morbidities.
- In addition to existing staff of sub center, after upgradation of Health and Wellness center will have one more health staff in the form **Community Health Officer** (mid-level Healthcare provider) who will be posted after training for six months.
- **List of services to be provided under CPHC are as follows:**
  - Care in pregnancy and child-birth.
  - Neonatal and infant Healthcare services
  - Childhood and adolescent Healthcare services.
  - Family planning, Contraceptive services and Other Reproductive Healthcare services
  - Management of Communicable diseases: National Health Programmes
  - Management of Common Communicable Diseases and General Out-patient care for acute simple illnesses and minor ailments
  - Screening, Prevention, Control and Management of Non-Communicable diseases
  - Screening and Basic management of Mental health ailments

- Care for Common Ophthalmic and ENT problems
- Basic Oral Healthcare
- Elderly and Palliative Healthcare services
- Emergency Medical Services

☐ AYUSHMAN Ambassadors: Health and Wellness Ambassadors will be School teachers (one male and one female) in public schools for prevention and promotion of diseases among school children.
☐ Every Tuesday will be celebrated as Health and Wellness Day in the schools
☐ These health promotion messages will also have bearing on improving health practices in the country and students will act as Health and Wellness Messengers in the society.

2. PRADHAN MANTRI JAN AROGYA YOJANA (PM-JAY)

☐ The second component under Ayushman Bharat is the Pradhan Mantri Jan Arogya Yojna or PM-JAY.
☐ This scheme was launched on 23rd September, 2018 in Ranchi, Jharkhand by the Hon'ble Prime Minister of India, Shri Narendra Modi.
☐ PM-JAY provides the States with the flexibility to choose their implementation model. They can implement scheme through assurance/trust model, insurance model or mixed model.
☐ PM-JAY was earlier known as the National Health Protection Scheme (NHPS). It subsumed the then existing Rashtriya Swasthya Bima Yojana (RSBY) which had been launched in 2008.
☐ PM-JAY is fully funded by the Government and cost of implementation is shared between the Central and State Governments.
☐ The inclusion of households is based on the deprivation and occupational criteria of the Socio-Economic Caste Census 2011 (SECC 2011) for rural and urban areas, respectively. This number also includes families that were covered in the RSBY but were not present in the SECC 2011 database.
☐ The SECC involves ranking of the households based on their socio-economic status.
☐ Rural households which are included are then ranked based on their status of seven deprivation criteria (D1 to D7). Urban households are categorised based on occupation categories.
☐ Out of the total seven deprivation criteria for rural areas, PM-JAY covered all such families who fall into at least one of the following six deprivation criteria (D1 to D5 and D7) and automatic inclusion (Destitute/living on alms, manual scavenger households, primitive tribal group, legally released bonded labour) criteria:
- D1: Only one room with kucha walls and kucha roof
- D2: No adult member between ages 16 to 59
- D3: Households with no adult male member between ages 16 to 59
- D4: Disabled member and no able-bodied adult member
- D5: SC/ST households
- D7: Landless households deriving a major part of their income from manual casual labour

Urban Beneficiaries: For urban areas, the following 11 occupational categories of workers are eligible for the scheme:
1. Rag picker
2. Beggar
3. Domestic worker

4. Street vendor/Cobbler/hawker/other street worker
5. Construction worker/Plumber/Mason/Labour/Painter/Welder/Security guard/Coolie and other head-load worker
6. Sweeper/Sanitationworker/Mali
7. Home-based worker/Artisan/Handicrafts worker/Tailor
8. Transport worker/Driver/Conductor/Helper to drivers and conductors/Cart puller/Rickshaw puller
9. Shop worker/Assistant/Peon in smallestablishment/Helper/Delivery assistant/Attendant/Waiter
10. Electrician/Mechanic/Assembler/Repair worker
11. Washerman/Chowkidar

Key Features of PM-JAY

- PM-JAY is the world's largest health insurance/ assurance scheme fully financed by the government.
- It provides a cover of Rs. 5 lakhs per family per year for secondary and tertiary care hospitalization across public and private empanelled hospitals in India.
- The benefits of INR 5,00,000 are on a family floater basis which means that it can be used by one or all members of the family.
- Over 10.74 crore poor and vulnerable entitled families (approximately 50 crore beneficiaries) are eligible for these benefits.
- PM-JAY provides cashless access to Healthcare services for the beneficiary at the point of service, that is, the hospital.
- PM-JAY envisions to help mitigate catastrophic expenditure on medical treatment which pushes nearly 6 crore Indians into poverty each year.
- It covers up to 3 days of pre-hospitalization and 15 days post-hospitalization expenses such as diagnostics and medicines.
- There is no restriction on the family size, age or gender.
- All pre-existing conditions are covered from day one.
- Benefits of the scheme are portable across the country, i.e., a beneficiary can visit any empanelled public or private hospital in India to avail cashless treatment.
- Services include approximately 1,393 procedures covering all the costs related to treatment, including but not limited to drugs, supplies, diagnostic services, physician's fees, room charges, surgeon charges, OT and ICU charges, etc.
- Public hospitals are reimbursed for the healthcare services at par with the private hospitals.

BIBLIOGRAPHY

1. https://pmjay.gov.in/

2.13 UNIVERSAL HEALTH COVERAGE

- It is State's responsibility to provide adequate food, appropriate medical care, safe drinking water, proper sanitation, education and health-related information for good health.
- The State should also address the wider determinants of health to effectively guarantee health security.

Healthcare Planning and Organization of Healthcare at Various Levels

- In October 2010, Planning Commission of India appointed "High Level Expert Group (HLEG)" for developing a framework of Universal Health Coverage (UHC) **(Fig. 2.6)**.
- It is for comprehensive health security to every Indian citizen.
- UHC entails ensuring all people have access to quality health services—including prevention, promotion, treatment, rehabilitation, and palliation—without incurring financial hardship.

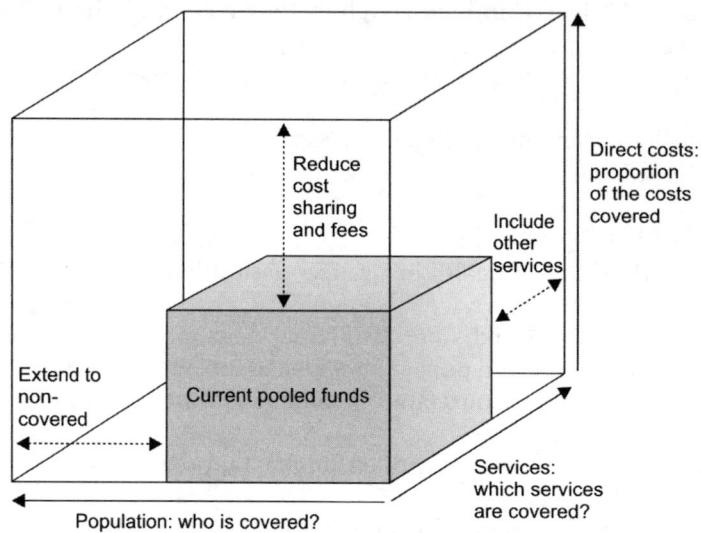

Fig. 2.6: Three dimensions of Universal Health Coverage.

- **Definition:** "Ensuring equitable access for all Indian citizens, resident in any part of the country, regardless of income level, social status, gender, caste or religion, to affordable, accountable, appropriate health services of assured quality (promotive, preventive, curative and rehabilitative) as well as public health services addressing the wider determinants of health delivered to individuals and populations, with the government being the guarantor and enabler, although not necessarily the only provider, of health and related services".
- India is committed to achieving Universal Healthcare for all by 2030, which is fundamental to achieving the other Sustainable Development Goals.
- The PMJAY was a step in this direction providing insurance cover to the poorest 40 per cent of the population.

Vision of UHC (Fig. 2.7)

- **Entitlement:** It is Universal to every citizen.
- **National health package:** It ensures access to all essential health services including in-patient and out-patient care which is provided free of cost (cashless) at all primary, secondary and tertiary level.
- **Choice of facilities:** People can select public sector or contracted in private sector.

Objectives: The concept covers three key elements—access, quality, and financial protection.
- Equity in access to health
- To ensure good quality of healthcare services
- Financial risk protection

Healthcare Planning and Organization of Healthcare at Various Levels

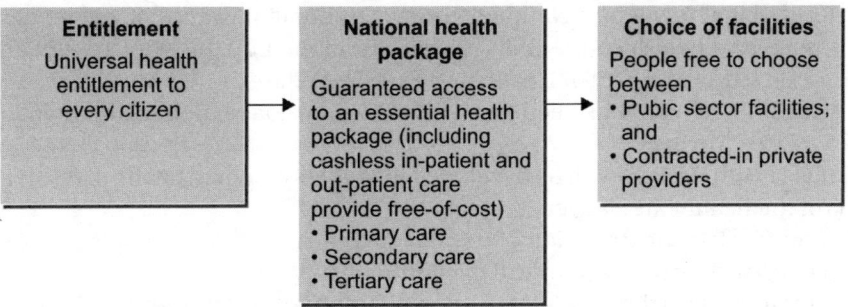

Fig. 2.7: Vision of Universal Health Coverage by 2022.

10 Guiding Principles of UHC
1. Universality
2. Equity
3. Non-Exclusion and Non-Discrimination
4. Comprehensive care that is rational and of good quality
5. Financial Protection
6. Protection of patients' rights that guarantee appropriateness of care, patient choice, portability and continuity of care
7. Consolidated and strengthened public health provisioning
8. Accountability and transparency
9. Community participation
10. Putting health in people's hands.

Expected outcomes of UHC
- Greater equity
- Improved health outcome
- Efficient accountable and transparent health system
- Poverty reduction
- Greater productivity
- Increased employment
- Financial protection

Areas of UHC
- **Health Financing and Financial Protection:**
  - It is targeted to increase the share of GDP for health from current 1.2% level to 2.5% by 2017 and to 3% of GDP by 2022.
  - There will be no fee under UHC but the fund for health will be generated from general taxation and in some case special health tax.
  - There will no private insurance company involvement under UHC.
  - Increase public spending on drug procurement to ensure availability of free essential medicines and at least 70% of all healthcare expenditures should account on primary healthcare.

- It is decided that it will be a National Health Entitlement Card that will replace all other cards related to health so the RSBY system developed by the Ministry of Labor will be transferred to the Ministry of Health and Family Welfare.
- Steps like PM-JAY card has been taken to realize the goal of financial protection.

❏ **Health Services Norms:**
- National Health Package will be developed that offers essential health services at different levels of the healthcare delivery system.
- Main Focus will be on provision of primary healthcare.
- Partnership with private sector will of contracting in type.
- Strengthen the District Hospitals and availability of functioning beds right from the second level of health system.

❏ **Human Resources for Health:**
- 4 million jobs will be created after implementation of UHC.
- It is needed to achieve WHO suggested ratio of 23 health worker per 10,000 population.
- To impart training there will be **District health knowledge institute**.
- **National council for human resources** will be established to prescribe and monitor the standards of health professional education.
- Strengthen existing State and Regional Institutes of Family Welfare.
- Good pay, incentives, and competency-based professional advancement related schemes must be adopted for better human resource practices.

❏ **Community Participation and Citizen Engagement:**
- VHSNC is going to be replaced by "PARTICIPATORY HEALTH COUNCILS".
- Under national health regulatory and development authority the "grievance redressal system"(Jan Sahayta Kendra) will be constituted.
- Elected representatives as well as Panchayati Raj institutions (in rural areas) and local bodies (in urban areas) should participate more actively.

❏ **Access to Medicines, Vaccines and Technology:**
- Essential Drugs List should be Revised and expanded.
- Essential drugs' price must be strictly regulated.
- Increase the capacity of domestic drug and vaccines industry to meet national needs.
- Rational use of drugs to prevent drug resistance
- Good pay, incentives, and competency-based professional advancement related schemes must be adopted for better human resource practices.

❏ **Management and Institutional Reforms:**
- For better and efficient management of public health it has been suggested under UHC that it should have **"All India and state level public health service cadres"** equivalent to IAS and IPS.
- Drug procurement and other issues related to drug will be handled by National drug regulatory authority.
- Following agencies to be formed under UHC:
  - National Health Regulatory and Development Authority (NHRDA)
  - National Drug Regulatory and Development Authority (NDRDA)
  - National Health Promotion and Protection Trust (NHPPT)

Note: Universal Health Coverage Day is celebrated on 12 December every year.

BIBLIOGRAPHY

2. Boerma T, Eozenou P, Evans D, Evans T, Kieny M-P, Wagstaff A (2014) Monitoring Progress towards Universal Health Coverage at Country and Global Levels. PLoS Med 11(9): e1001731. https://doi.org/10.1371/journal.pmed.1001731
3. http://www.ficci-heal.com/
4. http://www.searo.who.int/india/topics/universal_health_coverage/en/
5. https://phfi.org/wp-content/uploads/2018/05/UHC-ExecSummary.pdf

3

CHAPTER

Environmental Science, Environmental Health, and Sanitation

CHAPTER OUTLINE

3.1 Brief note: Natural resources, ecosystem and biodiversity
3.2 Concept of environment and health (house, water, air, noise, light)
3.3 Basics of different kinds of pollution
3.4 Climate Change and National Program on Climate Change and Human Health (NPCCHH)
3.5 Waste management
3.6 Acts related to environment
3.7 National Clean Air Program

3.1 BRIEF NOTE: NATURAL RESOURCES, ECOSYSTEM AND BIODIVERSITY

NATURAL RESOURCES

- India is rich in natural resources including human resources.
  - *Agriculture:* It is the main source of Indian economy. It provides employment to around 70% of India's population.
  - *Forestry:* It is a sources of timber, leaves, gum, bamboo, rubber, etc. Around 19.4% of area covered by forest.
  - *Minerals:* India is richly with minerals like iron, copper, coal, bauxite, diamond, gold, manganese, etc.
  - *Fisheries:* India has a vast sea-coast. The marine products earn foreign exchange.
  - *Manpower:* The greatest natural resource of the country is its Human Resource.
- Natural resources can be classified on the basis of availability into Renewable and Non-Renewable.
- Renewable resources can be renewed and sustainable in nature. Examples are Water, forest, wind, solar energy, etc.
- Non-renewable resources are limited in nature and cannot be renewed. Ex. Minerals, fossil fuels, coal, soil, etc.

Ecosystem

Concept: An ecosystem is defined as a community of lifeforms in concurrence with non-living components, interacting with each other. It is a chain of interactions between organisms and their environment.

Structure and Characteristics

- **Biotic components:** It includes autotrophs, heterotrophs and saprotrophs.
- Producers or autotrophs such as plants which can produce food through the process of photosynthesis. All other organisms higher up on the food chain rely on producers for food.
- Consumers or heterotrophs are organisms that depend on other organisms for food.
- Decomposers include saprophytes such as fungi and bacteria. They directly thrive on the dead and decaying organic matter. They are essential for the ecosystem as they help in recycling nutrients to be reused by plants.
- **Abiotic components:** It includes non-living component of an ecosystem. Examples are air, water, soil, minerals, sunlight, temperature, nutrients, wind, etc. **(Fig. 3.1)**.
- The four main components of an ecosystem are:
  - Productivity
  - Decomposition
  - Energy flow
  - Nutrient cycling (biochemical process)
- **Types**
  - **Terrestrial ecosystem**
    - Forest ecosystem
    - Mountain ecosystem
    - Grassland ecosystem
    - Desert ecosystem

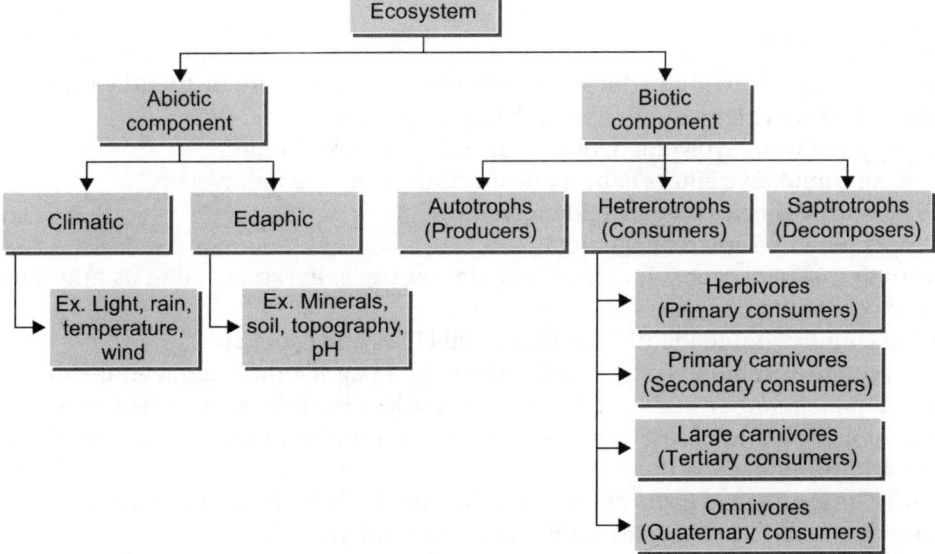

Fig. 3.1: Structure of ecosystem.

- **Aquatic ecosystem**
  - Fresh water ecosystem
  - Marine ecosystem.

Function: Maintain balance in the earth. Its important function is of the exchange of energy from one life form to others. It regulates ecological processes, supports life systems and stability.

Biodiversity

- Biodiversity: It means Bio (life) and diversity (variety).
- It means the number and variety of organisms found within a specified geographic region.
- It includes to the varieties of plants, animals and micro-organisms, the genes they contain and the ecosystems they form.
- Biodiversity is the result of evolution.
- Biodiversity is important for human existence. All forms of life are so closely interlinked that disturbance in one give rise to imbalance in the others.
- It can be divided into: (i) Genetic diversity; (ii) Species diversity; (iii) Ecosystem diversity.
- Genetic diversity is the variation in genes within species. It is essential for healthy breeding of population species.

Loss of Biodiversity

- Extensive Natural resources consumption increased due to population explosion which leads to loss of species in different parts of the world.
- Deforestation.
- Destruction of natural habitats leads to disaster in entire biosphere.
- Natural calamities like floods, earthquakes, volcanic eruption.
- Injudicious use of pesticides destroys some species.
- If any species of plants and animals become endangered, they cause degradation in the environment which is threaten the human existence.

Corrective Actions

- There is an urgent need to educate people to adopt environment-friendly practices and reorient their activities without damaging other species.
- It is only possible if involvement of an individual and community.
- Following cumulative efforts to be made for conservation of biodiversity:
  - Preserve the species that are endangered.
  - Proper planning and management.
  - Varieties of food crops, forage plants, timber trees, livestock, animals and their wild relatives should be preserved
  - Each country should identify habitats of wild lives and protection.
- Direct pressure on biodiversity is reduced by use of agriculture, aquaculture and forestry in sustainable manner, reduce the rate of forest loss by at least 50%, reduce overfishing, reduce pollution and excessive use of fertilizer, minimize choral reflow destruction and ocean acidification, etc.
- In 1972, Government of India passed the Wild Life (Protection) Act to protect, preserve and propagate the variety of species within natural boundaries.
- The biological diversity Act, 2002 provides conservation of biological diversity, sustainable use of its components.

Environmental Science, Environmental Health, and Sanitation

BIBLIOGRAPHY

1. https://neeriathome.neeri.res.in/biodiversity/whythisNew.php
2. https://www.weforum.org/agenda/2022/09/natural-resource-science-gives-us-immediate-steps-for-effective-biodiversity-governance/
3. https://ncert.nic.in/ncerts/l/kegy216.pdf
4. http://www.nbaindia.org/

3.2 CONCEPT OF ENVIRONMENT AND HEALTH (HOUSE, WATER, AIR, NOISE, LIGHT)

HOUSE AND HEALTH

- Standard of housing includes site, setback, rooms, kitchen, walls, roof, floor, windows, lighting, water supply, etc.
- **Site:**
  - Elevated from surrounding,
  - Surrounding pleasant environment,
  - Free from mosquito breeding places,
  - Away from nuisances such as noise, dust, smoke, etc.
  - Independent access to a street

According to census 2011, Pucca building may be treated as one which has its walls and roof made of the following material:

- **Wall material:** stones, galvanized iron/metal/asbestos sheets, burnt bricks, cement bricks, concrete.
- **Roof material:** machine made tiles, cement tiles, burnt bricks, stones, slate, GI/metal/Asbestos sheets, concrete.
- **Buildings:** The walls and/or roof of which are predominantly made of materials other than those mentioned above such as unburnt bricks, bamboos, mad, grass, thatch, plastic/polythene/loosely packed stone may be treated as kutcha building.
- **Set Back:**
  - The open space around the house which helps in having proper ventilation and lighting is called as **Set Back**.
  - In **rural areas** it is recommended that **two third** space of the plot should be left as set back it means the built up area should not more than **one-third** of the total area while for the **urban areas**, **one third** space of the plot should be left as set back it means the built-up area may be up to **two-third** of the total area.
  - The set back should be such that there is no obstruction to lighting and ventilation.
- **Floor:**
  - It should be impermeable so that it can be easily washed and kept clean and dry. Mud floors are prone to break up and create dust so they are not recommended.
  - There should be no cracks and crevices in the floor because they may be infested by insects **for example sand fly**.
  - The floors should be damp proof because it leads to skin problem (fungal infections) and allergic conditions (Asthma).
  - Plinth's height should be 2 to 3 feet (0.6 to 1 metre).

Environmental Science, Environmental Health, and Sanitation

- **Walls:** The characteristics of good wall is:
  - Strong
  - Low heat capacity means it should not absorb heat and conduct the heat
  - Weather Resistant
  - Unsuitable for Harborage of Rats and Vermin
  - Nine inch in thickness
  - Plastered (Smooth) and Colored (Cream or White Color)
- **Roof:**
  - The height of the roof should not be at least10 feet (3 m)
  - The roof should have a low heat transmittance coefficient.
  - Look over the roof to look for discarded items and collection of water and may be breeding of mosquitoes.
  - Check for any leakage.

Overcrowding: Overcrowding refers to the situation in which more people are living within a single dwelling than there is space for, so that movement is restricted, privacy secluded, hygiene impossible, rest and sleep difficult.

Minimum space for one adult person is 50 square feet.

The recommended standards with respect to overcrowding are as below:

- **Persons per room:** The degree of overcrowding can best be expressed as the number of persons per room, i.e., number of persons in the household divided by the number of rooms in the dwelling. The accepted standards are:
  - 1 room   : 2 persons
  - 2 rooms   : 3 persons
  - 3 rooms   : 5 persons
  - 4 rooms   : 7 persons
  - 5 or more rooms   : 10 persons (additional 2 for each further room)
- **Floor space:** The accepted standards are:
  - 110 sq ft (11 sq m.) or more : 2 persons
  - 90–100 sq ft (9–10 sq m)   : 1.5 persons
  - 70–90 sq ft (7–9 sq m)   : 1 person
  - 50–70 sq ft (5–7 sq m)   : 0.5 person
  - Under 50 sq ft (5 sq m)   : nil

(A baby under 12 months is not counted; children between 1 to 10 counted as **half a unit**).

Sex separation (psychological overcrowding): Overcrowding is considered to exist if 2 persons over 9 years of age, of opposite sexes who are not husband and wife, are obliged to sleep in the same room.

Hazards of Overcrowding

- Physical hazards: infectious diseases like TB, influenza, scabies spread rapidly under conditions of overcrowding
- Psychosocial: irritability, frustration, lack of sleep, anxiety
- Social hazards: violence and mental disorders.
- Public health hazards: higher morbidity and mortality

Other housing criteria: Continuous water supply is also required. Kitchen must be a separate. Sanitary privy should be available. Washing and batching facility should be available. Regularly garbage and refuse should be removed.

Water

- **Safe and wholesome water:**
  - Free from pathogenic agents
  - Free from harmful chemical substances
  - Pleasant to taste (free from color and odour)
  - Usable for domestic purposes

Water is said to be 'polluted' or 'contaminated' if it does not fulfill above criteria.

- **Water requirement:** Generally, it is recommended that 150 liters water per day per capita in urban area and 40 liters water per day per capita in rural area is required. As per the Jal Jeevan Mission, in urban area 135 liters per capita per day and for rural area 55 liters per capita per day water requirement is recommended.
- **Uses of water**
  - Domestic use: for drinking, cooking, bathing, washing and gardening, etc.
  - Agricultural purpose: irrigation
  - Public purposes: recreational purposes like swimming pools, public fountains, fire protection and public parks.
  - Industrial purposes: for processing and cooling
  - Power production from hydropower
  - Carrying away waste from all manner of establishments and institutions.

Hardness of Water

Classification

Level of hardness	mEq /liter
Soft water	Less than 1 (<50 mg/L)
Moderately hard	1–3 (50–150 mg/L)
Hard water	3–6 (150–300 mg/L)
Very hard water	6 (> 300 mg/L)

Types

Types	Contain
Temporary hardness	Calcium and Magnesium salts of Bicarbonates
Permanent hardness	Calcium and Magnesium salts of Sulfates, Calcium and Magnesium salts of Chlorides, Calcium and Magnesium salts of Nitrates

Measures to remove hardness of water (Fig. 3.2)

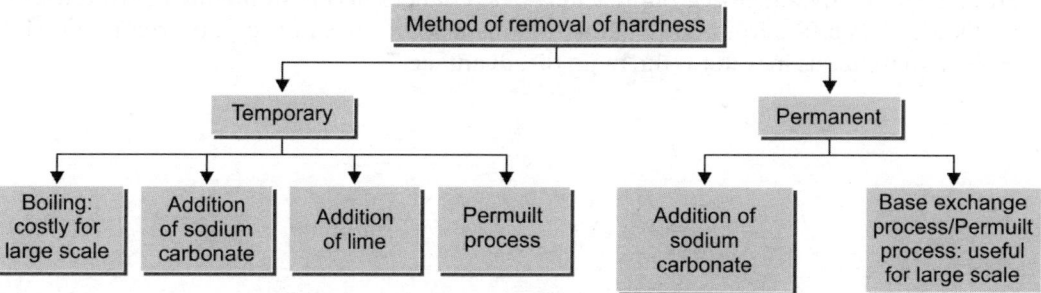

Fig. 3.2: Methods of removal of hardness of water.

Classification of Diseases having Relation with Water

Types disease	Remarks
Water-borne diseases	Occur due to drinking contaminated water, transmitted by feco-oral route. e.g., Cholera, typhoid, dysentery, viral hepatitis A and E
Water washed diseases	Include infections of the outer body surface which occur due to inadequate use of water or improper hygiene, e.g., Scabies, trachoma, bacillary dysentery, amoebic dysentery
Water based diseases	Infections transmitted through an aquatic invertebrate animal, e.g., Dracunculiasis (Guineaworm disease), Schistosomiasis
Water related diseases/ Water breeding diseases	Infections spread by insects that depend on water, e.g., Malaria, dengue, filariasis, yellow fever, onchocerciasis

Source of Water

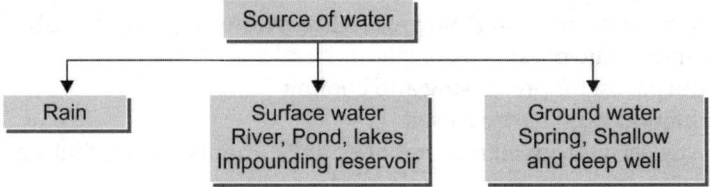

- **Rain:** It is a main source of water. Water is pure and soft. It became impure when suspended impurities like dust, gases such as sulphuric and nitric acid from environment react with atmospheric water and it leads to acid rain.
- **Surface water:** It is originating from rain water. Ex. River, lakes, tanks
  Main sources are: (1) river and streams, (2) tank and ponds (3) impounding reservoirs.
  - **Rivers:** The impurities in river are derived from industrial waste, sewage and sullage water and surface washings. Even pollution is also derived from the habits of the people like disposal of waste, bathing, animal washing, etc. Some amount of self-purification of water occur through natural method of water purification.
  - **Impounding reservoirs:** Artificial lake is constructed and water is stored. Drained area is known as catchment area. Generally, water is pure and soft. Impurities derives from catchment area which is affected by human habitation and animals.
  - **Tanks:** Water from tank is contaminated and aquatic vegetation also found in them. For prevention of tank contamination fence should be made, removal of weeds, periodically cleaning and elevated edges and platform of tank to prevent surface washing.
- **Ground water:** Sources: spring and wells. Types of wells: shallow well, deep well, dug well and tube well. Advantage of ground water—less chances of contamination in ground water that's why it is a free from pathogenic organism so, it does not require treatment. High content of minerals in water is the main disadvantage.

Difference between Deep Well and Shallow Well

	Deep well	Shallow well
Level	Below the first impervious layer	Above the first impervious layer
Bacteriological quality	Pure	Highly contaminated
Seasonal variation	Constant source	Dry in summer
Chemical	Hard	Moderately hard water
Remarks of deep well	**Saline intrusion**: when infiltration of sea water into deep wells develops brackish taste to the water and it is not useful for domestic purpose. **Artesian well**: when the water level rises above the ground level	

Dug wells

- It is common in rural area.
- Types:
  - **Pucca well/Masonry well**: it is an open well. It is made of stones /bricks
  - **Steps well**: when steps are constructed on pucca well known as step well. Chances of contamination is higher
  - **Kutcha well**: here hole is dug into water bearing stream.
  - **Masonry well**: handpump is installed in kutcha well and making the upper 10 feet or more of the lining water-tight, raising the lining one foot above the ground, and providing concrete slab cover at the top

Sanitary well
- Location: minimum distance required 15 m or 50 feet from the source of contamination
- Lining: to prevent the side entry of water cement lining should be built up to 6 m depth.
- Platform: cement concrete platform extending 1 m in all direction
- Parapet wall: 70–75 cm height wall
- Hand pump: it should be installed to drawn the water in sanitary way
- Drain: pucca drain should be installed to provide water upto consumer level
- Covering: it should be covered to prevent entry of pollution inside the well.

Tube well: Lifespan is long lasting.
- Location: minimum distance required 15 m or 50 feet from the source of contamination
- Hand pump: pipe installed into water bearing stratum and fitted with strained at the bottom and hand pump at the top level.
- Different engineering method used to make hundred feet deep tube well or bored well.

Water Distribution

- There are two **systems of water distribution**, the intermittent supply and the continuous supply.
- **The disadvantages of the intermittent system are:**
  - When the pipes are empty, there is negative pressure and by what is known as **back-siphoning**, bacteria and foul gases may be sucked in through leaky joints that are with nearby passing sewage pipe lines. A number of recorded outbreaks of typhoid and other diseases, have been traced back to the contamination of water in the intermittent piped water supplies.

- The pipes may be empty during times of emergency
- People need to store water in containers which may not be clean always and storage of water may be the source of mosquito breeding.

Key Guideline Aspects of WHO recommended Drinking Water Quality
- Color < 15 true color units (TCU)
- Turbidity < 5 nephlometric turbidity units (NTU)
- Hardness < 100–300 mg/litre calcium ion
- pH: 6.5–8.5
- Total dissolved solids (TDS) < 600 mg/litre
- Zero pathogenic microorganisms
- Zero infectious viruses
- Absence of pathogenic protozoa and infective stages of helminthes
- Fluorine < 1.5 ppm (0.5 – 0.8 ppm: Optimum level)
- Nitrates < 50 mg/litre
- Nitrites < 3 mg/litre
- Gross alpha radiological activity < 0.5 Bq/litre
- Gross beta radiological activity < 1.0 Bq/litre

Water Purification
Water purification is the process of removing contaminants from surface water or groundwater to make it safe and palatable for human consumption.

Purification of Water on a Large Scale
Components of typical water purification are:
- **Storage:** This is natural purification method in which all physical, chemical and biological mechanisms are involved.
  - **Physical:** About 90% of the suspended impurities settle down in 24 hours by gravity.
  - **Chemical:** Organic matter which is present in the water will be oxidized by the aerobic bacteria with the aid of dissolved oxygen. And due to this oxidation, the level of free ammonia is reduced and nitrates level increases.
  - **Biological**: Decrease bacteriological count. Up to 90% in first 5–7 days. It is the greatest benefit of storage.
- **Filtration:**
  - 98-99% bacteria are removed by filtration in addition to removal of the other impurities.
  - Two types of filters **(Fig. 3.3)**:
    1. Slow sand/biological filters
    2. Rapid sand/mechanical filters

Rapid Sand or Mechanical Filters
- Two types: Gravity type (Paterson's filter) and Pressure type (Candy's filter)
- After being pre-treated (coagulation and flocculation), fresh water flows through a sand and gravel bed.

Environmental Science, Environmental Health, and Sanitation

❏ **Steps:**
- Coagulation: Alum 5-40 mg/lit depending upon turbidity, color, pH
- Rapid mixing: In mixing chamber for a few minutes
- Flocculation: It consists of paddles which rotates at 2-4 rpm. This slow and gentle stirring results in formation of thick, copious, precipitate of aluminum hydroxide. In Flocculation chamber for 30 minutes
- Sedimentation: 2-6 hr at least 95% of flocculant precipitate needs to be removed.
- Filtration: Alum flock which is not removed by sedimentation, it forms a slimy layer comparable to zoogleal layer. It adsorbs bacteria from water and effect purification. When loss of head approaches 6-8 feet, filtration is stopped and backwashing start.

❏ **Backwashing:** It takes 15 minutes. Cleaning of the filter-bed every 24-72 hours. Backwashing water and sludge often toxic in nature so, treatment required.

Difference Between Rapid and Slow and Filtrations

S. No.	Characteristic	Rapid sand filter	Slow sand filter
1.	Requirement of space	Occupies little space	Large space
2.	Rate of filtration	200 m.g.a.d	2-3 m.g.a.d.
3.	Effective size of sand	0.4-0.7 mm	0.2-0.3 mm
4.	Preliminary treatment	Chemical coagulation and sedimentation	Plain sedimentation
5.	Washing method	By backwashing	By scraping the sand
6.	Skill requirement	Highly skilled	Less skilled
7.	Loss of head at	6-8 feet (2-2.5 m)	4 feet (1.5 m)
8.	Removal of turbidity	Good	Good
9.	Removal of color	Good	Fair
10.	Removal of microorganisms	98-99%	99.9-99.99%

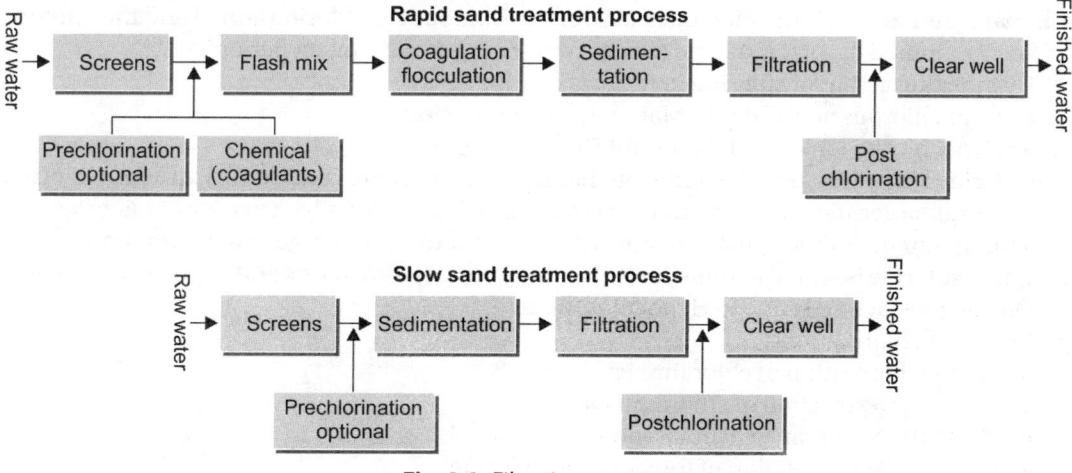

Fig. 3.3: Filtration process.

Disinfection

Types of disinfection
- ❐ Physical disinfection techniques include:
    - Boiling and
    - Irradiation with ultraviolet light.
- ❐ Chemical disinfection techniques include:
    - Chlorine
    - Bromine
    - Iodine, and
    - Ozone

Chlorination of Water (Fig. 3.4)

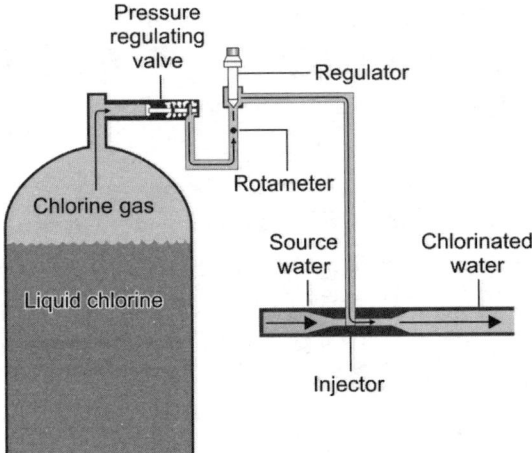

Fig. 3.4: Chlorination of water.

Chlorine demand: It is the difference between the amount of chlorine added and the amount of free, combined or total available chorine remaining at the contact period.
- ❐ Disinfecting action of chlorine in water is due to:
    - Hypochlorous acid (HOCl): Main role in disinfection
    - Hypochlorite ions (OCl): Minor role in disinfection
- ❐ Chlorine kills pathogenic bacteria, but has no effect on spores and certain viruses. Chlorine has residual germicidal effect (and not Ozone or UV rays): Provides a margin of safety against subsequent microbial contamination, as may occur during storage and distribution.
- ❐ When chlorine is added to water, there is formation of hydrochloric and hypochlorous acids. Disinfection action is due to Hypochlorous acid.
- ❐ Phases of chlorination:
    - Phase I: Formation of chloramines
    - Phase II: Destruction of chloramines
    - Phase III: Appearance of break-point
    - Phase IV: Accumulation of free residual chlorine.
- ❐ **Tests** for chlorination of water:
    - Orthotoluidine (OT) test: Measures
        - Free (residual) chlorine
        - Free and combined chlorine

- Orthotoluidine arsenite (OTA) test: Measures
  - Free chlorine
  - Combined chlorine
  - It can detect both free and combine chlorine separately.
- **Break point chlorination**: It is a chlorination point at which the residual chlorine appears and combined chlorines have been completely destroyed is the breakpoint chlorination.
- **Superchlorination**: It is required for heavily polluted water. During this process large amount of chlorine is added and removal of excess chlorine after disinfection.
- **Instrument Utility:**
  - Horrock's Apparatus: Chlorine demand estimation
  - Chlorinator/ Chloronome: Mixing or regulating dose of chlorine
  - Measuring residual level of chlorine: there are three methods:
    - Pool test kits (chloroscope is this type of instrument).
    - Color wheel test kit (use DPD tablet, water turns to pink if residual chlorine is present).
    - Digital colorimeters
  - Desirable level of chlorination:
    - At household level = 0.2 mg/L residual chlorine
    - In the distribution system = 0.5 mg/L residual chlorine
    - In swimming pool = 0.7 mg/L residual chlorine
    - During disaster = 1.0 mg/L residual chlorine

Side effect of excess chlorine in water: Mouth ulcer, gallstone, cancer

PURIFICATION OF WATER ON A SMALL SCALE

Household Purification of Water

A. Boiling

Advantages of boiling:
- Boiling kills all bacteria, spores, cysts and ova
- Removes temporary hardness

Limitation:
- Boiling has no residual effect, so it does not provide protection against the re-contamination
- Boiled water should be stored properly and used within a few days

B. Chemical Disinfection

Bleaching powder
- Bleaching powder or chlorinated lime is a white powder with pungent smell of chlorine.
- It contains about 33% of available chlorine.
- Unstable compound when exposed to air loses its chlorine content. So, mix with excess of lime. This is called "stabilized bleach".

Chlorine solution
If 4 kg of bleaching powder with 25% available chlorine mixed with 20 litres of water, it will give 5% solution of chlorine.

High test hypochlorite (HTH)
- HTH or perchloron is a calcium compound which contains 60–70% available chlorine.
- More stable than bleaching powder.

Chlorine tablet
- Available in market as trade name halozen tablet. But it is a costly.
- National environmental engineering research institute, Nagpur formulated tablet that is 15 times better than halogen tablet and it is less costly.
- A single tablet of 0.5 g is sufficient to disinfect 20 liters of water.

Iodine
- Used for emergency disinfection of water.
- Two drops of 2% ethanol solution of iodine will suffice for 1 liter of clean water.
- Contact time 20–30 min.
- Not react with organic compound but persist longer than chlorine.
- Disadvantage : high cost, physiological active (thyroid activity)

Potassium permanganate
- Powerful oxidizing agent, kills vibrio cholera
- But not useful due to altering color, smell and taste of water.

C. Filteration
- Ceramic filters such as Pasteur Chamberland filter, Berkefeld filter and Katadyn filter are used for domestic purpose.
- Candle is made of porcelain in chamberland type and infusorial earth in berkefeld type.
- In katadyn filter, surface coated with silver catalyst so bacteria killed by oligodynamic action of silver ions.
- Filter candle removes bacteria but not viruses.

D. Ultraviolet Irradiation
- Effective against bacteria, yeast, virus, fungi, algae, protozoa, etc.

Advantage
- Short period, No foreign matter introduce, no taste and odour produce

Disadvantage
- No residual effect, Expensive

Chlorination of Well
- Horrock's Apparatus is used to find bleaching powder requirement to disinfect 455 liters of water.
- First take 2 gm of bleaching powder with little water in black cup and make thin paste. Add some water is added to the circular mark and vigorous stirring is done to make a solution called as 'stock solution'.
- Then All 6 white cups are filled with the water which is to be tested.
- With help of pipette stock solution is added as follows: 1 drop to first cup, 2 drops to second cup, three drops to third cup and so on. Each glass is stirred with separate rod and left for half an hour as contact period.
- After that freshly prepared starch iodide indicator is added to all white cups by dropper and stirred.
- Development of blue color indicated the presence of free residual chlorine.
- If third cup showing blue color, it means $3 \times 2 = 6$ gm of bleaching powder is required to disinfect 455 liter of water. (2 gm is added amount of chlorine is multiplied with number of

cup which is first shows blue color to know the requirement of bleaching powder). If inside the well 11,77,500 liter water then amount of bleaching powder requirement: (well of 10 meter diameter with 15 meter depths of water)
455 liter of water requires – 6 gm of bleaching powder
Then 11,77,500 liter-how much?
  $= (6/455) \times 1,177,500$
  $= 70,65,000/455$
  $= 1,5527.5$ gm ≈ 15.5 kg

Roughly 15.5 kg of bleaching powder is required to disinfect the well water.

Summary of Water Purification Method

Process	Impurities removed
Aeration	Taste and odour
Screening	Floating matter
Clarifier+ flocculation	Dissolved matter
Filtration	Colloidal matter and living organisms
Chlorination	Living microorganisms

Ventilation

- The modern concept of ventilation implies not only supply of outdoor air in exchange of vitiated inside air, but also taking care of quality of incoming air in terms of temperature, humidity and purity.

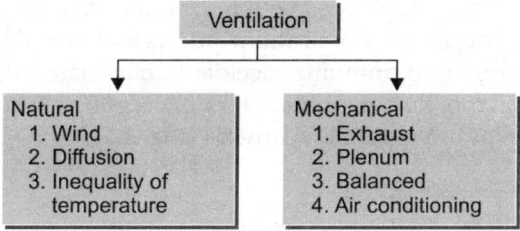

- **Sanitary ventilation:** The ventilation shall be called sanitary ventilation when it is combined with disinfectant aerosols in the room.
- **Cross ventilation:** Doors and windows facing each other provide cross ventilation. It is not necessary that they are just opposite but diagonally placed doors and windows also form the cross ventilation.
- **Standards of air change:** Direction of the air current in India is usually North West or East West. The air current shall help natural ventilation, if the living rooms are constructed with windows on east or north east or west side of the house.
  - In living room: 2-3 air change should be in one hour
  - Working room: 4-6 air change should be in one hour
  - More than 6 air change in one hour: not recommended

Assessment of Ventilation

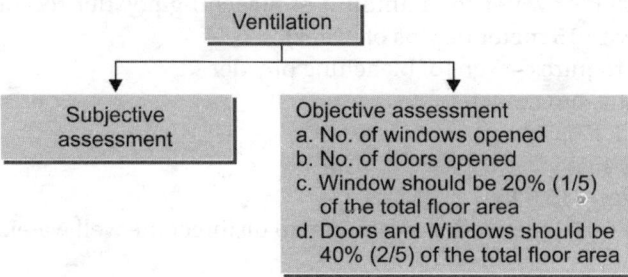

What are the Drawbacks of Poor Ventilation?
- Respiratory disease, Asthma
- Facilitate spread of disease
- Headache, uncomfortable, suffocation
- Bad odour
- Dampness and humidity: The degree of dampness shall vary with amount of sun light received in the rooms and with degree of ventilation. Dampness helps in the breeding and multiplication of disease producing germs and insects. Families living in damp houses suffer for longer period from respiratory, diarrheal and skin diseases.

Lighting Criteria
- Person should be able to read the suitable text from suitable distance in 2/3 portion of given room without aid of artificial light.
- Inadequate lighting is usually associated with inadequate ventilation.
- It also depends on the direction of doors and windows and direction of sunrise and sunset.
- Importance of adequate lighting: minimize accidents, eliminate lodgment ad multiplication of disease producing microorganisms and vectors, decreasing the humidity in the room, and avoid eye strain and helps in Vitamin D synthesis **(Fig. 3.5)**.

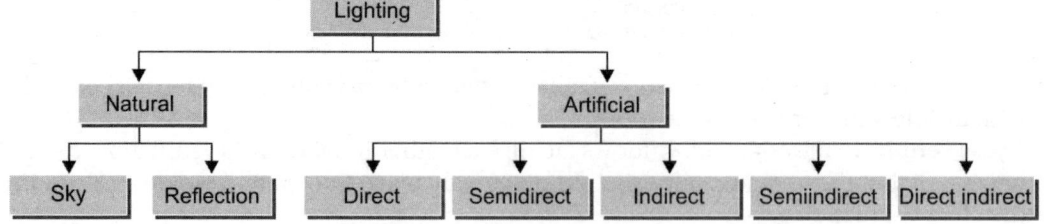

Fig. 3.5: Types of lighting.

For efficient vision, the following light factors are essential:
- It must be sufficient
- Evenly distributed
- Without glare
- Without sharp shadows
- It should be steady

Light Measurement Units

Description	Quantity measured	Recommended unit
• Brightness of point source	Luminous Intensity	Candela
• Flow of light	Luminous flux	Lumen
• Amount of light reaching surface	Illumination Illuminance	Lux
• Amount of light re-emitted by surface	Brightness Luminance	Lambert

Daylight Factor (DF): It is the ratio of light level inside house to the light level outside the structure.

$$\text{Daylight factor (DF)} = \frac{\text{Inside light level}}{\text{Outdoor light level}} \times 100$$

Daylight factor should be at least 8% in living room and 10% in kitchen.

Lux

Lux = SC + ERC + IRC
SC = Sky component
Toward Sunlight Window placement increases SC
ERC = externally reflected component
Increased by painting surrounding area
IRC = Internally reflected component
Increased by using light colors for room surface

Recommended Illumination (the IES Code)

Visual task	Illumination (lux)
For reading	100
For office work	400
Assembly	900
Very major tasks	1300–1200
Watch making industry	2000–3000

Hazards of Inadequate Lighting (Fig. 3.6)

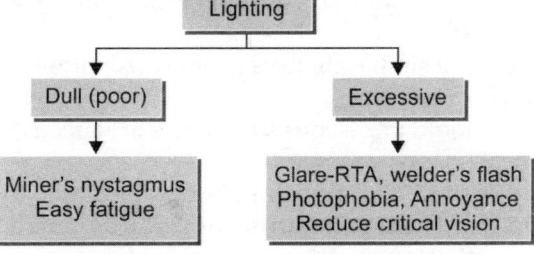

Fig. 3.6: Hazards of inadequate lighting.

Noise

- It is defined as "unwanted sound", but this definition is subjective because of the fact that one man's sound may be another man's noise.
- Another definition of noise is: "wrong sound, in the wrong place, at the wrong time".
- **Source**: Industries, automobiles, factories, air-crafts, etc. Use of pressure horns, recreational noise of loudspeakers with full volume during festivities particularly at night are other sources of noise production. The domestic noises from the Television, radios, transistors - all add to the quantum of noise in daily life.
- **Properties:** Frequency and intensity or loudness
- **Instrument** used for measurement:
  - Sound Level Meter: which measures the intensity of sound in db.
  - Octave Band Frequency Analyzer: which measures the noise in octave bands.
  - Audiometer: which measures the hearing ability.
- **Hazards**:

Auditory effect	Non-auditory effect
• Auditory fatigue: 90 dB • Deafness: Temporary hearing loss between 4000 to 6000 Hz • Permanent hearing loss when rupture of tympanic member occurs due to noise above 160 dB	• Annoyance • Interference with speech: more than 12 dB • Symptoms like headache, nausea, rise in blood pressure, heart rate, vision disturbance

BIBLIOGRAPHY

1. http://cpheeo.gov.in/upload/uploadfiles/files/Chapter%205_3.pdf
2. http://nwm.gov.in/
3. Mathur JS. A guidebook for family and field work in social and preventive medicine.
4. Park K. Park's Textbook of Preventive and Social Medicine (26th edition) Jabalpur: Banarsidas Bhanot-publishers 2021.
5. World health organization. Guideline for drinking water quality. 4th edition. Geneva: WHO; 2011.

3.3 BASICS OF DIFFERENT KINDS OF POLLUTION

DEFINITION

- Pollution is the introduction of substances (or energy) that cause adverse changes in the environment and living entities.
- Pollution is the effect of undesirable changes in our surroundings that have harmful effects on plants, animals and human beings.
- Pollutants include solid, liquid or gaseous substances produced due to human activity and have a detrimental effect on environment.
- From an ecological perspective pollutants can be classified as follows:
  - **Degradable or non-persistent pollutants:** These can be rapidly broken down by natural processes. E.g., domestic sewage, discarded vegetables
  - **Slowly degradable or persistent pollutants:** Pollutants that remain in the environment for many years in an unchanged condition and take decades or longer to degrade. E.g., DDT and most plastics.

- **Non-degradable pollutants:** These cannot be degraded by natural processes. Once they are released into the environment they are difficult to eradicate and continue to accumulate. E.g., toxic elements like lead or mercury.
- Types of pollution includes water pollution, air pollution, noise pollution, soil pollution. Besides these 4 types of pollution, other types exist such as light pollution, thermal pollution and radioactive pollution (least common but deadliest type).

Water Pollution

- **Definition of water pollution:** "When the quality or composition of water changes directly or indirectly as a result of man's activities such that it becomes unfit for any purpose it is said to be polluted".
- About 97% of the total water available on earth is found in oceans and is too salty for drinking or irrigation.
- The remaining 3% is fresh water. Of this, 2.997% is locked in ice caps or glaciers.
- Thus only 0.003% of the earth' total volume of water is easily available to us as soil moisture, groundwater, water vapour and water in lakes, streams, rivers and wetlands.
- Main reason for water pollution is urbanization and industrialization.
- The sources of pollution are: sewage, agriculture pollutants, industrial waste, radioactive substance and physical pollutant.
- Indicators used for testing pollution: BOD (Biological oxygen demand) at 20°C, total suspended solids, concentration of chlorides, nitrogen and phosphorus and absence of dissolved oxygen.
- Sometimes due to cross connection between water supply pipes and sewage drainage pipes, corrosion of pipe lines, leakage, etc., water pollution occur.
- Water pollution leads to disruption of the ecosystem, threats to marine life, water-borne diseases, increases toxic chemicals in water bodies and eutrophication.

Air Pollution

- Air pollution occurs due to the presence of undesirable solid or gaseous particles in the air in quantities that are harmful to human health and the environment.
- **Sources:** Natural events (for example, dust storms and volcanic eruptions) and human activities (emission from vehicles, industries, etc.).
- Types: (a) **Primary air pollutants**: (b) **Secondary air pollutants**
- **Primary Pollutants:** These are the pollutants that are emitted directly from the sources such as volcanic eruptions, combustion of fossil fuel, etc. These include nitrogen oxide, sulphur oxide, etc.
- There are five primary pollutants that together contribute about 90 percent of the global air pollution. These are carbon oxides (CO and CO_2), nitrogen oxides, sulfur oxides, volatile organic compounds (mostly hydrocarbons) and suspended particulate matter.
- **Secondary Pollutants:** These are the pollutants that are not directly emitted from the sources but are formed when primary pollutants react in the atmosphere. For example, ozone
- 'Smog' is the combination of smoke and fog.
- Major air pollutants: Particulate and Gaseous. Suspended particulate matter (SPM) include dust, smoke, fumes, etc. SPM generated by incomplete combustion of fossil fuels and production of particles of carbon or complex carbohydrates. Gaseous pollutant includes Sulphur dioxide, carbon monoxide, hydrocarbon, nitrogen dioxide.

- Hazards: Acute bronchitis, chronic bronchitis, asthma, respiratory allergy and lung cancer lead affect the neuropsychological development of the children.
- Environmental aspects hazard like corrosion of building and metals, destruction of plants life, etc.

Indoor Air Pollution

- Source: Combustion of solid fuel, indoors Tobacco smoking and outdoor air pollutant like CO, NO, SO_2, VOC, PCAH.
- Hazards of indoor air pollution: Pneumonia, COPD, lung cancer, stroke.
- There is also evidence of link between air pollution and LBW, TB, cataract and nasopharyngeal and laryngeal cancer.

Control Measures for Air Pollution

- Proper equipment in place which makes possible to collect the pollutants before they escape through use of dry and wet collectors, filters, electrostatic precipitators, etc.
- Providing a greater height to the stacks can help in facilitating the discharge of pollutants as far away from the ground as possible.
- Industries should be located in places so as to minimize the effects of pollution after considering the topography and the wind directions.
- Substitution of raw material that causes more air pollution.

Noise Pollution: Contributors to noise pollution include

- Industries: Heavy machines, mills, factories, etc.
- Transportation: Vehicles, aeroplanes, etc.
- Construction noises
- Noise from social events (loudspeakers, firecrackers, etc.)
- Household noises (such as mixers, TV, washing machines, etc.)

Auditory Effects

- *Auditory fatigue:* It appears in the 90 dB region and greatest at 4,000 Hz. It may be associated with side effects such as whistling and buzzing in the ears.
- *Deafness:* Temporary hearing loss results from a specific exposure to noise; the disability disappears after a period of time up to 24 hours following the noise exposure. It occurs in frequency range between 4,000 to 6,000 Hz.
- Permanent hearing loss occurs due to repeated or continuous exposure to noise around 100 decibels may result in a permanent hearing loss
- Exposure to noise above 160 dB may rupture the tympanic membrane and cause permanent loss of hearing.

Non-auditory effects

Decrease work efficiency, annoyance, interfere with speech, physiological changes like effect of heart rate, blood pressure, breathing, etc.

Soil Pollution

- Source: Industrial waste, garbage, sewage, pesticide including fertilizers, radioactive waste, hospital waste, oil spills, mining activities, etc.

- It makes soil unfit for agriculture.
- It affects the natural flora and fauna residing in the soil.
- It increases transmission of soil transmitted helminths infection like hookworm, round worm and *Trichuris trichuria*.
- Soil contaminated with animal excreta transmits Tetanus.
- Diarrheal disease can be transmitted indirectly by water which is passed through contaminated soil.

Radiation Pollution (Fig. 3.7)

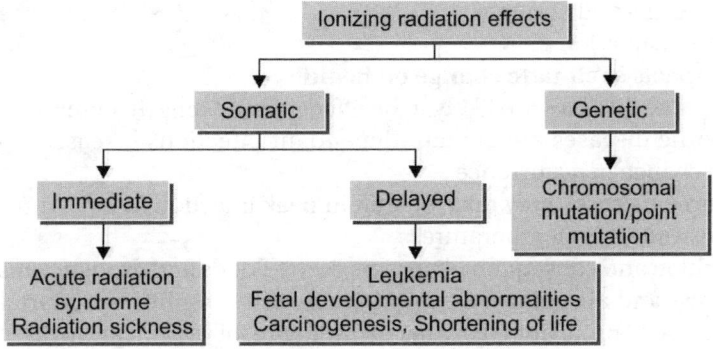

Fig. 3.7: Effects of ionizing radiation.

BIBLIOGRAPHY

1. https://cpcb.nic.in
2. https://moef.gov.in/en/
3. https://byjus.com/biology/types-of-pollution/
4. https://www.ugc.ac.in/oldpdf/modelcurriculum/Chapter5.pdf

3.4 CLIMATE CHANGE AND NATIONAL PROGRAM ON CLIMATE CHANGE AND HUMAN HEALTH (NPCCHH)

CLIMATE CHANGE

- The atmosphere transmits the incoming solar radiation but absorbs the majority of long wave radiation emitted upwards by the earth's surface. The gases that absorb long wave radiation are called Greenhouse gases (GHGs). This processes that warm the atmosphere are known as the greenhouse effect.
- The primary GHGs are carbon dioxide (CO_2), chlorofluorocarbons (CFCs), methane (CH_4), nitrous oxide (N_2O) and ozone (O_3).
- It refers to long-term shifts in temperatures and weather patterns.
- The main causes are:
  - Emission of greenhouse gases into the atmosphere
  - Deforestation
  - Exploitation of natural resources
  - Pollution caused by human activities and aerosol from volcanic eruptions

- Rich countries produce most of the world's greenhouse gases, but poor countries suffer the most. These occur either through direct effect (changes in temperature and precipitation and occurrence of heat waves, floods, droughts, and fires etc) or indirect effect (ecological disruptions resulting in crop failures, shifting patterns of diseases' vectors or displacement of populations, etc).
- The health effects may occur either due to direct or indirect causes of climate change or extremes of weather.
  - **Direct impacts of climate change on health:**
    - Heat- and Cold-Related Impacts
    - Floods, Storms and Drought
    - Ultraviolet Radiation
  - **Indirect impacts of climate change on health:**
    - Vector-borne diseases are likely to be affected by change in climate and weather
    - Waterborne diseases are climate-dependant infectious diseases and they are also likely to change in occurrence
    - Food borne diseases may raise or shift in peak infection rates as a response to rising global air and water temperatures
    - Malnutrition and consequent disorders due to floods and drought caused crop failure.
    - Heat stress and air pollution adversely affects morbidity and mortality particularly from non-communicable diseases including respiratory, cardiovascular, circulatory diseases.
  - **Positive impacts of climate change:**
    - Moderate reduction in cold-related morbidity and mortality in some cold extremes areas.
    - Geographical shifts in food production.
    - Reduced capacity of disease-causing vectors due to exceedance of thermal thresholds.
- These positive effects are very few and outweighed by the magnitude and severity of the negative effects of climate change.

Government of India has taken following steps to address the threat of climate change

- **The Make in India** campaign with **Zero Effect, Zero Defect (ZED)** is a policy initiative for quality control and pollution control through use of renewable energy.
- "We should manufacture goods in such a way that they carry zero defects and that our exported goods are never returned to us".
- "We should manufacture goods with zero effect that they should not have a negative impact on the environment".
- **Green Highways** (Plantation and Maintenance) Policy to develop 140,000 km long "tree-line" along both sides of national highways.
- **FAME India** is a incentives based scheme of the National Electric Mobility Mission Plan 2020 to promote **Faster Adoption and Manufacturing of Hybrid and Electric Vehicles**.
- Country's **fuel-efficiency standards** have set targets for new cars at the equivalent of 130 gCO_2/km and 113 gCO_2/km in 2016 and in 2021 respectively. These standards will reduce 50 million tons of CO_2 out of the atmosphere in 2030 alone.
- **National Bio-diesel Mission** has set an ambitious target of 20% blending of biofuels, for both bio-diesel and bio-ethanol. (Jatropha curcas as the most suitable tree-borne oilseed for bio-diesel production).

Environmental Science, Environmental Health, and Sanitation

- **National Air Quality Index** gives the status of air pollution in a particular city by giving One Number, One Color and One Description.

Adaptation strategies: strengthen societies' ability to deal with the impacts of climate change:
- **Soil Health Card Scheme**
- **Paramparagat Krishi Vikas Yojana**
- **Pradhan Mantri Krishi Sinchayee Yojana**
- **Neeranchal** is a new program for developing watershed in the country
- **National Mission for Clean Ganga** (**Namami Gange**)
- **India GHG (Green House Gas) Program** is voluntary program for the development of India-specific emission factors and to help corporates to measure their carbon footprints.
- **Smart Power for Environmentally-sound Economic Development (SPEED)** is a program for the electrification of rural areas by renewable energy system.
- **Green Co-Rating System** is based on 10 different parameters which is used to assess companies for their environmental performance.
- The **Small and medium-sized enterprises (SME) Cluster Programs** cover more than 150 clusters all over the country and has resulted in reduction in energy consumption and quality improvement.

Mitigation strategies: Reducing emissions strategies
- **India** has targeted to increase Renewable energy capacity from 35 GW (up to March 2015) to 175 GW by 2022.
- **National Solar Mission** has targeted to reach 100 GW from 20 GW by 2022. (World's first airport to fully run on solar power is the Kochi Airport in India).
- **Solar powered toll plazas** are planned to establish across country.
- **National Smart Grid Mission** is launched for efficient transmission and distribution network.
- **Smart Cities Mission:** It is an urban renewal and retrofitting program.
- **National Heritage City Development and Augmentation Yojana (HRIDAY)** launched to preserve the heritage character of each Heritage City by reasonable urban planning, economic growth and heritage conservation in an inclusive manner.
- **Atal Mission for Rejuvenation and Urban Transformation (AMRUT)**
- **Swachh Bharat Mission' (Clean India Mission)**

COP-21—Paris Agreement

- Paris agreement sets out a global action plan to avoid dangerous climate change by limiting global warming to well below 2°C.
- Paris agreement to come in force, at least 55 countries responsible for at least 55% of global emissions had to deposit their instruments of ratification.

COP-26 Glasgow, United Kingdom

Ministry of Environment Forest and Climate Change took part in the 26th Session of the Conference of Parties (COP-26) to the United Nations Framework Convention on Climate Change (UNFCCC) was held in Glasgow, United Kingdom for green net zero program. The National Statement in the World Leaders Summit was delivered by the Hon'ble Prime Minister at COP-26, which the following mainly discussed and highlighted during the summit:

- India's non-fossil energy capacity to reach 500 GW by 2030
- India will meet 50 percent of its energy requirements with renewable energy by 2030.
- India will reduce its total projected carbon emissions by one billion tonnes from now to 2030.
- India will reduce the carbon intensity of its economy by 45 percent by 2030, over 2005 levels.
- By 2070, India will achieve the target of net zero emissions.

National Program on Climate Change and Human Health

- The United Nations Framework Convention on Climate Change (UNFCCC) and its Kyoto Protocol in 1997 refers to the legal framework for climate change process internationally.
- The Conference of the Parties (COP) to the Convention meets annually to negotiate and discuss the international climate change agenda and related commitments from countries. The sustainable development Goal 13 (SDG 13) also emphasizes to "take urgent action to combat climate change and its impacts."
- India has undertaken some initiatives in pursuance to the obligation implied by UNFCCC like:
  - Identification of Ministry of Environment, Forest and Climate Change (MOEF and CC) as nodal ministry for matters related to Climate Change;
  - Formulation of National Environmental Policy 2006;
  - Formulation of Prime Minister's Council on Climate Change to advise proactive measures, facilitate interministerial coordination and guide policy in relevant areas.
  - The hon'ble Prime Minister of India office has released a National Action Plan on Climate Change in June 2008
- The plan identified eight national missions:
  1. National Mission on Sustainable habitat
  2. National Mission for Sustaining the Himalayan Ecosystem
  3. National Mission for Sustainable Agriculture
  4. National Solar Mission
  5. National Mission for Enhanced Energy Efficiency
  6. National Water Mission
  7. National Mission on Strategic Knowledge for Climate Change
  8. National Mission for "Green India"
- Executive Committee on Climate Change reviewed the progress of eight national missions on Climate Change and suggested formulation of four new missions viz.
  1. National Mission on Health
  2. National Mission on "Waste to Energy Generation"
  3. National Mission on India's Coastal areas
  4. National Wind Mission

In this background, **National Program on Climate Change and Human Health (NPCCHH)** initiated in February 2019.

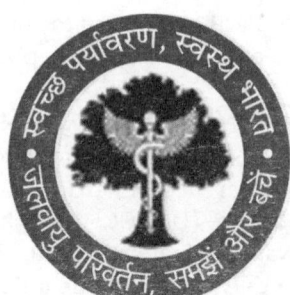

- **Vision:** Strengthening of healthcare services for all the citizens of India esp vulnerable like children, women and marginalized population against climate sensitive illnesses.
- **Goal**: To reduce morbidity, mortality, injuries, and health vulnerability due to climate variability and extreme weather conditions.
- **Objectives:**

- To create awareness among general population (vulnerable community), healthcare providers and Policy makers regarding impacts of climate change on human health.
- To strengthen capacity of healthcare system to reduce illnesses/ diseases due to variability in climate
- To strengthen health preparedness and response by performing situational analysis at national/state/district/below district levels.
- To develop partnerships and create synchrony/ synergy with other missions and ensure that health is adequately represented in the climate change agenda in the country
- To strengthen research capacity to fill the evidence gap on climate change impact on human health

❒ **Integration of different missions on climate change:** The possible of health impacts of other missions under NAPCC are forseen as follows (**Fig. 3.8**):

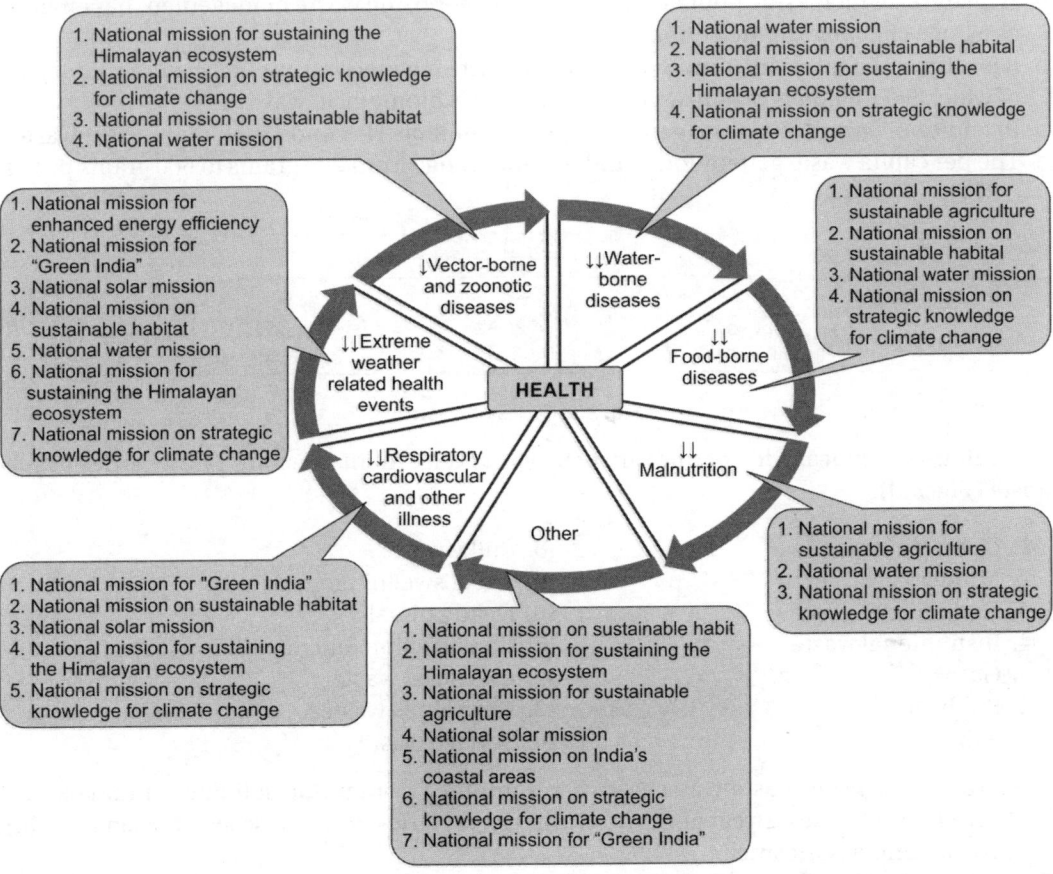

Fig. 3.8: Possible health impacts of intermission conversion under NAPCC.

BIBLIOGRAPHY

1. https://ncdc.gov.in/index1.php?lang=1andlevel=1andsublinkid=876andlid=660
2. http://nwm.gov.in/?q=climate-change
3. https://ncert.nic.in/textbook/pdf/kegy212.pdf
4. https://pib.gov.in/PressReleasePage.aspx?PRID=1786057

3.5 WASTE MANAGEMENT

WASTE

- With the ever increasing population and urbanization, the waste management has emerged as a huge challenge in the country.
- It is estimated that about 62 million tonnes of waste is generated annually in the country, out of which 5.6 million is plastic waste, 0.17 million is biomedical waste.
- In addition, hazardous waste generation is 7.90 million TPA and 15 lakh tonne is e-waste.
- The per capita waste generation in Indian cities range from 200 grams to 600 grams per day (2011).

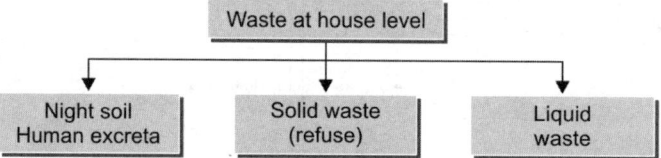

Fig. 3.9: Types of waste.

According to technical wing of ministry of urban development there are 14 categories of solid waste **(Fig. 3.9)**.

1. Domestic waste
2. Municipal waste
3. Commercial waste
4. Institutional waste
5. Garbage
6. Rubbish
7. Ashes
8. Bulky waste
9. Street sweepings
10. Dead animals
11. Construction and demolition waste
12. Industrial waste
13. Hazardous waste
14. Sewage waste

- **Sewage:** *Sewage* is waste water from a community, containing solid and liquid excreta, derived from houses, street and yard washings, factories and industries. It resembles dirty waste an unpleasant smell.
- The term **"sullage"** is applied to waste water which does not contain human excreta, e.g. waste from kitchens and bathrooms
- ***Refuse***: Solid waste generated from Street refuse, Market refuse, Domestic refuse, Industrial refuse, etc.

Environmental Science, Environmental Health, and Sanitation

- **Garbage:** Processed food waste generated from kitchen
- **Ash:** Residue from fire used for cooking and heating
- **Rubbish:** Paper, clothing, wood, metal, glass, dust
  - Urban areas in India generate more than 1,00,000 MT of waste per day. A large metro city like Mumbai generates about 7000 MT of waste per day while city like Ahmedabad generates in the range from 1,600–4,000 MT per day. It converts 600 grams daily per capita generation of solid waste.
  - Proper storage and collection play most important role to prevent hazards.
  - At household level waste should be collected in dust bin with close fitting cover.
  - At a large scale, public bins are used and kept on concrete platform to prevent flood water entering inside.
  - Waste ideally should be collected house to house. Refuse from public bean transported through refuse collection vehicle to the disposal place.

Health Hazard of Solid Waste
- It attracts rodent and fly breeding.
- It produces bad odours.
- Indirect food contamination can be occurred and also leads to soil and water pollution.

Integrated Solid Waste Management System Hierarchy (Fig. 3.10)

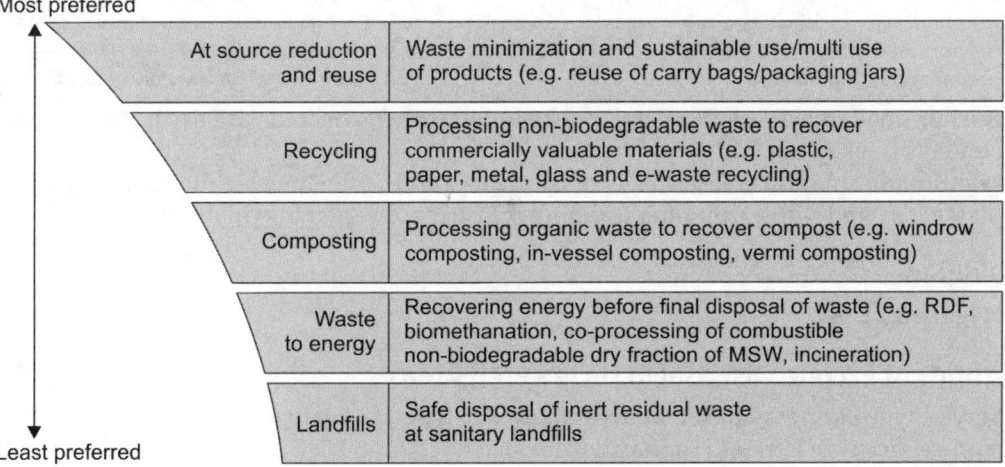

Fig. 3.10: Solid waste management system.

Methods of Solid Waste Disposal
- **Dumping:** Dry waste is converted into humus through bacterial action. Drawback of this method is source of nuisance, rodent, flies, pollution of surface and ground water.

- **Controlled tripping:** Also known as sanitary landfills. See below different methods:

Trench method	Ramp method	Area method
• Long trench is dug out. Per 1000 population one acre land is required. • Refuse is compacted and coverted with excavated earth.	• It is made available in moderately slopy area.	• Refuse is deposited in uniform layer up to 2-2.5 m and each layer is sealed with mud cover at least 30 cm. • Within one week temperature increase upto 60 deg C ; bacteriological and chemical changes occurred. It cools within 2 to 3 weeks. Decomposition of organic matter into innocuous mass in 6 months.

- **Incineration:** This method is useful for hospital refuse.
- **Composting:** Two methods available:

Banglore method	Mechanical composting
• It is an anaerobic method or hot fermentation process. • It is useful for town waste and nightsoil. Minimum distance from city is at least 800 m. • Alternate layer of refuse and nightsoil is spread in proportion of 15 cm and 5 cm respectively. It helps to prevent breeding of flies.	• It is an aerobic method. • In this method, initially refuse is cleared of different materials like metal, glass, rags, etc. then refuse is pulversied to reduce in size of article. Then this refuse mixed with sewage, nightsoil and sludge in machine and incubated.

- **Burial:** Small trench is formed and refuse is added then covered with earth. After 6-month contents is taken out.
- **Manure pits:** In rural area garbage, refuse, leaves and cattle dung are dumped into manure pit and covered with earth. After 6-month refuse is converted into manure.

F-Diagram
See **Figure 3.11.**

Methods of Excreta Disposal in Unsewered Areas
- Service type latrines (Conservancy system): Pail type/bucket type latrine
- Non-service type latrines (Sanitary latrines):
  - Bore hole latrine
  - Dug well or pit latrine
  - Water seal type latrines (at our house)
- PRAI (Planning Research Action Institute) type
- RCA (Research Cum Action) type
- Sulabh shauchalaya
  - Septic tank
  - Aqua privy
- Latrines suitable for camps and temporary use
  - Shallow trench latrine
  - Deep trench latrine

Environmental Science, Environmental Health, and Sanitation

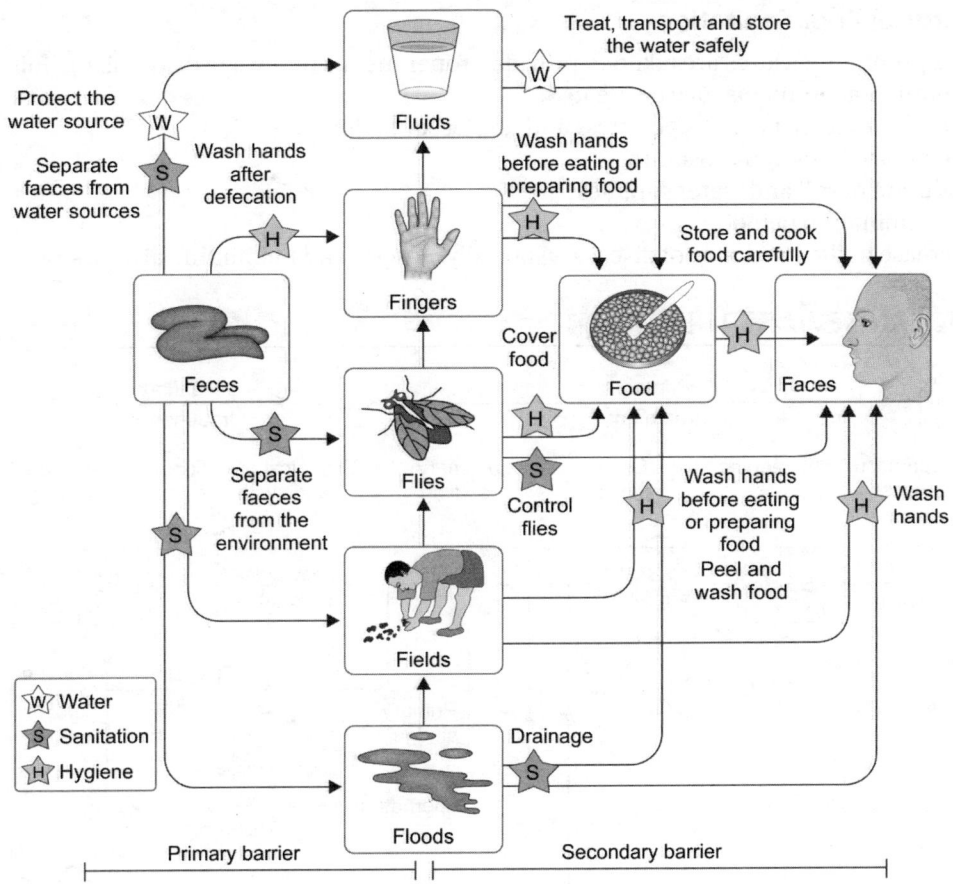

Fig. 3.11: F-diagram.

- Pit latrine
- Bore hole latrine.

Water Seal Performs Two Important Functions

1. It prevents access by flies. That is, the night soil is sealed off by a small depth of water contained in a bent pipe.
2. It prevents escape of odours and foul gases and thereby eliminates the nuisance from smell. Once the latrine is flushed, nightsoil is no longer visible.

Criteria for Sanitary Latrine

- Latrine should not allow the excreta to contaminate ground water
- Excreta should not be accessible to flies, rodents, or animals
- Should not allow to pollute soil
- Excreta should not create bad odor or ugly appearance.

Hazards of Poor Sanitation

Unless prompt measures are taken to provide proper means of sewage disposal, the following environmental problems may be created:
- Creation of nuisance, unsightliness and unpleasant odours.
- Breeding of flies and mosquitoes
- Pollution of soil and water supplies
- Contamination of food
- Increase in the incidence of disease, especially, enteric and helminthic diseases.

MODERN SEWAGE TREATMENT

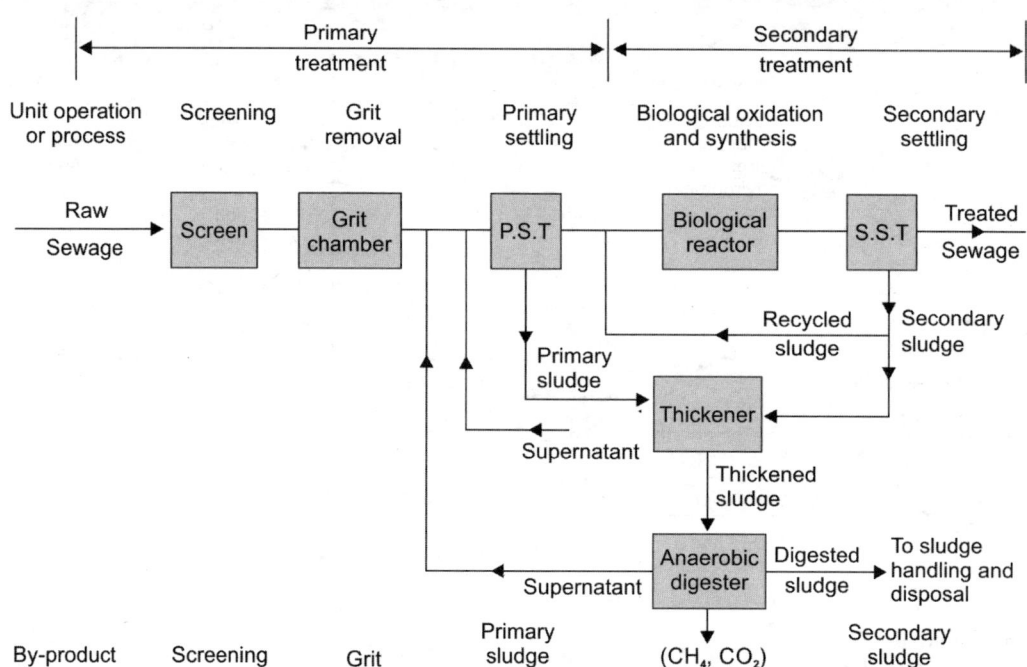

Fig. 3.12: Process flow sewage treatment plant

In modern sewage treatment plan treatment is divided into two process: Primary and secondary treatment **(Fig. 3.12)**.

Primary Treatment
- Screening: Removal of large floating objects.
- Grit chamber/Detritus chamber: Settlement of heavy solids at the bottom and it needs to be removed periodically. Chamber is 10-20 meters in length.
- Primary sedimentation: Sewage flow at a velocity of 1-2 feet per minutes in sedimentation tank. 30-40% of coliform organism is reduced in sewage after 6-8 hr in sedimentation tank. Sludge is an organic matter collected at the bottom.

Secondary Treatment

Aerobic oxidation of sewage further done by either activated sludge process or trickling filter method.
- Activated sludge process: It is a modern method of purifying sewage. Aeration is either done by mechanically or by forcing compressed air continuously in aeration tank. During this process organic matter oxidized into carbon dioxide, nitrates and water and destruction of cholera and typhoid bacteria.
- Trickling method: Effluent from primary sedimentation tank is sprinkled on the surface bed of stones. Zooglear layer is formed over the surface. Effluent pass through filter bed oxidized by bacteria present in zooglear layer.

Secondary sedimentation: Oxidized sewage from activated sludge process or trickling filter passed into secondary sedimentation tank. At the end of 2-3 hrs collected sludge is known as aerated sludge.

Sludge digestion and disposal of effluent: It is done in sludge digestion tank and methane gas is a by-product of this process. After the treatment disposal of effluent is done by either dilution in river, sea or in oxidation pond.

Biological oxygen demand (BOD): It is a measure of water quality. Amount of oxygen needed by bacteria and other organism to oxidize the organic matter present in a water at 20 degree C over a period of 5 days is known as BOD.

Chemical oxygen demand (COD): It is a chemical oxidation reaction. It measures majority of organic carbon which is not completely oxidized in reaction.

BIBLIOGRAPHY

3. http://cpheeo.gov.in/upload/uploadfiles/files/engineering_chapter5.pdf
4. https://mohua.gov.in/upload/uploadfiles/files/Part2.pdf
5. https://pib.gov.in/newsite/printrelease.aspx?relid=138591
6. https://wedcknowledge.lboro.ac.uk/resources/factsheets/FS009_FDI_A3_Poster.pdf
7. Park K. Park's Textbook of Preventive and Social Medicine (26th edition) Jabalpur: Banarsidas Bhanot-publishers 2021.

3.6 ACTS RELATED TO ENVIRONMENT

- **Ministry of Environment, Forest and Climate Change** (MoEFCC) serves as the nodal agency for the planning, promotion, making of environment laws and their enforcement in India.
- List of important agencies which help the MoEF in carrying out environment related activities:
  - Central Pollution Control Board
  - State Pollution Control Boards
  - State Departments of Environment
  - Union Territories (UT) Environmental Committees
  - The Forest Survey of India
  - The Wildlife Institute of India

- The National Afforestation and Eco-Development Board
- The Botanical and Zoological Survey of India, etc.

Environmental Laws and Rules are followed under following heads:
- Water pollution
- Air pollution
- Environment protection
- Public liability insurance
- National environment appellate authority
- National environment tribunal
- Animal welfare
- Wildlife
- Forest conservation
- Biodiversity
- Indian forest service

List of Public Health Important Environmental Legislation
- The Fisheries Act, 1897; Forest Act, 1927
- The Water (Prevention and Control of Pollution) Act, 1974
- The Water (Prevention and Control of Pollution) Cess Act, 1977
- The Air (Prevention and Control of Pollution) Act, 1981
- The Environment (Protection) Act, 1986
- The Hazardous Wastes (Management and Handling) Rules, 1989 and 2000.
- The Manufacture, Storage and Import of Hazardous Chemical Rules, 1989 and 2000.
- The Forest (Conservation) Act, 1980; Wildlife (Protection) Act 1972 and Wildlife (Protection) Amendment Act 1991.
- The Public Liability Insurance Act, 1991.
- The National Environment Tribunal Act, 1995, and Amendment 2010
- The Chemical Accidents (Emergency Planning, Preparedness and Response) Rules, 1996
- The Biomedical Wastes (Management and Handling) Rules, 1998 and Amendment, 2016
- The Recycled Plastic Manufacture and Usage Rules, 1999
- The Fly Ash Notification, 1999
- The Municipal Solid Waste (Management and Handling) Rule, 2000
- The Batteries (Management and Handling) (Draft) Rules, 2000.
- The Ozone Depleting Substance Rules, 2000
- The Energy Conservation Act, 2001
- The Biological Diversity Act, 2002
- The National Green Tribunal Act, 2010
- The Noise Pollution (Regulation and control) rules, 2010

Solid Waste Management Rules, 2016
Some of the Salient Features
- The Rules are now applicable beyond Municipal areas and extend to urban agglomerations, census towns, notified industrial townships, areas under the control of Indian Railways, airports, airbase, Port and harbour, defence establishments, special economic zones, State and Central government organizations, places of pilgrims, religious and historical importance.

- The source segregation of waste has been mandated to channelize the waste to wealth by recovery, reuse and recycle.
- Responsibilities of Generators have been introduced to segregate waste into three streams, Wet (Biodegradable), Dry (Plastic, Paper, metal, wood, etc.) and domestic hazardous wastes (diapers, napkins, empty containers of cleaning agents, mosquito repellents, etc.) and handover segregated wastes to authorized rag-pickers or waste collectors or local bodies.
- Integration of waste pickers/ragpickers and waste dealers/Kabadiwalas in the formal system should be done by State Governments, and Self Help Group, or any other group to be formed.
- No person should throw, burn, or bury the solid waste generated by him, on streets, open public spaces outside his premises, or in the drain, or water bodies.
- Generator will have to pay 'User Fee' to waste collector and for 'Spot Fine' for Littering and Non-segregation.
- Used sanitary waste like diapers, sanitary pads should be wrapped securely in pouches provided by manufacturers or brand owners of these products or in a suitable wrapping material and shall place the same in the bin meant for dry waste/non-bio-degradable waste.
- Bulk and institutional generators, market associations, event organizers and hotels and restaurants have been made directly responsible for segregation and sorting the waste and manage in partnership with local bodies.
- All hotels and restaurants should segregate biodegradable waste and set up a system of collection or follow the system of collection set up by local body to ensure that such food waste is utilized for composting / biomethanation.
- All Resident Welfare and Market Associations, Gated communities and institution with an area >5,000 sq m should segregate waste at source- into valuable dry waste like plastic, tin, glass, paper, etc. and handover recyclable material to either the authorized waste pickers or the authorized recyclers, or to the urban local body.
- The bio-degradable waste should be processed, treated and disposed of through composting or bio-methanation within the premises as far as possible. The residual waste shall be given to the waste collectors or agency as directed by the local authority.
- New townships and Group Housing Societies have been made responsible to develop in-house waste handling, and processing arrangements for bio-degradable waste.
- Every street vendor should keep suitable containers for storage of waste generated during the course of his activity such as food waste, disposable plates, cups, cans, wrappers, coconut shells, leftover food, vegetables, fruits, etc. and deposit such waste at waste storage depot or container or vehicle as notified by the local authority.
- The developers of special economic zone, industrial estate, industrial park to earmark at least 5% of the total area of the plot or minimum 5 plots/sheds for recovery and recycling facility.
- All manufacturers of disposable products such as tin, glass, plastics packaging, etc. or brand owners who introduce such products in the market shall provide necessary financial assistance to local authorities for the establishment of waste management system.
- All such brand owners who sale or market their products in such packaging material which are non-biodegradable should put in place a system to collect back the packaging waste generated due to their production.
- Manufacturers or brand owners or marketing companies of sanitary napkins and diapers should explore the possibility of using all recyclable materials in their products or they shall

provide a pouch or wrapper for disposal of each napkin or diapers along with the packet of their sanitary products.
- All industrial units using fuel and located within 100 km from a solid waste based RDF plant shall make arrangements within six months from the date of notification of these rules to replace at least 5% of their fuel requirement by RDF so produced.
- Non-recyclable waste having calorific value of 1,500 K/cal/kg or more shall not be disposed of on landfills and shall only be utilized for generating energy either or through refuse derived fuel or by giving away as feed stock for preparing refuse derived fuel.
- High calorific wastes shall be used for co-processing in cement or thermal power plants.
- Construction and demolition waste should be stored, separately disposed off, as per the Construction and Demolition Waste Management Rules, 2016
- Horticulture waste and garden waste generated from his premises should be disposed as per the directions of local authority.
- An event, or gathering organizer of more than 100 persons at any licensed/ unlicensed place, should ensure segregation of waste at source and handing over of segregated waste to waste collector or agency, as specified by local authority.
- Special provision for management of solid waste in hilly areas: Construction of landfill on the hill shall be avoided. A transfer station at a suitable enclosed location shall be setup to collect residual waste from the processing facility and inert waste. Suitable land shall be identified in the plain areas, down the hill, within 25 kilometers for setting up sanitary landfill. The residual waste from the transfer station shall be disposed off at this sanitary landfill.
- In case of non-availability of such land, efforts shall be made to set up regional sanitary landfill for the inert and residual waste.

Biomedical Waste Management (BMW) Handling Rules, 2016
Problem Statement
- In India the quantity of hospital waste is estimated to be 1-2 kg per bed per day in a hospital and 600 gm per day per bed in a clinic.
- Around 85% of the hospital waste is non-hazardous, 15% is infectious/hazardous.
- Mixing of non-hazardous waste with hazardous waste results in contamination and makes the entire waste hazardous.
- Hence there is necessity to segregate and treat and proper disposal.
- Improper disposal increases risk of infection, increase chances of the recycling of prohibited disposables and expired drugs.

BMW Management Rules, 2016
- Scope of the rule: These rules shall apply to all persons who generate, collect, receive, store, transport, treat, dispose, or handle biomedical waste in any form including hospitals, nursing homes, clinics, dispensaries, veterinary institutions, animal houses, pathological laboratories, blood banks, Ayush hospitals, clinical establishments, research or educational institutions, health camps, medical or surgical camps, vaccination camps, blood donation camps, first aid rooms of schools, forensic laboratories and research labs.

- These rules shall not apply to:
  - Radioactive wastes
  - Hazardous chemicals covered under the Manufacture, Storage and Import of Hazardous Chemicals Rules, 1989
  - Solid wastes covered under the Municipal Solid Waste Rules, 2000
  - The lead acid batteries
  - Hazardous wastes covered under the Hazardous Wastes Rules, 2008
  - E-Waste
  - Hazardous microorganisms, genetically engineered microorganisms and cells.

The major salient features of BMW Management Rules, 2016 include the following:
- The scope of the rules has been expanded to include vaccination camps, blood donation camps, surgical camps or any other healthcare activity.
- It is instructed to phase-out the use of chlorinated plastic bags, gloves and blood bags within two years.
- Pre-treatment of the laboratory waste, microbiological waste, blood samples and blood bags through disinfection or sterilization on-site in the manner as prescribed by WHO or NACO.
- Provide training to all healthcare workers and others involved in handling of biomedical waste at the time of induction and thereafter at least once in a year and immunize all health workers regularly especially for hepatitis and tetanus.
- Establish a Bar-Code System for bags or containers containing biomedical waste for disposal.
- Report major accidents that happen at any stage of bio medical waste management; and forward a report within twenty-four hours in writing regarding the remedial steps taken in Form I.
- Existing incinerators to achieve the standards for retention time in secondary chamber (retention time was 1 sec in BMW RULES 2011 that is now 2 seconds in BMW rules 2016) and Dioxin and Furans standards added for the first time in BMW rules and all these standards to be achieved within two years.
- These new standards for incinerator are more stringent and thus it will help to reduce the emission of pollutants in environment.
- Biomedical waste has been classified in to 4 categories instead 10 categories to improve the segregation of waste at place of origin.
- Procedure to get authorization for Bedded healthcare facilities (HCFs) been simplified.
- One time Authorization for Non-bedded HCFs also been made compulsory. (Non –beded hospitals were not needed to be registered in the earlier version of the BMW rules).
- State Government to provide land for setting up common biomedical waste treatment and disposal facility.
- No occupier shall establish on-site treatment and disposal facility, if a service of `common biomedical waste treatment facility is available within distance of seventy-five kilometer.
- Untreated human anatomical waste, animal anatomical waste, soiled waste and, biotechnology waste shall not be stored beyond a period of forty-eight hours:

Environmental Science, Environmental Health, and Sanitation

There are **4 schedules** and **five forms** in the BMW Act 1998, that are included with some changes in the BMW rules 2016 which are as follows:

Schedule I

Category	Type of waste	Type of bag or container to be used	Treatment and disposal options
Yellow	• Human Anatomical Waste	Yellow colored non-chlorinated plastic bags	Incineration or Plasma Pyrolysis or deep burial
	• Animal Anatomical Waste	Same as above	Same as above
	• Soiled Waste (ex. Blood or body fluids contaminated dressings, plaster cast or cotton swabs)	Same as above	If above facilities are not available then autoclaving or microwaving followed by shredding can be considered
	• Expired or discarded medicine	Same as above	Can be sent to pharmaceuticals companies for incineration or can be incinerated at common waste treatment plants
	• Chemical waste	Same as above	Disposed of by Incineration or Plasma Pyrolysis or encapsulation
	• Chemical liquid waste	Separate collection system leading to effluent treatment system	Chemical liquid must be pre-treated before mixing with other waste water
	• Microbiology, biotechnology and other clinical lab waste	Autoclave safe plastic bags or containers	Pre-treat first as per guidelines of NACO or WHO
Red	Contaminated waste red colored (recyclable)	Red colored non-chlorinated plastic bags or containers	Autoclaving or microwaving followed by shredding. Then this treated waste will be sent to authorized recyclers to make fuel or road
White	Sharp wastes including metals	Puncture proof, leak proof, tamper proof containers	Autoclaving or dry heat sterilization followed by shredding then disposal to iron foundries.
Blue	Glassware (ex. Medicine ampoules or vials)	Card board boxes with blue colored markings	Disinfection or autoclaving or microwaving then sent for recycling

Schedule II

Standards for Treatment and Disposal of Bio-medical Wastes

In this schedule standards have been given for incineration, microclaving, chemical disinfection, etc.

Schedule III

List of Prescribed Authorities and the Corresponding Duties

In this schedule authorities and duties right from the national level up to the district level has been mentioned for timely and correctly management of the biomedical waste and for the monitoring of the whole process.

Schedule IV

Schedule 4 has been divided into two parts:
1. **Part A:** Label for Bio-Medical Waste Containers or Bags
2. **Part B:** Label for Transporting Bio-Medical Waste Bags or Containers

List of the forms that to be filled for particular purpose as follows:
- Form—I: Accident Reporting
- Form—II : Application for authorization or renewal of authorization
- Form—III: Authorization
- Form—IV: Annual Report
- Form—V: Application for filing appeal against order passed by the prescribed authority

E-WASTE MANAGEMENT RULES, 2016

- The Ministry of Environment, Forest and Climate Change notified the E-Waste Management Rules, 2016 in supersession of the E-waste (Management and Handling) Rules, 2011.
- Twenty-one (21) types of electrical and electronic equipment (EEE) have been notified which includes product like Compact Fluorescent Lamp (CFL) and other mercury containing lamps.
- The responsibility of disposal of e-waste in a scientific and environmentally sound manner has been assigned to Producers of notified Electrical and Electronic Equipment (EEE) under the principle of Extended Producer Responsibility (EPR).
- Under EPR regime producers of EEE, have given annual e-waste collection and recycling targets based on the generation from the previously sold EEE or based on sales of EEE as the case may be.
- Deposit Refund Scheme has been introduced as an additional economic instrument wherein the producer charges an additional amount as a deposit at the time of sale of the electrical and electronic equipment and returns it to the consumer along with interest when the end-of-life electrical and electronic equipment is returned.
- The role of State Governments has been also introduced to ensure safety, health and skill development of the workers involved in dismantling and recycling operations.
- A provision of penalty for violation of rules has also been introduced.
- Urban Local Bodies (Municipal Committee/Council/Corporation) have been assigned the duty to collect and channelize the orphan products to authorized dismantlers or recyclers.
- Allocation of proper space to existing and upcoming industrial units for e-waste dismantling and recycling.

BIBLIOGRAPHY

1. http://qi.nhsrcindia.org/sites/default/files/Environmental%20Acts%20%26%20Rules-lecture2.pdf
2. https://moef.gov.in/en/rules-and-regulations/environment-protection/
3. https://pib.gov.in/newsite/printrelease.aspx?relid=138591
4. https://pib.gov.in/PressReleasePage.aspx?PRID=1805794
5. The gazette of India. The Bio-Medical Waste Management Rules, 2016.

3.7 NATIONAL CLEAN AIR PROGRAM

- It was launched by the **Ministry of Environment, Forest and Climate Change** (MoEFCC) in January 2019.
- It is the first-ever effort in the country to frame a national framework for air quality management with a time-bound reduction target.
- It seeks to cut the concentration of coarse (particulate matter of diameter 10 micrometer or less, or PM10) and fine particles (particulate matter of diameter 2.5 micrometer or less, or PM 2.5).

GOAL

The goal of the NCAP is to meet the prescribed annual average ambient air quality standards at all locations in the country in a stipulated timeframe (long-term).

TARGET

- Earlier national level target was 20%–30% reduction of PM 2.5 and PM10 concentration by 2024.
- Recently Government of India has set a new target of a 40% reduction in particulate matter concentration by 2026.
- This is keeping 2017 as the base year for the comparison of concentration.

OBJECTIVES

- To ensure stringent implementation of mitigation measures for prevention, control and abatement of air pollution.
- To augment and evolve effective and proficient ambient air quality monitoring network across the country for ensuring a comprehensive and reliable database.
- To augment public awareness and capacity-building measures encompassing data dissemination and public outreach programs for inclusive public participation and for ensuring trained manpower and infrastructure on air pollution.

NATIONAL AIR QUALITY INDEX

- **Definition**: An air quality index is defined as an overall scheme that transforms the weighed values of individual air pollution related parameters (for example, pollutant concentrations) into a single number or set of numbers (Ott, 1978).

- **There are two steps** in formulating an AQI:
  1. Formation of sub-indices (for each pollutant) and
  2. Aggregation of sub-indices to have an overall AQI.
- Air quality index provides a legal framework for air pollution control.
- The intention of having national air quality index is to protect public from adverse effects of air pollutants and to guide national/local authorities for pollution control decisions.
- Indian National Air Quality Standards (INAQS) includes following 12 parameters:

• Carbon monoxide (CO)	• Lead (Pb)
• Nitrogen dioxide (NO_2)	• Ammonia (NH_3)
• Sulphur dioxide (SO_2)	• Benzopyrene (bap)
• Particulate matter (PM) of less than 2.5 microns size ($PM_{2.5}$)	• Benzene (C_6H_6)
• PM of less than 10 microns size (PM_{10})	• Arsenic (As)
• Ozone (O_3)	• Nickel (Ni)

Objectives of AQI

- Main Objective of AQI is to quickly disseminate air quality information **(almost in real-time)** about the pollutants which have short-term impacts.
- Out of above mentioned 12 air quality standards only 8 have been considered in the proposed AQI system and Those 8 standards include **CO, NO_2, SO_2, $PM_{2.5}$, PM_{10}, O_3, NH_3** and **Pb**.

Classification of AQI Category with Range and Color Coding

AQI category	AQI range	Color
Good	0–50	Green
Satisfactory	51–100	Light green
Moderately polluted	101–200	Yellow
Poor	201–300	Orange
Very poor	301–400	Red
Severe	401–500	Maroon

Monitoring of air quality: (1) Automatic station (2) Manually

- There are **40 automated** air quality monitoring stations to record hourly, monthly or annual data about air quality standards.
- These stations **continuously** monitor parameters like PM_{10}, $PM_{2.5}$, NO_2, SO_2, CO, O_3, etc and they provide data about these parameters almost in real-time.
- There are **573 stations** where air quality is being monitored **manually** and these stations are overall under the National Air Monitoring Program (NAMP).
- At majority of the manually operated stations, only three pollutants namely PM_{10}, sulphur dioxide (SO_2) and nitrogen dioxide (NO_2) are measured while at some stations in addition to these three pollutants $PM_{2.5}$ and Pb are also measured.
- The frequency of monitoring is **twice a week**.

Relation of Level of AQI and Health Impact

AQI	Associated Health Impacts
Good (0–50)	**Minimal** Impact
Satisfactory (51–100)	Minor **breathing discomfort** to the sensitive people only
Moderately polluted (101–200)	May cause **breathing discomfort** to the people with lung and/or heart disease, children and older adults
Poor (201–300)	May cause breathing discomfort to the normal people on prolonged exposure and discomfort to people with heart disease
Very poor (301–400)	**May cause respiratory illness** to the people on prolonged exposure while Effect may be serious in people with lung and heart diseases
Severe (401–500)	May cause respiratory problems **even on healthy people** and **serious health impacts** on people with lung/heart diseases.

BIBLIOGRAPHY

1. Biswas DK, Pandey GK, (2002) "Strategy and Policy adopted in Air Quality Management in India" in Better Air Quality in Asian and Pacific Rim Cities, Hong Kong.
2. Govt. of India (2014), National Air Quality Index, central pollution control board, ministry of environment, forest and climate change, New Delhi.

CHAPTER 4

Nutrition Assessment and Nutrition Education

CHAPTER OUTLINE

4.1 Basics of nutrition
4.2 Nutrition assessment methods for individuals, families and community
4.3 Concept of meal and diet planning
4.4 Purpose, principles and methods of nutrition education
4.5 Overview of common nutritional disorders in India
4.6 National Nutritional Policy 1993
4.7 Different National Health Programs Related to Nutrition:
    4.7.1 Poshan Abhiyaan and Mission Poshan 2.0
    4.7.2 Pradhan Mantri Matru Vandana Yojana (PMMVY)
    4.7.3 Integrated Child Development Services Scheme (ICDS)
    4.7.4 Infant and Young Child Feeding (IYCF)
    4.7.5 Anemia Mukt Bharat (I-NIPI)
    4.7.6 Basics of Vitamin A and Nutritional Blindness
    4.7.7 Intensified Mission Indradhanush 4.0
    4.7.8 Intensified Diarrhea Control Fortnight
    4.7.9 Nutrition Rehabilitation Center
    4.7.10 Home Based Newborn Care and Home Based Care of Young Child
    4.7.11 Pradhan Mantri Poshan Shakti Nirman (PM POSHAN)
4.8 Brief Note on Food-related Diseases and Food Safety
4.9 Food Safety and Standards Act (FSSA), 2006 and Food Safety and Standards Rules, 2011
4.10 Consumer Protection Act,1986 and Amended in 2019

4.1 BASICS OF NUTRITION

Nutrition is the science of food and its relationship to health. It involves process of ingestion, digestion, absorption and metabolism.

Function of Food

Physiological function	Social function	Psychological function
It provides energy for body functions	Creates atmosphere for joyful eating.	Satisfying hunger and taste buds
Nutrients build and maintain body tissues	Used as offering to God in religious festivals and in fasts.	Providing enjoyment
Safeguarding body against diseases	Main component in any gathering or party.	Provides comfort in depressive mood
Regulating body functions	Means of communication and relationship.	Used as a reward or punishment, e.g., good or bad food
	Means of social prestige	

Foods are conventionally grouped as:
- Cereals, millets and pulses
- Vegetables and fruits
- Milk and milk products, egg, meat and fish
- Oils, fats, nuts and oilseeds

Major nutrients		Other nutrients
Energy rich foods	Carbohydrates and fats	Protein, fiber, minerals, calcium, iron and B-complex vitamins
	Whole grain cereals, millets	
	Vegetable oils, ghee, butter	Fat soluble vitamins, essential fatty acids
	Nuts and oilseeds	Proteins, vitamins, minerals
	Sugars	Nil
Body building foods	Proteins	
	Pulses, nuts and oilseeds	B-complex vitamins, invisible fat, fiber
	Milk and milk products	Calcium, vitamin A, riboflavin, vitamin B_{12}
	Meat, fish, poultry	B-complex vitamins, iron, iodine, fat
Protective foods	Vitamins and minerals	
	Green leafy vegetables	Antioxidants, fiber and other carotenoids
	Other vegetables and fruits	Fiber, sugar and antioxidants
	Eggs, milk and milk products and flesh foods	Protein and fat

Importance of diet during different stages of life

For being physically active and healthy.
Nutrient—dense low fat foods.

For maintaining health, productivity and prevention of diet-related disease and to support pregnancy/lactation.
Nutritionally adequate diet with extra food for child bearing/rearing

For growth spurt, maturation and bone development.
Body building and protective foods.

For growth, development and to fight infections.
Energy-rich, body building and protective foods (milk, vegetables and fruits).

For growth and appropriate milestones.
Breast milk, energy-rich foods (fats, sugar).

There are two types of nutrients: Macronutrients and Micronutrients. The macronutrients are protein, fat and carbohydrate while the micronutrients are vitamins and minerals.

Carbohydrates

- Carbohydrates are major sources of energy and they are either simple or complex in nature.
- Simple carbohydrates are: 1. Glucose, 2. Sucrose and 3. Fructose
- Source of Simple carbohydrates: glucose and fructose are found in fruits, vegetables and honey and sucrose in sugar and lactose in milk.
- Complex carbohydrates: Starches, cellulose, gums and pectins
- Starches are in cereals, millets, pulses and root vegetables and glycogen in animal foods.
- The other complex carbohydrates which are resistant to digestion in the human digestive tract are cellulose which are in vegetables and whole grains while gums and pectins are in vegetables, fruits and cereals, which constitute the dietary fiber component.
- Dietary fiber delays and retards absorption of carbohydrates and fats and increases the satiety value. Diets rich in fiber reduce glucose and lipids in blood and increase the bulk of the stools.
- Carbohydrate provides 4 Kcal/g of energy.
- Foods can also be categorized according to their **glycemic index**, a measure of how quickly glucose levels increase in the bloodstream after carbohydrates are consumed. For example, processed foods, white bread, white rice, and white potatoes have a high glycemic index. They quickly raise blood glucose levels after being consumed and also cause the release of insulin, which can result in more hunger and overeating. However, foods such as fruit, green leafy vegetables, raw carrots, kidney beans, chickpeas, lentils, and bran breakfast cereals have a low glycemic index. These foods minimize blood sugar spikes and insulin release after eating, which leads to less hunger and overeating. Eating a diet of low glycemic foods has been linked to a decreased risk of obesity and diabetes mellitus.

Proteins: There are Two Types

- Proteins are composed of carbon, hydrogen, oxygen, nitrogen and sulphur, phosphorus, iron and other elements in varying amounts.
- Protein is required for growth and development, for repair of body tissues and their maintenance and for synthesis of antibodies, enzymes and hormones.

Animal proteins	Vegetable proteins
High quality	Relatively poor quality
Provide all the essential amino acids	Low content of some of the essential amino acids.
Found in milk, meat, eggs, cheese, fish	Found in pulses (legumes) cereals, beans, nuts, oil-seed

Role	Examples	Functions
Digestive enzyme	Amylase, lipase, pepsin	Break down nutrients in food into small pieces that can be readily absorbed
Transport	Hemoglobin	Carry substances throughout the body in blood or lymph
Structure	Actin, tubulin, keratin	Build different structures, like the cytoskeleton
Hormone signaling	Insulin, glucagon	Coordinate the activity of different body systems
Defense	Antibodies	Protect the body from foreign pathogens
Contraction	Myosin	Carry out muscle contraction
Storage	Legume storage proteins, egg white (albumin)	Provide food for the early development of the embryo or the seedling

- **Amino acids** are the monomers that make up proteins. There are 20 types of amino acids commonly found in proteins.

Fats

- Dietary fat is concentrated source of energy as one gram of fat gives 9 kcal of energy.
- Vitamins A, D, E and K are fat-soluble vitamins.
- Essential fatty acids are needed for growth and maintenance of the integrity of the skin.
- Fats help in maintaining body temperature.
- Fats provide cushioning for many organs in the body (heart, kidney, intestine, etc.)
- Fats increase palatability of food.
- Fats could be saturated and unsaturated. Excessive consumption of saturated fat increases the risk of cardiovascular diseases.

There are two sources of dietary fats:
1. **Invisible fat**: It is the fat which is not extracted from the original source like present in cereals, pulses or even in animal foods.
2. **Visible** or added fats: It is the fat which is extracted from its original source like cooking oil.

Sources of fats: Animal sources: Ghee, butter, meat, fish oil, etc. and Vegetables sources are various vegetable oils such as groundnut, mustard, cottonseed, safflower, coconut oil, etc.
- It is recommended to use different sources of fat/oil.
- The vegetable oils contain very important substances like lignans (sesame oil), oryzanol (rice bran oil) which helps to reduce cholesterol level and also protect from the oxidant damage.
- Fatty acids are the primary constituents of all dietary fats. Based on their chemical nature, the fatty acids are broadly grouped as saturated (SFA), monounsaturated (MUFA) and polyunsaturated (PUFA) **(Table 4.1)**.

Table 4.1: Major types of fatty acids in fats and oils.

Saturated	Mono-unsaturated	Polyunsaturated		
			Linoleic (n-6)	α-Linolenic (n-3)
Coconut palm kernel/butter vonaspati	Red palm oil Palmolein groundnut ricebran sesame	Low	Red palm oil palmolein	Rapeseed, Mustard soyabean
		Moderate	Groundnut, Ricebran, Sesame	
		High	Salfflower, Sunflower Cottonseed, Corn, Soyabean	

- **Trans fats** are fats that have been altered through a hydrogenation process, so they are not in their natural state. Trans fats are found in processed foods, such as chips, crackers, and cookies, as well as in some margarines and salad dressings. Minimal trans fat intake is recommended because it increases cholesterol and contributes to heart disease.

Vitamins and Minerals

- Vitamins are required in small amounts.
- Most of the vitamins cannot be synthesized in the body that's why they must be supplied in the diet on daily basis.
- Fat-soluble vitamins can be stored in the body while water-soluble vitamins are not stored as they excreted in urine. That's why they must be supplied on daily basis in diet.

Classification

Fat Soluble Vitamins
- Vitamin A or retinol
- Vitamin D (caliciferol-D2, cholecalciferol D3)
- Vitamin E (Tocopherol)
- Vitamin K

Water Soluble Vitamins
- Thiamine (B1)
- Riboflavin (B2)
- Nicotinic acid (B3)
- Pantothenic acid (B5)
- Pyridoxine (B6)
- Folic acid (B9)
- Vitamin B12
- Ascorbic acid (vitamin C)

Vitamin A
- Function: It is very essential for eye, muscle, skin, immunity and reproductive system.
- Deficiency diseases: Xerophthalmia and night blindness
- Sources: Halibut fish liver oil (**richest source**), Cod liver oil, carrots, broccoli, eggs, fish, milk and milk products, sweet potatoes, kale, spinach, collard greens, cantaloupe melon, pumpkins, and apricots.

Vitamin D
- Function: It helps the body absorb calcium, thus aiding in the growth of bone tissues.
- Deficiency diseases: Osteomalacia and rickets
- Sources: This is the only nutrient among the types of vitamins that the human body can synthesize adequately from sunlight. It is also present in extremely minute portions in eatables like dairy products, fish, and fish oil.

Vitamin E
- Function: It is one of the types of vitamins that aid in the formation of red blood cells and reduces oxidative stress.
- Deficiency diseases: Hemolytic anemia in newborns and neuropathy
- Sources: Kiwis, eggs, wheat germ, almonds, nuts, vegetable oils, and leafy greens.

Vitamin K
- Function: This aids in blood coagulation or blood clotting post a wound formation.
- Deficiency diseases: Bleeding diathesis and hemorrhage
- Sources: Green and leafy vegetables, including broccoli, kale, spinach, and cabbage.

Vitamin B1
- Function: It aids in the production of the various enzymes responsible for converting carbohydrates into energy.

- Deficiency diseases: Beriberi (dry and wet)
- Sources: Cereal grains, oranges, yeast, pork, brown rice, sunflower seeds, whole grain rye, cauliflower, asparagus, kale, eggs, and potatoes.

Vitamin B2
- Function: It helps in the production of red blood cells and food metabolism.
- Deficiency diseases: Fissures and inflammation in the mouth (angular stomatitis), cheilitis
- Sources: Green beans, persimmons, okra, bananas, chard, milk and milk products, meat, eggs, fish, and asparagus.

Vitamin B3
- Function: It is important for cell growth and maintenance of healthy nerves and skin. It can also lower cholesterol at high doses.
- Deficiency diseases: Pellagra (4D: dermatitis, diarrhea, dementia and death)
- Sources: Lentils, chicken, salmon, beef, tomatoes, milk, eggs, leafy vegetables, carrots, nuts and seeds, broccoli, tofu, and tuna.

Vitamin B5
- Function: The human body needs it to produce hormones and energy.
- Deficiency diseases: Paresthesia (burning feet syndrome)
- Sources: Whole grains, avocados, broccoli, yoghurt, and meats.

Vitamin B6
- Function: It helps in the formation of red blood cells, the efficiency of body protein, and proper brain function.
- Deficiency diseases: Peripheral neuropathy and anemia
- Sources: Nuts, beef liver, squash, bananas, and chickpeas.

Vitamin B7
- Function: It helps in the metabolism of other nutrients, especially the structural protein keratin that aids in maintaining healthy nails, skin, and hair.
- Deficiency diseases: Dermatitis
- Sources: Cheese, egg yolk, broccoli, spinach, and liver.

Vitamin B9
- Function: It aids in the proper formation of DNA and RNA in fetuses and prevents carcinogenic transformation of these genetic units.
- Deficiency diseases: Megaloblastic anemia, neural tube defect.
- Sources: Sunflower seeds, leafy vegetables, select fortified grain products, legumes, liver, and peas.

Vitamin B12
- Function: It is also one of the types of vitamins in the human body that aid in healthy metabolism and maintenance of the central nervous system.

- Deficiency diseases: Megaloblastic anemia and neurological issues like SCDS (subacute combined degeneration of spinal cord)
- Sources: Fortified nutritional yeast, fish, meat, milk and milk products, shellfish, fortified cereals, fortified soy products, and eggs.

Vitamin C

- Function: Chemically called ascorbic acid, vitamin C has antioxidant and anti-aging benefits. This is because it promotes collagen formation, aiding in wound healing, strengthening blood vessels, bone formation, iron absorption and maintaining a strong immune system.
- Deficiency diseases: **Scurvy**
- Sources: Raw citrus fruits and vegetables like tomatoes, brussels, spinach, broccoli, and cabbage.

There are mainly two types of minerals:
1. **Macrominerals:** Sodium, potassium, calcium, phosphorus, magnesium and sulphur. They are typically measured in milligrams, grams, or milliequivalents.

Macromineral	Source	Function
Sodium	Table salt, spinach, and milk	Water balance
Potassium	Legumes, potatoes, bananas, and whole grains	Muscle contraction, cardiac muscle function, and nerve function
Calcium	Dairy, eggs, and green leafy vegetables	Bone and teeth development, nerve function, muscle contraction, immunity, and blood clotting
Magnesium	Raw nuts, spinach (cooked has higher magnesium content), tomatoes. and beans	Cell energy, muscle function, cardiac function, and glucose metabolism
Chloride	Table salt	Fluid and electrolyte balance and digestion
Phosphorus	Red meal, poultry, rice, oats, dairy, and fish	Bone strength and cellular function

2. **Microminerals:** Zinc, copper, selenium, molybdenum, fluorine, cobalt, chromium and iodine. They are needed in tiny amounts. They are also known as trace minerals.

Trace mineral	Source	Function
Zinc	Eggs, spinach, yogurt, whole grains, fish and brewer's yeast	Immune function, healing, and vision
Iron	Red meat, organ meats, spinach, shrimp, tuna, salmon, kidney beans, peas, and lentils (nonanimal forms are harder to absorb, so need more)	Hemoglobin production and collagen production
Chromium	Whole grains, meat and brewer's yeast	Glucose metabolism
Copper	Shellfish, fruits, nuts, and organ meats	Hemoglobin productlon, collagen, elastin, neurotransmitter production, and melan in production
Fluorine	Fluoridated water and toothpaste	Retention of calcium in bones and teeth

Nutrition Assessment and Nutrition Education

Trace mineral	Source	Function
Iodine	Iodized salt and seafood	Energy production and thyroid function
Manganese	Whole grain and nuts	Useful to metabolism of calcium and potassium
Molybdenum	Organ meats, green leafy vegetables, legumes, whole grains and dairy	Not fully understood, detoxification
Selenium	Broccoli, cabbage, garlic, whole grains, brewer's yeast, celery, onions, and organ meats	Not fully understood

Food Pyramid (Fig. 4.1)

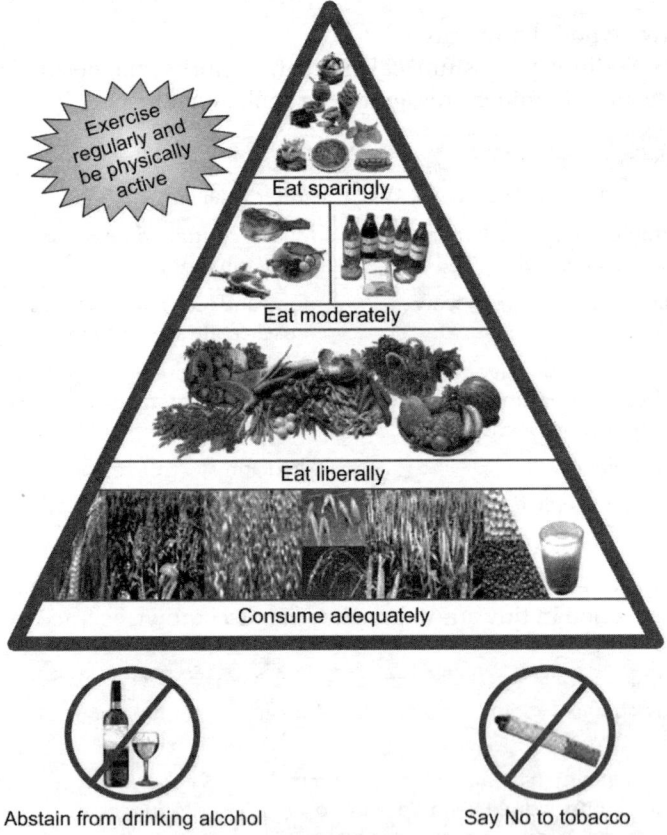

Fig. 4.1: Food pyramid.

BIBLIOGRAPHY

1. https://wtcs.pressbooks.pub/nursingfundamentals/chapter/14-2-nutrition-basic-concepts/
2. https://www.khanacademy.org/science/biology/macromolecules/proteins-and-amino-acids/a/introduction-to-proteins-and-amino-acids
3. https://www.nin.res.in/downloads/DietaryGuidelinesforNINwebsite.pdf

4.2 NUTRITION ASSESSMENT METHODS FOR INDIVIDUALS, FAMILIES AND COMMUNITY

RATIONALE FOR NUTRITION ASSESSMENT

- Epidemiological diet and nutrition data is significantly correlates with morbidity and mortality
- Nutrition data guides to know diet related problems like undernutrition, and non-communicable diseases like hypertension, diabetes, CVDs and some types of cancers, etc.
- High intake of fruits and vegetables (fiber diet) reduce the risk of gastro-intestinal disorders like constipation, colon cancer and others.
- Fish or soya consumption is also associated with low prevalence of breast cancer and CHD.
- It also helps to establish relation between a particular nutrient and morbidity.
- It may also help in the formation of various preventive strategies.

Common Nutritional Challenges

- Protein energy malnutrition (PEM)
- Low birth weight (LBW)
- Chronic energy deficiency (CED)
- Vitamin A deficiency (VAD)
- Iron deficiency anemia (IDA)
- Iodine deficiency disorders (IDD)
- Zinc deficiency
- Diet and nutrition related chronic diseases:
  - Overweight and obesity
  - Insulin resistance: Type 2 Diabetes
  - Cardiovascular diseases (CVD)
  - Cancers

Nutritional Assessment Methods: It may be Remembered as Acronym "ABCD"

- **A**nthropometric measurements
- **B**io-chemical estimations
- **C**linical examination
- **D**ietary intake methods

Other helpful methods include vital statistics and ecological studies.

1. Anthropometric Measurements

- Height (cm)
- Weight (kg)
- Head, chest, mid upper arm circumference (MUAC), waist and hip circumferences
- Measure of fat fold thickness at multiple sites (triceps, biceps, subscapular and supraliiac sites).
- **Merits:**
  - High specificity and sensitivity
  - Measures many variables of nutritional significance
  - Readings are numerical and gradable on standard growth charts.

- Readings are reproducible
- Non-expensive and needs minimal training
☐ **Demerits:**
  - Inter-observers' error in measurement
  - Limited nutritional diagnosis
  - Problems with reference standards
  - Based on Arbitrary statistical cut-off levels

2. Bio-chemical Estimations
☐ **More precise and accurate but expensive method**
☐ Useful in detecting nutritional deficiency at early stage, even before the appearance of overt clinical signs.
☐ Verification of other method can be done like salt intake with 24-hour urinary excretion.

3. Clinical Examination
☐ Clinical examination method usually helps in finding nutritional disorders like anemia, vitamin A deficiency, enlargement of thyroid, angular stomatitis, cheilosis, glossitis, phrynoderma, rickets, kwashiorkor, marasmus, obesity, etc.
☐ Clinical examination is done to see changes in hair (Sparse, discolored, easily pluckable), face (Moon face with edema), eye changes (Conjunctival xerosis, bitot spots, corneal xerosis, keratomalacia, corneal scar) nail changes (Koilonychia) gums (spongy bleeding), signs of rickets (knock knees/bow legs), etc.
☐ **Demerits:**
  - Malnutrition cannot be quantified on the basis of clinical signs
  - Many deficiencies are unaccompanied by physical signs
  - Lack of specificity and subjective nature of most of the physical signs

4. Dietary Intake Methods

Types of Diet Surveys:
☐ Family diet survey
☐ 24 hour recall method
☐ Institutional diet surveys
☐ Duplicate samples
☐ Food balance sheets

1. Family Diet Survey (Weighment Diet Survey)
☐ In this method all the raw foodstuffs must be weighed, before they are cooked (breakfast, lunch, evening snacks and tea and dinner). Food wastage and leftover also need to be taken care.
☐ Prior permission and assurance for cooperation from the participating family to be taken.
☐ Avoid fast and feast days during survey periods
☐ This survey usually done for 24 hours, 3 days or 7 consecutive days.
☐ The dietary intake is expressed in terms of consumption units (CU)/day
☐ Demographic particulars of all the individuals in a house-hold are needed
☐ Information on no. of guests/absentees/pet animals partaking the food needed

Nutrition Assessment and Nutrition Education

Merits:
- Accurate method
- Definite dietary consumption pattern can be studied at family level

Demerits:
- Time consuming procedure
- Data accuracy depends on the co-operation of participant
- It does not give the actual intake of an individual

2. 24 Hours Recall Method (OR) Oral Questionnaire (OR) Individual Diet Survey
- In this method Individual dietary intake is assessed
- Firstly, we need to know what food items prepared previous day and then we will ask to provide the total raw amounts used for each preparation and weighed.
- The total amount of each cooked food item and the actual amount consumed by each individual is assessed with the help of a set of standard cups (volumes known).
- Conversion factor for the intake of each food item (raw) of an individual is derived by:

$$\frac{\text{Raw quantity of item in each preparation}}{\text{Total quantity of cooked food item}} \times \text{Intake of cooked food}$$

3. Institutional Level Diet Survey
- Usually, this method is used in the set up like Hostels, Hospitals, Industrial Canteens, Jails and Orphanages
- There are two methods one is **Inventory method** and second one is **Weighment method** used for Institutional Level Diet Survey.

3.1 Inventory method:
- Inventory method: Food stock registers are verified for a week.
- The average intake/per person/day = (stocks at the beginning of week and stocks at the end of week)/Total number of inmates partaking × 7 days.
- Same calculation is to be done for every food item and estimation of nutrients also done.
- **Merits**: Less time consuming
- **Demerits:** It is only an estimate as no direct assessment involved.

3.2 Weighment method:
- All the raw and cooked foods items and individual plate servings are weighed and nutrients are derived.

4. Duplicate Samples
- The individual is required to save (in separate plate) a duplicate sample and the same to be sent to the laboratory for nutrient analysis.
- **It is most accurate method of diet survey.**

5. Food Balance Sheets
- Food balance sheet includes total food available/produced in the country as also the available buffer stocks.

$$\text{Per person per day of food availability} = \frac{\text{Beginning of the year stock (boys) + total food produced + imports} - \text{Stocks at the end of the years + exports + seeds + cattle/poultry feeds + wastages}}{\text{Total mid year population} \times 365 \text{ days}}$$

BIBLIOGRAPHY

1. http://www.ilsiindia.org/Workshop_National_Food_Consumption_Anthropometry_Physical_Activity_Survey/Methodology.pdf

4.3 CONCEPT OF MEAL AND DIET PLANNING

What is Meal Planning?

- It is use of seasonal foods which is economical and suits the taste and meets the desires of the individual eating it.
- It is done to ensure adequate nutrition for every member of the family within the availability of time, energy and money.
- It helps to meet the nutritional requirements of the family members by working 'daily food guide'.
- In short, meal planning helps us to make food nutritious, economical, address food preferences of the family members and save energy, time and money with help of use leftover food.

FACTORS AFFECTING MEAL PLANNING

- Nutritional adequacy
- Age
- Sex
- Physical activity
- Economic considerations
- Time, energy and skill considerations
- Seasonal availability
- Religion, region, cultural patterns, traditions and customs
- Variety in color and texture
- Likes and dislikes of individuals
- Satiety value

Steps of Meal Planning

- In first step, we need to consider a person's age, sex and physical activity during whole day from morning to night.
- Meal Planned is to be done for three major meals (breakfast, lunch and dinner) and 1–3 small meals for one full day.
- There should be gap of 2–3 hours between main and small meals and of 4–6 hours between two main/major meals.
- Timing of breakfast at 8–10 AM, lunch at 2–3 PM, and dinner at 8–9 PM.
- Use the food pyramid/food groups for selection of groups.
- Each main meal should contain one to two items from each food group like energy providing, body building and protective food groups. The fourth food group of fat/sugar should be included in moderation.

Nutrition Assessment and Nutrition Education

- Each meal should contribute approximately one-third of the nutritional requirements.
- As minor or small meal single food preparation or fruit is sufficient. Even minor meals should not be calorie-rich/energy-dense but should be nutrient-dense foods.
- Selection of food items must be based on income, season and food preferences.
- Write the menu plan for each meal giving the name of the food preparation along with quantity in house-hold measures.
- Food selection should be done in a way that the food preparation/meal gives variety in color, flavour and taste, and texture. It should also suit the daily routine/pattern of the individual and occasion.

Modification of family meal requires in following situations:
- Adult woman
- Pregnant woman
- Lactating mother
- Infant
- Preschooler
- School-going child
- Adolescent
- Elderly

Concept of Diet Planning

Balanced diet: A balanced diet should provide around 50–60% of total calories from carbohydrates, preferably from complex carbohydrates, about 10–15% from proteins and 20–30% from both visible and invisible fat.

A Healthy Diet Includes the Following

- Fruit, vegetables, legumes (e.g., lentils and beans), nuts and whole grains (e.g., unprocessed maize, millet, oats, wheat and brown rice).
- At least 400 g (i.e., five portions) of fruit and vegetables per day excluding potatoes, sweet potatoes, cassava and other starchy roots.
- Less than 10% of total energy intake from free sugars which is equivalent to 50 g (or about 12 level teaspoons), but ideally is less than 5% of total energy intake for additional health benefits.
- Less than 30% of total energy intake from fats. Unsaturated fats (found in fish, avocado and nuts, and in sunflower, soybean, canola and olive oils) are preferable to saturated fats (found in fatty meat, butter, palm and coconut oil, cream, cheese, ghee and lard) and *trans*-fats of all kinds, including both industrially-produced *trans*-fats (found in baked and fried foods, and pre-packaged snacks and foods, such as frozen pizza, pies, cookies, biscuits, wafers, and cooking oils and spreads) and ruminant *trans*-fats (found in meat and dairy foods from ruminant animals, such as cows, sheep, goats and camels). It is suggested that the intake of saturated fats be reduced to less than 10% of total energy intake and *trans*-fats to less than

1% of total energy intake. In particular, industrially-produced *trans*-fats are not part of a healthy diet and should be avoided.
- Less than 5 g of salt (equivalent to about one teaspoon) per day.
- Salt should be iodized.

Principles of Diet Planning

The six basic principles of diet planning are adequacy, balance, calorie control, density, moderation and variety.
- **Adequacy:** Maintaining adequate levels of energy, nutrients, movement and rest for optimal health
- **Balance:** Balancing different food groups, and consuming foods in the right proportion
- **Calorie control:** Consuming the appropriate number of calories to maintain a healthy weight depending on your metabolism and exercise levels
- **Density:** Focusing on creating a diet that is nutrient dense without being high in calories
- **Moderation:** Learning how to be moderate with foods that are higher in fat or sugar
- **Variety:** Exploring a varied diet that provides all the nutrients necessary for good health

Types of modification of a normal diet: Modifications can be done in:
- Consistency of the diet
- Nutrient content of the diet
- Interval and frequency of feeding

Modifications in Diet Consistency

- In some diseases the thickness of the food has to be changed. The food can then be served in two consistencies:
  1. Liquid
  2. Semisolid
- Sometimes, it becomes difficult to eat normal food. For example, in diarrhea and fever you serve a liquid diet. This liquid diet includes milk, fruit juices, coconut water, nimbu-pani, tea, lassi, soups, cold drinks, etc. When one is little better you can serve khichdi, curd, custard, fruits, bread, cooked vegetables, etc.

Modifications in Nutrient Content

Depending on the nature of the diseases, modifications may need to be made in one or more nutrients in the diet. The modifications can be in terms of an increase or decrease in amount of the nutrient. For example, salt has to be reduced in high blood pressure, intake of carbohydrates has to be restricted in case of diabetes and fluid intake has to be increased in the case of diarrhea.

Modifications in Interval and Frequency of Feeding

- Normally you eat 3–4 meals a day, that is, breakfast, lunch, tea and dinner. In sickness, you find it difficult to eat the amount you usually eat at one time. However, your body must get all the nutrients in correct amounts. Small amounts of food at intervals of 2–3 hours and as many as 8–10 small meals in a day instead of 3–4 meals facilitates speedy recovery.

Diet in Specific Diseases

Diseases	Modifications in			Food to be	
	Diet consistency	Nutrient content	Interval and frequency of feeding	Taken	Avoided
Diarrhea	Liquid/semi solid	Low fiber	Frequent meals, intervals of 1–2 hrs	Soup, banana biscuits sago khichdi, potato, boiled egg, curd, dals, refined cereals	Whole cereals, chillies, whole pulses, fried food, guava, fruit with skin, leafy vegetables, pastries, milk
Fever	Semisolid diet	High calorie, high protein	Frequent meals at 2–3 hours intervals	Milk, egg, chicken, fish, juices, fruits, soups, lassi, dalia, kheer	Whole cereals, chillies whole pulses, fried food, guava, fruit with skin, leafy vegetables, pastries, milk
Diabetes	No change	Normal diet with no sugar	Meals taken at fixed time take six small meals/day	Vegetables, roti, dal, milk, curd, fruit, egg	Sugar sweet, honey, jam, jellies, cakes, pastries, sweetened fruits, cold drinks, tinned fruit
Hypertension	No change	Low calorie Low cholesterol Low salt	No change	Roti, dal, vegetables, milk, fruits	Food rich in cholesterol and salt like cheese butter, egg yolk pickles, chutneys, papads, sauces
Jaundice	Starts wilh liquids slowly go to a normal diet	Low fat	Small frequent meals at 1–2 hrs, intervals	Roti, vegetable, dal, skimmed milk, fruit, sugar	Fried food-puri, pakoda, samosa
Constipation	No change	High fiber drink lots of water	No change	Atta with husk, whole pulses green leafy vegetables, guava	Refined foods like suji, rice, candies, bread, maida

BIBLIOGRAPHY

1. https://cpch.in/Course%20Module/BNS-041%20Foundations%20of%20Community%20health%20-%20%20Block-2.pdf
2. https://www.nios.ac.in/media/documents/srsec321newE/321-E-Lesson-5.pdf
3. https://www.who.int/news-room/fact-sheets/detail/healthy-diet

4.4 PURPOSE, PRINCIPLES AND METHODS OF NUTRITION EDUCATION

- Nutrition education must provide adequate information, skills and motivation to procure and to consume appropriate diets.
- It also ensures efficient utilization of available food and economic resources to provide nutritious diets and better care for the most vulnerable groups.
- Nutrition education should be directed to proper food selection, consumption and lifestyle to affluent people as well.
- Nutrition education programs should include at least following three components:
  1. Increasing the nutrition knowledge and awareness of the public and of policy-makers
  2. Promoting desirable food behavior and nutritional practices
  3. Increasing the diversity and quantity of family food supplies
- **Increasing the nutrition knowledge and awareness of the public and of policy-makers:** This can be achieved by providing information on:
  - Relationship between diet and health
  - Relationship between nutritional and health status and individual productivity and national development
  - Nutritional needs of the population and of individuals
  - Importance of ensuring the quality and safety of the food supply
  - Causes and consequences of nutritional disorders
  - Benefits of food labelling and legislation.
- **Promoting desirable food behavior and nutritional practices:** This can be achieved by providing information on:
  - Nutritional value of foods
  - Components of an adequate diet
  - Making appropriate food choices and purchases from available resources
  - Hygienic food preparation and handling of food
  - Storage, processing and preservation of food and
  - Equitable intrahousehold food distribution according to the nutritional needs of family members.
- **Increasing the diversity and quantity of family food supplies:** This can be achieved by providing information on:
  - Methods of improving food production
  - Crop selection and diversification
  - Proper storage, preservation and processing
  - Conservation of nutrients during food preparation and
  - Prevention of food waste.

Goal and Purposes of Nutrition Education

- To create positive attitudes toward good nutrition and physical activity and provide motivation for improved nutrition and lifestyle practices conducive to promoting and maintaining the best attainable level of wellness for an individual.
- To provide adequate knowledge and skills necessary for critical thinking regarding diet and health so the individual can make healthy food choices from an increasingly complex food supply.

- To assist the individual to identify resources for continuing access to sound food and nutrition information.
- Consumer issues, including the management of food purchasing power to obtain maximum food value for the money spent.
- Information on physical activity.
- Information on the roles of nutrition and physical activity in maintaining health and independence, and preventing or managing chronic diseases such as diabetes, heart disease, high blood pressure, osteoporosis, and arthritis.
- Nutrition education provides people with correct information on the nutritional value of foods, food quality and safety, methods of preservation, processing and handling, food preparation and eating to help them make the best choice of foods for an adequate diet.

Successful Nutrition Education Often Entails

- Active participation of the people, their awareness of their nutrition problems and their willingness to change
- Intersectoral collaboration
- Well-planned communication strategy
- Strong political and government support
- External funding
- The strengthening of local managerial and community capacities.

Nutrition Education Approaches

Conventional Approach

- Conventional strategies use didactic methods of education and one-way transfer of information. Common examples of this approach are telling mothers to eat more green vegetables or to breastfeed their children.
- This approach usually less effective because:
  - It uses only one channel of communication (i.e., face-to-face)
  - It addresses mainly women but their husbands and other family members often influence decisions regarding food purchasing and food allocations within the family
  - It focuses on the promotion of individual behavior change rather than active community participation
  - It pays little attention to people's social and cultural context.

Current Approaches

Social Marketing Approach

- Social marketing is defined as the promotion of socially responsible products, behavior and ideas. It is based on strategies to change human behavior through the application of commercial marketing principles.
- An important part of the strategy is audience segmentation. Instead of addressing an audience as a single unit, social marketing specialists divide a community into various groups with similar interests in relation to the behavior under consideration.
- There is combined use of interpersonal communication and mass media (radio, television and the printed press).

- Then development and pre-testing followed by monitoring and evaluation is very essential step of this approach.
- This approach has been successful in childhood immunization, breastfeeding and the use of oral rehydration solution.
- However, social marketing also has limitations, as reliance on mass media has not always led to sustained behavioral changes.

Community-based Approach

- It is increasingly recognized that unless people are offered the opportunity to participate actively in seeking solutions for their nutritional problems, the long-term impact of an intervention will be marginal.
- The community-based approach to nutrition education, which encompasses the best elements of the two approaches, emphasizes the importance of active community participation in making decisions and finding solutions for nutritional problems.
- With a strong participatory approach, the nutrition educator acts as a facilitator who assists the community in identifying and examining the factors that influence malnutrition and helps people to suggest solutions and implement actions to overcome nutritional problems.
- In the community-based approach the communication strategy involves face-to-face group interaction between the nutrition educators and the community members, yet learning is not restricted to the moment of delivery of the message; it also takes place in the context of many other activities. The involvement of the community members with nutrition educators in planning and carrying out these activities is an important part of the learning process. An example would be a feeding program to care for children while a group of mothers engage in income-generating activities such as production of vegetables or other foods to sell or consume.
- Nutrition education needs to be comprehensive and coordinated for effectiveness, to be participatory and to encourage ownership by the community.

Planning a Community Nutrition Education Program (Fig. 4.2)

- Nutrition education is effective only when it is based on adequate analysis of the nutritional problems and clear and concise definition of the objectives and the methods of communications.
- Nutrition education program should ideally be developed by a multidisciplinary team consisting of a nutrition educator, a communication specialist, a community leader and representatives of the beneficiary groups. It also requires collaboration among non-governmental organizations (NGOs), government ministries and institutions, the private sector and external assistance agencies.
- Planning and developing a nutrition education program should begin with the systematic

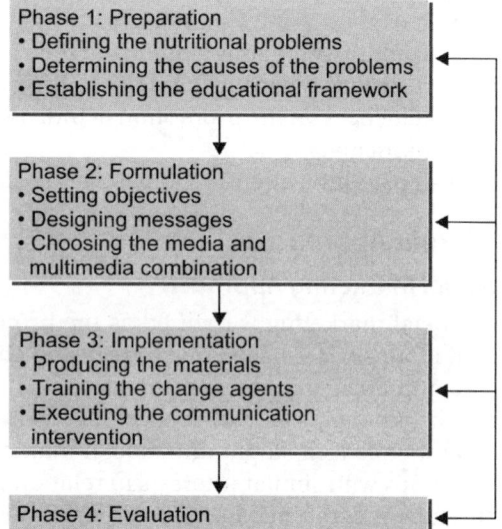

Fig. 4.2: A schema for planning nutrition education programs.

analysis of nutrition and health-related problems in a community. Methods for situation analysis methods include literature review, nutrition surveys and participatory nutrition appraisal.
- Once the factors and behavior patterns on which action needs to be taken have been identified and discussed with the community, the next step is to formulate an action plan and a communication strategy.
- To plan a strategy, it is necessary to define clear objectives.
- The nutrition education team determines the goals and objectives of a communication campaign, which should be defined for each group of beneficiaries. During this stage messages are designed, materials are field tested, and the media are selected.
- A multimedia plan is formulated in which all communication activities are integrated.
- Once the materials and training have been established and ensured, communication with the people can begin.
- The evaluation should be conducted with the participation of the beneficiary population and the field workers or change agents, as the actions to be evaluated concern them directly and the evaluation may help them improve their performance. Government representatives should also participate so they can see the impact of the activities they have promoted and consider further expansion of the program.

Beneficiary Groups for Nutrition Education

- The primary group: whose behavior is to be modified
- The secondary group: who acts as intermediaries and they deliver the message to the first group, such as health workers, nutritionists, horticulturists, agricultural extension officers, teachers, broadcasters and journalists.
- The tertiary group: who can help to make the program a success through their influence and authority. These may include community leaders, financial donors and politicians, together with members of the extended family of the at-risk child.

BIBLIOGRAPHY

1. https://wcd.nic.in/sites/default/files/integrated%20nutrition%20education-%20a%20handbook.pdf
2. https://egyankosh.ac.in/bitstream/123456789/44241/1/Unit-20.pdf
3. https://www.fao.org/3/w0078e/w0078e10.htm

4.5 OVERVIEW OF COMMON NUTRITIONAL DISORDERS IN INDIA

PROTEIN-ENERGY MALNUTRITION (PEM)

- It is caused by inadequate intake of the macronutrients (energy and protein).
- It is assessed by evaluating the anthropometric measurements (weight, height, head and chest circumference, etc.).
- Nutritional status of children of under 5 years of age at national level:

Indicator	NFHS-4	NFHS-5
Stunting	38.4%	35.5%
Wasting	21.0%	19.3%
Severely wasted	7.5%	7.7%
Overweight	2.1%	3.4%

Micronutrient Deficiencies

- If energy and protein intake is not sufficient then its very likely that intake of micronutrients viz. minerals and vitamins will not be sufficient.
- Micronutrient deficiency is also known as "hidden hunger".
- Description of common micronutrient deficiencies are here.

Iron-deficiency Anemia (IDA)

- It is the most common nutritional disorder globally.
- Women in child-bearing age, adolescent girls, pregnant women and school age children are the most vulnerable groups.
- Current status of anemia at National level:

Age group	NFHS-4	NFHS-5
Children (6-59 months) (Hb <11.0 g/dL)	58.6%	67.1%
Non-pregnant women (15–49 years) (Hb <12.0 g/dL)	53.2%	57.2%
Pregnant women (Hb <11.0 g/dL)	50.4%	52.2%
Girls (15–19 years) (Hb <13.0 g/dL)	54.1%	59.1%
Boys (15–19 years) (Hb <13.0 g/dL)	29.2%	31.1%

Note: More details of IDA is given in Ch. 4.7.5.

Vitamin A Deficiency (VAD)

- Vitamin A is necessary for maintenance of healthy epithelium, normal vision, growth and immunity.
- Deficiency of vitamin A results in night blindness which progresses to complete blindness if corrective measures are not taken.
- Details provided in Chapter 4.8.6.

Iodine Deficiency Disorders (IDD)

- Iodine is required for normal mental and physical growth and development.
- IDD is an ecological phenomenon, largely due to deficiency of iodine in the soil.
- Some of the states in India where IDD is common are—Jammu and Kashmir to Arunachal Pradesh in the Himalayan belt, Andhra Pradesh, Karnataka, Kerala, Maharashtra and Madhya Pradesh.
- The term 'Iodine Deficiency Disorders' refers to a spectrum of disabling conditions that affect the health of humans, from fetal life through adulthood due to inadequate dietary intake of iodine.
- Deficiency of iodine results in insufficient amount of thyroid hormone which is synthesized by the thyroid gland.

Government of India is implementing various schemes and programs to prevent malnutrition which are as follows:

- Infant and Young Child Feeding (IYCF) practices: for early initiation of breastfeeding, exclusive breastfeeding till 6 months of age and timely introduction of complementary feeding.
- "MAA-Mothers' Absolute Affection" program: to promote and support breastfeeding.
- Vitamin A supplementation (VAS) for children till the age of 5 years.
- "Intensified National Iron Plus Initiative or Anemia Mukt Bharat" has been launched as an effective strategy for supplementation and treatment of anemia in children, adolescents, pregnant and lactating women.
- National Deworming Day is a fixed day strategy to administer Albendazole tablets to all the children in the age group of 1–19 years through the platform of AWCs and Schools.
- Intensified Diarrhea Control Fortnight (IDCF): To increase awareness about the use of ORS and Zinc in diarrhoea with the ultimate aim of 'zero child deaths due to childhood diarrhea'.
- Incentives are provided to ASHA for tracking of low birth weight babies.
- Promotion for intake of iodized salt and monitoring salt quality through testing under National Iodine Deficiency Disorders Control Program.
- Under the Rashtriya Bal Swasthya Karyakram (RBSK), systematic efforts are undertaken to detect nutrition deficiency among children and adolescents respectively.
- Mission Indradhanush: Launched on 25th December, 2014 with the objective to ensure high coverage of children with all vaccines in identified districts with the goal of reaching the unreached to achieve 90% full immunization coverage in India. Now it is called as Intensified Mission Indradhanush 4.0.
- Rashtriya Bal Swasthya Karyakram (RBSK) provides child health screening for 30 common health conditions by expanding the reach of mobile health teams at block level and establishment of district early intervention centres (DEICs) at the districts for early interventions services.
- Village Health and Nutrition Days and Mother and Child Protection Card are the joint initiative of the Ministry of Health and Family welfare and the Ministry of Woman and Child Development for addressing the nutrition concerns in children, pregnant women and lactating mothers.
- Under Umbrella ICDS scheme of MWCD Supplementary Nutrition Program for addressing under-nutrition in pregnant and lactating women, under-6 children and out-of-school adolescent girls.
- National Nutrition Mission under MWCD for addressing malnutrition status of the country in a comprehensive manner.

BIBLIOGRAPHY

1. https://ncert.nic.in/textbook/pdf/lehe103.pdf
2. https://www.nhp.gov.in/healthlyliving/healthy-nutrition

4.6 NATIONAL NUTRITIONAL POLICY 1993

INTRODUCTION

- Malnutrition includes both overnutrition and undernutrition. We as country having both issues but still undernutrition is bigger scourge.
- Undernutrition results from inadequate intake of food or more essential nutrient(s) resulting in deterioration of physical growth and health.
- Undernutrition results in:
  - Reduces work capacity and productivity amongst adults
  - Enhances mortality and morbidity amongst children.
  - Reduced earning capacity, leading to further poverty, and the vicious cycle goes on as shown in **Figure 4.3**.

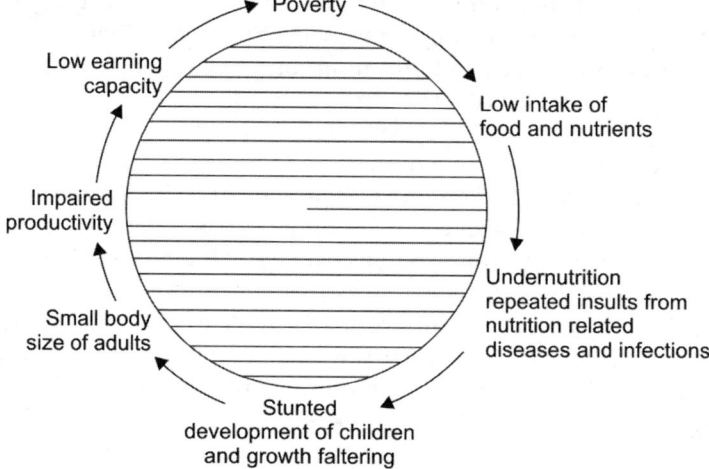

Fig. 4.3: Vicious cycle of poverty-malnutrition.

The major nutrition problems of India can be classified as follows:
- Undernutrition resulting in:
  - Protein energy malnutrition (PEM)
  - Iron deficiency
  - Iodine deficiency
  - Vitamin "A" deficiency
  - Low birth weight
- Seasonal dimensions of nutrition
- Natural calamities and the landless
- Market distortion and disinformation
- Urbanization
- Special nutritional problems of industrial workers, migrant workers, and other special categories
- Problems of overnutrition, overweight and obesity.

Key Findings of NFHS-5
- Stunting (low height-for-age) has declined from 38% to 36%
- Wasting (low weight-for-height) has declined from 21% to 19%
- Underweight (low weight-for-age) has declined from 36% to 32%
- Anemia has increased from 58.6 to 67% in under-5 children, from 53.1 to 57% in women and from 22.7 to 25% in men.
- Prevalence of overweight or obesity is 24% among women and 23% among men.

NUTRITION POLICY INSTRUMENTS

Strategy
Nutrition is a multi-sectoral issue and needs to be tackled at various levels. Nutrition affects development as much as development affects nutrition. It is therefore important to tackle the problem of nutrition both through direct nutrition intervention for specially vulnerable groups as well as through various development policy instruments which will create conditions for improved nutrition.

Direct Intervention: Short Term
- Nutrition intervention for especially vulnerable groups
- Fortification of essential foods
- Popularization of low-cost nutritious food
- Control of micronutrient deficiencies amongst vulnerable groups.

Indirect Policy Instruments: Long Term
- Food security
- Improvement of dietary pattern through production and demonstration
- Policies for effecting income transfers so as to improve the entitlement package of the rural and urban poor
- Land reforms
- Health and family welfare
- Basic health and nutrition knowledge
- Prevention of food adulteration
- Nutrition surveillance
- Monitoring of nutrition programs
- Research
- Equal remuneration
- Communication
- Minimum wage administration
- Community participation
- Education and literacy
- Improvement of the status of women

BIBLIOGRAPHY
1. https://wcd.nic.in/sites/default/files/National%20Nutrition%20Policy_0.pdf

4.7 DIFFERENT NATIONAL HEALTH PROGRAMS RELATED TO NUTRITION

4.7.1 POSHAN ABHIYAAN AND MISSION POSHAN 2.0

- **POSHAN:** Prime Minister's Overarching Scheme for Holistic Nutrition
- Earlier known as National Nutrition Mission.
- Poshan Abhiyaan (National Nutrition Mission) is India's flagship program to improve nutritional outcomes for children, pregnant women and lactating mothers through use of technology, a targeted approach and convergence, strives to reduce the level of stunting, undernutrition, anemia and low birth weight in children, as also, focus on adolescent girls, pregnant women and lactating mothers, thus holistically addressing malnutrition.

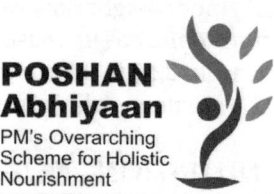

- Launched on 8th March 2018
- NNM is based on lifecycle approach, by adopting a synergized and result oriented approach.
- The NNM is set to work as governing body to monitor all various nutrition related programs and schemes across the other departments and ministries.
- Mapping of various nutrition related schemes will be done.
- Convergence of all the activities at grass root level.
- Strong monitoring
- Incentivizing States/UTs for better performing in terms of achieving targets and Anganwadi Workers (AWWs) also will be given incentives for using information technology in their routine work.
- Well-researched, designed and tested communication plan and IEC materials have been developed and intensive mass media campaign is conducted through various mass media channels like radio, television and social media.

Expected Impact

Reduction in the level of stunting, undernutrition, anemia and low birth weight.

Objectives and Targets

S. No.	Objective	Target
1.	Prevent and reduce Stunting in children (0–6 years)	@ 2% pa
2.	Prevent and reduce undernutrition (underweight prevalence) in children (0–6 years)	@ 2% pa
3.	Reduce the prevalence of anemia among young Children (6–59 months)	@ 3% pa
4.	Reduce the prevalence of anemia among Women and Adolescent Girls in the age group of 15–49 years	@ 3% pa
5.	Reduce low birth weight (LBW)	@ 2% p.a.

Note: Although the target to reduce Stunting is at least 2% pa, Mission would strive to achieve reduction in Stunting from 38.4% (NFHS-4) to 25% by 2022 (Mission 25 by 2022).

Mission Poshan 2.0

- Mission Poshan 2.0 is an Integrated Nutrition Support Program.
- It seeks to address the challenges of malnutrition through a strategic shift in nutrition content and delivery, by creation of a convergent eco-system to develop and promote practices that nurture health, wellness and immunity.

- Poshan 2.0 will seek to optimize the quality and delivery of food under the Supplementary Nutrition Program.
- Mission Poshan 2.0 will contribute to human capital development of the country; address malnutrition challenges; promote nutrition awareness and good eating habits for sustainable health and well-being and address nutrition related deficiencies through key strategies.
- Under the program, nutritional norms and standards, quality and testing of take home ration (THR) will be improved and greater stakeholder and beneficiary participation will be promoted besides traditional community food habits.
- Poshan 2.0 will bring 3 important programs/schemes under its ambit, viz., Anganwadi Services, Scheme for Adolescent Girls and Poshan Abhiyaan.
- Poshan 2.0 shall focus on Maternal Nutrition, Infant and Young Child Feeding Norms, treatment of MAM (Moderate Acute Malnourished)/SAM (Severe Acute Malnourished) and wellness through AYUSH.
- It will rest on the pillars of convergence, governance, and capacity-building.
- Poshan Abhiyan will be the key pillar for Outreach and will cover innovations related to nutritional support, ICT interventions, media advocacy and research, community outreach and Jan Andolan.
- Mission Poshan 2.0 will integrate several key strategies to fulfil its objectives, viz., corrective strategies, nutrition awareness strategies, communication strategies and creation of green ecosystems.
- Digital infrastructure under the "Poshan Tracker" will strengthen and bring about transparency in nutrition delivery support systems. Technology under Poshan Tracker is being leveraged for (i) dynamic identification of stunting, wasting, underweight prevalence among children; (ii) last mile tracking of nutrition service delivery. 'Poshan Tracker' is being linked with the RCH Portal (Anmol) of MoHFW.

The Objectives of POSHAN 2.0
- To contribute to human capital development of the country
- Address challenges of malnutrition
- Promote nutrition awareness and good eating habits for sustainable health and well being
- Address nutrition related deficiencies through key strategies.

Poshan Maah
- Month of September is celebrated as Poshan Maah since 2018.
- It includes a month-long activities focussed on antenatal care, optimal breastfeeding, Anemia, growth monitoring, girls education, diet, right age of marriage, hygiene and sanitation and eating healthy (Food Fortification).
- Similarly, in/around March every year, Poshan Pakhwada is celebrated.

POSHAN Vatika
For leveraging convergence for food and nutrition, Poshan Vatikas (kitchen gardens and nutri-gardens) shall be set up at or near Anganwadi Centers, wherever possible and in Government led schools and Gram Panchayat lands where benefits can easily be provided to women and children.

BIBLIOGRAPHY

1. http://icds-wcd.nic.in/nnm/NNM-Web-Contents/LEFT-MENU/Circulars/Rename_NNM_POSHAN_Abhiyaan.pdf
2. https://pib.gov.in/PressReleasePage.aspx?PRID=1794595
3. https://www.drishtiias.com/daily-updates/daily-news-analysis/poshan-2-0
4. https://wcd.nic.in/sites/default/files/Final%20Saksham%20Guidelines%20with%20covering%20letter%20%281%29.pdf

4.7.2 PRADHAN MANTRI MATRU VANDANA YOJANA (PMMVY)

- **Ministry:** Women and Child Development
  - **Launched date:** 01.01.2017
  - Initially this scheme was launched as Indira Gandhi Matritva Sahyog Yojana (IGMSY)—a Conditional Maternity Benefit Scheme in 2010–2011.
  - It is centrally sponsored scheme.

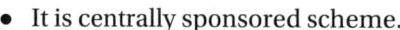

- **Objectives**
  - To improve the health and nutrition status of pregnant and lactating women and their young infants thus provide partial compensation for the wage loss so that the woman is not under compulsion to work till the last stage of pregnancy and can take adequate rest before and after delivery.
  - To improve health seeking behavior amongst the pregnant women and lactating mothers.
- **Beneficiaries**
  - Under PMMVY, a cash incentive of Rs. 50,00*/- is provided directly to the Bank/Post Office Account of Pregnant Women and Lactating mothers for **first living child** of the family subject to fulfilling specific conditions relating to Maternal and child health.
  - Women who are either employee of state/central government or receiving benefits of any such other scheme would not be eligible for the PMMVY.
  - Private hospitals directly cannot avail the benefit of the scheme. However, if the requisite conditions are duly certified by a government doctor or officer/functionary of the Health Department not below the rank of ANM, the beneficiary can claim maternity benefit under PMMVY.
- **Benefits under the Scheme:**

Instalment	Conditions	Documents required	Amount (in ₹)
First instalment	• Register her pregnancy in the MCP card along with required documents within 150 days from LMP.	• Duly filled Application Form 1A • Copy of MCP Card • Copy of Identity Proof • Copy of Bank/Post Office Account Passbook	₹ 1,000
Second instalment	• At least one antenatal check-up • Can be claimed post 180 days of Pregnancy	• Duly filled Application Form 1 B • Copy of MCP Card	₹ 2,000

*Additional Rs 1,000 given if child birth takes place at hospital and mother is beneficiary of JSY scheme.

Instalment	Conditions	Documents required	Amount (in ₹)
Third instalment	• Child birth is registered • Child has received first cycle of immunizations of Hepatitis B birth dose, BCG, OPV (0 and 1,2 and 3, DPT and Hepatitis B or Pentavalent 1,2 and 3. • Aadhaar is mandatory in all states except for J and K, Assam, Meghalaya	• Duly filled Application Form 1C • Copy of MCP Card • Copy of Aadhaar ID • Copy of child birth registration certificate	₹ 2,000

- In Gujarat State, there is one more similar scheme known as Kasturba Poshan Sahay Yojna (KPSY), in which Rs 6,000 is given to the beneficiaries when they fulfilled almost same criteria which are applicable in PMMVY. As they are similar schemes, benefit of both schemes would not be given and so, at the time of first child, 5,000 Rs from PMMVY and 1,000 Rs from KPSY will be given to all BPL families while for Non-BPL families at the time of first child, benefits of only PMMVY as Rs 5,000 will be given. Benefits of KPSY will continue to only BPL families as Rs 6000 for second and third child birth.
- Pradhan Mantri Matru Vandana Yojana Common Application Software (PMMVY-CAS) is used to maintain all the details of the beneficiaries and for DBT as well.

BIBLIOGRAPHY

1. https://wcd.nic.in/schemes/pradhan-mantri-matru-vandana-yojana
2. https://wcd.nic.in/sites/default/files/PMMVY%20Scheme%20Implementati n%20Guidelines%20-%20 MWCD%20%281%29_0.pdf

4.7.3 INTEGRATED CHILD DEVELOPMENT SERVICES SCHEME (ICDS)

- Integrated Child Development Services (ICDS) Scheme launched on 2nd October, 1975 as one of the flagship programs of the Government of India under the Ministry of Women and Child Development (MOWCD) **(Table 4.2)**.
- It is one of the world's largest and unique programs for early childhood care and development.
- It is the symbol of country's commitment to its children and nursing mothers, as providing pre-school non-formal education on one hand and breaking the vicious cycle of malnutrition, morbidity, reduced learning capacity and mortality on the other.
- **The beneficiaries under the scheme are**:
  - Children in the age group of 0–6 years
  - Pregnant women
  - Lactating mothers
  - Adolescent girls

Objectives

- To improve the nutritional and health status of children in the age-group 0–6 years;
- To lay the foundation for proper psychological, physical and social development of the child;
- To reduce the incidence of mortality, morbidity, malnutrition and school dropout;
- To achieve effective coordination of policy and implementation amongst the various departments to promote child development; and
- To enhance the capability of the mother to look after the normal health and nutritional needs of the child through proper nutrition and health education.

Table 4.2: Details about services along with target group and service providers.

Services	Target group	Service provided by
• Supplementary Nutrition	Children below 6 years, Pregnant and Lactating Mothers (P and LM)	Anganwadi Worker and Anganwadi Helper [MWCD]
• Immunization*	Children below 6 years, Pregnant and Lactating Mothers (P and LM)	ANM/MO [MOHFW]
• Health Check-up*	Children below 6 years, Pregnant and Lactating Mothers (P and LM)	ANM/MO/AWW [MOHFW]
• Referral Services	Children below 6 years, Pregnant and Lactating Mothers (P and LM)	AWW/ANM/MO [MOHFW]
• Pre-School Education	Children 3–6 years	AWW [MWCD]
• Nutrition and Health Education	Women (15–45 years)	AWW/ANM/MO [MOHFW and MWCD]

* AWW assists ANM in identifying the target group.

ICDS Team

- The ICDS team comprises the Anganwadi Workers, Anganwadi Helpers, Supervisors (Mukhyasevika), Child Development Project Officers (CDPOs) and District Program Officers (DPOs).
- Anganwadi Worker, selected from the local community, honorary worker of the ICDS Program. She is also an agent of social change, mobilizing community support for better care of young children, girls and women.
- Besides, the medical officers, Auxiliary Nurse Midwife (ANM) and Accredited Social Health Activist (ASHA) form a team with the ICDS functionaries to achieve convergence of different services.

Revised Nutritional Norms in ICDS

Beneficiaries	Calories	Protein (g)
Children (6 months to 72 months) In case of 6 months to 3 years as part of take home ration while for 3 to 6 years as part of morning snacks and hot cooked meal.	500	12–15
Severely malnourished children (SAM) (6 months–72 months)	800	20–25
Pregnant women and lactating mothers	600	18–20

Example of take home ration (THR) in Gujarat state is given below **(Fig. 4.4)**.

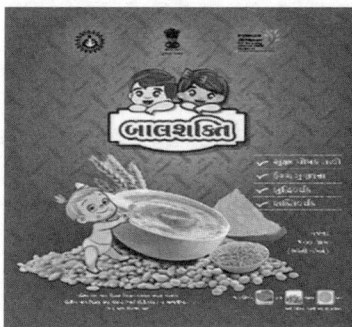 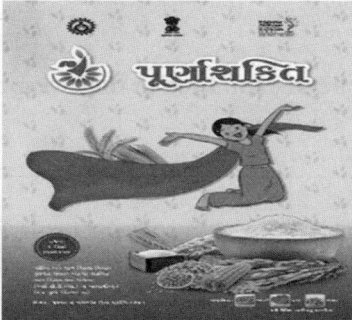 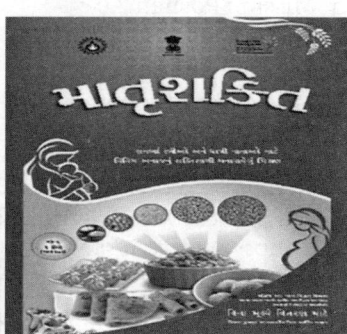

Fig. 4.4: THR packets and packging.

Packging and Quantity of Take Home Ration

Sr. No.	Type of beneficiaries	Quantity per day (gm)	Quantity per month (kg)	Nos of packets (500 gm each packet)
1.	6 M–3Y of normal children	125	3.5	7 packets
2.	6 M–3Y of SUW children	185	5.0	10 packets
3.	3Y–6Y SUW children	72	2.0	4 packets
4.	Adolescent girls, pregnant and lactaing mothers	145	4.0	4 packets

Population Norms for Anganwadi

For AWCs in Rural/Urban project	
400–800	1 AWC
800–1600	2 AWCs
1,600–2,400	3 AWCs
Thereafter in multiples of 800	1 AWC
For Mini-AWC	
150–400	1 Mini-AWC
For Tribal/Riverine/ Desert, Hilly and other difficult areas/projects	
300–800	1 AWC
For Mini-AWC	
150–300	1 Mini-AWC

Major Schemes of MOWCD

- Anganwadi Services
- Pradhan Mantri Matru Vandana Yojana
- National Creche Scheme
- POSHAN Abhiyaan

- Scheme for Adolescent Girls
- Mission Poshan 2.0
- Mission Shakti
- Mission Vatsalya

Details of these schemes have been explained in their respective chapters.

BIBLIOGRAPHY

1. https://icds-wcd.nic.in/icds.aspx
2. https://wcd.nic.in/sites/default/files/AR%202017-18%20Chapter%203.pdf

4.7.4 INFANT AND YOUNG CHILD FEEDING (IYCF)

- WHO/UNICEF have emphasized the first 1,000 days of life, i.e., the 270 days in-utero and the first two years after birth as the critical window period for nutritional interventions.
- Infant and Young Child Feeding (IYCF) is a set of recommendations to achieve appropriate feeding of newborn and children under two years of age so that they achieve optimal nutrition outcomes.
- Core Recommendations under IYCF guidelines are:
  - **Initiating breastfeeding within one hour of birth**: Breastfeeding must be initiated for all normal newborns as early as possible after birth, ideally within first hour for vaginal delivery and within 4 hours for cesarean section. Colostrum, the milk secreted in the first 2–3 days, must not be discarded but should be fed to newborn as it contains high concentration of protective immunoglobulins and cells. No pre-lacteal fluid should be given to the newborn.

    The principles of feeding HIV exposed and infected infants are:
    - All HIV positive pregnant women should have PPTCT interventions provided from early stages of pregnancy, as far as possible. The interventions include either maternal or infant ARV prophylaxis for the duration of breastfeeding.
    - Exclusive breastfeeding is the recommended infant feeding choice for the first 6 months, irrespective of whether mother or infant is provided with ARV drugs for the duration of breastfeeding.
    - Mixed feeding should not be practiced.
    - Only in situations where breastfeeding cannot be done or on individual parents' informed decision, replacement feeding may be considered.
  - **Exclusive breastfeeding for the first six months of life:** It means an infant receives only breast milk from his or her mother or expressed breast milk, and no other liquids or solids, not even water. The only exceptions include administration of oral rehydration solution, oral vaccines, vitamins, minerals supplements or medicines. Exclusive breastfeeding prevents diarrhea like conditions.
  - **Initiation of appropriate complementary feeding from the age of 6 months:** It means complementing breast milk with introduction of solid/semi-solid food with after child attains age of six months. It should be timely, adequate and safe.

Nutrition Assessment and Nutrition Education

Meeting nutritional need as the child grows

	6 months up to 9 months	9 months up to 12 months	1 year up to 2 years	2 year up to 5 years
Food	Thick porridge; fruit and dark green vegetables, rich in vitamin A and iron and animal source foods (meat, fish, eggs, and curd or other dairy products)	Fruit and dark green vegetables, rich in vitamin A and iron; and animal source foods	Greater variety of fruit and dark green vegetables, rich in vitamin A and iron; and animal source foods	Greater variety of family foods, including fruit and dark green vegetables rich in vitamin A and iron and animal source foods
Quantity, how much at each meal	Start with 2–3 spoons increase to 1/2 katori of food	1/2 katori	3/4 katori	1 katori
Frequency, how often meals	2 to 3 meals each day	3 or 4 meals each day	3 or 4 meals each day	3 or 4 meals each day
Snacks	1 or 2 snacks	1 or 2 snacks	1 or 2 snacks	1 or 2 snacks
Consistency, how it is prepared for child to eat	Mashed, thicks consistency that stay on spoon	Mashed, or finely chopped; some chewable items that the child can hold	Mashed, or chopped; some items the child can hold	Prepared as the family eats (with own serving)

- Continued breastfeeding for two years or beyond.
- Mother should communicate, look into the eyes, touch and cares the baby while feeding. Practice responsive feeding.
- WHO Growth Charts recommended for monitoring growth.

Strategies to Promote IYCF

- Mother's Absolute Affection (MAA) Program
- IMS Act [Infant Milk Substitutes Feeding Bottles, and Infant Foods (Regulation of Production, Supply and Distribution) Act 1992, and Amendment Act 2003]
- VHND Days (ANM as main service provider while AWW, ASHA, LHV and ICDS supervisor as supportive role in strengthening IYCF practices).
- NRC
- HBNC (ASHA)

Benefits of Infant and Young Child Feeding (Figs. 4.5 and 4.6)

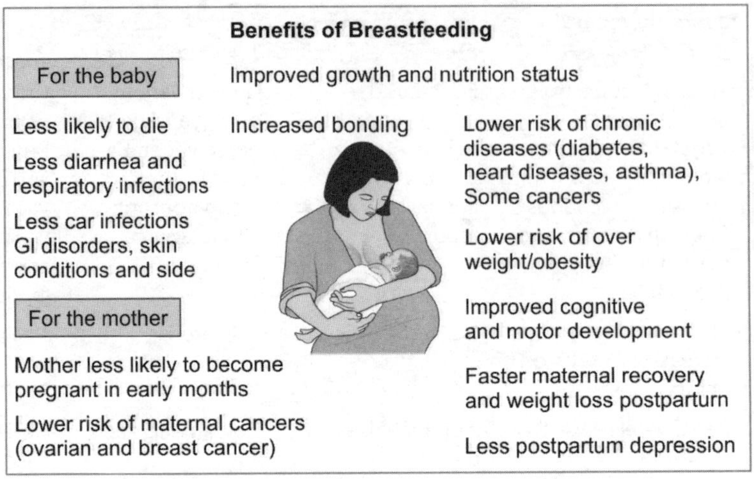

Benefits of Breastfeeding

For the baby:
- Improved growth and nutrition status
- Less likely to die
- Increased bonding
- Less diarrhea and respiratory infections
- Less car infections GI disorders, skin conditions and side
- Lower risk of chronic diseases (diabetes, heart diseases, asthma), Some cancers
- Lower risk of over weight/obesity
- Improved cognitive and motor development

For the mother:
- Mother less likely to become pregnant in early months
- Lower risk of maternal cancers (ovarian and breast cancer)
- Faster maternal recovery and weight loss postparturn
- Less postpartum depression

Fig. 4.5: Benefits of breastfeeding to baby and mother.

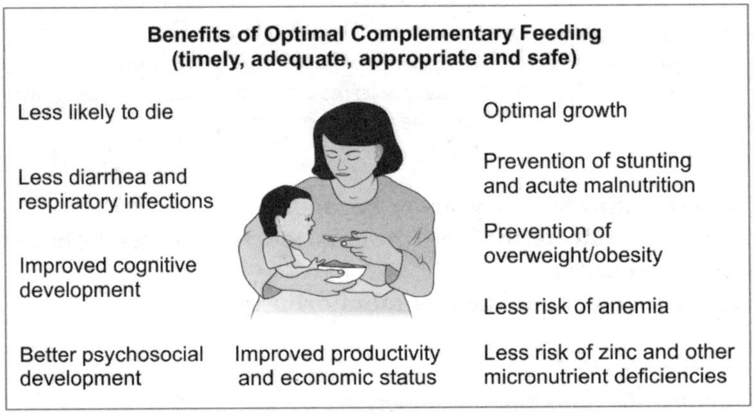

Benefits of Optimal Complementary Feeding (timely, adequate, appropriate and safe)

- Less likely to die
- Less diarrhea and respiratory infections
- Improved cognitive development
- Better psychosocial development
- Improved productivity and economic status
- Optimal growth
- Prevention of stunting and acute malnutrition
- Prevention of overweight/obesity
- Less risk of anemia
- Less risk of zinc and other micronutrient deficiencies

Fig. 4.6: Benefits of complementary feeding to baby.

BIBLIOGRAPHY

1. http://www.nrhmorissa.gov.in/writereaddata/Upload/Documents/Operational%20Guide%20IYCF.pdf
2. https://wcd.nic.in/sites/default/files/nationalguidelines.pdf
3. http://naco.gov.in/sites/default/files/Paedia%20Nutrition%20national%20guidelines%20NACO.pdf

4.7.5 ANEMIA MUKT BHARAT (I-NIPI)

- As per the NFHS-5 (2019–21), anemia among children aged 6–59 months was highest 67.1 percent **(Tables 4.3 and 4.4)**.
- Pregnant women aged 15–49 years, 52.2 percent were anemic.
- There is considerably high disparity of anemia prevalence among rural and urban areas.

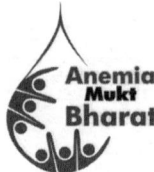

- It is also seen that disadvantaged groups (particularly scheduled tribes) and children and women in households in the lower wealth quintiles have higher prevalence of anemia.

Table 4.3: Hemoglobin levels to diagnose anemia (g/dL).

Population	Anemia		
	Mild	Moderate	Severe
Children 6–59 months of age	10–10.9	7–9.9	<7
Children 5–11 years of age	11–11.4	8–10.9	<8
Children 12–14 years of age	11–11.9	8–10.9	<8
Non-pregnant women (15 years of age and above)	11–11.9	8–10.9	<8
Pregnant women	10–10.9	7–9.9	<7
Men (15 years of age and above)	11–12.9	8–10.9	<8

Source: WHO–Nutrional Anemia: Tools for Effective Prevention and Control, 2017.

Table 4.4: Comparison of anemia prevalence for NFHS-4 and 5 (India).

Prevalence of anemia	NFHS-4	NFHS-5
Women (15–49 years)	53.1%	57%
Pregnant Women 1 (15–49 years)	50.4%	52.2%
Adolescent Women (15–19 years)	54.1%	59.1%
Children (6–59 months)	58.6%	67.1%
Adolescent boys (15–19 years)	29.2%	31.1%

- India's National Health Policy (2017) emphasizes on a need for intensifying efforts to address all causes of anemia for accelerating decline in anemia prevalence, in a mission mode using a unified multi-pronged strategy rather than multiple programs.
- Government of India has also made a commitment to Global World Health Assembly target of 50% reduction of anemia among women of reproductive age by 2025 and the Poshan Abhiyaan (2018–2022) also sets ambitious target to reduce prevalence of anemia among children 6–59 months, adolescents and women of reproductive age 15–49 years by 3 percentage points per year.
- Apart from NIPI, there are other programs which are dealing with other causes of anemia (other than iron deficiency) like:
  - National Deworming Day (NDD) for deworming
  - National Vector-borne Disease Control Program (NVBDCP) for malaria and special efforts to reach out to populations affected with hemoglobinopathies
  - National Program for Prevention and Control of Fluorosis.
- Simultaneously, behavior change communication programs to promote the consumption of iron-rich foods along with vitamin C, adopting of sanitation-hygiene practices and promoting the consumption of iron folic acid fortified foods are also carried out.

Nutrition Assessment and Nutrition Education

❏ In this context, based on the technical and operational evidence from National Iron Plus Initiative (NIPI) and Weekly Iron and Folic Acid (WIFS) programs, the Anemia Mukt Bharat [Intensified National Iron Plus Initiative (I-NIPI)] strategy has been designed.

❏ **Milestones of Anemia Control Program:**
   - There is mechanism of giving rank to the states on the basis of AMB score.
   - Anemia Mukt Bharat strategy providing preventive and curative mechanisms through a 6 × 6 × 6 strategy including **(Fig. 4.7)**:
     ▪ **6 target beneficiaries**
     ▪ **6 interventions**
     ▪ **6 institutional mechanisms.**

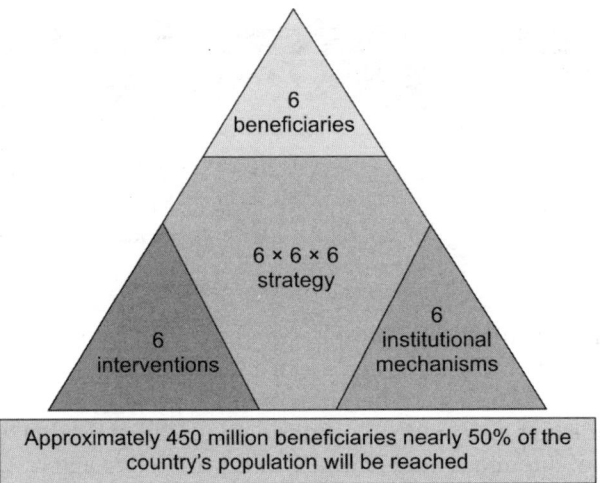

Fig. 4.7: 6 × 6 × 6 strategy of Anemia Mukt Bharat.

The strategy also included newer initiatives such as use of advanced methods of hemoglobin estimations like digital hemoglobinometers, and point of care management of anemia among in-school adolescents and pregnant women.

Six Target Beneficiaries
1. Children (6–59 months)
2. Adolescent girls (15–19 years)
3. Adolescent boys (15–19 years)
4. Women of reproductive age
5. Pregnant women
6. Lactating women

Six Interventions

1. **Prophylactic iron and folic acid supplementation (Table 4.5):**

Table 4.5: Prophylactic dose and regime for iron folic acid supplementation.

Age group	Dose and regime
Children 6–59 months of age	Biweekly, 1 mL iron and folic acid syrup Each mL of iron and folic acid syrup containing 20 mg elemental Iron + 100 mcg of folic acid Bottle (50 mL) to have an auto-dispenser and information leaflet as per MoHFW guidelines in the mono-carton (see Note 1)
Children 5–9 years of age	Weekly, 1 iron and folic acid tablet Each tablet containing 45 mg elemental Iron + 400 mcg folic acid, sugar-coated, pink color
School-going adolescent girls and boys, 10–19 years of age Out-of-school adolescent girls, 10–19 years of age	Weekly, 1 iron and folic acid tablet Each tablet containing 60 mg elemental iron + 500 mcg folic Acid, sugar-coated, blue color (See Note 2)
Women of reproductive age (non-pregnant, non-lactating) 20–49 years	Weekly, 1 iron and folic acid tablet Each tablet containing 60 mg elemental iron + 500 mcg folic acid, sugar-coated, red color (See Note 2)
Pregnant women and lactating mothers of 0–6 months child	Daily, 1 iron and folic acid tablet starting from the fourth month of pregnancy (that is from the second trimester), continued throughout pregnancy (minimum 180 days during pregnancy) and to be continued for 180 days, postpartum Each tablet containing 60 mg elemental iron + 500 mcg folic acid sugar-coated, red color

Note 1: Prophylaxis with iron should be withheld in case of acute illness (fever, diarrhoea, pneumnia, etc.), and in a known case of thalassemia major/history of repeated blood transfusion. In case of SAM children, IFA supplementation should be continued as per SAM management protocol.

Note 2: All women in the reproductive age group in the pre-conception period and up to the first trimester of the pregnancy are advised to have 400 mcg of Folic Acid tablets, daily, to reduce the incidence of neural tube defects in the fetus.

2. **Deworming:** Albendazole (400 mg) biannually ½ tablet to children 12-24 months and 1 tablet to children 24–59 months. Other age group receive 1 tablet biannually and pregnant women in the second trimester.

3. **Intensified year-round behavior change communication campaign** (Solid Body, Smart Mind) focusing on four key behaviours:
    1. Improving compliance to iron folic acid supplementation and deworming
    2. Appropriate infant and young child feeding practices
    3. Increase in intake of iron-rich food through diet diversity/quantity/frequency and/or fortified foods with focus on harnessing locally available resources and
    4. Ensuring delayed cord clamping after delivery (by 3 minutes) in health facilities.

4. **Testing and treatment of anemia**, using digital methods and point of care treatment, with special focus on pregnant women and school-going adolescents.

Treatment of iron deficiency anemia among pregnant women

Hb level	First level of treatment	Follow-up and referral
10–10.9 g/dL (mild anemia)	Two tablets of Iron and Folic Acid tablet (60 mg elemental Iron and 500 mcg Folic Acid) daily, orally	• Every 2 months • 1 g/dL increase per month in Hb is expected. • Hemoglobin levels have come up to normal level, discontinue the treatment and continue with the prophylactic IFA dose
7–9.9 g/dL (moderate anemia)	Two tablets of Iron and Folic Acid tablet (60 mg elemental Iron and 500 mcg Folic Acid) daily, orally Parental iron (IV Iron Sucrose or FCM) may be considered as the first line of management in pregnant women who are detected to be anemic late in pregnancy or in whom compliance is likely to be low.	Follow-up every two months. If no improvement in hemoglobin (<1 g/dL increase) after two month of treatment, refer to First Referral Unit (FRU)/District Hospital (DH) where further investigations for cause of anemia and can be managed with IV Iron Sucrose/FCM
5.0–6.9 g/dL (severe anemia)	IV Iron Sucrose/Ferric Carboxy Maltose (FCM) will be administered by the medical officer	Follow-up will be on monthly basis. severely anemic pregnant women with hemoglobin less than 5 g/dL, immediate hospitalization irrespective of period of gestation where round-the-clock specialist care is available

5. Mandatory provision of **Iron and Folic Acid fortified** foods in government funded public health programs.
6. Intensifying awareness, screening and treatment of **non-nutritional causes of anemia** in endemic pockets, with special focus on malaria, hemoglobinopathies and fluorosis.

Six Institutional Mechanisms

1. Intraministerial Coordination
2. National Anemia Mukt Bharat Unit
3. National Centre of Excellence and Advanced Research on Anemia Control (NCEAR-A)
4. Convergence with other Ministries
5. Strengthening Supply Chain and Logistics
6. Anemia Mukt Bharat Dashboard and Digital Portal – One-Stop Shop on Anemia

BIBLIOGRAPHY

1. https://anemiamuktbharat.info/#/
2. https://anemiamuktbharat.info/home/institutional-mechanisms/
3. https://iasscore.in/data-story/data-story-anaemia

4.7.6 BASICS OF VITAMIN A AND NUTRITIONAL BLINDNESS

Introduction
- Vitamin A is a fat-soluble vitamin.
- It is essential for growth and differentiation of cells like retina (vision pigment), respiratory epithelium lining, gastrointestinal tract and immune system **(Fig. 4.8)**.
- Vitamin A is found in two forms—retinol and carotenes.
- Sources of retinol form: Milk, liver and egg
- Sources of beta carotene form: Green leafy vegetables, carrot, yellow fruits.
- Richest source of vitamin a is halibut fish liver oil.
- RDA of Vitamin A is:
  - Men: 1000 µg/d;
  - Women: 840 µg/d;
  - Pregnant women: 900 µg/d;
  - Lactating women: 950 µg/d;
  - Infants (0–12m): 350 µg/d;
  - Children (1–3 y): 390 µg/d; (4–6 y): 510 µg/d

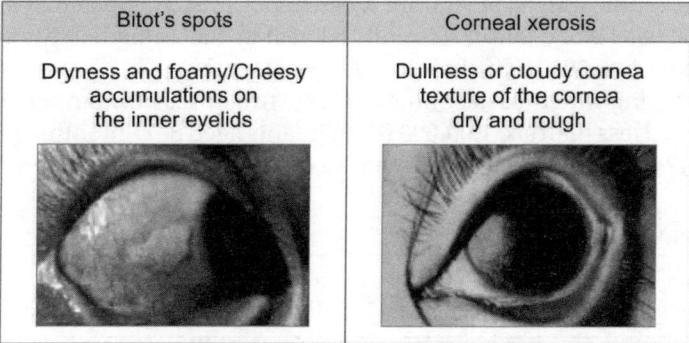

Fig. 4.8: Signs of vitamin A deficiency.

Classification of Xerophthalmia
- Night blindness (XN): First symptom
- Conjunctival xerosis (X1A): First sign
- Bitot spots (X1B)
- Corneal xerosis (X2)
- Corneal ulceration/keratomalacia < ⅓ corneal surface (X3A)
- Corneal ulceration/keratomalacia ≥ ⅓ corneal surface (X3B)
- Corneal scar (XS)
- Xerophthalmic fundus (XF)

Prevalence criteria for determining the public health significance of xerophthalmia and vitamin A deficiency in children aged 6 months to 6 years:

Indicator	Minimum prevalence, %
Night blindness (XN)	>1
Bitot spots (X1B)	>0.5
Corneal xerosis/corneal ulceration/keratomalacia (X2/X3A/X3B)	>0.01
Corneal scar (XS)	>0.05

Prophylactic Vitamin A as per the following Dosage Schedule
- 1,00,000 IU at 9 months with measles immunization
- 2,00,000 IU at 16–18 months, with DPT booster
- 2,00,000 IU every 6 months, up to the age of 5 years in total, 17 Lakh IU vitamin A to be given by 5 years of age [1 Lakh in first year of age and rest 16 Lakh (2 Lakh every 6 months so, 2 Lakh × 8 = 16 Lakh) in 1–5 years age]
  - Vitamin A bottle once opened should be consumed within 8 weeks.
  - Vitamin A also can be tried as fortified food.

Treatment of Vitamin A Deficiency
- All children with clinical signs of vitamin A deficiency must be treated as early as possible
- Administer 2,00,000 IU of vitamin A to child >1 year of age immediately after diagnosis
- To be followed by 2,00,000 IU of vitamin A 1–4 weeks later
- All children suffering with measles should receive two doses of vitamin A, one dose (50,000 IU for infants aged less than six, 1,00,000 IU for infants aged 6–11 months, and 2,00,000 IU for children aged 12 months) on the day of measles diagnosis and one dose on the following day.

BIBLIOGRAPHY
1. https://www.nin.res.in/RDA_short_Report_2020.html
2. https://www.aiims.edu/aiims/departments_17_5_16/ccm/vitamin%20A%20book-1.pdf

4.7.7 INTENSIFIED MISSION INDRADHANUSH 4.0
- The Universal Immunization Program (UIP) was launched in 1985 to protect children from vaccine-preventable diseases.
- Currently, the program caters to a birth cohort of around 2.6 crore infants and 2.9 crore pregnant women every year.
- The program provides protection against 12 life-threatening diseases including diphtheria, pertussis, tetanus, polio, tuberculosis, measles, rubella, hepatitis B, meningitis, rotavirus diarrhea and pneumococcal pneumonia at the national-level while Japanese encephalitis at the subnational level.
- A steady fall in the Infant Mortality Rate reflects Government of India's dedicated efforts under UIP to reduce child mortality and morbidity.
- The Full Immunization Coverage (FIC) among children aged 12–23 months of age has increased from 62% (NFHS-4) to 76.4% (NFHS-5).
- The Government of India is committed to improve immunization coverage and achieve full immunization coverage of 90 percent.

Nutrition Assessment and Nutrition Education

- In line with the commitment to improve immunization coverage and address equity issues, the flagship program Mission Indradhanush (MI) was launched in December 2014. The mission targeted unvaccinated and partially vaccinated children less than 2 years of age to reach >90% full immunization coverage and unvaccinated pregnant women.
- Intensified Mission Indradhanush (IMI) launched in October 2017 for reaching the drop-out and left-out children for immunization.
- Yet there are Challenges, like gaps in health systems, issues of inequities, awareness-gap among parents regarding immunization services, and the fear of side-effects of immunization.
- To boost the RI coverage in the country, Government introduced Intensified Mission Indradhanush 2.0 (IMI) to ensure reaching the unreached with all available vaccines and accelerate the coverage of children and pregnant women in the identified districts and blocks from December 2019-March 2020.
- IMI 3.0 was launched in 2021. Focus of the IMI 3.0 was the children and pregnant women who had missed their vaccine doses during the COVID-19 pandemic. There were two rounds.

IMI 4.0

- The achievements made in the past were offset by the COVID-19 pandemic, with an estimated 2.3 crore children under the age of 1 year left unvaccinated with basic vaccines and 1.7 crore have not received even their 1st dose of DTP vaccine globally. About 62% of those missed children are in ten countries, of which India ranks first, with the highest number of missed children. The DTP coverage in India dropped from 91% in 2019 to 85% in 2020.
- This coupled with other inequities in immunization based on wealth, education, urban-rural setting, etc., has further contributed to the immunization gap.
- As the COVID-19 pandemic has disrupted essential immunization services due to multiple reasons, the possibility of un/partially vaccinated children being exposed to the risk of vaccine-preventable diseases is very high. As the poorly vaccinated cohort increase in an area/pocket, there is a high risk of disease outbreaks.
- Thus, to catch up on gaps that might have emerged due to the pandemic, Intensified Mission Indradhanush 4.0 planned to reach out to unvaccinated and partially vaccinated children and pregnant women.
- The target beneficiaries for the mission are unvaccinated/partially vaccinated pregnant women and children up to 2 years of age.
- The available data utilized to for selection of the areas for IMI-4.0 in 2022 include:
  - Number of children not vaccinated with age-appropriate Penta-1, MCV-2 and fIPV-2 vaccine doses
  - Full Immunization coverage as per NFHS-5 survey
  - Reduction in number of RI sessions conducted
  - Incidence of Measles, Rubella and Diphtheria cases
  - Non-Measles Non-Rubella discard rate
  - Demographic risk factor (s)
- Based on the above criteria, districts have been identified where the number of missed children is high. Three rounds of intensified Mission Indradhanush have been conducted in the identified districts as per the following schedule:
  - Round 1: 7th February 2022 onwards
  - Round 2: 7th March 2022 onwards
  - Round 3: 4th April 2022 onwards
- Each round of IMI 4.0 will be spread over seven days may include RI days, Sundays, and public holidays.

Changes in IMI 4.0 from Previous IMI

- **Focus areas:** In addition to the focus on high-risk areas, this IMI will focus on areas where RI sessions were impacted due to COVID-19 pandemic and in the urban areas
- **Head count survey:** Will be conducted in the entire district that has been selected based on the parameters defined above. The HTH (House to House Survey) survey to be conducted during the upcoming Polio NID could be used in these districts for identifying children who may be missed out or left out. Sessions will be planned based on the number of missed children and pregnant women identified.
- **Session timings:** Flexible session timings will be followed. "On demand vaccination timings" in consultation with the community will ensure better turn-out of beneficiaries.

BIBLIOGRAPHY

1. https://imi2.nhp.gov.in/documents/operationalGuideline

4.7.8 INTENSIFIED DIARRHEA CONTROL FORTNIGHT

Problem Statement

- Childhood diarrheal diseases continue to be a major killer among under-five children in many states, contributing to 6.4 percent of under five deaths in the country.
- It means around 0.62 lakhs children die due to diarrhoea every year.
- Most of the Diarrheal deaths are clustered around summer and monsoon seasons and the worst affected are children from poor socio-economic situations.
- At the national level, ORS coverage improved from 50.6 percent (2015–16, NFHS 4) to 60.6 percent (2019–21 NFHS 5) and Zinc coverage from 20.3 percent (2005–06) to 30.5 percent (2015–16).
- However, the coverage of both ORS and Zinc need to reach the target of 90 percent by 2025 as per the India Action Plan for Pneumonia and Diarrhea (IAPPD).

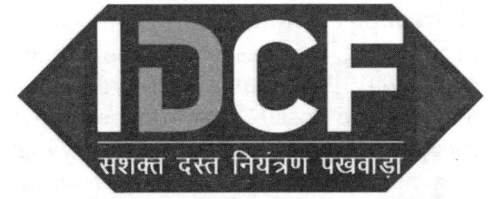

Current Available Interventions for Prevention and Control of Diarrhea

- ORS
- Zinc supplementation
- Immunization for the prevention (e.g., Rota vaccine)
- Breastfeeding
- Infant young child feeding practice (IYCF)
- Handwashing and Sanitation

IDCF

- IDCF launched in 2014 with aim of zero child death due to diarrhea.
- In view of the high prevalence of diarrhea, this fortnight is organized especially during summer/monsoon so that preventive measures can be taken.
- IDCF program was implemented from 13th June to 27th June, 2022.

Goal: Zero death due to childhood diarrhea.

Objectives

- To improve usage of ORS and Zinc for childhood diarrhea
- Facility level strengthening to manage cases of dehydration
- To complement awareness activities (including Swachh) for the prevention of management of diarrhea in <5 years of age.

Strategy

- Improved availability and use of ORS and zinc at the community.
- Facility level strengthening in the management of the dehydration and diarrhea.
- Enhanced advocacy and communication on prevention and control of diarrhea through IEC campaign.

The Target Beneficiaries for the Campaign Include

- All under-five children including their care-givers/mothers for community mobilization (for pre-positioning ORS/Zinc)
- Under 5 years children suffering from diarrhea (for treating diarrhea).

Activities

- **ORS distribution and counselling-home visits by ASHAs:**
  - ASHA to distribute ORS sachets to all families with under five children and demonstration for the preparation of the ORS solution by gathering of members from 4–8 households.
  - She also educates the people about hygiene and sanitation.
  - ASHA will report all diarrheal deaths during the fortnight.
  - At the end of Fortnight a report will be submitted by ASHA→ANM→BMO→ DCM →State Health Society.
  - ASHA will visit 10 under-five children in a day and would be provided an incentive of Rs. 1 per ORS packet distributed to a family with under five children.
- **IPC activities by ANM on sanitation and hygiene along with management of diarrhea:**
  - ANM should carry out Participatory learning technique on sanitation and hygiene.
  - ANM should conduct IDCF meeting in her subcenter village to disseminate information on prevention and control of diarrhea.
  - **Key messages for awareness generation:**
    - Give ORS and extra fluids to child immediately at the onset of diarrhea and continue till diarrhea stops.
    - Giving Zinc for 14 days for children suffering from diarrhea, even if diarrhea stops.
    - Safe and quick disposal of child's faeces.

- Continue feeding, including breastfeeding in those children who are being breastfed and give extra feeds during and after illness.
- Use clean drinking water after safe handling.
- Mother should wash her hands with soap before preparation of food, before feeding the child and after cleaning stool of child.
- Return to the health worker/centre if the child develops the following during treatment: · Child becomes sicker · Not able to drink or breastfeed · Blood in stool · Drinking poorly · Develops a fever.

❏ **Handwashing demonstration in schools:**
- Before mid-day-meal, all children should be taught to wash hands following the steps in the poster with water and soap.
- Prabhat pheri or rally by primary and middle school children on topic of handwashing should be carried out.

❏ **Establishment of ORS-zinc corners for treatment of diarrhea (at facility level):**
- ORS-zinc corner should be established for the treatment of diarrhea preferably in an easily noticeable area near the entrance of following facilities:
  - Medical colleges
  - District hospital
  - Block CHC/PHC
  - Subcenter
  - Anganwadi centers
  - Urban health posts/health centers
  - Private medical practitioners
- There will be demonstration of ORS preparation along with zinc regimen and also display of IEC material for awareness generation.

❏ **Multi-sectoral involvement:** Departments such as WCD, drinking water and sanitation, Rural development, Panchayati Raj and Education along with IAP will be involved.

The below mentioned protocols is for treatment of all diarrhea cases managed at both public and private health facilities routinely and during IDCF:

❏ Diarrhea cases with no dehydration to be treated with ORS, extra oral fluids and zinc as per IMNCI Plan A.

❏ Diarrhea cases with some dehydration to be managed for rehydration with ORS under observation as per IMNCI Plan B; then shifted either to IMNCI Plan A to C.

❏ Diarrhea cases with severe dehydration to be admitted and rehydrated with IV Ringer Lactate in wards (IMNCI Plan C), once rehydrated will shift to Plan A (ORS, extra oral fluids and Zinc).

BIBLIOGRAPHY

1. Govt. of India, Operational Guidelines Intensified Diarrhoea Control Fortnight (IDCF 2016), Ministry of Health and Family Welfare, New Delhi.
2. https://nhm.assam.gov.in/frontimpotentdata/intensified-diarrhoea-control-fortnight-idcf
3. https://www.learning4impact.org/content/927531429.pdf

4.7.9 NUTRITION REHABILITATION CENTER

- As per the recent report of NFHS-5 (2019–21), the nutrition indicators for children under 5 years have improved as compared with NFHS-4 (2015–16). Stunting has reduced from 38.4% to 35.5%, Wasting has reduced from 21.0% to 19.3% and Underweight prevalence has reduced from 35.8% to 32.1%.
- There are two major approaches to address children with SAM:
  - Facility/hospital-based care for children with SAM and medical complications
  - Home/community-based care for children with SAM but without medical complications
- Almost 90% of SAM children are not having any medical complications so they can be managed at home or community based care.
- Effective management of SAM must be based on the basic principle of "Continuum of Care" from the home and community, to the health center /health facility and back again.
- The NRCs should be established at Medical College Hospitals and District Hospitals. Sub-District Hospitals and Community Health Centres can be considered where facilities are geared to manage paediatric emergencies and complications in children with SAM.
- **Nutrition rehabilitation center (NRC)** is in a health facility where children with Severe Acute Malnutrition (SAM) and Medical Complications are admitted and managed.

Objectives

- To provide clinical management and reduce mortality among children with severe acute malnutrition, particularly among those with medical complications
- To promote physical and psychosocial growth of children with severe acute malnutrition (SAM)
- To build the capacity of mothers and other caregivers in appropriate feeding and caring practices for infants and young children
- To identify the social factors that contributed to the child slipping into severe acute malnutrition.

Services

- 24 hour care and monitoring of the child
- Treatment of medical complications
- Therapeutic feeding
- Providing sensory stimulation and emotional care
- Social assessment of the family to identify and address contributing factors
- Counseling on appropriate feeding, care and hygiene
- Demonstration and practice-by-doing on the preparation of energy dense child foods using locally available, culturally acceptable and affordable food items
- Follow-up of children discharged from the facility.

Human Resource

Staff position	Numbers for 10 bedded unit	Number for 20 bedded unit
Medical officer	One	Two
Nursing staff	Four	Eight
Nutrition counsellor	One	Two
Cook cum caretaker	One	Two
Attendant/cleaners	Two	Two
Medical social worker	One	One

Nutrition Assessment and Nutrition Education

Case Identification Algorithm (Fig. 4.9)

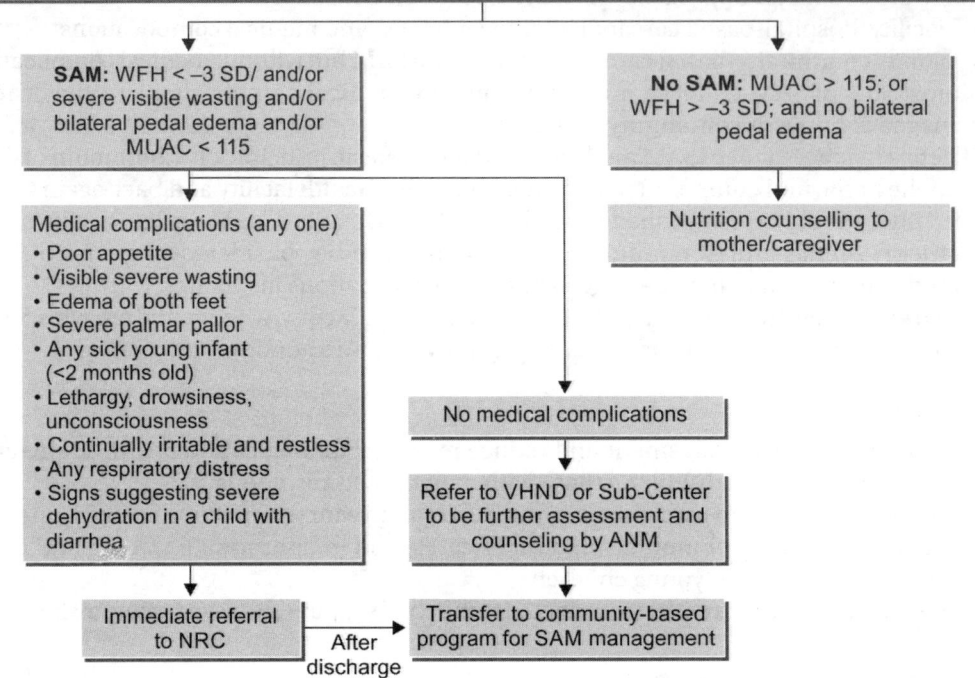

Fig. 4.9: Case identification algorithm.

Admission and Discharge Criteria

Children less than 6 months of age

Admission Criteria:	**Discharge Criteria**
• Problem of breastfeeding: The infant is too weak to suck 　▪ And/Or • Bilateral pitting edema 　▪ And/Or • Visible severe wasting 　▪ And/Or • W/H or W/L <–3 Z score	Discharge the infant from the facility when gaining weight for 5 days and has no medical complications.

For children <6 months of age suffering from severe acute malnutrition, emphasis is laid on supporting and sustaining breastfeeding through counselling and re-establishment of lactation in mothers with lactation failure using supplementary suckling technique (SST).

Children age 6 months up to 60 months

Admission Criteria:	Discharge Criteria:

• W/H or W/L <−3 Z score
  ▪ And/Or
• MUAC <11.5 cm
  ▪ And/Or
• Presence of bilateral edema
• With any medical complications as mentioned in above algorithm.
	• Edema has resolved
	• Child has achieved weight gain of >15% and has satisfactory weight gain for 3 consecutive days (>5 gm/kg/day)
	• All infections and other medical complications have been treated

The principles of management of SAM are based on 3 phases: Stabilization Phase, Transition Phase and Rehabilitative Phase.

Stabilization Phase

- Children with SAM without an adequate appetite and/or a major medical complication are stabilized in an in-patient facility.
- This phase usually lasts for 1–2 days.
- Starter diet (F75) is used during this phase which promotes recovery of normal metabolic function and nutrition-electrolytic balance.
- All children must be carefully monitored for signs of overfeeding or over hydration in this phase.

Transition Phase

- This phase usually lasts for 2–3 days.
- The transition phase is intended to ensure that the child is clinically stable and can tolerate an increased energy and protein intake.
- The child moves to the transition phase from stabilization phase when there is:
  - At least the beginning of loss of edema AND
  - Return of appetite AND
  - No nasogastric tube, infusions, no severe medical problems AND
  - Is alert and reactive
- There is gradual transition from Starter diet (F75) to Catch up diet (F100).
- The quantity of Catch up diet (F100) given is equal to the quantity of Starter diet (F75) given in stabilization Phase.

Rehabilitation Phase

- Once children with SAM have recovered their appetite and received treatment for medical complications, they enter Rehabilitation Phase.
- The aim is to promote rapid weight gain, stimulate emotional and physical development and prepare the child for normal feeding at home.
- The child progresses from Transition Phase to Rehabilitation Phase when:
  - She/he has reasonable appetite
  - Finishes >90% of the feed that is given, without a significant pause
  - Major reduction or loss of edema
  - No other medical problem

Wage compensation: is to be given to the mother/caregiver for the duration of the stay at NRC, as per the basic daily wages in the state. Mother or the caregiver staying with the child should be provided food from the health facility.

ASHA incentives: Incentives of Rs. 50 for accompanying the child to the NRC and motivating the mother to stay for at least 7 days till the child is stabilized and has started to eat. Additional incentive of Rs. 50 for each follow-up visit by the child up to a maximum of three visits.

BIBLIOGRAPHY

1. http://www.nrcmis.mp.gov.in/NRCConcept.aspx
2. https://nhm.gujarat.gov.in/images/pdf/nrc_guidelines.pdf
3. https://rajswasthya.nic.in/MTC%20Guideline-%20MOHFW.pdf

4.7.10 HOME BASED NEWBORN CARE AND HOME BASED CARE OF YOUNG CHILD

- Home Based Newborn Care (HBNC) comprising of six home visits in case of institutional delivery (Days 3, 7, 14, 21, 28 and 42) and seven visits in case of home delivery (Days 1, 3, 7, 14, 21, 28 and 42).
- ASHA gets INR 250/- after completing all these 6 or 7 visits with provided that baby and mother are healthy, baby's birth weight is measured and mentioned, birth registration done and vaccination of 1.5 months of age is done.
- **The major objective of HBNC is to decrease neonatal mortality and morbidity through:**
  - The provision of essential newborn care to all newborns and the prevention of complications
  - Early detection and special care of preterm and low birth weight newborns
  - Early identification of illness in the newborn and provision of appropriate care and referral
  - Support the family for adoption of healthy practices and build confidence and skills of the mother to safeguard her health and that of the newborn.

The Key Activities in HBNC

- Care for every newborn through a series of home visits in the first six weeks of life.
- Information and skills to the mother and family of every newborn to ensure better health outcomes.
- An examination of every newborn for prematurity and low birth weight.
- Extra home visits for preterm and low birth weight babies by the ASHA or ANM, and referred for appropriate care as defined in the protocols.
- Early identification of illness in the newborn and provision of appropriate care at home or referral as defined in the protocols.
- Follow up for sick newborns after they are discharged from facilities.
- Counselling the mother on postpartum care, recognition of postpartum complications and enabling referral
- Counselling the mother for adoption of an appropriate family planning method.

Nutrition Assessment and Nutrition Education

Home Based Care for Young Child

- HBYC is a Joint Initiative of Ministry of Health and Family Welfare and Ministry of Women and Child Development.
- It aims to reduce child mortality and morbidity and improve nutrition status, growth and early childhood development of young children through additional home visits by our community health worker, the ASHA and Anganwadi worker.
- Five additional home visits by ASHA in coordination with AWW starting from 3rd month and extending into 2nd year of life (in 3rd, 6th, 9th, 12th and 15th months) are done as part of HBYC **(Figs. 4.10 and 4.11)**.
- Additional incentive of INR 250/- for these five additional visits is given under NHM.

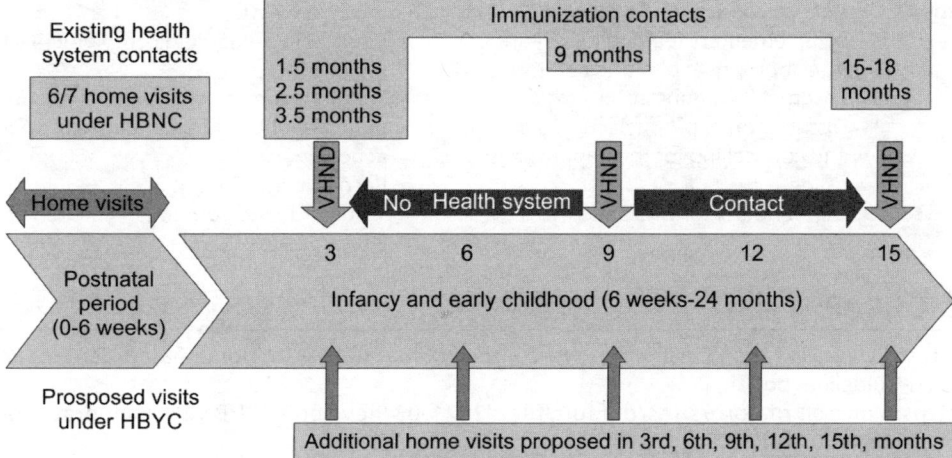

Fig. 4.10: Schedule of visits under HBYC.

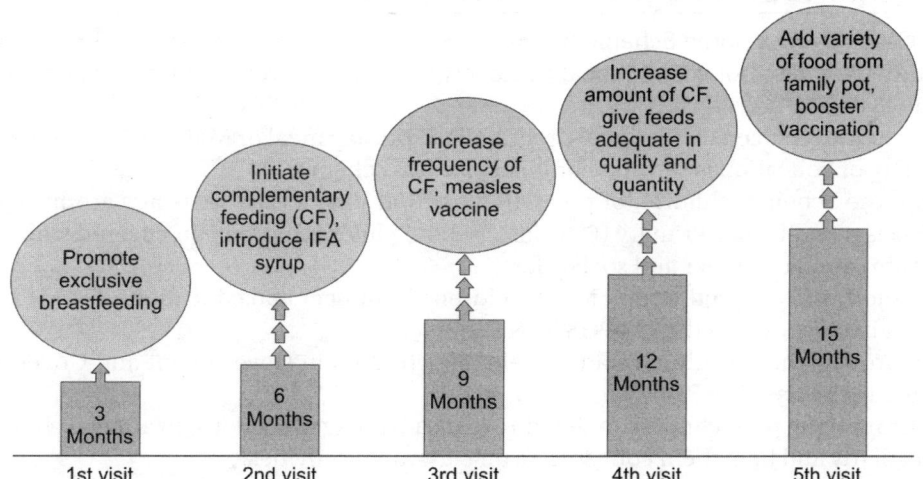

Fig. 4.11: Age-appropriate interventions to be promoted during HBYC home visits.

Brief Description of Activities to be done under HBYC at the Time of Home Visit

Home visits	ASHA	AWW
At 3rd Month	• Support for exclusive breastfeeding • Counsel on handwashing practices • Appropriate play and communication • Check immunization status • Check weight recording in MCP card; identify growth faltering	• Monthly weighing of infants • Weight recording and plotting on growth chart • Detect underweight children and take further action • Counsel mother for exclusive breast feeding
At 6th, 9th, 12th and 15th Months	All above activities PLUS • Counsel on initiation of complementary feeding and continued breastfeeding • Age appropriate and adequate complementary feeding for children • Age appropriate play and communication • Ensure full immunization • Distribution of prophylactic IFA and ORS and counselling for their appropriate usage • Depot holder for ORS and Zinc	• 'Take Home Ration' and nutrition specific counselling to mothers • Monthly weighing and supplementary food from AWC • Counselling regarding complementary feeding • Weight recording on growth chart; detect underweight children and take further action • Record length/height • Counsel for deworming of children above 1 year of age

BIBLIOGRAPHY

1. https://www.aspirationaldistricts.in/wp-content/uploads/2019/02/Home-Based-Care-for-Young-Child-Guidelines.pdf
2. https://nhsrcindia.org/sites/default/files/2021-03/Revised%20HBNC%20Operational%20Guidelines%202014%20English.pdf

4.7.11 PRADHAN MANTRI POSHAN SHAKTI NIRMAN (PM POSHAN)

- It is Centrally Sponsored Scheme 'Pradhan Mantri Poshan Shakti Nirman (PM POSHAN)' for providing one hot cooked meal in Government and Government-aided Schools from 2021–22 to 2025–26.
- The scheme replaced the national program for Mid-day meal or Mid-day Meal Scheme.
- Ministry of Education is the nodal ministry for this scheme.
- Under the Scheme, children of pre-schools or Bal Vatika (3–5 years age group) Primary (1–5 class) and Upper Primary (6–8 class) school children have been covered without any discrimination of gender and social class.
- It is to address two major problems of children viz. hunger and education.
- The main objectives of the PM POSHAN Scheme:
  - Improving the nutritional status of eligible children in Government and Government-aided schools
  - Encouraging poor children, belonging to disadvantaged sections, to attend school more regularly and help them concentrate on classroom activities.

KEY INITIATIVES

- **Tithi Bhojan:** As community participation initiative, people provide special food to children on special occasions/festivals.

- School Nutrition Gardens
- Social Audit
- **Supplementary nutrition** items to children in aspirational districts and districts with high prevalence of Anemia.
- **Cooking competitions** to promote ethnic cuisine and innovative menus based on locally available ingredients and vegetables.
- **Vocal for Local**: Involvement of Farmers Producer Organizations (FPO) and Women Self Help Groups in implementation of the scheme will be encouraged.
- Monitoring through field visits

Nutritional Norms Per Child

Item	Primary	Upper primary
Calorie	450	700
Protein	12 gm	20 gm

BIBLIOGRAPHY

1. https://pib.gov.in/Pressreleaseshare.aspx?PRID=1812421

4.8 BRIEF NOTE ON FOOD-RELATED DISEASES AND FOOD SAFETY

- Food-borne diseases, including food-borne intoxications and food-borne infections, are terms applied to illnesses acquired through consumption of contaminated food.
- The global burden of infectious diarrhea involves 3–5 billion cases and nearly 1.5 million deaths annually, mainly in young children, due to diarrheal disease caused by contaminated food and water.
- The WHO South East Asia Region having the second highest burden of food-borne diseases per population and contributes to one third of the global deaths due to diarrhea in children under five years of age among WHO regions.
- The pathogenic organisms transmitted through contaminated foods are bacteria, viruses, protozoa and helminths.
- *Staphylococcus aureus, Vibrio sp, Salmonella sp, E. coli, Yersinia enteroclitica* are some important microbial pathogens responsible for food-borne illnesses.
- *Salmonella* is the most common cause of food-borne illnesses.
- *Staphylococcus aureus* bacteria grow in food and produce toxins that cause staphylococcal food poisoning.
- Cholera, although primarily a water-borne disease, may have a food source if contaminated water is used.
- Different foods implicated in food-borne outbreaks in India are milk and milk products, meat, poultry, fish, fowl, sea food such as prawns; cooked and uncooked rice and cooked as well as uncooked vegetables.
- Chemical contamination of food may result from various sources. Industrial or agricultural practices such as use of pesticides, fertilizers lead to entry of heavy metals such as cadmium, lead and mercury into the food chain.

- Mycotoxins are produced by several fungi in foodstuffs, often under warm and humid conditions. Mycotoxins such as aflatoxins, ochratoxin A, fumonisins, trichothecenes, ergot alkaloids and zeralenone are of public health importance. In India, mouldy maize, sorghum and wheat flour are associated with outbreaks of mycotoxicosis.
- Food poisoning from consumption of poisonous wild mushrooms has been reported frequently.
- Difference between infections vs intoxications:

Infections versus Intoxications		
	Infections	Intoxications
Cause	Bacteria/Viruses/Parasites	Toxin
Mechanism	Invade and/or multiply within the lining of the intestines	No invasion or multiplication
Incubation period	Hours to days	Minutes to hours
Symptoms	Diarrhea Nausea / Vomiting Abdominal cramps ± Fever	Vomiting, nausea, diarrhea, double vision, weakness, respiratory failure, numbness, sensory and motor dysfunction
Transmission	Can be spread from person-to-person via the feco-oral route	Not communicable
Factors related to food contamination	Inadequate cooking Cross-contamination Poor personal hygiene Bare hand contact	Inadequate cooking Improper holding temperatures

- Chemical food poisoning can also occur through adulteration of food by adding prohibited substances to partly or wholly substitute healthy ingredients or to artificially create the impression of freshness in stale food.

Brief About Food Adulteration

Name of disease	Normal food	Adulterant	Toxin	Clinical features	Detection and solution
Neuro-lathyrism	Red gram dhal	L. sativus (Khesari Dal)	BOAA (Beta Oxalyl Amino Alanine)	Spastic paralysis of lower limbs. There are five stages of diseases extending from latent stage to crawler stage	There are three main solutions: 1. Banning of crop 2. Removal of toxin by steeping method and Paraboiling. 3. Vitamin C prophylaxis
Epidemic Dropsy	Mustard oil	Argemona Mexicana oil	Sanguinarine	Due to blockage of Krebs Cycle leads to B/L lower limb edema (non-inflammatory), diarrhea, cardiac failure, glaucoma and even death	Tests: Nitric acid test and paper photo chromatography

Endemic Ascites	Millet "Pancium miliare" (Gondhli)	Crotalaria seeds (Jhunjhunia)	Pyrrolizdine alkaloids (Hepatotoxins)	Ascites	Education and Deweeding of Jhunjhunia plants
Ergotism	Cereals	Claviceps fusiformis	Clavin Alkaloids	Nausea, vomiting, drowsiness, in long-term cramp in limb and peripheral gangrene can develop	Ergot infested grain can be easily treated by floating them in 20% salt water. Hand picking and air floatation can be tried
Aflatoxicosis	Groundnut, Cereals	Apergilius flavus and parasiticus	Aflatoxin (B1 and G1 are the most potent hepatotoxins)	Diarrhea, vomiting	Proper dry storage to avoid fungal contamination. Moisture content should be less than 10%

PATHOGENESIS

☐ Food-borne illness is typically caused by microorganisms or their toxins, and most often manifests with gastrointestinal symptoms, which can vary in severity and duration. In addition to food-borne pathogens (bacteria, viruses and parasites), food-borne disease may also be caused by contaminants like heavy metals, chemicals, pesticides and toxic substances present naturally in food like toxic mushrooms, plants, fish or shellfish.
☐ The food-borne diseases due to infectious causes form the majority of cases, and are largely dependent on the inoculum size or the infective dose of the pathogen.
☐ Food may become contaminated during food production and processing or during food preparation and handling, or during storage.

Food Production and Processing

Foods, such as fruits and vegetables, may be contaminated if washed or irrigated with water that is contaminated with pathogens from animal or human faeces. During slaughter, meat and poultry carcasses can become contaminated if they are exposed to small amounts of intestinal contents.

Food Preparation and Handling

☐ *Infected individuals*—most food-borne pathogens are shed in the faeces of infected persons and these pathogens may be transferred to others through food via the faecal-oral route. Bacteria present in infected lesions and normal nasal flora may also be transmitted from an infected food-handler to ready-to-eat foods **(Table 4.6 to Table 4.8)**.
☐ *Cross-contamination*—pathogens naturally present in one food may be transferred to other foods during food preparation if same cooking equipment and utensils are used without washing and disinfecting in between, especially in case of ready-to-eat foods.
☐ *Inadequate cooking temperature*—with insufficient cooking, bacteria can multiply and produce toxins within the food. Many bacterial toxins are heat stable and may not be destroyed by cooking.

Food Storage

Improper storage: Food being held or stored at warm (10–50°C) temperature allows multiplication of pathogens and is an important cause of food-borne outbreaks.

Table 4.6: Mechanisms of food poisoning.

Mechanism	Location	Illness	Stool M/E	Examples
Non-inflammatory (enterotoxin)	Proximal small intestine	Watery diarrhea	No fecal leukocytes	Vibrio cholerae, Enterotoxigenic E. coli (ETEC), Enteroaggregative Escherichia coli (EAggEC), Cl. perfringens, Bacillus cereus, Staph aureus, rotavirus, norovirus, enteric adenoviruses, Giardia lamblia, Cryptosporidium, Cyclospora, Microsporidia
Inflammatory (invasion/cytotoxin)	Colon/distal small intestine	Dysentery/inflammatory diarrhea	PMN fecal leukocytes	Shigella, Salmonella, C. jejuni, Enterohemorrhagic E. coli (EHEC), EIEC, Y. enterocolitica, Vibrio parahemolyticus, Cl. difficile, E. histolytica
Penetrating	Distal small intestine	Enteric fever	Mono-nuclear fecal leukocytes	Salmonella typhi, Y. enterocolitica, Campylobacter fetus

Table 4.7: Bacterial food poisoning.

Incubation period	Cause	Symptoms	Common foods
1–6 hours	Staph aureus	Nausea, vomiting, diarrhea	Ham, poultry, potato/egg salad, mayonnaise, cream Pastries
	Bacillus cereus	Nausea, Vomiting, Diarrhea	Fried rice
8–16 hours	Cl. perfringens	Abdominal cramps, diarrhea (vomiting rare)	Beef, poultry, legumes, gravies
	B. cereus		Meats, vegetables, dried beans, cereals
>16 hours	Vibrio cholerae	Watery diarrhea	Shell-fish
	Enterotoxigenic E. coli (ETEC)	Watery diarrhea	Salad, cheese, meats, water
	Enterohemorrhagic E. coli (EHEC)	Bloody diarrhea	Beef, salami, raw milk/vegetables, apple juice
	Salmonella sp	Inflammatory diarrhea	Beef, poultry, eggs, diary products
	Campylobacter jejuni	Inflammatory diarrhea	Poultry, raw milk
	Shigella sp	Dysentery	Potato/egg salad, lettuce, raw eggs
	V. parahemolyticus	Dysentery	Sea food—Molluscs, crustaceans

Table 4.8: Major food-borne hazards: Clinical features and samples.

Time to onset of symptoms	Predominant symptoms	Associated organism or toxin	Samples from cases (and food-handlers)
Upper gastrointestinal tract symptoms (nausea, vomiting) occur first or predominate			
<1 hour	Nausea, vomiting, unusual taste, burning of mouth.	Metallic salts	Vomit, urine, blood, stool
1–2 hours	Nausea, vomiting, cyanosis, headache, dizziness, dyspnea, trembling, weakness, loss of consciousness	Nitrites	Blood
1–6 (mean 2–4) hours	Nausea, vomiting, retching, diarrhea, abdominal pain, prostration	*Staphylococcus aureus* and its enterotoxins	Stool, vomit, (swabs from nostril, skin lesions)
8–16 hours (2–4 hours if emesis predominant)	Vomiting, abdominal cramps, diarrhea, nausea	*Bacillus cereus*	Rectal swab, stool
6–24 hours	Nausea, vomiting, diarrhea, thirst, dilation of pupils, collapse, coma	Mycotoxins (*Amanita phalloides* Fungi)	Urine, blood (SGOT, SGPT), vomit
12–48 (median 36 hours)	Nausea, vomiting, watery non-bloody diarrhea, dehydration	Norovirus	Stool
Lower gastrointestinal tract symptoms (abdominal cramps, diarrhea) occur first or predominate			
2–36 (mean 6–12) hours	Abdominal cramps, diarrhea (putrefactive diarrhea - *Clostridium perfringens*), sometimes nausea and vomiting	*Clostridium perfringens*, *Bacillus cereus*	Rectal swabs, stool
6–96 hours (usually 1–3 days)	Fever, abdominal cramps, diarrhoea, vomiting, headache	*Salmonella spp*, *Shigella*, *Aeromonas*, Enteropathogenic *E. coli*	Rectal swabs, stool
6 hours to 5 days	Abdominal cramps, diarrhea, vomiting, fever, malaise, nausea, headache, dehydration (sometimes bloody or mucoid diarrhea, cutaneous lesions associated with *Vibrio vulnificus*)	*Vibrio cholerae (O1 and non- O1)*, *V. vulnificus*, *V. fluvialis*, *V. parahemolyticus*	Stool
1–10 (median 3–4) days	Diarrhea (often bloody), abdominal pain, nausea, vomiting, malaise, fever (uncommon with *E. coli* O157)	Enterohaemorrhagic *E. coli* (including *E. coli* O157), *Campylobacter*	Stool, rectal swabs
3–5 days	Fever, vomiting, watery non-inflammatory diarrhea	Rotavirus, astrovirus, enteric adenoviruses	Stool, vomit
3–7 days	Fever, diarrhea, abdominal pain (can mimic acute appendicitis)	*Yersinia enterocolitica*	Stool

Time to onset of symptoms	Predominant symptoms	Associated organism or toxin	Samples from cases (and food-handlers)
1–6 weeks	Mucoid diarrhea (fatty stools) abdominal pain, flatulence, weight loss	Giardia lamblia	Stool
1 to several weeks	Abdominal pain, diarrhea, constipation, headache, drowsiness, ulcers, variable – often asymptomatic	Entamoeba histolytica	Stool
3–6 months	Nervousness, insomnia, hunger pains, anorexia, weight loss, abdominal pain, sometimes gastroenteritis	Taenia saginata, T. solium	Stool, rectal swab

Most food-borne infections are diagnosed through the identification of the pathogen in stool collected from infected persons. Vomitus has also been used to detect certain organisms and confirm the etiology. Blood samples are recommended for cases with systemic involvement.

Stool Specimens: Stool samples should be collected in clean, dry, leak-proof screw cap container and tape Proper collection and transport of stool specimens requires the appropriate transport medium (modified Cary-Blair medium), and encouraging ill persons to submit a stool specimen.

Vomitus/gastric aspirate can also be tested for organisms and toxins, and should be collected as soon as possible after onset of illness. Instruct the patient to vomit directly into a sterile specimen container, such as a screw-capped bottle (or a urine specimen container). If this is not possible, ask the patient to vomit in a clean container, bowl or plastic bag and transfer the vomitus to the screw-capped container with a clean spoon. Place the cap securely on the container and seal the lid with tape.

Food specimens: Microbiological analysis of food supports the epidemiological investigation of a food-borne disease outbreak. The purpose of testing is to isolate and identify pathogenic microorganisms in food samples, which have been implicated in the outbreak.

Food samples must be collected using aseptic techniques and appropriate containers. Samples must be refrigerated during storage and transport and must arrive at the food microbiology laboratory within three days of collection. Samples collected frozen should be stored and transported frozen on dry ice.

TREATMENT

Initial treatment of patients with food-poisoning should focus on assessment and reversal of dehydration, either through oral rehydration therapy (ORT) especially in children, or through IV fluids in seriously dehydrated cases.

The earlier standard Oral Rehydration Salts (ORS) provided a solution containing 90 mEq/L of sodium with a total osmolarity of 311 m Osm/l. In 2003, the **"improved" ORS having lower osmolarity** was formulated by reducing the solution's glucose and salt concentrations. Because of the improved effectiveness of reduced osmolarity ORS solution, especially for children with acute, non-cholera diarrhea, WHO and UNICEF now recommend that countries use and manufacture the following formulation in place of the previously recommended ORS solution (**Table 4.9**).

Table 4.9: Reduced osmolarity ORS formulation.

Formula	g/L	Constituents	mmol/L
Sodium chloride	2.6	Sodium	75
Glucose, anhydrous	13.5	Chloride	65
Potassium chloride	1.5	Glucose, anhydrous	75
Trisodium citrate, dihydrate	2.9	Potassium	20
		Citrate	10
		Total Osmolarity	245

Food Safety

- Food safety is an area of public health action to protect consumers from the risks of food poisoning and food-borne diseases, acute or chronic (WHO).
- Food safety is now the need of the hour because of the following factors:
  - Nowadays people started to eat more outside than home prepared foods.
  - Increased consumption of processed and packaged foods
  - Quality of raw material and even spices and condiments also a big concern
  - Mass production and time lag in usage and distribution could affect the food quality
  - Trade and travel expansion
  - Pollution and Pesticides injudicious usage
  - Irrational usage of preservatives, colors, flavoring agents
- Food safety is a continuum with its scope extending from farm to plate. The health risks impact the whole food supply chain, starting from input supply to the farm to the consumer table.
- Key strategies to ensure food safety include:
  - having a clear food safety policy and regulations
  - effective surveillance system for food-borne diseases
  - food control and inspection systems with analytic capacity and adoption of quality assurance systems such as HACCP
  - Food safety education for food-handlers and the community about proper practices in cooking and storage of food, and personal hygiene. Handwashing is one of the key interventions, not just by food handlers, but also by the community at large.
  - Environmental measures include discouraging sewage farming for growing vegetables and fruits.

Five Keys to Safer Food

1. **Keep Clean**
   - Wash your hands before handling food and often during food preparation
   - Wash your hands after going to the toilet
   - Wash and sanitize all surfaces and equipment used for food preparation
   - Protect kitchen areas and food from insects, pests and other animals

Nutrition Assessment and Nutrition Education

2. **Separate raw and cooked food**
   - Separate raw meat, poultry and seafood from other foods
   - Use separate utensils such as knives and cutting boards for handling raw foods
   - Store food in containers to avoid contact between raw and prepared foods
3. **Cook thoroughly**
   - Cook food thoroughly, especially meat, poultry, eggs and seafood
   - Bring foods like soups and stews to boiling to make sure that they have reached 70°C
   - Reheat cooked food thoroughly
4. **Keep food at safe temperatures**
   - Do not leave cooked food at room temperature for more than 2 hours
   - Refrigerate promptly all cooked and perishable food (preferably below 5°C)
   - Keep cooked food piping hot (more than 60°C) prior to serving
   - Do not store food too long even in the refrigerator
   - Do not thaw frozen food at room temperature
5. **Use safe water and raw materials**
   - Use safe water or treat it to make it safe
   - Select fresh and wholesome foods
   - Choose foods processed for safety, such as pasteurized milk
   - Wash fruits and vegetables, especially if eaten raw
   - Do not use food beyond its expiry date

Pasteurization of Milk

- **Pre-pasteurization test: Methylene blue reduction test** to assess the level of contamination of milk.
- **Pasteurization:**

Sr. No	Method	Process
1	Holder/Vat	Milk is heated at 63–66 degree C for at least 30 minutes and then quickly cooled for 5 degree C
2	High temperature short time (HTST)	Milk is heated at 72 degree C for at least 15 seconds then cooled to 4 degree C
3	Ultra high temperature (UHT)	Milk is heated at 125 degree C for few seconds only

- **Postpasteurization Tests: To assess the efficacy of pasteurization**
  - **Standard Plate count**
  - **Coliform count**
  - **Phosphatase test:** Most widely used test.

Food Safety Regulation

In order to ensure that foods are safe and of good quality, across the world various governments and international bodies have laid down food standards that manufacturers/suppliers are expected to adhere to.

International Organizations and Agreements in the Area of Food Standards, Quality, Research and Trade:

- **Codex Alimentarius Commission (CAC):** The document published by the CAC is Codex Alimentarius which means 'Food Code' and is a collection of internationally adopted Food Standards. The document includes Standards, Codes of Practice, Guidelines and other recommendations in order to protect consumers and ensure fair practices in food trade. Different countries use Codex Standards to develop national standards
- **International Organization for Standardization (ISO):** It is a worldwide, non-governmental federation of national standards bodies (ISO member bodies). The mission of ISO is to promote the development of standardization and related activities in the world with a view to facilitate the international exchange of goods and services, and to develop cooperation in the spheres of intellectual, scientific, technological and economic activity. Adoption of these standards is voluntary.
- **World Trade Organization:** WTO was established in 1995. The main objective of WTO is to help trade flow smoothly, freely, fairly and predictably, by administering trade agreements, settling trade disputes, assisting countries in trade policy issues. The WTO Agreement covers goods, services and intellectual property.

Food Safety Standards in India

- Mandatory: Food Safety and Standards (FSS)
- Voluntary: AGMARK, BIS certification

Food Safety and Standards (FSS)

- Prior to 2006 in India, food-related issues were managed by various departments and ministries through a number of central acts. These included the Prevention of Food Adulteration Act 1954, Fruit Products Order 1955, Meat Food Products Order 1973, Vegetable Oil Products (Control) Order 1947, and the Edible Oils Packaging (Regulation) Order 1988, among others.
- In 2006, these orders were consolidated and brought under one overarching act, the Food Safety and Standards (FSS) Act, 2006.
- The Food Safety and Standards Authority of India (FSSAI) is an autonomous statutory body created for defining science-based standards for articles of food, and regulating the manufacture, storage, distribution, sale and import of food items to ensure the availability of safe and wholesome food for human consumption.
- The Ministry of Health and Family Welfare, Government of India is the Administrative Ministry for the implementation of FSS Act.
- Enforcement and execution of the act is done at the central level by the Food authority and at the state level by Food Safety Commissioners. At the local level Food Safety Officers are the licensing authority and municipal corporations and gram panchayats are the registering authority.

BIS Certification

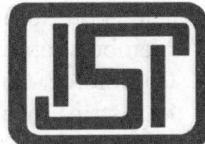

BIS certification scheme is voluntary and aims at providing quality, safety and dependability to the ultimate consumer. Presence of certification mark known as Standard Mark on a product is an assurance of conformity to specifications. The activities of Bureau of Indian Standards (BIS) are formation of Indian Standards in the processed food sector and the implementation of standards through promotion, voluntary and third party certification systems. In general these standards cover raw materials and their quality parameters, hygienic conditions under which products are manufactured and packaging and labeling requirements. Manufacturers complying with standards laid down by the BIS can obtain the ISI Mark that can be exhibited on product packages.

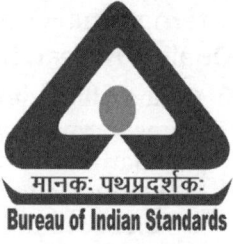
Bureau of Indian Standards

AGMARK

- The word Agmark is derived from Agricultural Marketing. The DMI under the Department of Agriculture and Co-operation in the Ministry of Agriculture enforces the Agricultural Products (Grading and Marketing) Act 1937.
- Under this Act Grade standards are prescribed for agricultural and allied commodities.
- Agmark grading means grading of an article in accordance with grade/standards prescribed under the provisions of the act. These are known as AGMARK standards.
- Grading under the provision of this Act is voluntary.
- Manufacturers who comply with standard laid down by DMI are allowed to use "AGMARK" labels on their products.

BIBLIOGRAPHY

1. https://ncert.nic.in/textbook/pdf/lehe106.pdf
2. http://ecoursesonline.iasri.res.in/mod/page/view.php?id=1034
3. WHO, 2016. Burden of foodborne diseases in the South-East Asia Region.

4.9 FOOD SAFETY AND STANDARDS ACT (FSSA), 2006 AND FOOD SAFETY AND STANDARDS RULES, 2011

- FSSA, 2006 is an Act enacted to keep with changing requirements of time and to consolidate the laws relating to food and to establish the Food Safety and Standards Authority of India.
- The Act was needed to establish a single statutory body for standards setting and enforcement of food laws, so no confusion in the minds of consumers, traders, manufacturers and investors which was due to multiplicity of food laws.
- The priorities of the FSSAI is laying down science based standards for articles of food and to regulate their manufacture, storage, distribution, sale and import, to ensure availability of safe and wholesome food for human consumption.
- The Food Authority consists of a Chairperson and 22 members out of which 7 ex-officio members represent the Ministries or Departments of Central Government viz. Agriculture, Commerce, Consumer Affairs, Food Processing, Health, Legislative Affairs, Small Scale Industries; two representatives from food industry; two representative from consumer organizations; three eminent food technologists or scientists; five members to represent

the States and the Union Territories on rotation basis; two persons to represent farmers "organizations and one person to represent retailers" organizations.

The following Acts are under the umbrella of the Food Safety and Standards Act, 2006:
- The Prevention of Food Adulteration (PFA) Act 1954
- The Fruit Products Order, 1955
- The Meat Food Products Order, 1973
- The Vegetable Oil Products (Control) Order, 1947
- The Edible Oils Packaging (Regulation) Order, 1998
- The Solvent Extracted Oil, De oiled Meal, and Edible Flour (Control) Order 1967
- The Milk and Milk Products Order, 1992
- Any other order under essential commodities Act, 1955 relating to food.

Commissioner of Food Safety

Qualification: No person below the rank of "Commissioner and Secretary" to State Government shall be eligible to be appointed as the Commissioner of Food Safety.
- He prohibits manufacture, storage, distribution or sale of any adulterated food articles.
- He conducts training programs.
- He sanctions prosecution for offences punishable with imprisonment under this act.

Designated Officer

- There shall be a Designated Officer for each district.
- Full time Officer, not below the rank of Sub-Divisional Officer or equivalent
- Receive food samples from food safety officer and get them analyzed.
- suspension, cancellation or revocation of the license of the Food Business Operator in case any threat or grave injury to public, has been noticed in the report of the Food Analyst.
- He can sanction prosecution and gives recommendations (within 14 days) to the food safety commissioner.

Food Safety Officer

- To inspect, as frequently as may be prescribed by the Designated Officer, all food establishments licensed for manufacturing, handling, packing or selling of an article of food within the area assigned to him.
- He can take samples of food for testing.
- He can seize any adulterated food or food which is unsafe or sub-standard or mis-branded or containing extraneous matter.
- He may seal the premises for investigation after taking a sample of such adulterant or food for analysis.

Food Analyst

- The Food Analyst shall analyse the article of food sent to him for analysis.
- Food Safety Officer shall analyse the sample and send the analysis report mentioning method of sampling and analysis within fourteen days to Designated Officer with a copy to Commissioner of Food Safety.
- Food Analyst shall send his report to the Purchaser of article of food as well if requested.

Licensing and Registration Procedure Under this Act

- The person who desirous to commence any food business shall apply for a licence to the designated officer along with fees.
- Petty retailer, hawker, vendor or temporary stall holders don't need to get the license but they shall have registration with food safety officer or designated officer.
- If licence is not issued within two months of application, the applicant may start his food business.
- If registration is not done within one month of application, the applicant may start his food business.
- FSSAI issues three types of license based on the nature of the food business and turnover:
  - Registration: For Turnover less than ₹12 Lakh
  - State License: For Turnover between ₹12 Lakh to ₹20 Crore
  - Central License: For Turnover above ₹20 Crore
- **Provision of punishment for unsafe food under this act:**
  - Penalty for selling food not of the nature or substance or quality demanded: liable to a penalty not exceeding five lakh rupees
  - Penalty for sub-standard food: liable to a penalty which may extend to five lakh rupees
  - Penalty for misbranded food: liable to a penalty which may extend to three lakh rupees
  - Penalty for misleading advertisement: liable to a penalty which may extend to ten lakh rupees
  - Penalty for food containing extraneous matter: liable to a penalty which may extend to one lakh rupees
  - Penalty for failure to comply with the directions of Food Safety Officer: liable to a penalty which may extend to two lakh rupees
  - Penalty for unhygienic or unsanitary processing or manufacturing of food: liable to a penalty which may extend to one lakh rupees
  - Penalty for possessing adulterant: (i) where such adulterant is not injurious to health, to a penalty not exceeding two lakh rupees; (ii) where such adulterant is injurious to health, to a penalty not exceeding ten lakh rupees
  - Punishment for unsafe food:

Type of injury	Imprisonment	Fine	Compensation to consumer
No Injury	6 months	1 lakh	—
Nongrievous injury	1 year	3 lakhs	1 lakh
Grievous injury	6 years	5 lakhs	3 lakhs
Death	7 years or may be life time	10 lakhs	5 lakhs

- Dealing food business without license liable for punishment with imprisonment for a term which may extend to six months and also with fine may extend to 5 lakh rupees.

BIBLIOGRAPHY

1. http://www.fssai.gov.in/Portals/0/Pdf/FAQ.pdf
2. http://www.slideshare.net/Adrienna/fssai-act-presentation
3. https://fssai.gov.in/upload/uploadfiles/files/FOOD-ACT.pdf

4.10 CONSUMER PROTECTION ACT (CPA), 1986 AND AMENDED IN 2019

- **Rights of the consumer:**
  - The right to safety
  - The right to be informed
  - The right to choose
  - The right to be heard
  - The right to redress
  - The right to consumer education
  - The right to clean and healthy environment
  - The right to basic needs
- First 6 rights have been addressed in CPA.
- It's part of Ministry of Consumer Affairs, Food and Public Distribution
- CPA came into force on 15th April 1987.
- CPA has been amended in 2019.

CPA, 2019 key features

- There is three tier judicial machinery under this Act.
  - While the **District consumer disputes redressal forum** District CDRC (comprised of one district judge and two members) will entertain complaints when the value of goods or service is up to Rs 1 crore. (earlier it was up to 20 lakhs). Complaints should be filed within 30 days to state forum.
  - The **State consumer disputes redressal forum** (comprised of high court judge and two members) State CDRC will entertain consumer complaints when the value is more than ₹ 1 crore but less than ₹ 10 crore. (earlier the limit was from 20 lakh to 1 crore). Complaints should be filed within 30 days to national forum.
  - The **National consumer disputes redressal forum** (National CDRC) will entertain complaints worth more than ₹ 10 crores. Earlier it is used to give decision over disputes of the money more than 1 crore.
  - Final appeal should be filed within 30 days to Supreme Court.
  - If culprit fails to comply with order of any above mentioned forum then he/she is punishable with imprisonment for a term not less than one month which may extend to 3 years or fine not less than ₹ 2,000 or both.
  - It covers transactions through all modes including offline, and online through electronic means, teleshopping, multi-level marketing or direct selling.
  - There is provision of Establishment of the Central Consumer Protection Authority (CCPA).
  - The CCPA may impose a penalty of up to INR 1,000,000 (Indian Rupees One Million) on a manufacturer or an endorser, for a false or misleading advertisement.
  - The CCPA may also sentence them to imprisonment for up to 2 (two) years for the same.
  - In case of a subsequent offence, the fine may extend to INR 5,000,000 (Indian Rupees Five Million) and imprisonment of up to 5 (five) years.
  - The CCPA can also prohibit the endorser of a misleading advertisement from endorsing that particular product or service for a period of up to 1 (one) year. For every subsequent offence, the period of prohibition may extend to 3 (three) years.

- Whoever, by himself or by any other person on his behalf, manufactures for sale or stores or sells or distributes or imports any product containing an adulterant shall be punished, if such act:
    - Does not result in any injury to the consumer, with imprisonment for a term which may extend to six months and with fine which may extend to one lakh rupees;
    - Causing injury not amounting to grievous hurt to the consumer, with imprisonment for a term which may extend to one year and with fine which may extend to three lakh rupees;
    - Causing injury resulting in grievous hurt to the consumer, with imprisonment for a term which may extend to seven years and with fine which may extend to five lakh rupees; and
    - Results in the death of a consumer, with imprisonment for a term which shall not be less than seven years, but which may extend to imprisonment for life and with fine which shall not be less than ten lakh rupees.
- The offences under clauses (c) and (d) shall be cognizable and non-bailable.

❏ **CPA and medical profession**:
- Supreme Court declared that doctors should be treated just like other providers of the services and therefore they are under the same obligation under CPA Act.
- A person who treated free of cost at either government or charitable trust run hospital is not considered as consumer under this Act.
- Hospitals are liable for redressal for both temporary and permanent staff members' faults.
- Complaints should be filed within 2 years from the date of incidence.
- But in recent amendment the word "healthcare" has been dropped.

BIBLIOGRAPHY

1. http://ncdrc.nic.in/bare_acts/Consumer%20Protection%20Act-1986.html
2. http://www.medindia.net/indian_health_act/consumer_protection_act_and_medical_profession_introduction/list-of-acts.htm
3. https://consumeraffairs.nic.in/sites/default/files/CP%20Act%202019.pdf
4. https://www.mondaq.com/india/Consumer-Protection/838108/Consumer-Protection-Act-2019-Key-Highlights
5. https://www.jagranjosh.com/general-knowledge/meaning-and-features-of-consumer-protection-act-2019-1578557665-1

CHAPTER 5

Concepts of Communication in Health Education

CHAPTER OUTLINE

5.1 Behavior change: Concept, steps, techniques and models
5.2 Basic methods of communication
5.3 Barriers to effective communication
5.4 Social and behavior change communication
5.5 Basics of health education and health promotion

5.1 BEHAVIOR CHANGE: CONCEPT, STEPS, TECHNIQUES AND MODELS

- Behavior is acquired and amenable to change.
- It is an observable action.
- It is reaction to specific circumstances or stimuli.
- It is affected by factors like genetic, social, cultural, attitude, emotions, perceived risk and benefits.

CATEGORIES OF HEALTH BEHAVIOR

- **Preventive health behavior:** Any activity undertaken by an individual who believes himself (or herself) to be healthy, for the purpose of preventing or detecting illness in an asymptomatic state.
- **Illness behavior:** Any activity undertaken by an individual who perceives himself to be ill, to define the state of health, and to discover a suitable remedy.
- **Sick-role behavior:** Any activity undertaken by an individual who considers himself to be ill, for the purpose of getting well. It includes receiving treatment from medical providers, generally involves a whole range of dependent behaviors and leads to some degree of exemption from one's usual responsibilities.

STEPS OF CHANGE IN BEHAVIOR

- **Knowledge:** Person gains knowledge about new behavior through recalling messages and understands their meanings.
- **Approval:** After discussing with professionals, colleagues and family members, person approves the new behavior and responds favourably to messages.
- **Intention:** Once the person understands the benefits of changing behavior, they intend to consult the provider to discuss the strategies to adopt these practices in future.
- **Practice:** The person goes to provider of information/supplies/services. One then attempts new behavior and continues to practice.
- **Advocacy:** One can then promote the new behavior through their social or professional networks as a satisfied practitioner. For example, A hypertensive person develops habit of regular monitoring of blood pressure which helped in controlling blood pressure, will tell other hypertensive persons to do so.

Techniques of Behavior Change

- **Information:** It is used with the assumptions that audience do not have the required information. Usually required information then delivered in the one-way kind of communication.
- **Education:** It focuses on applying knowledge through techniques like demonstrations which builds confidence and makes behaviors convenient.
- **Motivation:** It is useful only after information is established. Motivation works as driving force to bring behavior change. Motivation can be done through rationale appeal, emotional appeal, threat/fear appeal, joy/fun appeal.
- **Reinforcement:** It is used to sustain behavior change.
- **Social Pressure:** When person in need of health services not willing to undergo treatment is encouraged by near and dear ones to avail health services.

Glimpse of some of the Theories and Models of Behavior Change

- **The rational model** also known as the "knowledge, attitudes, practices model" (KAP), is based on the premise that increasing a person's knowledge will prompt a behavior change.
- **The health belief model** which explains human health decision-making and subsequent behavior is based on the following six constructs: perceived susceptibility, severity, benefits and barriers, cues to action and self-efficacy.
- **The transtheoretical model of change** in which behavior change is viewed as a progression through a series of five stages: pre-contemplation, contemplation, preparation, action and maintenance.
- **The theory of planned behavior:** The theory holds that intent is influenced not only by the attitude towards behavior but also the perception of social norms (the strength of others' opinions on the behavior and a person's own motivation to comply with those of significant others) and the degree of perceived behavioral control.
- **The activated health education model:** This is a three-phase model that actively engages individuals in the assessment of their health (experiential phase); presents information and creates awareness of the target behavior (awareness phase); and facilitates its identification and clarification of personal health values and develops a customized plan for behavior change (responsibility phase).

Concepts of Communication in Health Education

- **Social cognitive theory:** According to this theory, three main factors affect the likelihood that a person will change health behavior: self-efficacy, goals and outcome expectancies. If individuals have a sense of self-efficacy, they can change behavior even when faced with obstacles.
- **Communication theory:** This theory holds that multilevel strategies are necessary depending on who is being targeted, such as tailored messages at the individual level, targeted messages at the group level, social marketing at the community level, media advocacy at the policy level and mass media campaigns at the population level.
- **Diffusion of innovation theory:** This theory holds that there are five categories of people: innovators, early adopters, early majority adopters, late majority adopters and laggards; and the numbers in each category are distributed normally: the classic bell curve. By identifying the characteristics of people in each adopter category, health educators can more effectively plan and implement strategies that are customized to their needs.

Details of the Important Models and Theories
Health Belief Model (1950)
- The Health Belief Model (HBM) was developed to understand the failure of people to adopt disease prevention strategies like screening tests and later on for patients' responses to symptoms and compliance with medical treatments.
- The HBM derives from psychological and behavioral theory with the two components:
  1. The desire to avoid illness, or conversely get well if already ill; and,
  2. The belief that a specific health action will prevent, or cure, illness.
- There are six constructs of the HBM:
  1. Perceived susceptibility
  2. Perceived severity
  3. Perceived barriers
  4. Perceived benefits
  5. Cue to action
  6. Self-efficacy

  Example:

Construct	Message example
Perceived susceptibility	So, you don't think dengue is a real problem. It is here in our community now. Young and old get sick with dengue
Perceived severity	It is (dengue) a killer!
Perceived barriers	Little time to do a clean-up to reduce mosquito breeding sites. No problem. Use the action plan checklist. Use it once a week
Perceived benefits	If everyone spends just a few minutes each week to clean-up stagnant water, throwaway unneeded containers, or cover them, it will... reduce dengue fever

Limitations of Health Belief Model
- It does not account for a person's attitudes, beliefs, or other individual determinants that dictate a person's acceptance of a health behavior.

- It does not take into account behaviors that are habitual and thus may inform the decision-making process to accept a recommended action (e.g., smoking).
- It does not take into account behaviors that are performed for non-health related reasons such as social acceptability.
- It does not account for environmental or economic factors that may prohibit or promote the recommended action.
- It assumes that everyone has access to equal amounts of information on the illness or disease.
- It assumes that cues to action are widely prevalent in encouraging people to act and that "health" actions are the main goal in the decision-making process.
- The HBM is more descriptive than explanatory, and does not suggest a strategy for changing health-related actions.

Theory of Planned Behavior
- The Theory of Planned Behavior (TPB) started in 1980.
- The key component to this model is behavioral intent.
- It suggests that behavioral achievement depends on both motivation (intention) and ability (behavioral control).
- It distinguishes between three types of beliefs—behavioral, normative, and control.
- The TPB is comprised of six constructs:
  1. Attitudes
  2. Behavioral intention
  3. Subjective norms
  4. Social norms
  5. Perceived power
  6. Perceived behavioral control.

Limitations of the Theory of Planned Behavior
- It assumes the person has acquired the opportunities and resources to be successful in performing the desired behavior, regardless of the intention.
- It does not account for other variables that factor into behavioral intention and motivation, such as fear, threat, mood, or past experience.
- It does not take into account environmental or economic factors that may influence a person's intention to perform a behavior.
- It assumes that behavior is the result of a linear decision-making process, and does not consider that it can change over time.
- It does not say anything about actual control over behavior.
- It does not address the time frame between "intent" and "behavioral action".

The TPB has shown more utility in public health than the Health Belief Model, but it is still limiting in its inability to consider environmental and economic influences.

Diffusion of Innovation Theory
- Diffusion of innovation (DOI) theory was developed by EM Rogers in 1962.
- Adoption means that a person does something differently than what they had previously and it is possible when person perceives the idea, behavior, or product as new or innovative.

- Researchers have found that people who adopt an innovation early have different characteristics than people who adopt an innovation later.
- There are five established adopter categories and for promoting an innovation, there are different strategies used to appeal to the different adopter categories.
- Categories:
  - **Innovators:** These are people who want to be the first to try the innovation.
  - **Early Adopters:** These are people who represent opinion leaders. They enjoy leadership roles, and embrace change opportunities.
  - **Early Majority:** These people are rarely leaders, but they do adopt new ideas before the average person.
  - **Late Majority:** These people are skeptical of change, and will only adopt an innovation after it has been tried by the majority.
  - **Laggards:** These people are bound by tradition and very conservative. They are very skeptical of change and are the hardest group to bring on board.

Limitations of Diffusion of Innovation Theory
- Much of the evidence for this theory did not originate in public health.
- It does not foster a participatory approach to adoption of a public health program.
- It works better with adoption of behaviors rather than cessation or prevention of behaviors.
- It does not take into account an individual's resources or social support to adopt the new behavior (or innovation).

The Transtheoretical Model (Stages of Change)
- Transtheoretical model (TTM) (also called the Stages of Change Model), developed by Prochaska and DiClemente in the late 1970s.
- It was used first time for the people who wanted to quit smoking.
- It is focused on the decision-making of the individual and is a model of intentional change. The TTM operates on the assumption that change in behavior occurs continuously through a cyclical process.
- The TTM is not a theory but a model based on different behavioral theories.
- The TTM posits that individuals move through six stages of change (**Fig. 5.1**):
  1. **Precontemplation:** In this stage, people do not intend to take action in the foreseeable future (defined as within the next 6 months). People are often unaware that their behavior is problematic or produces negative consequences. People in this stage often underestimate the pros of changing behavior and place too much emphasis on the cons of changing behavior.
  2. **Contemplation:** In this stage, people are intending to start the healthy behavior in the foreseeable future (defined as within the next 6 months). People recognize that their behavior may be problematic, and a more thoughtful and practical consideration of the pros and cons of changing the behavior takes place, with equal emphasis placed on both. Even with this recognition, people may still feel ambivalent toward changing their behavior.

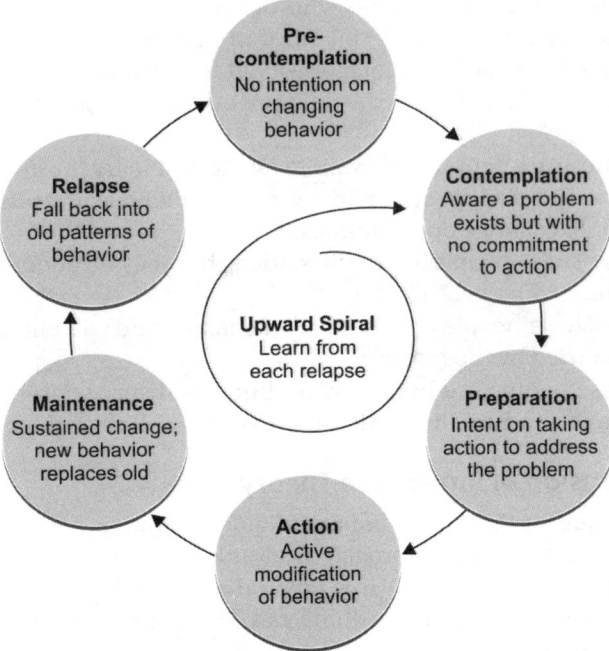

Fig. 5.1: Stages of behavior changes.

2. **Preparation (Determination):** In this stage, people are ready to take action within the next 30 days. People start to take small steps toward the behavior change, and they believe changing their behavior can lead to a healthier life.
3. **Action:** In this stage, people have recently changed their behavior (defined as within the last 6 months) and intend to keep moving forward with that behavior change. People may exhibit this by modifying their problem behavior or acquiring new healthy behaviors.
4. **Maintenance:** In this stage, people have sustained their behavior change for a while (defined as more than 6 months) and intend to maintain the behavior change going forward. People in this stage work to prevent relapse to earlier stages.
5. **Termination:** In this stage, people have no desire to return to their unhealthy behaviors and are sure they will not relapse. Since this is rarely reached, and people tend to stay in the maintenance stage, this stage is often not considered in health promotion programs.

Limitations of the Transtheoretical Model

- The theory ignores the social context like SES and income.
- The lines between the stages can be arbitrary with no set criteria of how to determine a person's stage of change.
- There is no clear sense for how much time is needed for each stage, or how long a person can remain in a stage.
- The model assumes that individuals make coherent and logical plans in their decision-making process when this is not always true.

BIBLIOGRAPHY

1. http://www.ogelk.net/dersnot/tip/healthbehaviorders.pdf
2. https://applications.emro.who.int/dsaf/EMRPUB_2012_EN_1362.pdf
3. https://egyankosh.ac.in/bitstream/123456789/48007/1/Unit-1.pdf
4. https://sphweb.bumc.bu.edu/otlt/mphmodules/sb/behavioralchangetheories/BehavioralChange Theories_ print.html
5. Jeffrey LL. (2005). The Use of the Health Belief Model in Dengue Health Education. WHO Regional Office for South-East Asia. https://apps.who.int/iris/handle/10665/164117
6. McDonnell BP, Regan C. Smoking in pregnancy: pathophysiology of harm and current evidence for monitoring and cessation. The Obstetrician & Gynaecologist. 2019;21:169–75. https://doi.org/10.1111/tog.12585
7. Pacheco I. The Stages of Change (Prochaska & Diclemente). 2012. [http://socialworktech.com/2012/01/09/stages-of-change-prochaska-diclemente/]
8. Prochaska JO, DiClemente CC. Stages and processes of self-change of smoking: toward an integrative model of change. J Consult Clin Psychol. 1983;51:390–5.

5.2 BASIC METHODS OF COMMUNICATION

INTRODUCTION

- Communication can be regarded as a two-way process of exchanging or shaping ideas, feelings and information.
- Communication is a two-way interaction between two or more people. Good communication means both good verbal communication (words and tone of voice) and good non-verbal communication (body language).
- Communication is more than mere exchange of information.
- It is a process necessary to pave way for desired changes in human behavior, and informed individual and community participation to achieve predetermined goals.
- Communication strategies can enhance learning.
- Communication is helpful to provide education, information, counselling, motivation, health development and persuasion.
- The ultimate goal of all communication is to bring about a change in the desired direction of the person who receives the communication.

Level	Domain
Cognitive	Knowledge
Affective	Attitude
Psychomotor	Skills

- Communication is part of our normal relationship with other people. Our ability to influence others depends on our communication skills, e.g., speaking, writing, listening, reading and reasoning. These skills are much needed in health education.
- It is said that without communication an individual could never become a human being, without mass communication, he could never become a part of modern society.

The communication process: It has the following main components.

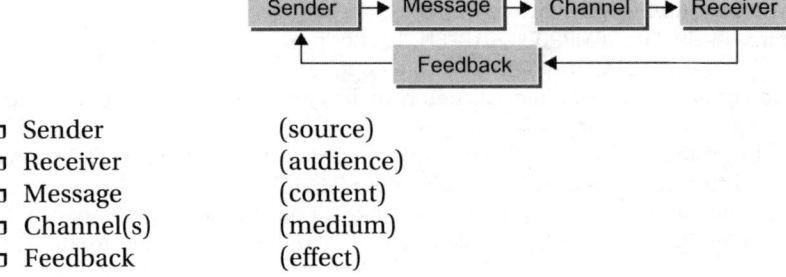

- Sender (source)
- Receiver (audience)
- Message (content)
- Channel(s) (medium)
- Feedback (effect)

1. Sender
- The sender (communicator) is the originator of the message.
- Effective communicator must be knowing objectives, audience, audiences' interest and needs, channels of communication, own professional abilities and limitations.
- The impact of the message will depend on communicator's (sender's) knowledge and prestige in the community.

2. Receiver
- As audience it may be a single person or a group of people.
- It is this element of audience and their frame of mind (e.g., opinions, attitudes, prejudices) which lends meaning to all the different types of communication.
- Controlled (homogeneous) audience is always better than uncontrolled (free) audience to have greater chances of an effective communication.

3. Message
- Communicator transmits message may be in the form of words, pictures or signs to the audience to receive, understand, accept and act upon.
- Message must be clear, understandable, timely, culturally and socially appropriate, in line with the objective and based on felt needs of the audience.
- Transmitting the right message to the right people at the right time is a crucial factor in successful communication.

4. Channels of Communication
- By channel is implied the "physical bridges" or the media of communication between the sender and the receiver.
- The total communication effort is based on three media systems:
  1. Interpersonal communication
  2. Mass media
  3. Traditional or folk media
     - Interpersonal communication:
       - The most common channel of communication is the interpersonal or face-to-face communication.

- Being personal and direct it is more persuasive and effective than any other form of communication.
- Interpersonal communication is particularly important in influencing the decisions of the undecided persons.
- Mass media:
  - In mass communication, the channel is one or more of the following "mass media", viz TV, radio, printed media, etc.
  - Mass media have the advantage of reaching a relatively larger population in a shorter time than is possible with other means.
  - Being one-way channels of communication, mass media carry messages only from the center to the periphery; feedback mechanisms are poorly organized.
  - Being impersonal media, they are usually not effective in changing established modes of behavior.
- Folk media:
  - Every community has its own network of traditional or folk media.
  - These are important channels of communication close to the cultural values of the rural population.
  - Health messages may be communicated through these traditional media.

5. Feedback

- It is the flow of information from the audience to the sender.
- It is the reaction of the audience to the message.
- If the message is not clear or otherwise not acceptable the audience may reject it outright.
- The feedback thus provides an opportunity to the sender to modify his message and render it acceptable.
- Feedback is generally obtained through opinion polls, attitude surveys and interviews.
- It can rectify transmission errors.
- Since effective communication is made by uses a variety of methods to help people understand their own situations and choose actions that will improve their health.

7Cs: It is tool of effective communication:
1. **Clarity:** It is message with clear ideas and in a language that is easy to understand.
2. **Completeness:** It should convey all the necessary information required by audiences thus it brings the desired response.
3. **Conciseness:** Communicating message with least possible words thus it is time saving. It means complete and brief.
4. **Concreteness:** Communication which is specific based on facts and figures.
5. **Correctness:** No grammatical error in the communication and accuracy in stating facts. It has greater impact on audience.
6. **Consideration:** Before putting any message in front of receiver consider their problems from their points of view.
7. **Courtesy:** Courtesy means the message must have sender's expression as well as must have the respect for the receiver. Courtesy strengthen the relations.

Types of Communication

One-way communication (Didactic Method)	• Communication is "one-way" from the communicator to the audience. Ex. Lecture • As its imposing of knowledge in authoritative manner with little audience participation and in the absence of feedback usually does not influence human behavior.
Two-way communication (Socratic method)	• Two-way method of communication in which both the communicator and the audience take part. • Audience usually have active participation. • It is an active and democratic way of learning. • It is more likely to influence human behavior.
Verbal communication	• Refers to the words used in the communication and the tone in which they are delivered. • It is largely conscious and is controlled by the individual speaking. • Direct verbal communication is more persuasive than non-direct written communication.
Non-verbal communication	• Its communication through it includes a whole range of bodily movements, postures, gestures, facial expressions (e.g., smile, raised eyebrows, frown, staring, gazing, etc.). • It is largely unconscious and often reveals to the observant the real feelings or message being conveyed. • Silence is non-verbal communication. • It can speak louder than words.
Formal communication	• It is the communication done in the line of authority.
Informal communication	• It is the gossip kind of communication which exists in every organization and sometimes it is more active than formal channels.
Visual communication	It comprises of charts and graphs, pictograms, tables, maps, posters, etc.
Telecommunication	It is the process of communicating over distance using electromagnetic instruments. Mass mode: Radio, TV and internet, etc. Point to Point (IPC type): telephone

BIBLIOGRAPHY

1. http://gmch.gov.in/sites/default/files/documents/Communication%20&%20Health.pdf.

5.3 BARRIERS TO EFFECTIVE COMMUNICATION

☐ Presence of communication barrier between the communicator and community often lead to failure of health education.
☐ Barrier could be physiological, psychological, environmental and cultural.

Concepts of Communication in Health Education

Type of barrier	Example
Physiological	Difficulties in hearing and speech Difficulties in expression
Psychological	Emotional disturbances Neurosis (e.g., anxiety) Level of intelligence
Environmental	Noise, invisibility, congestion
Cultural	Illiteracy, custom, belief, religion, attitude, language and sociol class differences
Others	Jargon, slang and acronyms

Ways to Overcoming Barriers to Communication
- Reduce outside noise
- Listen carefully
- Speak clearly and slowly
- Display clear signs
- Use interpreters
- Improve lighting
- Adapt to the person's needs

Listening LADDER for Good Listener
- **L**ook at the person speaking to you
- **A**sk question
- **D**on't interrupt
- **D**on't change the subject
- **E**xtend the conversation
- **R**espond verbally and non-verbally

Communication Can be Improved by the Following Factors (Fig. 5.2)

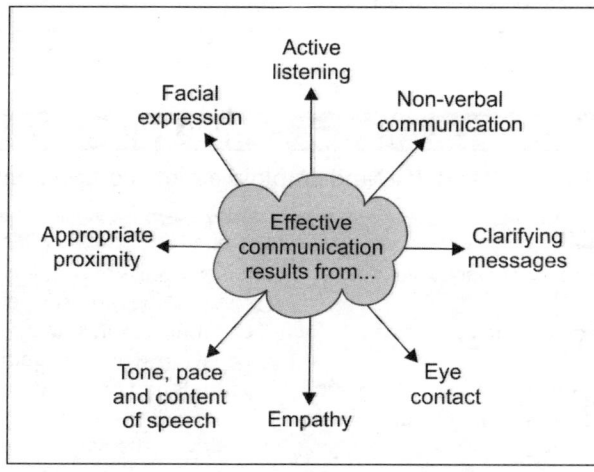

Fig. 5.2: Communication improving factors.

Verbal Communication Skills

- Active listening
- Verbal encouragement
- Positive tone of voice
- Using simple language
- Giving feedback
- Empathy
- Being non-judgemental

Positive Non-verbal Cues

- Leaning towards the client
- Smiling, not showing tension
- Presenting facial expressions which show interest and concern
- Maintaining eye-contact
- Nodding

Negative Non-verbal Cues

- Reading from a chart
- Glancing at one's watch
- Yawning or looking elsewhere
- Frowning
- Fidgeting

BIBLIOGRAPHY

1. Eisenhart C. Oral Language Development: The Foundation for Literacy, PHD dissertation, The University of Virginia, 1990.
2. http://cghealth.nic.in/dhs/NEW%20OFFERINGSFP%20GUIDELINES/Handbook%20for%20RMNCH%20Counsellors.pdf
3. https://resources.collins.co.uk/free/BTECHSCunit1.pdf

5.4 SOCIAL AND BEHAVIOR CHANGE COMMUNICATION

- SBCC has evolved from IEC and BCC and employs a more comprehensive approach.

IEC	BCC
• Information—Useful and representative data on a related issue. • Education—The process of transferring and embedding information. • Communication—A process through which two or more people share transfer of information, and which is complete only after compliance by both the parties on whether the information and education have been perceived in the same way as transmitted.	• It is a process of working with individuals, communities and societies to develop communication strategies to promote positive behaviors which are appropriate to their settings and provide a supportive environment which will enable people to initiate and sustain positive behaviors. • It clears all doubts and misconception and ensures change of the behavior from the negative to positive side.

Concepts of Communication in Health Education

IEC	BCC
• It is a process of working with individuals, communities and societies to develop communication strategies to promote positive behaviors which are appropriate to their settings. • It is made with assumption that one size fits all. • It tells how to behave. • It lacks pre-testing, methodology and taken for granted that merely awareness automatically leads to action. • IEC is the part of BCC. • Example: poster, leaflets, radio, TV advertisement.	• It enables to behave in intended way. • BCC builds on IEC. • BCC does not take into consideration the interaction of social factors with biological factors. Example: flipbook, pocketbook

- SBCC is the systematic application of interactive, theory and research driven communication processes and strategies that address change at individual, community and societal levels.
- SBCC is "use of communication to change behaviors, including service utilization, by positively influencing knowledge, attitude, and social norms" (Johns Hopkins University).
- SBCC refers to both social change and behavior change. Social change includes changes in social order and institutions, social behaviors and norms while behavior change includes changes in human behavior.
- SBCC looks at a problem from multiple sides by analyzing personal, societal, and environmental factors to facilitate healthy norms and choices and remove barriers to them.

SBCC encompasses three core elements:
- **Communication** uses channels and themes accessible and acceptable to an intended audience based on their needs and preferences;
- **Behavior change** makes efforts to simplify specific health actions, make them feasible so as to protect or improve health outcomes; and
- **Social change** brings about shifts in operationalization of an issue, community mobilization, public policies, and gender norms and relations.

Characteristics of SBCC: SBCC has Three characteristics: 1. Process, 2. Socio-ecological model, 3. Three key strategies
- SBCC is a process:
  - It is interactive, researched, planned, and strategic.
  - It aims to change social conditions and individual behaviors.
  - The SBCC process includes five steps shown in the **Figure 5.3**.
- SBCC applies a comprehensive, socio-ecological model to identify effective tipping points for change by examining:

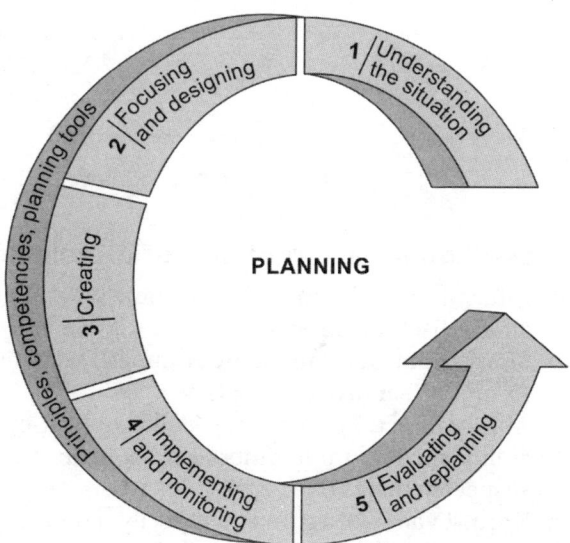

Fig. 5.3: C-Planning process.

- Individual knowledge, motivation, and other behavior change communication concepts.
- Social, cultural, and gender norms, skills, physical and economic access, and legislation that contribute to an enabling environment.
- A socio-ecological model examines several layers of influence to provide greater insight into the causes of problems.
❏ The levels of analysis (represented by the rings) are:
  - Innermost ring: the individual most affected by the issue (or self)
  - Next ring: Direct influencer as the interpersonal: partners, family, and peers
  - Next ring: Direct influencer as the community: organizations, service structures, providers, as well as products available.
  - Next ring: Indirect influences make up the outer enabling environment. Components may facilitate or hinder change, and include national policies and legislation, political forces, prevailing economic conditions, the private sector, religion, technology, and the natural environment

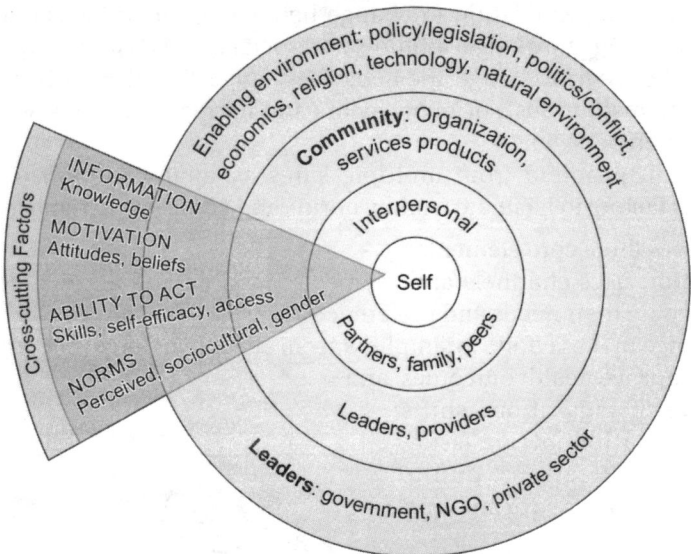

Fig. 5.4: Socio-ecological model for change.

Cross-Cutting Factors of the Socio-Ecological Model (Fig. 5.4)

❏ **Information:** Information that is timely, accessible, and relevant. Example, lack of knowledge about HIV transmission.
❏ **Motivation:** Determined by attitudes and beliefs about the issues we are trying to change. Example, fear of acquiring HIV
❏ **Ability to act:** For example, skills and self-efficacy. Example, lack of confidence in one's ability to stand up to others who may be stigmatizing or discriminating against someone suspected to be HIV+.
❏ **Norms:** Values of a group that specify actions expected by society, including perceived norms, socio-cultural norms, and gender norms. Example, socio-cultural and religious norms, gender norms, pervasive culture of stigma and discrimination toward these individuals.

Concepts of Communication in Health Education

❑ **SBCC uses three key strategies (Fig. 5.5):**

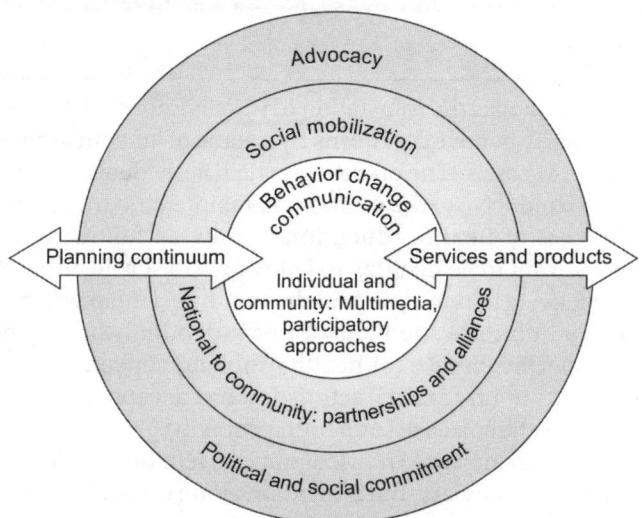

Fig. 5.5: Key strategies of SBCC.

- **Advocacy:** To raise resources as well as political and social leadership commitment to development actions and goals
- **Social mobilization:** For wider participation, coalition building, and ownership, including community mobilization
- **Behavior change communication:** For changes in knowledge, attitudes, and practices among specific audiences.

Ten Principles of SBCC

❑ Principle 1: Follow a systematic approach (e.g., C-Planning).
❑ Principle 2: Use research, not assumptions to drive your program.
❑ Principle 3: Consider the social context.
❑ Principle 4: Keep the focus on your audience(s).
❑ Principle 5: Use theories and models to guide decisions (e.g., the socioecological model).
❑ Principle 6: Involve partners and communities throughout.
❑ Principle 7: Set realistic objectives and consider cost-effectiveness.
❑ Principle 8: Use mutually reinforcing materials and activities at many levels.
❑ Principle 9: Choose strategies that are motivational and action-oriented.
❑ Principle 10: Ensure quality at every step.

BIBLIOGRAPHY

1. https://c-changeprogram.org/sites/default/files/sbcc_module0_intro.pdf
2. https://egyankosh.ac.in/bitstream/123456789/57206/1/Unit7.pdf
3. McKee, Neill, Erma Manoncourt, Chin Saik Yoon, Rachel Carnegie, (Editors) 2000. Involving people, evolving behavior. New York: UNICEF; Penang: Southbound.
4. McKee, Neill. 1992. Social mobilization & social marketing in developing communities: Lessons for communicators. Penang: Southbound

5.5 BASICS OF HEALTH EDUCATION AND HEALTH PROMOTION

HEALTH EDUCATION

- Definition: "Health education is the translation of what is known about health, into desirable individual and community behavior patterns by means of an educational process".
- Definition given by John M Last is "The process by which individuals and groups of people learn to behave in a manner conducive to the promotion, maintenance or restoration of health".
- The dynamic definition of health education is now as follows: "a process aimed at encouraging people to want to be healthy, to know how to stay healthy, to do what they can individually and collectively to maintain health, and to seek help when needed".
- Strategies designed to influence the behavior of individuals or groups will vary greatly depending upon the specific disease (or health problem) concerned and its distribution in the population as well as upon the characteristics and acceptability of available methods preventing or controlling that disease (or health problem).
- Health education can help to increase knowledge and to reinforce desired behavior patterns.
- It is clear that education is necessary, but education alone is insufficient to achieve optimum health. The target population must have access to proven preventive measures or procedures.

Emphasis of health education has been shifted from
- Prevention of disease to promotion of health
- The modification of individual behavior to modification of "social environment" in which the individual lives
- Community participation to community involvement; and
- Promotion of individual and community "self reliance".

Aims and Objectives
- To encourage people to adopt and sustain health promoting lifestyle and practices;
- To promote the proper use of health services available to them;
- To arouse interest, provide new knowledge, improve skills and change attitudes in making rational decisions to solve their own problems; and
- To stimulate individual and community self-reliance and participation to achieve health development through individual and community involvement at every step from identifying problems to solving them.

Role of Healthcare Providers
- To provide opportunities for people to learn how to identify and analyse health and health-related problems, and how to set their own targets and priorities;
- To make health and health-related information easily accessible to the community.
- To indicate to the people alternative solutions for solving the health and health-related problems they have identified; and
- To ensure people must have access to proven preventive measures.

Approach to Health Education

There are 4 well-known approaches to health education:
1. Regulatory approach or coercive approach
2. Service approach
3. Health education approach
4. Primary healthcare approach

1. Regulatory Approach or Coercive Approach

- Regulation may be defined as any governmental intervention, direct or indirect, designed to alter human behavior.
- Regulations may take many forms ranging from prohibition to imprisonment.
- The coercive or regulatory approach acts through a variety of external control or laws like the Cigarettes (Regulation of Production, Supply and Distribution) Act or the use of compulsory seat belts.
- This approach seems simplest ad quickest to improve health or to being desired behavior change but not the case in reality as lots of failure have been observed in different laws.
- This approach has highest applicability and usefulness during emergency situations.
- Possible reasons for the failure of this approach could be:
  - Only legislation cannot eradicate the cause of the disease.
  - Legislation has very limited role in the areas where people's personal choice matters, for example legislation cannot force people to adopt healthy lifestyle. Legislation can be successful when the majority of people are in favor of it and if it does not interfere with the rights of the individual.

2. Service Approach

- It was used earlier in 1960 as part of basic services where services were provided at people's doorstep without considering felt needs assessment which resulted in failure of this approach.
- Even today in some pockets of the country it has been observed that people still are not using sanitary latrine even though latrines have been built by government free of cost. It means any service which is provided even free of cost may not be utilized unless it is based on people felt needs.

3. Health Education Approach (Table 5.1)

- Health education approach have been successful in many solving many problems like cessation of smoking, use of safe water supply, fertility control.
- This approach basically based on principle of making individual well informed, educated and encouraged to make right decision on their own.
- Results of this approach could be slow but are enduring.
- This approach is useful when applied among young generation as behavior pattern sets in early age as once, they are formed then difficult to change.

Concepts of Communication in Health Education

Table 5.1: Propaganda and health education.

Propaganda	Health education
• It is a passive process of instillation of knowledge in the minds of the people. • It prevents the creative thinking by providing readymade slogans. • It develops common way of behavior according to mould used. • It hits to people's emotion. • It is information oriented.	• It is an active process of acquiring knowledge and skills by the people. • It enables people think more wisely. • It promotes self-expression and individuality of behavior. • It advocates reasoning. • It is action oriented.

4. Primary Healthcare Approach
- This the new approach and fundamental shift from the earlier approaches.
- This is the most effective approach based on two principles of primary healthcare namely community participation and intersectoral coordination.
- Main objective is to make individuals self-reliant in matters of health.
- In this approach we need to ensure that people receive the necessary guidance from health care providers in identifying their health problems and finding workable solutions.

Models of Health Education
- **Medical Model:**
  - It explains disease and illness information with medical facts.
  - Knowledge and behavior gap is not reduced.
- **Motivational Model:** After the awareness of information; individual gets interest in particulate matter. Motivation includes evaluation and decision making. Evaluation is a mental exercise after that individual takes decision to accept or reject the idea.
- **Social Intervention Model:** It is based on fact that individual can easily accept new idea if it is already followed or approved by their known people.

Principles of Health Education
- **Credibility:** It is the degree to which the message is perceived as trustworthy by the receiver and it must be consistent and compatible with scientific knowledge and also with the local culture, educational system and social goals.
- **Interest:** It is a very obvious that people are likely to listen to those things which are of their interest. We must find out the "felt needs", that is needs the people feel about themselves. And whenever any health program is based on "felt needs" people will gladly participate in the program; and only then it will be a people's program.
- **Participation:** Community participation is a key in health education.
- **Motivation**: In health education context, Awakening desire to learn is called motivation. There are two types of motives—primary (internal) and secondary (external). Primary motives (e.g., sex, hunger, survival) are inborn desires while secondary motives are praise, love, rivalry, rewards and punishment, and recognition.
- **Comprehension:** In health education, the level of understanding, education and literacy of people are very important factors. Communication always to be done in the language people understand and with consideration of the mental capacity of the audience.

Concepts of Communication in Health Education

- **Reinforcement:** Repetition at intervals is necessary otherwise there is very possibility of the individual going back to the pre-awareness stage.
  - **Learning by doing:** The Chinese proverb : "If I hear, I forget; if I see, I remember; if I do, I know" illustrates the importance of learning by doing.
  - **Known to unknown:** In health education, it is recommended to proceed "from the concrete to the abstract"; "from the particular to the general"; "from the simple to the more complicated;" "from the easy to more difficult"; and "from the known to the unknown".
  - **Setting an example:** The health educator should set a good example like he /she must be nonsmoker before advising quitting smoking.
  - **Good human relations:** Building good relationship with people makes sharing of information, ideas and feelings much easier.
  - **Feedback:** For effective communication, feedback is very important as it helps to modify the message of health education and to make it more effective.
  - **Leaders:** Psychologists have shown and established that we learn best from people whom we respect and regard.

Methods in Health Communication (Fig. 5.6 and Table 5.2)

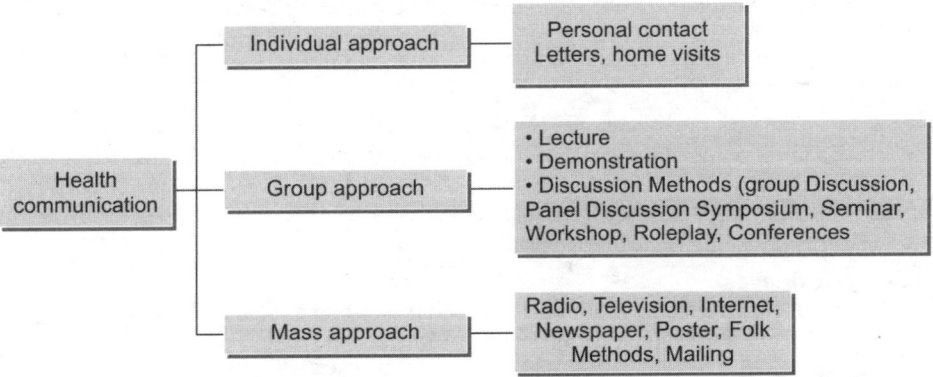

Fig. 5.6: Methods in health communication.

Individual approach: Advantage of this approach is one to one interaction is possible and person can discuss their thought and ask the question.

Group approach: Effective way of educating particular group like mother, child, old age, etc.

Mass approach: It is a one-way method but wide approach to educate the general public.

Table 5.2: Tools of health education.
Group Approach
Lecture • It is a carefully presentation of facts with organized thoughts and ideas by a qualified person. • The "chalk" is the visual component. • The talk is based on a topic of needs of the group. • The group should not be more than 30 members and the talk should not exceed 15 to 20 minutes.
Demonstration • It is based on principles of "seeing is believing" and "learning by doing". • It is a presentation to show how to perform a skill or procedure. • Procedure is explained step by step.

Group Approach

Symposium
- It is a series of speeches on a selected subject.
- Each expert presents the subject briefly.
- There is no discussion among the symposium members
- In the end of the session, audience can raise questions.

Group discussion
- A "group" is an "aggregation of people interacting in a face-to-face situation".
- Very effective method of health communication.
- It allows the participants to learn by freely exchanging their knowledge, ideas and opinions.
- It provides a wider interaction.

Panel discussion
- 4 to 8 persons who are qualified to talk about the topic sit and discuss a given problem/ topic, in front of a large group or audience.
- It is composed of a chairman or moderator and 4 to 8 speakers.
- It is started with chairman who opens the meeting, welcomes the group and introduces speakers and topic briefly and invites them to present their points of view.
- There is no specific agenda, no order of speaking and no set speeches.
- Audience is also allowed to take part.
- The discussion should be spontaneous and natural.
- It is extremely effective method.

Workshop
- It consists of a series of meetings, usually four or more, with emphasis on individual work, within the group, with the help of consultants and resource personnel.
- The total workshop may be divided into small sessions.
- It provides an opportunity to each participant.

Role play/ Socio drama
It is useful to discuss the problems of human relationship. Sometimes some values cannot be expressed in words. It is effective if situation is dramatized by the group of people.

Conferences and seminars
It is organized either state level or national level and length is either day or week.

Mass approach

- **Television:** It is a popular method. It is raising levels of understanding and helping people familiarize with things they have not seen before.
- **Radio:** It covers more audience and more cheaper method.
- **Internet:** It is a computer-based advanced and instant method. Health related literature is also available on this platform. Direct mailing is also effective.
- **Newspapers and printed material:** Most widely disseminated of all forms of literature. They reach only literates group of people.
- **Health museums and exhibitions** provide mass communication to large number of people. Photographic panels and three dimensional models with lighted visuals are effective way. Personal communication is also possible through workers who explain each item on the exhibit.
- **Folk media:** Mass communication also done by this method. It includes folk songs, dramas, dances, katha, puppet shows.

Concepts of Communication in Health Education

Audiovisual aids: To makes effective way of communication audiovisual aids are used.
- Auditory aids: Radio, microphones, amplifiers, tape-recorder, etc.
- Visual aids
  - Without projection: Charts, posters, chalk-board, flannel graph, exhibits, models, specimens, leaflets, etc.
  - Requiring projection: Slides, film strips.
- Combined AV aids: Television, cinema, etc.

Planning of Health Education (Fig. 5.7)

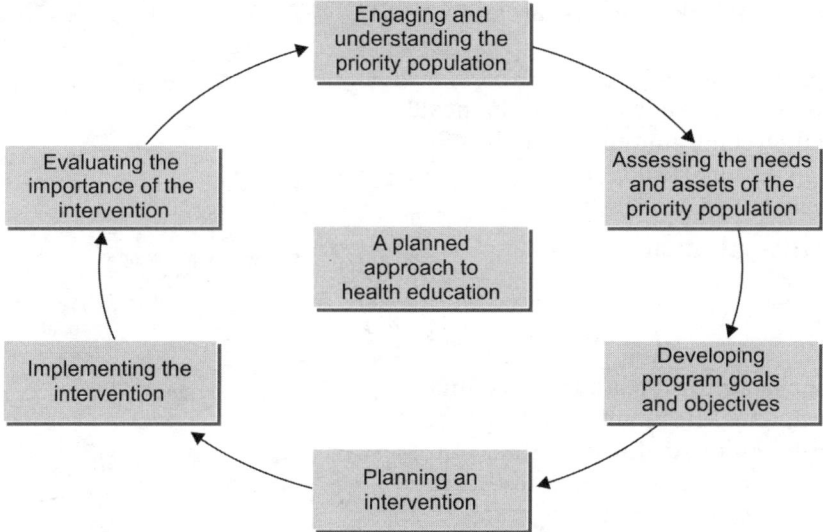

Fig. 5.7: Health education planning.

The specifics of a health education strategy in a local community have to be formulated in accordance with their needs and its socio-cultural, psycho-social, political, economic and situational characteristics.

The main steps in scientific health planning:
- Collecting information on specific problems as seen by the community
- Identification of the problem
- Deciding on priorities
- Setting goals and measurable objectives
- Assessment of resources
- Consideration of possible solutions
- Preparation of a plan of action: What will be done?, When? and By whom?
- Implementing the plan

Health Promotion

- Definition: "The process of enabling people to increase control over, and to improve, their health."

- Health promotion comprises three overlapping components: health education, health protection and prevention **(Fig. 5.8)**.

Ottawa Charter for Health Promotion

- International Conference on Health Promotion which was held in Ottawa, Canada, in 1986 **(Fig. 5.9)**.
- The logo has a circle with 3 wings.
- It represents five key action areas in health promotion:
  1. Build healthy public policy
  2. Create supportive environments for health
  3. Strengthen community action for health
  4. Develop personal skills, and
  5. Re-orient health services

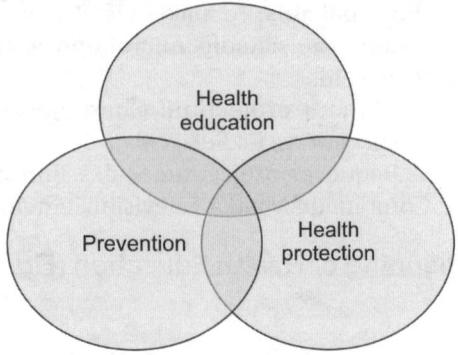

Fig. 5.8: Components of health promotion.

Three basic HP strategies:
1. To enable,
2. Mediate, and
3. Advocate

Advocacy for health to create the essential conditions for health; enabling all people to achieve their full health potential; and mediating between the different interests in society in the pursuit of health.

Principles of Health Promotion

- Health promotion involves the population as a whole in the context of their everyday life, rather than focusing on people at risk from specific diseases.

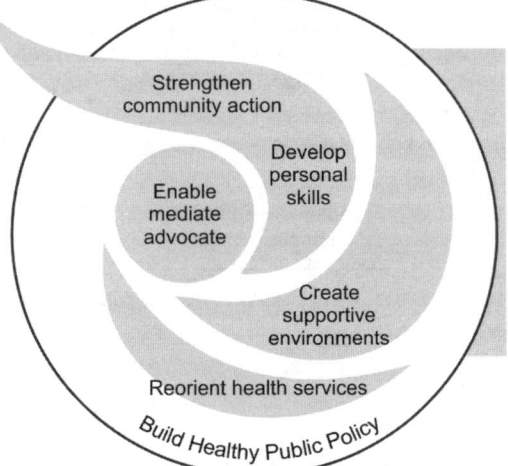

Fig. 5.9: The Ottawa Charter for health promotion.

- Health promotion is directed towards action on the determinants or cause of health. This requires a close cooperation between sectors beyond healthcare reflecting the diversity of conditions which influence health.
- Health promotion combines diverse but complementary methods or approaches including communication, education, legislation, organizational change, community change, and community development.
- Health promotion aims particularly at effective and concrete public participation. This requires the further development of problem defining and decision-making life skills both individually and collectively and the promotion of effective participation mechanisms.
- Health promotion is primarily a societal and political venture and not medical service although health professionals have an important role in advocating and enabling health promotion **(Fig. 5.10)**.

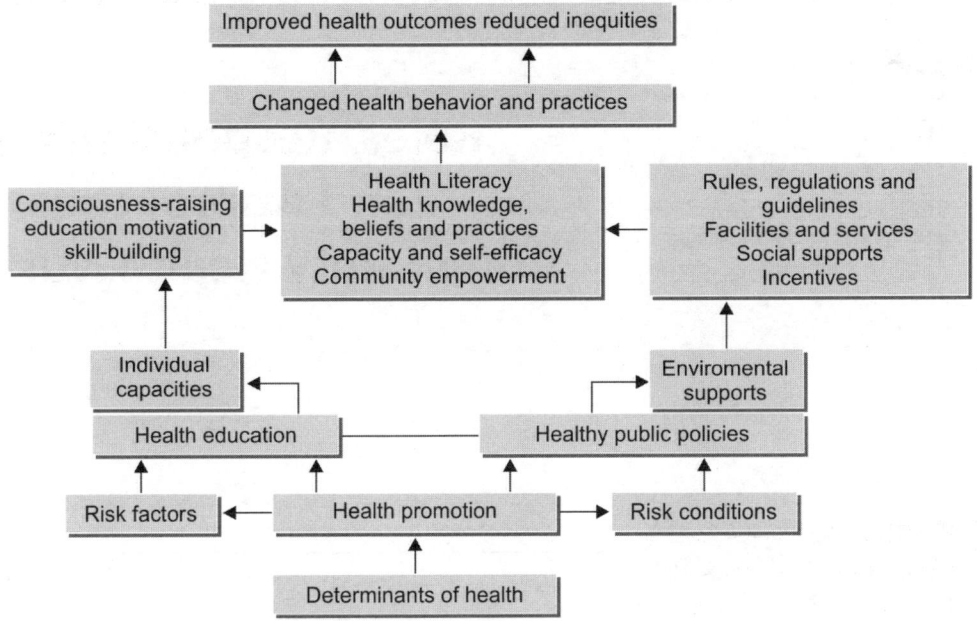

Fig. 5.10: Relationship between major health concepts.

Intervention in Health Promotion

- **Health education:** It is a cost effective method to prevent many diseases.
- **Nutritional intervention:** It includes nutritional education, food fortification, child feeding education, etc.
- **Environmental modification:** It includes non-clinical measures like hygiene and sanitation, safe water, insect control, etc. many infectious diseases can be prevented by this method.
- **Lifestyle and behavioral changes:** It is helpful to control the progress of disease.

Tones Formula Based on O'Byrne's Distinction

Health promotion = health education × healthy public policy

BIBLIOGRAPHY

1. https://applications.emro.who.int/dsaf/EMRPUB_2012_EN_1362.pdf
2. https://www.who.int/teams/health-promotion/enhanced-wellbeing/first-global-conference
3. http://ndl.ethernet.edu.et/bitstream/123456789/79382/5/Unit%201%20Introduction%20to%20health%20education%20and%20health%20promotion.pdf

CHAPTER 6

Roles, Responsibilities and Approaches of Community Health Nurse

CHAPTER OUTLINE

- 6.1 Community health nursing approaches
- 6.2 Role and responsibilities of community health nurse in family health services (MCH)
- 6.3 Role and responsibilities of community health nurse during home visit (including bag technique)
- 6.4 Basics of counseling
- 6.5 Role and responsibilities of community health nurse in supportive supervision and training

6.1 COMMUNITY HEALTH NURSING APPROACHES

TYPES OF APPROACHES

- Nursing process
- Problem solving approach
- Epidemiological approach
- Evidence-based approach
- People empowerment approach

Nursing Process

- Community health nursing process is a systematic way of determining a client health status, isolating health problems, developing the plan, initiate actions to implement the plan and evaluating the appropriateness of plan in problem resolution.
- Nursing process commonly consists of five phases:
  1. **Community assessment:** Identification of client, collection of data as subjective and objective information, organization of data and accurate documentation of data.
  2. **Community nursing diagnosis:** Classification, analysis, interpretation of data as human response patterns/functional status patterns, identification of actual/potential problems, validation and documentation of diagnostic statement.

3. **Planning:** Prioritizing the nursing diagnoses development of expected outcomes/possible solutions for the clients, possible interventions and documentation of the nursing care plan.
4. **Implementation:** Preparation phase, action or intervention phase, documentation of care as nurses notes, problem-oriented records using Subjective Objective Assessment Planning Implementing Evaluating Reassessing (SOAPIER) format, flowsheets lesson plans and computer-assisted records.
5. **Evaluation:** Evaluation is an ongoing process in which reassessment of clients status, making judgement about achievement of expected outcomes (progress) is done. Once the basis of judgement, revision in the nursing care plans are made. Nurses need to communicate their observations, challenges and innovations with their co-professionals, while solving unique problems of their clients.

Problem Solving Approach

The problem process involves:
- The systematic identification of a problem
- Determination of goals related to the problem
- Identification of possible solutions to achieve these goals
- Implementation of selected solutions
- Evaluation of goal achievement.

Epidemiological Approach

- Epidemiological analysis and measurement allow researchers to measure health status and measurement of disease occurrences in a population.
- Surveillance of disease yields epidemiological intelligence data by providing systematic count of disease frequency.
- These data can be in turn used to estimate the magnitude (size or amount) of health problems in the community, detect epidemics and understand natural history of a disease or detect potential emerging infectious disease threats.
- Another use of this approach is case finding to identify health status of people who are at risk.

Evidence-based Approach

- A way of providing nursing care that is guided by the integration of the best available scientific knowledge with nursing expertise.
- This approach requires nurses to critically assess relevant scientific data or research evidence, and to implement high-quality interventions for their nursing practice.

People Empowerment Approach

- Health of the individuals living in a defined community is not only their right but also their responsibility to take care of their own health and of the community at large.
- Without people's help, participation or cooperation, it is neither possible to make health care services accessible and acceptable to them nor it is feasible to achieve community health goals and aims.
- Community involvement and participation is recognized as one of the crucial supportive approach for successful implementation of community healthcare services.

- The extent of community involvement may vary from one community to another. It may depend upon their socioeconomic andcultural aspects, health attitude, health knowledge, etc.
- It ranges from true or active participation (i.e., people are knowledgeable and have a positive attitude and get involved in planning and implementing their healthcare) to passive recipient of care provided, i.e., the major responsibility of community involvement lies with health personnel who directly deal with people at the community level.
- They need to encourage and promote them for their participation.
- Community health nurse working with individuals, families, groups within the community as a whole for community health nursing services need to mobilize, encourage, organize and prepare them to take greater interest and responsibilities, develop self-reliance for their own health matters.

Other Approaches

- **The persuasive approach** implies convincing people through dialogue and educate them to change or modify their health behavior.
- **The enforcement approach** implies the use of more coercive (obligatory) measures such as use of legislation (like COTPA act for tobacco) to being intended positive healthy behavioral change.
- **Team approach** much crucial as community health is a problem solving process and a team approach is very necessary to deal with varied and complex health needs and problems at large.

BIBLIOGRAPHY

1. https://holyfamily.libguides.com/c.php?g=610214andp=4236305
2. https://nur.uobasrah.edu.iq/images/pdffolder/3.Approaches%20to%20community%20health.pdf
3. https://www.peoplesuniversity.edu.in/Nursing/wpcontent/uploads/2018/08/GNM-Vol-I-Community-Health-Nursing-Part-1-min.pdf

6.2 ROLE AND RESPONSIBILITIES OF COMMUNITY HEALTH NURSE IN FAMILY HEALTH SERVICES (MCH)

- Family health services defined as help in prevention of disease, promotion of health status and to rehabilitate the health of family and to achieve the optimum health status of family.
- **Factor related to family health services:**
  - Socioeconomic condition of the family: It is necessary to know as we can have idea about family budget and we can give idea how to improve financial condition of family like having small family, taking benefit of all government schemes.
  - Education status: Literacy is very important for understanding health problems and adopting healthy behavioral practices.
  - Culture and environment: Cultural and environmental factors could have very profound effect on overall health of family.
  - Availability of health services.
  - Family composition.

- **Aims of family health services:**
  - Reducing maternal morbidity and mortality
  - Family planning
  - Providing help in solving the problem of malnutrition in family
  - Providing health education to the family.
- **Principles of family health services:**
  - Community Health Nurse should have good relations with every family and should encourage the families to have good relation with each other and in the community.
  - Community health nurse should have the knowledge about all basic facts about the family like family size, occupation, customs, rituals and status of literacy, etc.
  - Problems should be identified and assigned the priority level.
  - Problems should be discussed with the family for finding the solution of the problems, opinion of the family members should be considered and the information about the available health and development facilities should be given to them.
  - Cooperation of the family members should be obtained to implement the desired plan of action.
  - Family should be encouraged to be self-sufficient to fulfill their needs and to pay attention to nutrition, health and family welfare.
  - At every contact/visit, a message should be given that is important from the point of view of family health.
  - Participation of family members is essential in family health nursing services.
- **Function of community health nurse in family health services:**
  - To do family health survey includes collecting demographic facts through preparing the list of houses along with location. Data related to number of pregnant women, infant, children and eligible couple must be gathered.
  - To motivate the family to adopt small family norms by explaining the importance and necessity of family planning and also education related to available various techniques of contraceptives including permanent methods.
  - To manage special clinics
  - To organizing family planning camps
  - To maintain records
  - To liaise the work.

FAMILY HEALTH NURSING PLAN

- Family health nursing process refers to a series of planning steps and intervention directed to meet the health needs and solving the problems of the family. Family health nursing process is the core of family healthcare.
- Steps of family health nursing plan:
  - **Family health assessment:** It is always desirable that nurse first takes the head of the family into confidence before starting assessment. Assessment mainly focuses on collecting the baseline information about the family and its environment. Tools like interviews (structured and nonstructured), questionnaires, observation (participant observation methods), anecdotal reports and review of available family records can be used to collect following data related to family:
    - *Family composition:* Family size, education, marital status, occupation, socioeconomic status, division in terms of role, labor and power.

- *Family environment:* Residence, neighborhood, community, housing, etc.
- *Family process:* Communication, patterns, decision-making, problem solving, etc.
- *Family function:* Physical, social, emotional, etc.
- *Family coping:* Conflict, life changes, family satisfaction, etc.
- Family health status
- *Family resources:* Support group, friends, financial, institutional, NGOs, etc.

☐ **Nursing diagnosis:** Nursing diagnosis is the clinical judgment about family's actual or potential health problems, which is based upon the data obtained from the family health assessment.

☐ **Planning:** Planning phase includes problems prioritization and establishing goal-objectives. Problem prioritization depends on:
- Family awareness about the problem
- Motivation of family members
- Nurse ability to influence
- Availability of resources
- Severity of the consequence (if the problem is unresolved)

After problem prioritization objectives are set nursing action are planned and family nursing care plan is prepared.

☐ **Implementation:** It refers to putting the nursing care plan into action.

☐ **Evaluation:** Evaluation is the process of measuring the extent to which goal or objectives of family care has been met. The effectiveness of implementation (care plan) is ascertained by noting the family responses and examining the outcomes, evaluation can be done as formative (evaluation during implementation phase) or as summative. The results of evaluation success or failure are utilize for further family health nursing processes. In case of failure appropriate modification. Each step of family health nursing care plan needs to be properly documented.

Main areas family health services are:
☐ Maternal and child health
☐ Family planning
☐ Family life education of parents
☐ Nutrition
☐ Healthy environment in the home
☐ Immunization services
☐ Care of the sick, aged person and handicapped in home.

☐ **Maternal and child health:** The main objectives of MCH services are:
- Protection from infection
- Promote growth and development of children up to 5 years
- Promote reproductive and safe motherhood
- Help to reduce malnutrition
- Improve health status of child and mother by health education
- Reduce infant and maternal mortality and morbidity rate

☐ **Family planning:**
- Family planning is considered to be one of the basic human rights and as necessary for better quality of life. Child spacing is important for, family health and mother health too. In family planning with help of GATHER approach, nurse educate community people

regarding different services and areas, e.g., proper spacing, diagnosis of reproductive tract disease, premarital examination, sex education, genetic counseling, adoption services, etc.

- **Family life education of parents:**
  - Community health nurse has many opportunities to help parents to build a good family life and to help their children to develop good personality.
  - Family life education is necessary to increase health status of each family member.
- **Nutrition of the family:**
  - Community health nurse should work with the family to improve their diet and nutritional status.
  - Community health nurse explains the importance of nutrition as it is main factor to improve immunity system and overall building healthy family.
  - Healthy habit of eating keeps body healthy.
- **Immunization services:**
  - Community health worker should give knowledge and immunization services to community people for protection, prevention and promotion of health of children and pregnant women.
  - Immunization program has important role In control of spread of communicable disease. Immunization program boost up body immune system.
- **Healthy environment in the home:** There are some points for health full environment at home are as follow:
  - Promote removal and proper disposal of all refuse, sullage water, and excreta by making sanitary latrine and composite pit.
  - Safe drinking water with water purification method suitable at home, e.g., boiling of water at 100°C.
  - Safe food by keep flies away from food and rat proof bins for storing grains.
  - Good ventilation by proper window at home and smokeless chulla or use of LPG stove.
- **Care of sick, aged person and handicap in home:**
  - **Care of sick:**
    - Community health nurse provide care to sick people and health education to community people regarding maintain of body hygiene.
    - Knowledge regarding good ventilation, rest and sleep, proper diet, etc. also given during home visit.
  - **Care of aged person:**
    - The aged person usually having problems like poor eyesight, hearing problem, lack of teeth, poor memory, etc. so, while providing care in a family, these all factors must be kept in mind.
    - Community health nurse provides knowledge to family member regarding check up of eyesight, ear and use of denture, etc.
    - Community health worker provides health education regarding proper nutrition for healthy body or maintain healthy immune system.
  - **Care of the handicapped person**
    - The community health nurse can help families to think and discuss the problem related to handicapped person at their home.
    - A nurse should educate people regarding all schemes and all services started by government of India for ease of handicapped peoples' life.

BIBLIOGRAPHY

1. https://www.peoplesuniversity.edu.in/Nursing/wpcontent/uploads/2018/08/GNM-Vol-I-Community-Health-Nursing-Part-1-min.pdf
2. https://www.glocaluniversity.edu.in/files/eContent/eNursing/family%20health%20services.pdf

6.3 ROLE AND RESPONSIBILITIES OF COMMUNITY HEALTH NURSE DURING HOME VISIT (INCLUDING BAG TECHNIQUE)

- **Definition:** Home visit as part of comprehensive healthcare in which health services are provided to individuals and families in their place of residence for the purpose of promoting maintaining or restoring health or of maximizing the level of independence while minimizing the effect of disability and illness, including terminal illness.
- Home visit is one of the oldest types of health services.
- Home environment is the most effective ways of increasing family's understanding and involvement in health problems.
- Home visit gives comprehensive picture of the family health status.
- Home health service refers to all the services and products provided to clients in their home, to maintain, restore, or promote their physical, mental, and emotional health.

PURPOSE OF HOME VISIT

- Afford the opportunity to gain more accurate assessment of the family structure and behavior in the natural environment.
- Provide opportunity to make observations of the home environment and to identify both barriers and supports for reaching family health promotion work.
- Meeting the family on their home ground may also contribute to family's sense of control and active participation in meeting their health needs.

OBJECTIVES OF HOME VISITING

- To create close relationship with communities and families
- To discover the condition in which the family lives and to identify how these conditions affect their health.
- To promote family health by providing family members with health education adapted to their levels of growth and development.
- To monitor the use of skill learned in health education.
- To demonstrate to the family how to administer healthcare needed by others family members.
- To refer to appropriate specialized services.

Advantages of Home Visit

- Familiar atmosphere makes communication easier than at hospital or clinic.
- All family members can be seen and assessed by one person at one visit.

- Can have better understanding about local problems, priorities, customs, difficulties, and resources.
- High risk families can be identified and visited as a priority.
- The health workers, can observe, assess, and act up on obvious and latent health problems. Health workers can follow these problems at subsequent visit.'
- Much can be assessed at one time. Example, personal hygiene, water supply, sanitation, waste disposed, food storage.
- More accurate assessment is done.
- Better understanding and good relationship is established with the family members.
- Advice will be practical and suited to the family's needs.

Limitations of Home Visit
- Time consuming
- Limited equipment can only be carried to home
- Appointment might be not kept
- Sometimes houses may be geographically not reachable.

Types of Home Care
- **Home for the aged:** For the elder greater than 65 years of age, who need a minimum care which is often characterized as "supervized living or residential care."
- **Basic home:** It is a home for those individuals who need assistance in activity of daily living (ADL), such as eating, breathing or routine nursing care including administration of medication.
- **Skilled home:** It is a home for those individuals with serious health problems who need 24 hours nursing care or supervision.

Phases and Activities of Home Visit
- **Initiation phase:** To clarify purpose of home visiting and share information to family member
- **Pre-visit phase:** To initiate contact with family and determine family willingness. Also, to prepare schedule of home visit and review records
- **On home phase:** Introduction him/her self-warm greeting-social interaction (to develop trusting r/s -implement nursing process.
- **Termination phase:** Review visit with family-plan for future visit
- **Post visit phase:** Record visit-plan for next visit.

Areas (Points) to be Assessed During Home Visit
- General cleanliness
- Solid waste disposal
- Sanitation facilities
- Personal hygiene
- Vaccination of infant
- Vaccination of women
- ANC
- Feeding of children <2 years
- Family planning

- Presence of insects/rodents in the house
- Presence of sick person in the house and action taken.

Basics of Bag Technique

- Definition: A specially prepared bag for carrying supplies to the field a clean and orderly way.
- Purposes
  - Helps the nurse to give service effectively in homes
  - Reduces the danger of spreading infections
  - Provides the necessary items needed in the field
  - Identifies the nurse in the field because a home visiting bag is a part of the uniform
- Contents of the bags can be grouped into: A. General supplies, B. Equipment and C. Others

A. General Supplies

- Soap and soap dish
- Plastic apron
- Plastic square to put the bag on
- Aluminum cup for water
- One or two small towels to dry the hand

B. Equipment/Instrument and Drugs

- Thermometer
- Fetoscope
- Scissors
- Artery forceps
- Tape measure
- Plaster
- Cotton
- Gauze
- Applicator
- Bandage
- Antiseptic solution
- Syringe and needle
- Gentian violet
- Tetracycline eye ointment
- Kidney dish
- Vaseline
- Tongue depressor,
- Disposable gloves
- Cord tie
- Anti pain
- Ergometrine tablets
- Ferrous sulphate
- Vitamin, A
- Test tube
- Baby scale
- Chloroquine
- Mebendazole
- BBL
- Pocket
- Small towel
- Soap and soap dish
- Plastic square
- Newspaper for placement of the gag
- Match

Responsibilities of Nurses

- Change inner lining of bag as needed
- Refill supplies as needed
- Use the bag correctly and do not put your properties on the bag
- Keep the bag clean and orderly
- Labe bottles
- Pay attention for broken equipment

- Report all broken equipment
- Do not miss equipment
- Go through nursing process and form family focused nursing.

BIBLIOGRAPHY

1. Daniel Mengistu and Equlinet Misganaw. Community Health Nursing: Lecture Notes for Nursing Students. Incollaboration with the Ethiopia Public Health Training Initiative, The Carter Center, the Ethiopia Ministryof Health, and the Ethiopia Ministry of Education, 2006.

6.4 BASICS OF COUNSELING

Counseling	Advice
It is a face to face communication through which a person is helped to make decision	It is a guidance regarding a decision
It is a non-judgmental method	It is a judgmental method
Choice is given to clients.	Choice to clients is not given.
Open ended questions are asked.	Close ended questions are asked.
It is a problem solving approach, bidirectional in nature	Unidirectional in nature
It is a active process	It is a passive process
It is a democratic in nature	It is a autocratic in nature

What is counseling
- Counseling is a two-way communication between a health care worker and a client, for the purpose of confirming or facilitating a decision by the client, or helping the client address problems or concerns.

Key components of counseling
- Mutual trust is established between client and provider. The provider shows respect for the client and identifies and addresses her/his concerns, doubts, and fears.
- The client and service provider give and receive relevant, accurate, and complete information that enables the client to make a decision.

Tasks involved in counseling
- Helping clients assess their own need for a range of health services, information and emotional support
- Providing information appropriare to clients' identified problems and needs
- Assisting clients in making their voluntary and informed decisions
- Helping clients develop the skills they will need to carry out the decision.

Benefits of counseling
Good counseling results in higher client satisfaction

Counseling should be CLEAR:
- Communicate clearly
- Listen
- Encourage and Empathize
- Ask
- Respect

Desired characteristics and skills of effective counselor

Counselor characteristics

An effective counselor:
- Believes in and is committed to the basic values and principles of family planning and client rights
- Is accepting, respectful, non-judgmental, and objective when dealing with clients
- Is aware of her/his own values and biases and does not impose them on clients
- Understands and is sensitive to cultural and psychological factors (such as family or community pressures) that may affect a client's decision to adopt family planning
- Always maintains client's privacy and confidentiality

Counselor skills

An effecrive counselor possesses strong technical knowledge:
- Knows all technical aspects of concerned service thoroughly
- Is prepared to answer questions comfortably on subjects such as myths, rumors, sexuality, reproductive and personal concerns
- Is able to use visual aids and explain technical information in language (that the client understands)
- Is able to recognize when to refer the client to a specialist or other provider

GATHER approach for counseling

G: Greet
- Empress respect and friendliness
- Give clients your full attention as soon as you meet them
- Be polite, friendly and respectful: Greet clients introduce yourself, and offer them seats
- Ask how you can help. Determine purpose of visit
- Explain what will happen during the visit
- Assure the client that all information discussed will be confidential
- Talk in a private place, where no one else can hear

A: Ask
- Ask about their problems as well as listening to any measures they have already taken to solve the problem
- Ask them how they believe that you can help them
- Ask for all the information needed to complete client records
- Listen to the answers to these questions which will guide the provider/counselor to methods most of appropriate for the clients' current needs
- Help clients express their feelings needs, wants and any doubts, concerns or questions
- Keep questions open, simple, and brief
Look at your client as you speak
- Show your interest and understanding at all time. Express empathy, Avoid judgments and opinions

T: Tell
- Tell the client about the available methods and possible choices that would best meet the client's current needs based on their reponses to the questions asked above
- Information should be personalized—that is put in terms of the clients own life
- Ask if the client wants to learn more and answer client concerns and questions

H: Help
- Help them to make their own decisions and guide them to look at various alternatives
- Help them to choose solutions which best fit their own personal circumstances
- Help client think about the results of each possible choice
- Ask if the clients wants anythings made clearer. Reword and repeat information as needed
- Check whether the client has made a clear decision. Specifically ask, "What have you decided to do? Wait for the client to answer

E: Explain
- Explain any misunderstandings.
- Ask some questions in order to check your understanding for important key points and repeat those key points in their own words if necessary
- If the method or services cannot be given at once, tell the client how, when, and where they will be provided
- Explain how to use the method
- Describe possible side effects and what to do if they occur
- Explain when to come back for routine follow-up or more supplies, if needed
- Explain any medical reasons to return

R: Return • Schedule and carry out return visit and follow-up of client At a follow-up visit: • Ask if the client has any questions or anything to discuss. Treat all concerns seriously • Ask if the client is satisfied. Have there been problems • Help the client handle any problems	• Ask if any health problems have come up since the last visit. Check if these problems make it better to choose another method or treatment. Refer clients who need care for health problems • Check if the client is using the method or treatment correctly • If a follow-up visit is not appropriate then you should give them the name of someone they can contact if they need help

- Counseling is a means of assisting people to understand and cope more effectively with their problems, improve health seeking behavior, bring about lifestyle modifications, etc.
- Counseling is an important means to share information related disease management, enabling treatment compliance, educate individuals and families for primary and secondary prevention and support in necessary health promotion.
- Few examples where counselling is most commonly required are:
  - Antenatal Care (ANC), Postnatal Care (PNC), Essential Newborn Care, Infant Young Child Feeding (IYCF), Nutrition counseling, Iron Folic acid tablet (IFA) use, Water Sanitation and Hygiene (WASH), Childhood Immunization, enabling Early Childhood Development (ECD), registration in government sponsored Maternity benefit schemes, etc.
  - Prevention of Reproductive Tract Infections (RTIs) and Sexually Transmitted Infections (STIs), health risk behaviors related to-substance abuse, diet, exercise, injury, violence, sexual and reproductive health, hygienic practices, social drop outs, menstrual hygiene, etc., in adolescents.
  - Adoption of Contraceptive for specific case, and facilitation for safe abortion services, post abortion follow-up care.
  - Prevention, of vector-borne diseases, prevention of infectious diseases such as TB, Leprosy, HIV/AIDS, STI/RTIs, etc., and for self-care, treatment compliance, identification of complications related to each of these conditions.
  - Lifestyle modification, addressing risk factors and treatment for NCDs.
  - Psychosocial support for mental health, awareness and stigma reduction activities and address the myths related to mental/neurological illnesses.

BIBLIOGRAPHY

1. http://cghealth.nic.in/dhs/NEW%20OFFERINGS-FP%20GUIDELINES/Handbook%20for%20RMNCH%20Counsellors.pdf
2. http://www.nrhmorissa.gov.in/writereaddata/Upload/Documents/Induction%20Training%20Module%20for%20CHOs.pdf

6.5 ROLE AND RESPONSIBILITIES OF COMMUNITY HEALTH NURSE IN SUPPORTIVE SUPERVISION AND TRAINING

IMPORTANCE OF SUPERVISION

- It provides opportunity for learning to fill the gaps in the knowledge or skills of the service provider.
- It helps in understanding ground realities and challenges.
- It motivates the health worker.
- Supervision helps in team building.
- Supervision also helps in making the workers aware of new guidelines.
- Supervision helps the workers relate better to the community.

The differences between supervision and monitoring:

Supervision	Monitoring
• Supervision is overseeing or watching over an activity or task being done by someone and ensuring that it is performed correctly. • Supervision deals with the performance of the people working within the programme including giving them support and assessing conditions in the health facility. • supervision usually having component of monitoring	• Monitoring is the continuous review of programme implementation to identify and solve problems so that activities can be implemented correctly and effectively. • Monitoring involves regular collection and analysis of information/data on aspects of the programme's activities. • Monitoring does not often or automatically have a supervisory element.

Types of Supervision Approach

Control approach	Supporting approach
• Focus on finding faults with individuals. • Supervisor is like a policeman. Episodic problem-solving. Little or no follow-up. • Punitive actions intended.	• Focus on improving performance and building relationships. • More like a teacher, coach, mentor. • Use local data to monitor performance and solve problems. Follow up regularly. • Only support provided.

Supportive Supervision

- Supportive supervision is a process of helping staff to improve their own work performance continuously. It is carried out in a respectful and non-authoritarian way with a focus on using supervisory visits as an opportunity to improve knowledge and skills of health staff.
- Supportive supervision encourages open, two-way communication, and building team approaches that facilitate problem-solving.
- It focuses on monitoring performance towards goals, and using data for decision-making, and depends upon regular follow-up with staff to ensure that new tasks are being implemented correctly.
- Supportive supervision is helping to make things work, rather than checking to see what is wrong.

Steps of Supportive Supervision

Steps of supportive supervision are seen in **Figure 6.1**.

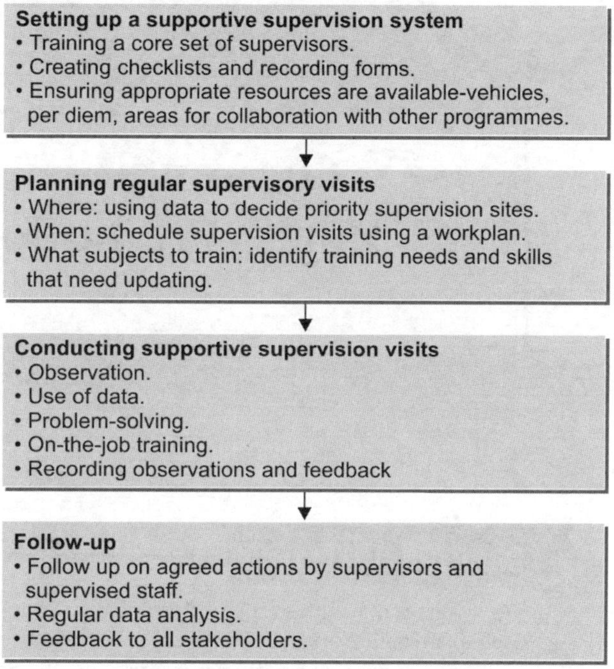

Types of Training in NHM

- **Induction training:** At the time of entry into service, Induction Training of at least four weeks duration must be made mandatory for all categories of health care workers. This must have components of requisite skill enhancement, management and knowledge about the drugs/equipment and services offered at all levels of health care. This must be completed in a fixed time frame.
- **In-service training:** It must be provided to all categories of health care workers to upgrade their knowledge and skills in technical and management fields at least once every two years.
- **Refresher training:** Refresher training and system of continuous education for health providers needs to be institutionalised. Knowledge and skills of every health provider should be upgraded after every two years.

Setting up a supportive supervision system
- Training a core set of supervisors.
- Creating checklists and recording forms.
- Ensuring appropriate resources are available-vehicles, per diem, areas for collaboration with other programmes.

↓

Planning regular supervisory visits
- Where: using data to decide priority supervision sites.
- When: schedule supervision visits using a workplan.
- What subjects to train: identify training needs and skills that need updating.

↓

Conducting supportive supervision visits
- Observation.
- Use of data.
- Problem-solving.
- On-the-job training.
- Recording observations and feedback

↓

Follow-up
- Follow up on agreed actions by supervisors and supervised staff.
- Regular data analysis.
- Feedback to all stakeholders.

Fig. 6.1: Supportive supervision.

BIBLIOGRAPHY

1. http://www.nihfw.org/doc/NCHRC-Publications/Module%20-%204.pdf
2. https://nhm.gov.in/images/pdf/guidelines/nrhmguidelines/national_training_strategy_final.pdf
3. Training for mid-level managers (MLM). Module 4: supportive supervision. Geneva: World Health Organization; 2008, republished 2020 under the licence: CC BY-NC-SA 3.0 IGO.

CHAPTER 7

Community Health Nurse's Role in Health Promotion and Maintenance

CHAPTER OUTLINE

7.1 Assessment of health status (anthropometry, BP and temperature measurement, breast self-examination and lab tests like Hb, urine sugar and albumin)
7.2 Provision of primary health care (routine health check up, immunization, counseling, management of common health problems)
7.3 Record keeping
7.4 Social issues affecting health and development of the family (women empowerment, child abuse, abuse of elders, female feticide, commercial sex workers, substance abuse)
7.5 Brief introduction of community resources (old age homes, orphanages, palliative care centers, hospice care centers)

7.1 ASSESSMENT OF HEALTH STATUS (ANTHROPOMETRY, BP AND TEMPERATURE MEASUREMENT, BREAST SELF-EXAMINATION AND LAB TESTS LIKE Hb, URINE SUGAR AND ALBUMIN)

ANTHROPOMETRY

Height Recording

- Keep the stadiometer (height measuring scale) on the floor against wall. Identify how much is each division.
- Ask the person to stand straight on the stadiometer and holding the head upright.
- Tell them to place the legs together, bringing the ankles and knees together.
- Read and record the scale.

Weight Recording

- Keep the weighing scale on a hard, flat surface and check for zero error before taking the weight
- Ask the person to stand straight on the weighing scale
- Read and record the scale from the top

Blood Pressure Recording

- Person rest at 5 minutes before measurement
- Select the type of blood pressure instrument
- Check that the bulb is properly attached to the tubing and there are no cracks or leakage
- Ask the person to sit on a chair or lie down on his/her left side or slightly tilt to the left on a flat surface
- Place the apparatus on a horizontal surface at the level of the person's heart
- Note any zero error, and replace with a functional sphygmomanometer
- Tie the cuff 3 cm above the elbow, placing both the tubes in front
- Raise the pressure of the cuff to 30 mm Hg above the level at which pulse is no longer felt
- Release pressure slowly and listen with stethoscope keeping it on brachial artery at the elbow
- Note the reading where the sound is heard (systolic pressure)
- Follow the sound and note reading where the sound disappears (diastolic)
- Deflate and remove the cuff; close the mercury column knob
- Record the reading.

Electronic BP Apparatus

Tie the cuff in the same way and keep the arms stable. Press the ON button and both systolic and diastolic pressure will be displayed automatically on the screen.

Temperature Recording

- Wash your hands.
- Take the thermometer and wipe it with cotton swab from bulb towards the tube
- Shake the thermometer with strong wrist movements until the mercury line falls to at least 95°F (35°C).
- Be sure the client's axilla is dry. If it is moist, pat it dry gently before inserting the thermometer.
- Place the bulb of thermometer in hollow of axilla at anterior inferior with 45 degree or horizontally.
- Keep the arm flexed across the chest, close to the side of the body.
- Hold the glass thermometer in place for 3 minutes.
- Remove and read the level of mercury of thermometer at eye level.
- Shake mercury down carefully and wipe the thermometer from the stem to bulb with spirit swab.

Breast Self-examination (BSE)

Best time to do:
- Once a month.
- 10 days after menstrual period.
- If not menstruating, select certain day-such as the first day of each month.
- If taking hormones then do it 1-2 days after withdrawal bleeding.

Steps

Step 1
Stand in front of the mirror with shoulders straight and arms on hips and look towards both breasts for:
- At their usual size, shape, and color
- That they are evenly shaped without visible distortion or swelling

Consult doctor if there is:
- Redness, rash, or swelling of the breasts
- Dimpling, puckering, or bulging of the skin
- Changed position or an inverted nipple (pushed inward instead of sticking out)
- Redness, rash, or swelling of the breasts.

Step 2
- Gently squeeze each nipple between finger and thumb
- Consult doctor if nipple discharge is milky or yellow fluid or blood.

Step 3
- Lie down and use right hand to feel left breast and then left hand to feel right breast.
- Use a firm, smooth touch with the first few fingers of hand, keeping the fingers flat and together.
- Cover the entire breast from top to bottom, side to side—from your collarbone to the top of your abdomen, and from your armpit to your cleavage.
- Be sure to feel all the breast tissue:
- Follow a pattern to be sure that cover the whole breast. Begin at the nipple, moving in larger and larger circles until reach the outer edge of the breast. Also move fingers up and down vertically, in rows.

Begin examining each area just beneath skin with a very soft touch, and then increase pressure so that you can feel the deeper tissue, down to your ribcage using fingers only.

Step 4
- Feel your breasts while you are standing or sitting.
- It is easier to feel the breasts when their skin is wet while taking bath.

Hemoglobin Estimation

Necessary items: Sahli's hemoglobinometer, N/10 HCl, gloves, spirit swabs, lancet, distilled water and dropper, puncture-proof container, 0.5% chlorine solution
- Wash hands and wear gloves
- Clean the Hb tube and pipette
- Fill the Hb tube with N/10 HCl up to 2 g with the dropper
- Clean tip of the person's ring finger with the spirit swab
- Prick the ring finger with the lancet and discard the first drop of blood
- Allow a large blood drop to form on the fingertip
- Suction with the pipette up to the 20 mm 3 mark (connect pipette to syringe and pull the barrel instead of mouth suctioning by pipette)
- Take care that air does not enter while suctioning the blood
- Wipe the tip of the pipette and transfer the blood to the Hb tube containing N/10 HCl

- Rinse the pipette 2–3 times with N/10 HCl.
- Leave the solution in the test tube for 10 mins
- After 10 mins, dilute the acid by adding distilled water drop by drop and mix it with a stirrer
- Match with the color of the comparator
- Note down the reading (lower meniscus)
- Dispose of the used lancet in a puncture-proof container
- Immerse the used gloves in 0.5% chlorine solution

Urine Testing

Necessary items: Urine specimen collection bottles/containers and dipsticks
Check the expiry date on the kit and carefully read the instructions before use.
- Remove one strip from the bottle and screw the cap tightly
- Completely immerse the reagent area of the strip in the urine and remove it immediately
- Remove the strip of the urine and tap at the edge of container to remove excess urine
- For glucose: compare the blue reagent area against the color chart area on the bottle and record the finding (time as per manufacturer's instruction)
- For urine albumin: compare the yellow reagent area against the color chart area on the bottle and record the finding (time as per manufacturer's instruction)
- Dispose of strip and urine as per Government of India (GOI) protocol.

BIBLIOGRAPHY

1. Daksh Skills Lab training manual RMNCH+A services for participants, https://nhm.gov.in/images/pdf/programmes/maternalhealth/guidelines/SKILLS_LAB_TRAINING_MANUAL_Participant%20.pdf
2. National Programme on Prevention and Control of Cancer, Diabetes, CVD and Stroke,https://nhm.gov.in/index1.php?lang=1andlevel=2andsublinkid=1048andlid=604
3. www.mohfw.nic.in

7.2 PROVISION OF PRIMARY HEALTH CARE (ROUTINE HEALTH CHECK-UP, IMMUNIZATION, COUNSELING, MANAGEMENT OF COMMON HEALTH PROBLEMS)

ROUTINE HEALTH CHECK-UP

Purpose
- To identify the patient's response to health and illness
- To determine the nursing care needs of the patient
- To evaluate outcomes of healthcare and patient progress
- To identify risk factors.

Preparation
- Infection control: It includes hand hygiene, use standard precautions, use personal protective equipment (gloves, mask, etc.), utilize clean instruments.

- Preparation of environment: Adequate lighting, examination tables, adequate privacy
- Preparation of equipment: Arrange all equipment for easy access, check functioning, warm equipment before use, if required. Equipment usually collected are sphygmomanometer, stethoscope, thermometer, cotton balls, tongue depressor, reflex hammer, swab stick, tuning fork, etc.
- Preparation of the patient: Ensure physical comfort, position, dress and drape appropriately, assist patient for sample collection.
- Psychological preparation of the patient: Explain the procedure and clarify doubts to reduce anxiety.

Physical Assessment

- **General appearance, mental status, anthropometric measurements and vital signs:**
  - General appearance and mental status: Physical assessment begins with observation of the patient's general appearance, level of comfort, and mental status.
  - Anthropometric measurements: Measurement of height, weight and BMI.
  - Vital signs: The pulse, blood pressure, bodily temperature and respiratory rate.
- **Assessment of the integumentary system:**
  - The color of the skin, the quality, distribution and condition of the bodily hair, the size, the location, color and type of any skin lesions are assessed and documented, the color of the nail beds, and the angle of curvature where the nails meet the skin of the fingers are also inspected.
  - Palpation: The temperature, level of moisture, turgor and the presence or absence of any edema or swelling on the skin are assessed.
- **Assessment of the head and neck**
  - **Face and skull inspection:** The size, shape and symmetry of the face and skull, facial movements and symmetry are inspected. The presence of any lumps, soreness, and masses are assessed.
  - **Eyes inspection:** Pupils in reference to their bilateral equality, reaction to light and accommodation, the presence of any discharge, irritation, redness and abnormal eye movement are assessed. **Standardized testing:** The Snellen chart for visual acuity.
  - **Ears inspection:** The auricles are inspected in terms of color, symmetry, elasticity and any tenderness or lesions; the external ear canal is inspected for color and the presence of any drainage and ear wax; and the tympanic membrane in terms of color, integrity and the lack of any bulging is also assessed. **Standardized testing:** The Rinne test and the Weber test for the assessment of hearing can be done using a tuning fork.
  - **Nose inspection:** The color, size, shape, symmetry, and any presence of drainage, flaring, tenderness, and masses are assessed; the nasal passages are assessed visually using an otoscope of the correct size for an infant, child and adult; the sense of smell is also assessed. The sinuses are assessed for any signs of tenderness and infection.
  - **Mouth and throat inspection:** The lips are visualized for their symmetry and color; the buccal membranes, the gums and the tongue are inspected for color, any lesions and their level of dryness or moisture; the tongue is inspected for symmetry of movement; teeth are inspected for the presence of any loose or missing teeth; the uvula is assessed for movement, position, size and color; the salivary glands are examined for signs of inflammation or redness; the oropharynx, tonsils, hard and soft palates are also inspected for color, redness and any lesions. Lastly, the gag reflex is assessed. The mouth and the throat are assessed using a tongue blade and a light source.

- **Neck inspection:** The neck and head movement is visualized; the thyroid gland is inspected for any swelling and also for normal movement during swallowing. Palpation: The neck, the lymph nodes, and trachea are palpated for size and any irregularities.
- **Assessment of the breast and axillae inspection:** The breasts are visualized to assess the size, shape, symmetry, color and the presence of any dimpling, lesions, swelling, edema, visible lumps and nipple retractions. The nipples are also assessed for the presence of any discharge, which is not normal for either gender except when the female is pregnant or lactating. *Palpation:* The nurse performs a complete breast examination using the fingertips to determine if any lumps are felt. The lymph nodes in the axillary areas are also palpated for any enlargement or swelling.
- **Assessment of respiratory system:**
  - Assessment of the Thorax Inspection: The anterior and posterior thorax is inspected for size, symmetry, shape and for the presence of any skin lesions and/or misalignment of the spine; chest movements are observed for the normal movement of the diaphragm during respirations. *Palpation:* The posterior thorax is assessed for respiratory excursion and fremitus. *Percussion:* It is done to assess normal and abnormal sounds over the thorax.
  - Assessment of the Lungs Auscultation: The assessment of normal and adventitious breath sounds. *Percussion:* It is done to identify for normal and abnormal sounds. Normal breath sounds like vesicular breath sounds, bronchial breath sounds, bronchovesicular breath sounds are auscultated and assessed in the same manner that adventitious breath sounds like rales, wheezes, friction rubs, rhonchi, and abnormal bronchophony, egophony, and whispered pectoriloquy are auscultated, assessed and documented.
- **Assessment of the cardiovascular system (heart) inspection:** Pulsations indicating the possibility of an aortic aneurysm are identified by inspection. *Auscultation:* Listening to systolic heart sounds like the normal S1 heart sound and abnormal clicks, the diastolic heart sounds of S2, S3, S4, diastolic knocks and mitral valve sounds, all of which are abnormal with the exception of S2 which can be normal among patients less than 40 years of age.
- **Assessment of the abdomen inspection:** The abdomen is visualized to determine its size, contour, symmetry and the presence of any lesions. As previously mentioned, the abdomen is also inspected to determine the presence of any pulsations that could indicate the possible presence of an abdominal aortic aneurysm. *Auscultation:* The bowel sounds are assessed in all four quadrants which are the upper right quadrant, the upper left quadrant, the lower right quadrant and the lower left quadrant. *Palpation:* Light palpation, which is then followed with deep palpation, is done to assess for the presence of any masses, tenderness, and pain, guarding and rebound tenderness
- **Assessment of the male and female genitalia inspection:** The skin and the pubic hair are inspected. The labia, clitoris, vagina and urethral opening are inspected among female patients. The penis, urethral meatus, and the scrotum are inspected among male patients. *Palpation:* The inguinal lymph nodes are palpated for the presence of any tenderness, swelling or enlargements. A testicular examination is done for male patients.
- **Assessment of the rectum and anus inspection:** The rectum, anus and the surrounding area are examined for any abnormalities. Palpation: With a gloved hand, the rectal sphincter is palpated for muscular tone, and the presence of any blood, tenderness, pain or nodules.
- **Assessment of the musculoskeletal system inspection:** The major muscles of the body are inspected by the nurse to determine their size, and strength, and the presence of any tremors, contractures, muscular weakness and/or paralysis. All joints are assessed for their full range of motion. The areas around the bones and the major muscle groups are also inspected

to determine any areas of deformity, swelling and/or tenderness. Palpation: The muscles are palpated to determine the presence of any spasticity, flaccidity, pain, tenderness, and tremors.
- **Assessment of the peripheral vascular system inspection:** The extremities are inspected for any abnormal color and any signs of poor perfusion to the extremities, particularly the lower extremities. While the patient is in a supine position, the nurse also assesses the jugular veins for any bulging pulsations or distention. *Auscultation:* The nurse assesses the carotids for the presence of any abnormal bruits. *Palpation:* The peripheral veins are gently touched to determine the temperature of the skin, the presence of any tenderness and swelling. The peripheral vein pulses are also palpated bilaterally to determine regularity, number of beats, volume and bilateral equality in terms of these characteristics.
- **Assessment of the neurological system:** The neurological system is assessed with: Inspection balance, gait, gross motor function, fine motor function and coordination, sensory functioning, temperature sensory functioning, kinesthetic sensations and tactile sensory motor functioning, as well as all of the cranial nerves are assessed.

Immunization

- Immunization is the process whereby a person is made immune or resistant to an infectious disease, typically by the administration of a vaccine.
- As health worker, you play a very important role in providing immunization services to mothers and children.
- Responsibilities of nursing staff:
  - Planning for immunization
  - Cold chain management
  - Vaccine carrier and logistics management at the immunization session site
  - Preparing and conducting the immunization session
  - Communicating with caregivers
  - Recording, reporting and tracking of dropouts
  - Capacity building of ASHAs and AWWs to perform their roles in UIP
  - Coordination with ICDS supervisor.

Planning for Immunization

- Prepare area map under SC with names of villages, urban areas including all hamlets, sub-villages, sector, mohalla, hard to reach areas, etc.
- House to house survey and head counting for beneficiary count
- Ensure and confirm list of high risk areas, nomads, construction site etc.
- After every RI session: Review for due list, identify dropout/left-out beneficiaries, ensure follow-up visits to beneficiaries to identify minor vaccine reactions or AEFIs.

Managing the Cold Chain: It is required if pharmacist is not available.

Vaccine carrier and logistics management at the immunization session site:
- Ensure that vaccines are brought in a vaccine carrier with 4 well-sealed conditioned ice packs;
- Ensure vaccine carriers are kept in shade and are not opened frequently;
- Check the labels for expiry date and VVM of the vaccine vials before use;
- Ensure Open Vial Policy applicable vaccine vials have readable labels with date and time of opening/reconstitution;

- Check that T-Series and Hep B vaccines are not frozen;
- Follow the guidelines for use of open vaccine vials;
- Check that required diluents are placed in separate bag and in cold chain; Required number of syringes are available;
- AEFI/Anaphylaxis kit contains all needed items as per checklist.

Preparing and Conducting the Immunization Session
- Prepare for the session by selecting appropriate site; arranging for required equipment and supplies; with the help of AWW and ASHA
- Assess infants for vaccination and possible contraindications before vaccinations;
- Use aseptic technique to prepare and reconstitute vaccines;
- After reconstitution, write the date and time of reconstitution on the label of vaccine vial;
- Use Auto Disable Syringe (ADS) for each injection;
- Explain to the caregiver the correct positioning to keep the child still and the caregiver and vaccinator comfortable;
- Administer the vaccines by using correct technique;
- After the session, store opened vials based on open vial policy guidelines;
- Ensure separate packing of used vials with Session site name and date;
- Pack the vaccine carrier and return vaccines to the ILR;
- Follow immunization waste disposal as per guidelines.

Communicating with Caregivers
- **At the start of session:** Greet the caregiver and thank them for coming for vaccination
- Ask the caregiver if they have any questions and answer them politely.
- **During assessment and after vaccination:** Key messages:
  - Explain what vaccine(s) will be given and the disease it prevents;
  - Explain the importance of waiting for 30 minutes after vaccination;
  - Mention possible adverse events (minor AEFIs) and explain how to handle them; and explain the need for the child to return
  - Write the date for the next vaccination on the immunization card and tell the caregiver; Remind the caregiver to bring the immunization card when they bring the child back for the next vaccination.

Counseling: Kindly refer Chapter 6.4

Management of Common Health Problems
Management at Community Level
- Symptomatic care for fevers, URIs, LRIs, bodyaches and headaches, with referral as needed
- Identify and refer in case of skin infections and abscesses
- Preventive action and primary care for water-borne disease, like diarrhea (cholera, other enteritis) and dysentery, typhoid, hepatitis (A and E)
- Creating awareness about prevention, early identification and referral in cases of helminthiasis and rabies
- Preventive and promotive measures to address musculoskeletal disorders—mainly osteoporosis, arthritis and referral or follow-up as indicated
- Providing symptomatic care for aches and pains—joint pain, back pain, etc.

Management at Health and Wellness Center Level
- Identification and management of common fevers, ARIs, diarrhea, and skin infections (scabies and abscess)
- Identification and management (with referral as needed) in cases of cholera, dysentery, typhoid, hepatitis and helminthiasis
- Management of common aches, joint pains, and common skin conditions (rash/urticaria).

Management at Referral Site
- Diagnosis and management of all complicated cases (requiring admission) of fevers, gastroenteritis, skin infections, typhoid, rabies, helminthiasis, hepatitis acute
- Specialist consultation for diagnostics and management of musculo-skeletal disorders, e.g., arthritis.

BIBLIOGRAPHY
1. https://www.indiannursingcouncil.org/uploads/pdf/1653647581794.pdf
2. https://nhm.gov.in/New_Updates_2018/NHM_Components/Immunization/Guildelines_for_immunization/Immunization_Handbook_for_Health_Workers-English.pdf
3. https://www.nhm.gov.in/New_Updates_2018/NHM_Components/Health_System_Stregthening/Comprehensive_primary_health_care/letter/Operational_Guidelines_For_CPHC.pdf

7.3 RECORD KEEPING
- Every organization and every department in the hospital have its own records.
- Medical record is a legal document of a specific case.
- It is useful to identify each patient and evaluate both patient and hospital progress.
- As per the area of work of nursing, as an administrator, practitioner, researcher, educator need to maintain different records.
- Nursing record is a clinical, scientific, administrative and legal document is written sequence of events to justify the nursing diagnosis, the treatment and end results of care.
- Record is a piece of information or evidence or essential facts in order to maintain a continuous history of events over a period of time. It is a format and register in which data is collected with details of OPD, IPD, treatment, referral, follow-up, etc.
- Reporting is giving account of something, talking about something.
- Oxford defined "Record is piece of information or evidence constitutive account of something that has occurred preserved in writing."
- Dugas defined "Records are the means of communicating essential facts in writing in order to maintain a continuous history of events over a period of time."

PURPOSES OF RECORDS
- To understand the comprehensive needs of the patients and their problems.
- It is essential to make immediate diagnosis and nursing intervention.
- To coordinate the work of nursing staff with other personnel.
- It serves as legal documents.

- To assess the health situation and need of the community.
- Useful as a tool of communication between health worker and family.
- Useful for research and also used as teaching reference and evaluation tool.

Principles of Recording
- Having specific purpose
- Simple and understandable
- Essential for efficiency and uniformity of services
- Confidential
- Provide summary and follow the progress.

Characteristic of Good Documentation
- Have specific objective and purpose
- Complete, accurate, authentic, comprehensive, brief, written with legibility, clear, appropriate and in chronological order as per date and time
- Based on specific classification system
- Minimum in number and content
- Easily retrievable and cost effective.

Importance of Records
- Helps in effective communication
- Useful for evaluate performance and planning
- Provides information about the treatment and follow-up
- To check the quality and quantity of work
- Statistics helps to track present, past and future trends
- Assessing the health situation in the SHC-HWC
- Decision making
- Management of HWC by enabling planning, organizing and reviewing healthcare services at the local level.

Types of Records (Table 7.1)
- **Clinical records**
  - Information is provided by doctor and nurse for this record. All the events of patient from illness to recovery is properly recorded and maintained.
  - Useful for scientific and legal.
  - Provide the evidence of patient's care.
  - Study of record is useful to evaluate actual need, challenges and to identify solution.
- **Admission records**
  - This record is useful for legal and the diagnostic point of view.
  - Admission Record includes a full description of symptoms, both related and unrelated to the condition for which he/she was admitted and also observation of the patient's condition like swelling, rash, bleeding, etc.
- **Nurses notes**

  It is useful to maintain condition and observation of patients accurately timely manner.

Community Health Nurse's Role in Health Promotion and Maintenance

- **Nursing chart**
  - It is useful for vital signs/symptoms chart, nursing care plan, in-take out-put chart, progress report of the patient.
  - Names of patient and doctor must be complete and correctly spelt on each sheet. It should be chronological order and up to date. Needs to ensure uniformity, accuracy, specificity and objectivity of their format.
- **General records**
  - It is depending upon the ward or unit-wise equipment, instrument record, work of nursing staff, etc.
- **Familyrecord**
  - For each family separate family folder is prepared. It contains all family member's records, social, environmental factors which affect the health. And also record all the services like maternal, child, immunization, chronic disease etc.
  - Records are the registers and formats in which the data is collected with respect to details of pregnant women, OPD, eligible couples, referral and follow-up etc.

Table 7.1: Types of different registers in healthcare delivery system.

Sl. No.	Recording formats/registers	Entered by	Checked by	Signed by
1.	RCH register	MPW/CHO	CHO	CHO
2.	Births and deaths register	MPW	CHO	CHO
3.	Communicable diseases/epidemic/outbreak register	MPW/CHO	CHO	CHO/PHC-MO
4.	Passive surveillance registers for malaria cases	MPW	CHO	CHO
5.	Register for Janani Suraksha Yojana	MPW	CHO	CHO
6.	Register for Untied Funds	MPW/CHO	CHO	CHO/MPW
7.	Register for water quality and sanitation	MPW-male	CHO	CHO
8.	NCD-family folder and CBAC form	ASHA/MPW	CHO/MPW	CHO/MPW
9.	OPD register	CHO/MPW	CHO	CHO
10.	Stock register (drug, equipment, furniture and other accessories)	CHO/MPW	CHO	CHO
11.	Due list for pregnant women and children (immunization)	ASHA	MPW/CHO	CHO/MPW
12.	VHSND supportive supervision format	CHO	PHC-MO	Counter signed by MPW and ASHA
13.	NCD register	MPW/CHO	CHO	CHO
14.	Monthly meeting register	MPW	CHO	CHO
15.	Referral and follow-up register (NCD/others)	MPW/CHO	MPW/CHO	CHO

Reports

- It is prepared from records and submitted to the program manager.
- Oxford defined Report as "To bring back, give an account of anything especially a format or official account."
- Dugas defined "Reports are the effective methods of communication among the member of the team or group."
- A report summarizes the services of the person especially in fixed format. It is usually written daily, weekly, monthly or yearly.
- It can be classified as oral and written. Oral report is convenient and useful in emergency condition. It is also used at the shift time of duty to convey the information of patient to another nurse. Written report is more important than oral report. Written report gives description of patient's necessary condition, treatment, progress which is useful for future planning and decision-making.
- Depending upon the frequency like daily for IHIP (earlier was weekly in IDSP), monthly for maternal and child death, NPCDCS, VHND, National program, HMIS report, etc. are submitted.
- Example of Reporting at HWC level:

Daily Reporting	Online reporting on HWC portal
Weekly Reporting	S-form for outbreak reporting
Monthly Reporting	• HMIS sub-center reporting format • Maternal death reporting format • Child death reporting format • NPCDCS + reporting format-1 • HWC-SHC reporting format • VHSND reporting format • National Program Reports (NVBDCP, NACP, NLEP, RNTCP, blindness control, etc.) • VHSNC format
Annual Reporting	HMIS Annual reporting format

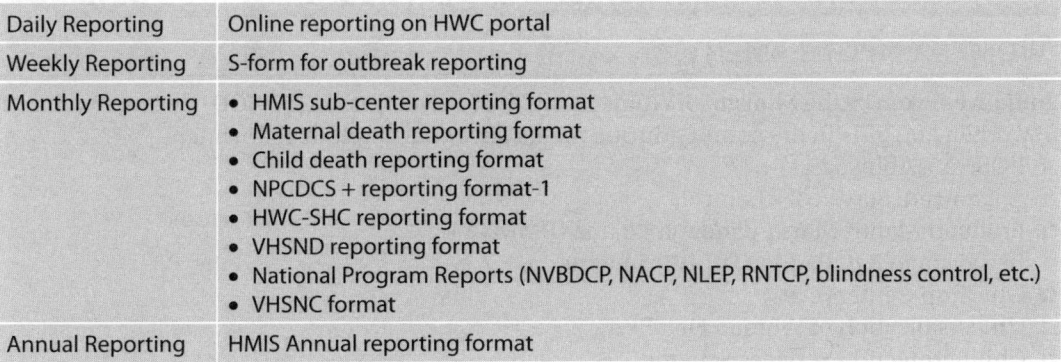

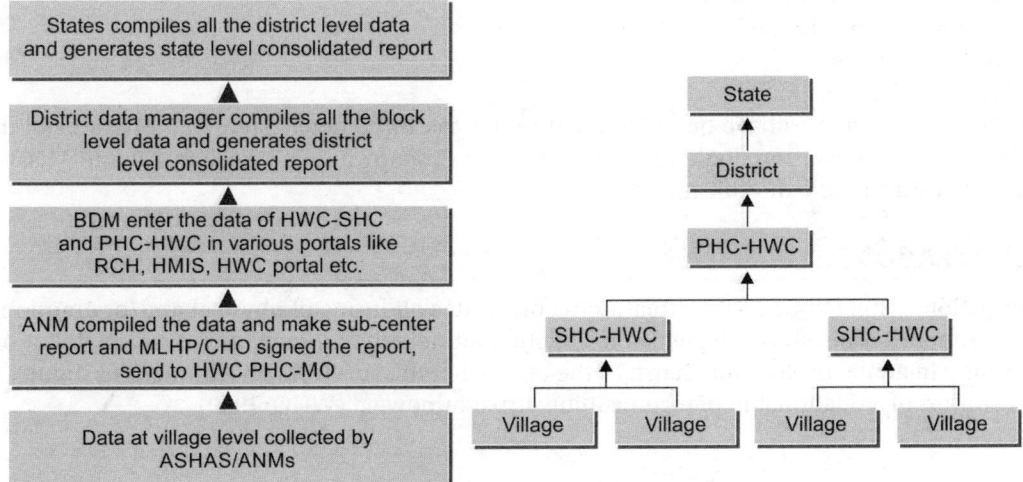

Fig. 7.1: Flow of data at various levels of healthcare system.

Example of IT platforms being used at HWC level for records and reports (Fig. 7.1)
- Health Management Information System (HMIS)
- Reproductive and Child Health Portal (RCH)
- ANM Online (ANMOL)
- CPHC-IT Application
- Health and Wellness Center Portal

BIBLIOGRAPHY

1. https://egyankosh.ac.in/bitstream/123456789/33218/5/Unit-3.pdf
2. http://164.100.161.63/91-records-and-reports-maintained-sub-health-centre-level
3. https://ab-hwc.nhp.gov.in/document/6

7.4 SOCIAL ISSUES AFFECTING HEALTH AND DEVELOPMENT OF THE FAMILY (WOMEN EMPOWERMENT, CHILD ABUSE, ABUSE OF ELDERS, FEMALE FETICIDE, COMMERCIAL SEX WORKERS, SUBSTANCE ABUSE)

WOMEN EMPOWERMENT

Initiatives taken by the Ministry of Women and Child Development (MWCD) for empowerment of women and girls in the country during the last five years include following:
- POSHAN Abhiyaan
- Anganwadi Services Scheme
- Pradhan Mantri Matru Vandana Yojana (PMMVY)
- Beti Bachao Beti Padhao (BBBP) Scheme
- One Stop Center (OSC)
- Universalization of Women Helpline
- Child Protection Services Scheme
- Scheme for Adolescent Girls (SAG)
- Swadhar Greh Scheme
- Ujjawala Scheme
- Working Women Hostel

The above schemes have been included under the three newly launched Missions of the Ministry namely Mission Shakti, Mission Saksham Anganwadi and Poshan 2.0 and Mission Vatsalya with suitable modifications.

CHILD ABUSE

Definition: "Child abuse or maltreatment constitutes all forms of physical and/or emotional ill-treatment, sexual abuse, neglect or negligent treatment or commercial or other exploitation, resulting in actual or potential harm to the child's health, survival, development or dignity in the context of a relationship of responsibility, trust or power." (WHO, 1999)

Risk Factors for Child Abuse

- **Community or society related factors:**
  - Poverty
  - Unemployment
  - High crime rate
- **Parents related factors:**
  - Personal history of sexual abuse
  - Teenage parents
  - Single parent
  - Substance abuse
  - Low self-esteem
  - Child from unwanted pregnancy
  - Lack of parenting skills
  - Domestic violence
- **Child related factors:**
  - Prematurity
  - Low birth weight
  - Handicap

Types of Child Abuse

- Physical abuse
- Sexual abuse ⎤
- Emotional or pyschological abuse ⎦ — act of commission
- Neglect ← act of omission.
- **Physical abuse**
  - It is any non-accidental injury to a child under the age of 18 by a parent or caretaker.
  - Example of injuries : beatings, burns, strangulation, or immersion in scalding water with resulting bruises, fractures, scars, burns, internal injuries or any other injuries.
  - **"Battered Child Syndrome"** is the form of serious physical abuse in young children and **"The shaken infant"** is a form of abuse seen in very young children (less than 1 year).
  - Physical abuse generally results as part of punishment.
- **Emotional abuse:** Emotional abuse is defined as the failure of a caregiver to provide an appropriate and supportive environment and acts (like restricting a child's movements, discrimination, rejection, threats) that have an adverse effect on the emotional health and development of a child.
- **Neglect:**
  - Neglect means the failure of a parent to the basic needs of the child like **health, education, emotional development, nutrition, shelter and safe living conditions** despite of parent's affordability.
  - There is a difference between poverty and neglect as neglect can occur only when reasonable resources are available to the family or caregiver.
  - **Subtypes of neglect include:** Supervisory neglect, medical neglect, emotional neglect, educational neglect, and abandonment.

- **Sexual abuse:**
  - Child sexual abuse is the exploitation of a child or adolescent for the sexual gratification or for the financial gain.
  - There are main 4 types: Penetrative sexual assault, nonpenetrative sexual assault, sexual harassment and pornography.

Health Consequences of Child Abuse (Fig. 7.2)

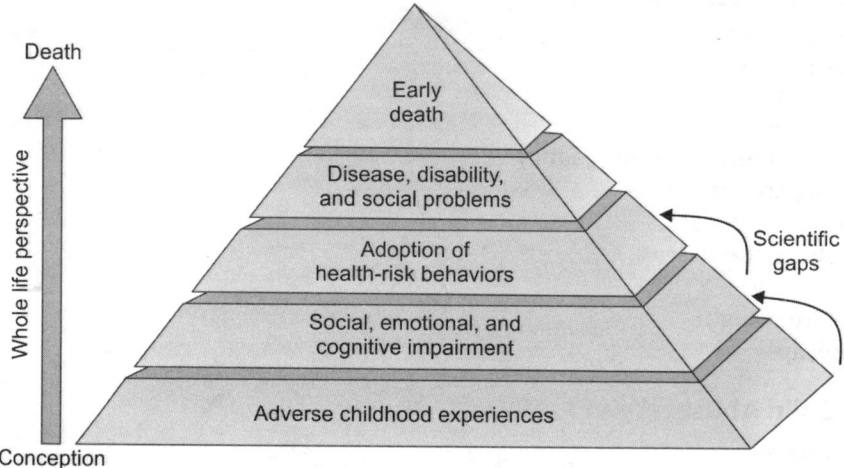

Fig. 7.2: Health consequences of child abuse.

- **Physical**: Injury, disability, burns, fractures.
- **Sexual and reproductive**: Sexual dysfunction, STI, unwanted pregnancy.
- **Psychological and behavioral**: PTSD, depression, anxiety, drug abuse, feeling guilt, cognitive impairment
- The POCSO Act, 2012 provides protection to the children from the offences of sexual assault, sexual harassment and pornography.

ABUSE OF ELDERS

- The abuse of older people is a single or repeated act, or lack of appropriate action, occurring within any relationship where there is an expectation of trust, which causes harm or distress to an older person.
- Abuse of older people can have serious physical and mental health, financial, and social consequences, including, for instance, physical injuries, premature mortality, depression, cognitive decline, financial devastation and placement in nursing homes.
- For older people, the consequences of abuse can be especially serious and recovery may take longer.
- Strategies for the prevention of abuse of elders include:
  - Caregiver interventions, which provide services to relieve the burden of caregiving;
  - Money management programs for older adults vulnerable to financial exploitation;
  - Helplines and emergency shelters; and
  - Multi-disciplinary teams, as the responses required often cut across many systems, including criminal justice, healthcare, mental healthcare, adults protective services and long-term care.

FEMALE FETICIDE

- Some of the reasons for female feticide are:
  - Son preference,
  - Low status of women,
  - Social and financial security associated with sons,
  - Socio-cultural practices including dowry and violence against women,
  - Small family norm and consequent misuse of diagnostic techniques with the intention of female feticide.
- Measures taken to prevent female feticide:
  - Pre-conception and Pre-natal Diagnostic Techniques (Prohibition of Sex Selection) Act, 1994: For prohibition of sex selection
  - Beti Bachao, Beti Padhao campaign
  - Awareness generation as well as programs for socio-economic empowerment of women.

COMMERCIAL SEX WORKERS

- Sex workers face an increased burden of sexually transmitted infections (STIs) and blood-borne infections.
- Globally, female sex workers are estimated to be 30 times more likely to be living with HIV than other women of reproductive age. In 2019, the Joint United Nations Programme on HIV/AIDS estimated a mean HIV prevalence of 36% among sex workers.
- The average reported prevalence of active syphilis among sex workers is 10.8% (range 5.8% to 30.3%).
- Sex workers face high levels of stigma and criminalization almost everywhere.

Some important interventions for welfare of commercial sex workers:

Health interventions	Structural interventions
• Prevention (condom, pre-exposure prophylaxis, etc.) • Harm reduction interventions (needle and syringe programs, opioid substitution therapy, naloxone) • Behavioral interventions • HIV testing services • HIV treatment and care • Prevention and management of tuberculosis, hepatitis and mental health • Sexual and reproductive health interventions	• Supportive legislation, policy and funding including decriminalization of behaviors (e.g. drug use and possession, sex work, same-gender sex) • Addressing stigma and discrimination • Available, accessible and acceptable health services • Community empowerment • Addressing violence

- The Ministry of Women and Child Development is implementing "Ujjawala"—a Comprehensive Scheme for Prevention of Trafficking and Rescue, Rehabilitation, Re-integration and Repatriation of Victims of Trafficking for Commercial Sexual Exploitation.
- Immoral Traffic (Prevention) Act, 1956.

SUBSTANCE ABUSE

- Substance abuse refers to the harmful or hazardous use of psychoactive substances, including alcohol and illicit drugs.

- The use of psychoactive substances causes significant health and social problems for the people who use them, and also for others in their families and communities. Substances of abuse include alcohol, opiates, cocaine, amphetamines, hallucinogens, prescription and over-the-counter drug abuse.
- Strategies for prevention:
  - National Action Plan for Drug Demand Reduction (NAPDDR)
  - Nasha Mukt Bharat Abhiyaan (NMBA)
  - The Narcotic Drugs and Psychotropic Substances Act.

BIBLIOGRAPHY

1. Childhelp (2016). The issues of child abuse, available at: https://www.childhelp.org/child-abuse/
2. Health consequences of child abuse; Division of Violence Prevention, Centers for Disease Control and Prevention
3. https://pib.gov.in/newsite/PrintRelease.aspx?relid=77845
4. https://www.nhp.gov.in/disease/non-communicable-disease/substance-abuse
5. https://www.who.int/news-room/fact-sheets/detail/abuse-of-older-people
6. McCoy ML, Keen SM (2013). "Introduction". Child Abuse and Neglect (2 ed.). New York: Psychology Press. pp. 3–22. ISBN 1-84872-529-9. OCLC 863824493. Retrieved 4 october 2016.

7.5 BRIEF INTRODUCTION OF COMMUNITY RESOURCES (OLD AGE HOMES, ORPHANAGES, PALLIATIVE CARE CENTERS, HOSPICE CARE CENTERS)

OLD AGE HOMES

- Demographic transition has been accompanied by changes in society and economy.
- It is true that family ties in India are very strong and an overwhelming majority live with their sons or are supported by them. Also, working couples find the presence of old parents emotionally bonding and of great help in managing the household and caring for children.
- However, due to the operation of several forces, the position of a large number of older persons has become vulnerable due to which they cannot take for granted that their children will be able to look after them when they need care in old age, especially in view of the longer life span implying an extended period of dependency and higher costs to meet health and other needs.
- This situation is more serious in rural areas where the children migrate to cities and towns, abroad in search of jobs and livelihoods leaving old parents behind in the village.
- Sometimes elders are unable to look after themselves. Even increase in the proportion of the elderly in the population have contributed to an increasing need for alternative arrangements for helping the old to find a place of rest in their later years.
- There are two types of old age home available—free and paid. When no one is available for care of old person, then free old age homes provide free shelter, cloth, food to old person. Whereas in paid home, fee should be paid.

Standard norms under Atal Vayo Abhyuday Yojana (AVYAY) to be followed by implementing agencies for running old age homes

- Land—the land for the old age home should be adequate to comply with the Floor-Area Ratio (FAR) as prescribed by Government.
- Living space-norms:
  - Area of bedroom/dormitory per resident (7.5 sq.mtr)
  - There shall be a separate bed for each resident
  - There shall be hygienic toilet and bath facilities @ one per 10 residents
  - The living area or carpet area per resident, i.e., including (i) above plus ancillary areas like kitchen, dining hall, recreation room, medical room, etc. but excluding verandahs, corridors, etc. (12 sq. mtr)
- Facilities—every institution shall have following facilities:
  - Rooms/dormitories—separately for men and women;
  - Adequate safe drinking water and for ancillary purposes
  - Electricity, fans and heating arrangement for residents (as necessary)
  - Kitchen-cum-store and office
  - Dining hall
  - Recreation facilities, television, newspaper and books
  - Activities for keeping the residents productively occupied;
  - First aid and primary healthcare facilities.
  - Should be barrier-free with provision of handrails and lifts etc.
- Operational standards—minimum standards required like:
  - Nutrition—adequate and good quality food containing an average of 1,700 calories and 50 grams protein to be provided to the beneficiaries, daily.
  - Medical facilities—the project should have first aid kit, glucometer, BP monitoring machine, weighing machine and medicines, as prescribed by a Doctor. As far as possible, the residence of the doctor should be near the project. Regular Health Camps to be organized. Arrangements is required with the nearest Government hospital for emergency medical care.
  - Recreation—at each center the implementing agency must provide Books, 3–4 Magazines, 2–3 newspapers (in regional/local language), outings at nearby places (2 in a month)- religious/cultural, games like caroms, chess, cards, one cable connection, one computer with internet connection. All projects should have a separate room for reading for the residents.
  - Implementing agencies shall ensure that the services of minimum staff as prescribed in the scheme are in available in each project.
  - Security—necessary security arrangements to be made in the projects by the implementing agencies.
  - Clothing—keeping in view local climate, weather conditions and traditional norms all the residents must be provided with 4 pairs of clothing in a year.
  - Rooms—properly ventilated rooms with sufficient space between the beds of the beneficiaries for their easy movement.
  - Bathrooms and toilets—each project should have separate toilets for females and males. There should be at least one toilet with western style fixed/removable commodes. Bathrooms and toilets must have anti-slippery tiles and railings for support.

- Hygiene and Sanitation—all the rooms, courtyard and kitchen must be cleaned at least 2 times a day. Bathrooms and toilets must be cleaned at least 3 times a day. Disinfectants must be used for infection control and ensure a sanitized environment. Handwashing facilities are prominently located. Hygiene measures (cleanliness of rooms, mosquito control measures) and waste segregation needs to be followed.

CHILDREN'S HOME

- Children's home shall be established for children in need of care and protection, treatment, education, training, development, and rehabilitation. Separate homes based on age, gender and special needs of children could be established.
- Special focus on children in child care institute who are not able to go to school due to physical or mental disabilities.
- Special provision is available like special educators or therapist and occupational therapy, speech therapy, verbal therapy, etc.

OPEN SHELTERS

- Open shelters registered by the state government shall be supported to look after runaway children, missing children, trafficked children, working children, children in street situation, child beggars, and child substance abusers, children affected by any natural disaster, children living in unauthorized areas/slums, children of migrant population, children of socially marginalized groups, and any other vulnerable group of children for the short-term based on the need assessment.
- These shelters will be used for educating, counseling and imparting life skills to children in difficult circumstances, so as to keep them away from a life in the streets.
- Open shelter may include the following:
  - **Observation homes** shall be established for temporary reception, care and rehabilitation of any child alleged to be in conflict with law, during the pendency of any inquiry under the Juvenile Justice (Care and Protection of Children) Act, 2015.
  - **Special homes** shall be established for providing long-term rehabilitation and protection of children who are found to have committed an offence and placed thereby an order of the Juvenile Justice Board.
  - **Place of safety** shall be established to host children between the ages of 16 to 18 years and are accused of or convicted for committing a heinous offence in conflict with law.

Non-institutional Care

- **Sponsorship:** Financial support may be extended to vulnerable children living with extended families/biological relatives for supporting their education, nutrition and health needs.
- **Foster care:** The responsibility of the child is undertaken by an unrelated family for care protection and rehabilitation of the child. Financial support is provided to biologically unrelated Foster Parents for nurturing the child.
- **Adoption:** Finding families for the children found legally free for adoption. Specialized Adoption Agencies (SAA) will facilitate the adoption program.
- **After care:** The children who are leaving a Child Care Institution on completion of 18 years of age may be provided with financial support to facilitate the child's re-integration into mainstream of society. Such support may be given from the age of 18 years up to 21 years, extendable up to 23 years of age to help her/him become self-dependent.

ORPHANAGES

- As per the Juvenile Justice (Care and Protection of Children) Act, 2015, orphan and destitute children in the country are "Children in need of care and protection (CNCP). Ministry of Women and Child Development is implementing a centrally sponsored Child Protection Services (CPS) Scheme for supporting the children in difficult circumstances.
- It is a residential institution for the care of children whose are deceased or unable to care for them.
- The financial norms for various components under ICPS (now "Child Protection Services"):
  - Maintenance grant for children in homes was enhanced to Rs.2160 per child per month,
  - Sitting allowance of Child Welfare Committee and Juvenile Justice Board's members has been enhanced from Rs. 1,000/- to Rs. 1,500/- in accordance with new JJ (Juvenile Justice) Model Rules, 2016 and
  - Programmatic allocation for Childline India Foundation Head office and four regional Centers, was increased by Rs. 9.70 Crore for protection services of CHILDLINE, to address expansion and emerging protection needs.

PALLIATIVE CARE

- Definition: It is an approach that improves the quality of life of patients and their families facing the problems associated with life-threatening illnesses, through the prevention and relief of suffering by means of early identification, impeccable assessment and treatment of pain and other problems, physical, psychosocial and spiritual.
- Provides relief from pain and other distressing symptoms;
- Affirms life and regards dying as a normal process;
- Intends neither to hasten or postpone death;
- Integrates the psychological and spiritual aspects of patient care;
- Offers a support system to help patients live as actively as possible until death;
- Offers a support system to help the family cope during the patients illness and in their own bereavement;
- Uses a team approach to address the needs of patients and their families, including bereavement counseling, if indicated;
- Improve the quality of life, and may also positively influence the course of illness; is applicable early in the course of illness, in conjunction with other therapies that are intended to prolong life, such as chemotherapy or radiation therapy, and includes those investigations needed to better understand and manage distressing clinical complications.
- The majority of adults in need of palliative care have chronic diseases such as cardiovascular diseases (38.5%), cancer (34%), chronic respiratory diseases (10.3%), AIDS (5.7%) and diabetes (4.6%). Patients with many other conditions may require palliative care, including kidney failure, chronic liver disease, rheumatoid arthritis, neurological disease, dementia, congenital anomalies and drug-resistant tuberculosis.

Components

- Physical: Assessment of symptoms and treatment, nursing care, appropriate analgesics, wound care, ensuring comfort in dying patient.

- ❏ Psychological: Communicating with the patient and families, providing emotional support, empowering patients to make choices about their treatment.
- ❏ Social: Helping patients against social stigmatization to live as normal life
- ❏ Spiritual: Helping patients and families cope with spiritual issues that may come up in the face of life limiting situations.
  - Palliative care can be delivered in a variety of ways including hospice care, in-patient care, outpatient care and home-based care.
  - Home-based palliative care services take care to the doorstep of the patient. This is where people are most comfortable at the end of their lives, surrounded by their loved ones. It is also well suited to conditions in India where a family member is usually available and willing to nurse the sick person.

Hospice

- ❏ Hospice care is end-of-life care.
- ❏ A team of Doctors, nurses and volunteers provides it.
- ❏ They give medical, psychological, and spiritual support to patient, caregiver and family.
- ❏ The goal of the care is to help people who are dying, have peace, comfort, and dignity. It is also aimed to empower and support a patient's family, so that they can take care of patient at home, if they wish to.
- ❏ It is aimed to "Add life to days and not days to life" of cancer patients of advanced stage of disease.

BIBLIOGRAPHY

1. https://pib.gov.in/PressReleasePage.aspx?PRID=1602395
2. https://nhsrcindia.org/sites/default/files/202106/Operational%20Guidelines%20for%20Palliative%20Care%20at%20HWC.pdf
3. https://www.gcriindia.org/Download/Hospice%20and%20Home%20Care%20Services.pdf
4. http://www.who.int/cancer/palliative/definition/en/

CHAPTER 8

Epidemiology Made Easy

CHAPTER OUTLINE

8.1 Epidemiology: Concept and definition
8.2 Basic tools of epidemiology
8.3 Uses of epidemiology
8.4 Theories of disease causation
8.5 Modes of disease transmission
8.6 Glimpse about important concepts of epidemiology
8.7 Classification of different epidemiological study designs
8.8 Cross-sectional study: Design, steps, analysis and interpretation
8.9 Case control study: Design, steps, analysis and interpretation
8.10 Cohort study: design, steps, analysis and interpretation
8.11 Randomized control trial (RCT) study: Design, steps, analysis and interpretation
8.12 Levels of prevention: Primordial, primary, secondary and tertiary
8.13 Outbreak investigation
8.14 Evidence-based public health
8.15 Screening

8.1 EPIDEMIOLOGY: CONCEPT AND DEFINITION

- Hippocrates in his book entitled "On Airs, Waters, and Places explained that disease occurrence is rational phenomenon and not a supernatural". Hippocrates suggested that environmental and host factors such as behaviors might influence the development of disease.
- In 1662, John Graunt, published a landmark analysis of mortality data.
- William Farr considered the father of modern vital statistics and surveillance, developed many of the basic practices used today in vital statistics and disease classification.

History of Evolution of Concepts of Epidemiology

Edward Jenner

- He invented smallpox vaccine (1st vaccine) on 14th May 1796 by inoculating James Phipps, an eight-year-old boy.
- Edward Jenner scraped pus from cowpox blisters on the hands of Sarah Nelmes, a milkmaid who had caught cowpox.
- Term vaccination was first coined by **Edward Jenner**.
- He is known as **Father of Immunology**.

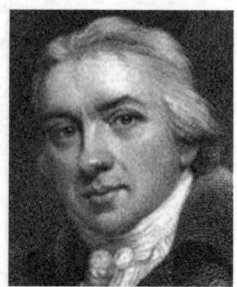

James Lind

- 1st ever clinical trial in the form of scurvy trial was conducted by James Lind.
- This experiment was done among 12 pairs naval officers of Britain.
- One group was given citrus fruits in addition to normal diet while another group was on normal diet.
- So due to having vitamin C in citrus fruits that group had a smaller number of officers who were suffering from the scurvy.

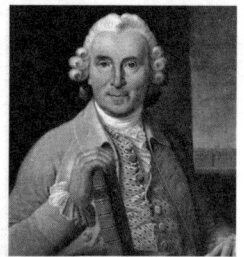

Ignaz Philipp Semmelweis

- He is known as saviors of mothers as he gave intense emphasis on handwashing which helped in the prevention of puerperal sepsis and thus maternal death.
- He proved his hypothesis in 1847 at Vienna General Hospital by collecting data about maternal deaths of two maternity division, in which one group of doctors always washed their hands before touching postnatal mothers while another group of doctors were used to directly came to the maternal ward from the autopsy room which lead to puerperal sepsis or child bed fever.
- He published his book on it as "etiology, concept and prophylaxis of childbed fever".

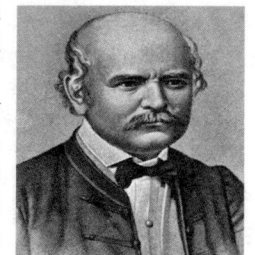

Edwin Chadwick

- He was the first personality to do research on sanitation.
- His report titled as "The Sanitary Condition of the Labouring Population (1843)" leads to Enactment of Public Health Act, 1848 in London.

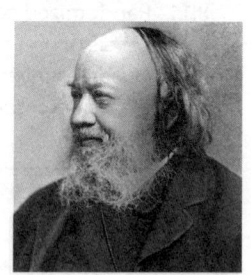

John Snow

- He is known as **Father of Modern Epidemiology**
- He discovered the mode of transmission of cholera and this discovery was a result of natural experiment
- He is also known for **"Shoe leather epidemiology"** (house to house survey)
- John Snow prepared spot map cholera outbreak in London, 1854.
- John Snow mapped the all 13 public wells and all the confirmed cholera deaths.

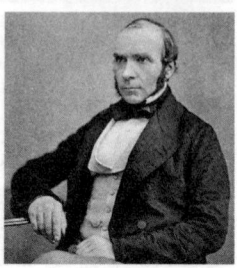

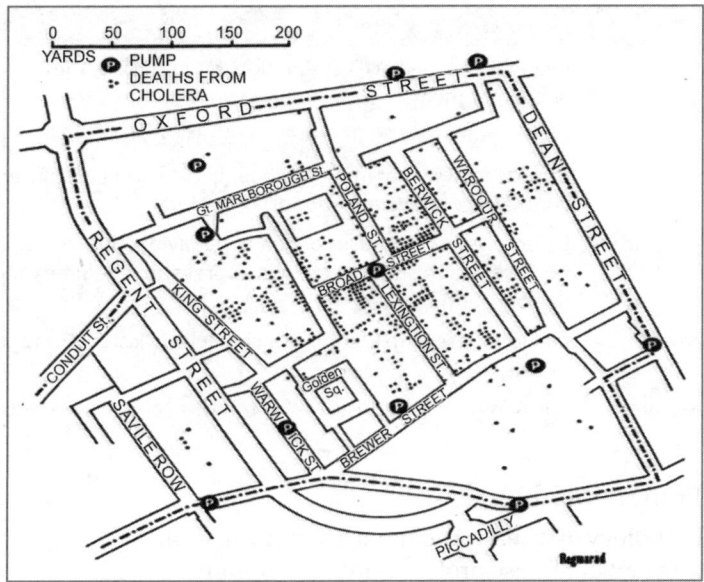

Fig. 8.1: Spot map of Broad Street cholera outbreak, 1854.

- On the basis of this mapping, he noted the spatial clustering of cases around one particular water pump on Broad Street **(Fig. 8.1)**.
- That's why he had removed the pump handle from the Broad Street pump and the outbreak subsided quickly.

Note: Cholera is known as **father of public health.**

Louis Pasteur

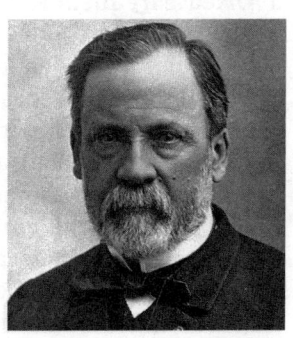

- Disproved spontaneous generation of diseases and established germ theory of the diseases
- He coined the term vaccine.
- Invented method of pasteurization
- Invented vaccine for rabies and anthrax

So based on above findings, we can summarize that epidemiology has evolved from findings modes of transmission like in case of cholera and childbed fever to preventive trial in the form scurvy prevention and smallpox vaccination.

Causative aspect was better explained with cohort study like Framingham Heart Study on risk factors for cardiovascular diseases.

Thus, epidemiology as science has evolved from merely observational studies to till date in the more of systematic reviews and meta-analysis.

The word epidemiology comes from the Greek words *epi*, meaning on or upon, *demos*, meaning people, and *logos*, meaning the study of.

Definition of Epidemiology

Epidemiology is the **study** of the **distribution** and **determinants** of **health-related states or events** in **specified populations**, and the **application** of this study to control of health problems (John M Last, 1988).

Term	Explanation
Study	Includes: surveillance observation, hypothesis testing, analytic research and experiments
Distribution	Refers to analysis of: times persons, places and classes of people affected.
Determinants	Include factors that influence health: bioiogical, chemical, physical, social, cultural, economic genetic and behavioral
Health-related states and events	Refer to: diseases causes of death, behaviors such as use of tobacco, positive health states, reactions to preventive regimes and provision and use of health services
Specified populations	Include those with identifiable characteristics, such as occupational groups
Application to prevention and control	The aims of public health—to promote, protect, and restore health

Objectives of Epidemiology

- Investigate the etiology of disease and modes of transmission
- Determine the extent of disease problems in the community
- Study the natural history and prognosis of disease
- Evaluate both existing and new preventive and therapeutic measures and modes of health care delivery
- Provide a foundation for developing public policy and regulatory decisions.

Components of Epidemiology

- **Disease frequency**: It is the quantification of disease. It measures morbidity and mortality of given disease. For this we use rate, ratio or proportions which are collectively called as basic tools of epidemiology.
- **Distribution of disease:**
  - It gives answers of three very important questions like who are affected (person), where happened (place) and when occurred (time).
  - This is called as person, place and time (PPT) distribution which collectively called as descriptive **epidemiology**.
- **Determinants of disease:**
  - Hypothesis will be tested by various epidemiological study designs to know the determinants (risk factors or causes) of the disease.
  - Analytic epidemiology studies help us to know "Why" and "How" any health event occurs.

SUMMARY

Epidemiology is the study (scientific, systematic, data-driven) of the distribution (frequency, pattern) and determinants (causes, risk factors) of health-related states and events (not just diseases) in specified populations (patient is community, individuals viewed collectively), and the application of (since epidemiology is a discipline within public health) this study to the control of health problems.

BIBLIOGRAPHY

1. https://www.cdc.gov/csels/dsepd/ss1978/SS1978.pdf
2. https://www.bbc.co.uk/history/historic_figures/jenner_edward.shtml
3. https://www.britannica.com/biography/James-Lind
4. https://www.thehindu.com/children/know-the-scientist-ignaz-semmelweis/article33986506.ece
5. https://www.lshtm.ac.uk/aboutus/introducing/history/frieze/sir-edwin-chadwick
6. https://www1.udel.edu/johnmack/frec682/cholera/
7. https://www.revolvy.com/main/index.php?s=John%20Snow%20(physician)&item_type=topic
8. https://www.lshtm.ac.uk/aboutus/introducing/history/frieze/louis-pasteur
9. https://www.cdc.gov/csels/dsepd/ss1978/lesson1/section1.html

8.2 BASIC TOOLS OF EPIDEMIOLOGY

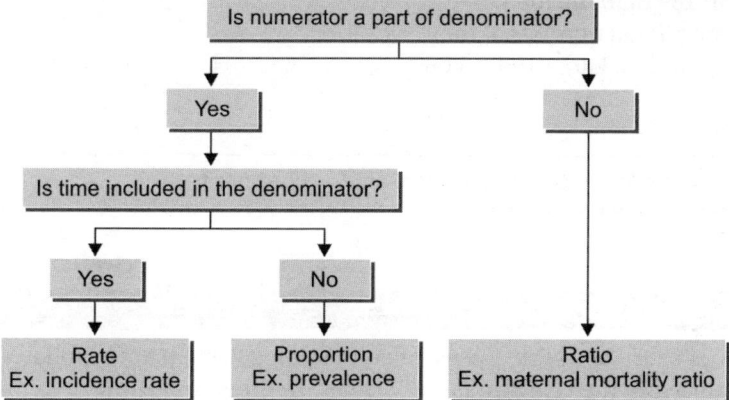

- ❏ **Rate:**
  - Numerator is part of the denominator.
  - Usually, it is calculated for specific disease for given population and during particular time period.
  - Multiplier could be 1,000, 10,000 ... so on.
  - Rate is measure of risk
  - It tells about the speed of disease occurrence. For example, 70 new cases of breast cancer per 1,000 women per year. This measure conveys a sense of the speed with which disease occurs in a population.
  - Example: Death rate, IMR, incidence.
- ❏ **Ratio:**
  - Numerator is **not** part of the denominator.
  - Usually, it is calculated to know relation of one entity with other.
  - Ratio can be used in descriptive statistics (e.g., sex ratio, maternal mortality ratio) while in analytical statistics it is used as odds ratio or risk ratio.
  - Example: A city of 40,000 population has 50 clinics. Calculate the ratio of clinics per person.
    50/40,000 = 0.00125 clinics per person.

❑ **Proportion:**
  - Numerator is always part of the denominator, e.g., the number of apples divided by the number of oranges is not a proportion, but the number of apples divided by the total number of fruits of all kinds is a proportion.
  - Usually it is calculated for specific disease for given population and during particular time period.
  - Multiplier is generally 100 and so prevalence is usually presented in percentage. (For example, prevalence of LBW is 28%).
  - A proportion can be expressed as a fraction, a decimal, or a percentage.
  - It tells about the extent or fraction of the population that affected by particular disease or situation.
  - Example: Case fatality rate (it is not rate but proportion), prevalence (it is also not rate but proportion)
  - Sum: Calculate the proportion of diabetic men among total men.
  - Numerator: 189 diabetic men
  - Denominator: Total number of men = 3,340
  - Proportion: (189/3,340) × 100 = 5.66%

BIBLIOGRAPHY

1. https://www.cdc.gov/csels/dsepd/ss1978/lesson3/section1.html

8.3 USES OF EPIDEMIOLOGY

Major Jerry Morris described seven 'uses' of epidemiology which are as follows:
1. **To study historically the rise and fall of disease in the population**
2. **Community Diagnosis**
3. **Planning and Evaluation**
4. **Evaluation of individual's risks and chances**
5. **Syndrome Identification**
6. **Completing the natural history of disease**
7. **Searching for causes and risk factors**

❑ **To study historically the rise and fall of disease in the population:** In *historical study* of the health of the community and of the rise and fall of diseases in the population; useful 'projections' into the future may also be possible.

❑ **Community diagnosis:** Community diagnosis generally refers to the identification and quantification of health problems in a community in terms of mortality and morbidity rates and ratios, and identification of their correlates for the purpose of defining those individuals or groups at risk or those in need of healthcare.

Quantification of health problems:
  - Helps in laying down priorities in disease control and prevention.
  - Can serve as a benchmark for the evaluation of health services.
  - The quantification of health problems can be a source of new knowledge about disease distribution, causation and prevention.
  - We should try to find answers of the following questions:

- What are the actual and potential health problems in the community?
- Where are they occurring?
- Who are at increased risk?
- Which problems have declined over time and which ones are increasing or have the potential to increase?
- How do these patterns relate to the level and distribution of public health services available?

☐ **Planning and evaluation:** To study the *workings of health services*. This begins with the determination of needs and resources, proceeds to analysis of services in action and, finally, attempts to appraise. Such studies can be comparative between various populations.

☐ **Evaluation of individual's risks and chances:** To estimate, from the common experience, *the individual's chances* and risks of disease.

Our day-to-day decisions like decide to quit smoking, climb the stairs rather than using an elevator, eat a salad rather than a cheeseburger, they may be influenced, knowingly or unknowingly, are based on epidemiologic findings.

☐ **Syndrome identification:** In *identifying syndromes* from the distribution of clinical phenomena among sections of the population.

☐ **Completing the natural history of disease:** To *help complete the clinical picture* by including all types of cases in proportion; by relating clinical disease to the subclinical; by observing secular changes in the character of disease, and its picture in other countries.

☐ **Searching for causes and risk factors:** In the *search for causes* of health and disease, starting with the discovery of groups with high and low rates, studying these differences in relation to differences in ways of living; and, where possible, testing these notions in the actual practice among populations.

BIBLIOGRAPHY

1. https://academic.oup.com/ije/article-pdf/30/5/1146/18479125/301146.pdf

8.4 THEORIES OF DISEASE CAUSATION

INTRODUCTION

☐ To know the cause of the disease is very essential to find the cure for the same.
☐ Every medical system has tried to find the reason of diseases and based on their understanding they develop models of treatment.
☐ For example, field of biomedicine understands pathogen as root cause of disease and deals with use of antibiotics and antivirals. Ayurveda believes the disturbances in tridosha as cause of diseases and they try to bring back the harmony of tridosha to treat the diseases.
☐ Every model of treatment is different in the terms of concept but ultimate aim is to provide rational treatment and they all doing effort to bring homeostasis (balance) with one's surroundings based on their medical philosophy to extend a healthy state to the sick and tackle diseases.

FACTORS OF DISEASE CAUSATION

- **Predisposing factors:** These are the factors making host vulnerable by increasing the susceptibility, e.g., age, gender, and history of illness.
- **Enabling factors:** These are the factors either responsible for the development of disease or even in recovery, e.g., living conditions, socio-economic status.
- **Precipitating factors:** These are the factors are associated with immediate exposure to the disease agent or onset of disease, e.g., drinking contaminated water, close contact with a case of pulmonary TB.
- **Reinforcing factors:** These are factors which aggravate an already existing disease, e.g., malnutrition.
- **Risk factors:** These are the factors whose presence increases the chances of an individual to have, develop or be adversely affected by a disease process. The risk factor need not necessarily cause the disease but does increase the probability that the person exposed to the factor may get the disease easily.

Different Theories on Causation of Diseases

Theories of Premodern (Ancient) Era

The demonic theory: This theory is based on following different concepts:
- The evil spirit entering the body directly and pursuing nefarious actions.
- The evil spirit as a messenger of God giving warnings in the form of diseases.
- Human enemy with supernatural powers, send evil spirits to harm.
- The souls of dead ancestors influencing their family members.

The Punitive Theory

Since ancient times and even today some sector of society believes that disease has been considered as punishment by an outraged God for any bad deed done by the individual or the race.

Miasmatic Theory

Miasmatic theory is based on the inference that the air arising from certain kinds of ground, especially low, swampy areas, was a cause of disease.

Humoral Theory

- As per Greek philosophy, the matter is made up of four elements—Earth, Air, Fire and Water which are represented in the body by four humors—*phlem, yellow bile, black bile and blood.*
- According to this theory, the equilibrium among these humors characterizes health *(eucrasia),* and disequilibrium *(dyscrasia)* characterizes disease.
- Hippocrates rejected the super natural theories and considered disease as a natural process.
- Hippocrates moved medicine from magic and metaphysics to give it a scientific basis. He introduced logic into medical thinking, elaborated the theory of humors and recognized the importance of the environment in health. He also suggested that an excess of one of the humors would result in various idiosyncrasies—hematic, phlegmatic, choleric and melancholic.

- The Ayurveda believes that the imbalance of the three doshas (tridosha) is the reason behind disease causation.
- Chinese medicine considers a discrepancy between the male (yang) and female (yin) principle resulting in disease.

Contagion Theory

- Girolamo Fracastoro (1478–1553), an Italian physician, contended that there is a large class of diseases caused by contagion rather than humoral imbalances.
- He observed that person could contract infections even if humors are normally balanced.
- He described how contagion can occur by direct contact, by indirect contact via clothes and other substances, and by long-distance transmission.
- In addition, he stated that diseases can arise within an individual spontaneously.
- His theory is being superseded by a fully developed germ theory.

Theories of Modern Era

Germ Theory

- Germ theory was proposed by Louis Pasteur (1822–1895).
- Germ theory postulates that every human disease is caused by a microbe or germ, which is specific for that disease and one must be able to isolate the microbe from the diseased human being.
- Germ theory brought drastic shift in the understanding of disease causation.
- The germ theory implies the causal effect is one-to-one, i.e., a single microorganism is the culprit behind a specific disease, e.g., *Mycobacterium tuberculosis* bacteria and the occurrence of tuberculosis.
- But that seldom is the case, as many diseases cannot be explained by this one-to-one causal relation but in reality, an interaction of various other contributory factors.

Epidemiological Triad

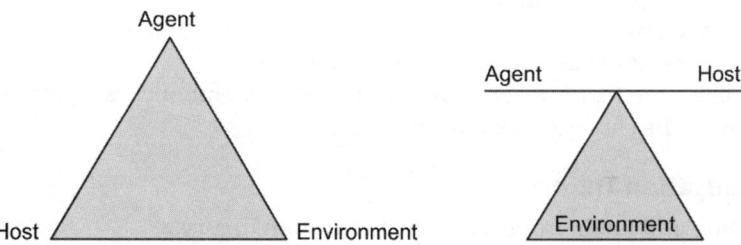

- Triad theory explains that an external agent can cause diseases on a susceptible host when there is a conducive environment
- **Agent** originally referred to an infectious microorganism or pathogen: a virus, bacterium, parasite, or other microbe. Generally, the agent must be present for disease to occur; however, presence of that agent alone is not always sufficient to cause disease. A variety

of factors influence whether exposure to an organism will result in disease, including the organism's pathogenicity (ability to cause disease) and dose.
- Over time, the concept of agent has been broadened to include chemical and physical causes of disease or injury.
- **Host** refers to the human who can get the disease. A variety of factors intrinsic to the host, sometimes called risk factors, can influence an individual's exposure, susceptibility, or response to a causative agent. Opportunities for exposure are often influenced by behaviors such as sexual practices, hygiene, and other personal choices as well as by age and sex. Susceptibility and response to an agent are influenced by factors such as genetic composition, nutritional and immunologic status, anatomic structure, presence of disease or medications, and psychological makeup.
- **Environment** refers to extrinsic factors that affect the agent and the opportunity for exposure. Environmental factors include physical factors such as geology and climate, biologic factors such as insects that transmit the agent, and socioeconomic factors such as crowding, sanitation, and the availability of health services.

Epidemiological triangle: In addition to agent, host and environment, the time factor is added. Here, Time factor depicts incubation periods, life expectancy of the host or pathogen and duration of the illness.

Dever's Epidemiological Model
- This model highlights the interplay of four factors namely: Human biology, Lifestyle, Environment and Health system.
- All of which can have a positive or a negative effect.

Multifactorial Theory
- Germ theory alone is not sufficient to explain the causation of all the diseases and thus need of multifactorial theory arises.
- Pettenkofer proposed multifactorial theory.
- Germ theory was relatively good in explaining communicable diseases but rise in non-communicable diseases needed another explanation.
- Factors like genetic, nutritional, immunological, metabolic, cytological factors have been identified as the cause for specific diseases.

Web of Causation Theory
- MacMahon and Pugh proposed web of causation theory.
- Ideally suited in the study of chronic disease, where the agent is often not known and disease is the outcome of interaction of multiple factors.

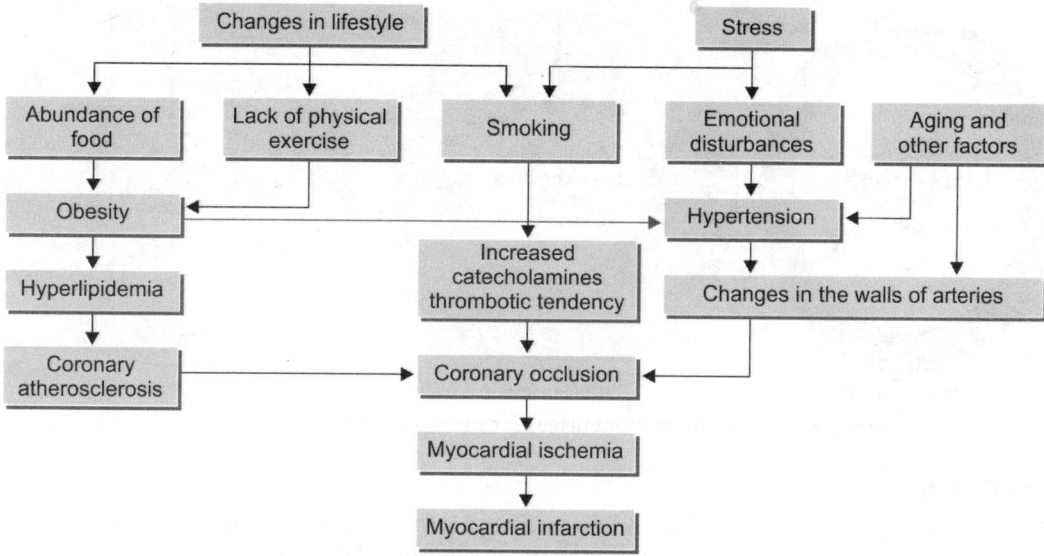

Fig. 8.2: Web of causation for myocardial infarction.

- The various factors, (e.g., hypercholesterolemia, smoking, hypertension) are like an interacting web of a spider, Each factor has its own relative importance in causing the final departure from the state of health, as well as interacts with others, modifying the effect of each other (Fig. 8.2).
- Once we have more factor interacting with each others this will increase the risk of developing chronic disease.
- For example, smoking might increase the risk of developing ischemic heart disease, but if smoker is under stress and they are hypertensive as well the will increase that risk way more than before.

Wheel Theory

- Mausner and Kramer proposed wheel theory in 1985.
- This theory explores the "genetic" and the "environmental" factors in causation of disease.
- The theory visualizes human disease in the form of a wheel, which has a central hub representing the genetic components and the peripheral portion representing the environmental component which is further divided into 3 subcomponents, representing the social, biological and physical component (Figs. 8.3 and 8.4).

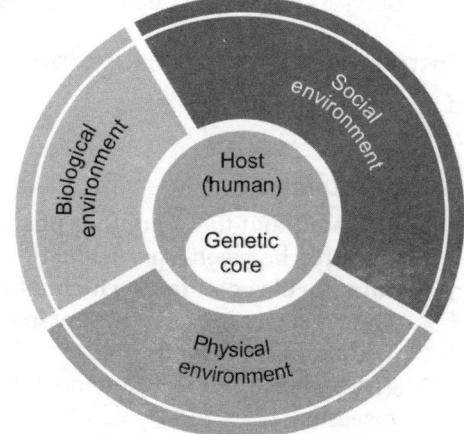

Fig. 8.3: The wheel of disease causation.

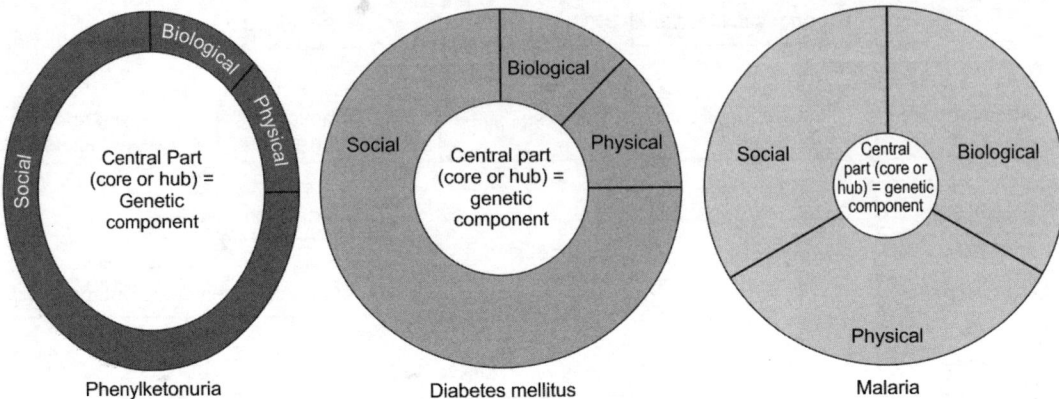

Fig. 8.4: Example of different diseases causation based on wheel theory.

BEINGS Theory

BEINGS concept postulates that human diseases and its consequences are caused by a complex interplay of nine different factors. By coining the first letters of these factors the theory is called BEINGS theory. These are:
1. **B**iological factors innate in a human being,
2. **B**ehavioral factors concerned with individual lifestyles,
3. **E**nvironmental factors as physical, chemical and biological aspects of environment,
4. **I**mmunological factors,
5. **N**utritional factors,
6. **G**enetic factors,
7. **S**ocial factors,
8. **S**piritual factors and
9. **S**ervices factors, related to the various aspects of healthcare services.

Postulates of Diseases Causation
- Koch's postulate
- Hill's criteria

Koch's Postulates
- Koch stated that there are four postulates which all four should be met to accept causal relationship between a particular disease agent (e.g., bacteria) and the disease.
- All **four koch's postulates which** must be fulfilled are as below:
  1. The organism must be present in every case of the disease;
  2. The organism must be able to be isolated and grown in pure culture;
  3. The organism must, when inoculated into a susceptible healthy host, cause the specific disease;
  4. The organism must then be recovered from the diseased experimental host subjects and cultured and identified the original causative agent.

Limitations of Koch's Postulate
- Not useful for noncommunicable disease
- One to one relation is rare in biology.
- Disease production may require cofactors.
- Viruses cannot be cultured like bacteria because viruses need living cells in which to grow (Ex. Mycobacterium leprae and rabies virus)
- Pathogenic microbes may be present without clinical disease (subclinical infections, carrier states).

Hill's Criteria (1965)
- Temporal relationship
- Strength of the association
- Biologic plausibility
- Dose-response relationship
- Replication of the findings
- Effect of removing the exposure
- Extent to which alternate explanations have been considered
- Specificity of the association
- Consistency with other knowledge

Temporal relationship:
- Most important criterion that must be met.
- Exposure precedes outcome (disease) development with adequate elapsed incubation period (in case of communicable disease) and latent period (in case of noncommunicable disease).
- Study designs which can establish temporal relationship are cohort, case-control, and RCT.

Strength of the association:
- Strength of association can be established with help of RR (cohort study) and odds ratio (case control study).
- Stronger the association more likely to be causal and weak association is least likely be causal.

Biological plausibility:
- It answers the question that does the association makes the sense biologically and is it consistent with current biological knowledge about the given condition.
- Lack of plausibility may simply reflect lack of scientific knowledge.
  Example: Smoking causes lung cancer because inhaled smoke directly comes in contact with lung parenchyma and triggers carcinogens.

Dose-response relationship:
- If risk increases with increasing dose of exposure, it supports principle of causal association.
- However, the absence of dose-response does not exclude causal association.

Replication of the findings (coherence):
It is supportive of causal association if the same finding can be replicated in different populations and/or by using various study designs.

Effect of removing the exposure (cessation of the exposure):
- Similar to the dose-response relationship, the presence of this criterion supports the notion of causal association.
- However, the absence does not preclude it.

Extent to which alternate explanations have been considered

Specificity of association:
- Specificity of the association suggests that one exposure is specific to one disease.
- This criterion is not applicable to all exposure-disease associations because a disease may be caused by several exposures, and an exposure may cause several diseases.
- An exposure, such as smoke from cigarette smoking, is comprised of many smaller chemical components and out of these which is the main cause of lung cancer is difficult to find out.

Consistency with other knowledge:
- In vitro studies
- Animal studies
- Other studies such as ecological studies, cross-sectional studies
- Other types of data such as sales data, time trend
- Meta-analysis is very good method for testing consistency.
- It summarizes odds ratios from various studies.

BIBLIOGRAPHY

1. https://www.nhp.gov.in/causation-of-diseases_mtl
2. https://www.sciencedirect.com/topics/immunology-and-microbiology/germ-theory-ofdisease. Last accessed on 20.08.2022.
3. https://medicopublication.com/index.php/ijfmt/article/download/12923/11906/24684
4. https://ksumsc.com/download_center/Archive/3rd/436/Females/First%20semester/community%20Medicine/4-%20Natural%20History%20of%20Disease%20%20and%20concepts%20of%20prevention%20and%20control.pdf

8.5 MODES OF DISEASE TRANSMISSION

Concept of chain of infection: Disease transmission occurs when the agent leaves its **reservoir** or host through a **portal of exit**, is conveyed by some **mode of transmission**, and enters through an appropriate **portal of entry** to infect a **susceptible host** (Fig. 8.5).

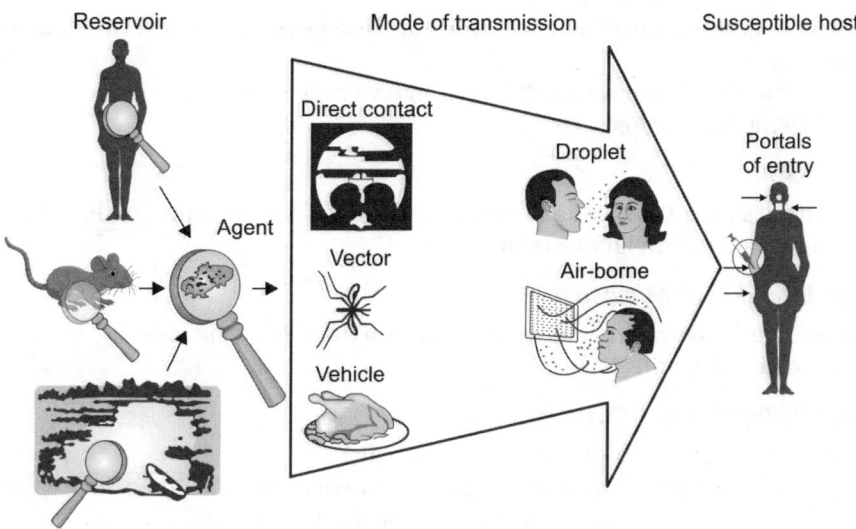

Fig. 8.5: Chain of infection.

DIFFERENT MODES OF DISEASE TRANSMISSION

Direct Transmission
- Direct contact
- Droplet infection
- Contact with soil
- Inoculation into skin or mucosa
- Transplacental (vertical)

Direct Contact
- Direct and immediate transfer of infectious agents from the reservoir or source to a susceptible individual, without an intermediate agency.
- It occurs through skin to skin (by touching), mucosa to mucosa and mucosa to skin of the same or another person.
- Reduces the period for which the organism will have to survive outside the human host and ensures a larger dose of infection.
- Example: Leprosy, leptospirosis, skin and eye infections and STD including HIV.

Droplet Infection
- Droplet spread refers to spray with relatively large, short-range aerosols produced by sneezing, coughing, or even talking.
- Droplet spread is classified as direct because transmission is by direct spray over a few feet, before the droplets fall to the ground.
- Expelled droplets may impinge directly upon the conjunctiva, oro-respiratory mucosa or skin of a close contact.
- Particles of 10 microns or greater in diameter are filtered off by nose while those 5 microns or less can penetrate deeply and reach the alveoli.
- The droplet spread is limited to a distance of 30–60 cm between source and host.

- Transmission gets increased in conditions of close proximity, overcrowding and lack of ventilation.
- Example: Pertussis (whooping cough), meningococcal meningitis, eruptive fevers, common cold, diphtheria, tuberculosis, etc.

Contact with Soil

Direct exposure of susceptible tissue to the disease agent in soil, compost or decaying vegetable matter. Example: hookworm larvae, tetanus, etc.

Inoculation Into Skin or Mucosa

- The disease agent may be inoculated directly into the skin or mucosa.
- Example: Rabies, Hepatitis B.

Transplacental (or Vertical) Transmission

- Disease agents can be transmitted transplacentally.
- Example: TORCH agents (Toxoplasma gondii, rubella virus, cytomegalovirus and herpes virus), varicella virus, syphilis, hepatitis B, Coxsackie B and AIDS.
- Some of the non-living agents (e.g., thalidomide, diethylstilbestrol) can also be transmitted vertically.
- In these cases, the disease agent produces malformations of the embryo by disturbing its development.

Indirect Transmission

- Vehicle-borne
- Vector-borne
  - Mechanical
  - Biological
- Air-borne
  - Droplet nuclei
  - Dust
- Fomite-borne
- Unclean hands and fingers

Indirect: Indirect transmission refers to the transfer of an infectious agent from a reservoir to a host by suspended air particles, inanimate objects (vehicles), or animate intermediaries (vectors).

- This embraces a variety of mechanisms including the traditional 5 F's—**"flies, fingers, fomites, food and fluid"** (for more detail on F-diagram is given in Chapter 3.5).
- The infectious agent must be capable of surviving outside the human host in the external environment and retain its basic properties of pathogenesis and virulence till it finds a new host.
- Depends upon the characteristics of the agent, the inanimate object and the influence of environmental factors such as temperature and humidity.
- Drug resistance further facilitate its spread.

1. Vehicle-borne
- Transmission of the infectious agent through the agency of water, food, blood, serum, plasma or other biological products such as tissues and organs.
- Water and food are the most frequent vehicles of transmission.
- The infectious agent may have multiplied or developed in the vehicle (e.g., *S. aureus* in food) before being transmitted or only passively transmitted in the vehicle (e.g., hepatitis A virus in water).
- Example: Acute gastroenteritis, typhoid fever, cholera, polio, hepatitis A, food poisoning and intestinal parasites, hepatitis B, malaria, syphilis, brucellosis, trypanasomes (Chaga's disease), infectious mononucleosis and cytomegalovirus infection.

2. Vector-borne
It is an arthropod or any living carrier (e.g., snail) that transports an infectious agent to a susceptible individual.

Epidemiological classification of vector-borne diseases
I. By vector
- Invertebrate: Flies, mosquitoes, fleas, cockroaches, sucking lice, bugs, ticks, mites, cyclops
- Vertebrate: Mice, rodents, bats.

II. By methods in which vectors transmit agent
- Biting
- Regurgitation
- Scratching-in of infective feces
- Contamination of host with body fluids of vectors.

III. By transmission chain
Three principal patterns:
1. Man and a non-vertebrate host
   - Man-arthropod-man (malaria)
   - Man-snail-man (schistosomiasis).
2. Man, another vertebrate host, and a non-vertebrate host
   - Mammal-arthropod-man (plague)
   - Bird-arthropod- man (encephalitis).
3. Man and 2 intermediate hosts
   - Man-cyclops-fish-man (fish tapeworm)
   - Man-snail-fish-man (*Clonorchis sinensis*)

IV. By methods in which vectors are involved in the transmission and propagation of parasites
- ***Mechanical transmission:*** The infectious agent is mechanically transported by a crawling or flying arthropod through soiling of its feet or proboscis; or by passage of organisms through its gastrointestinal tract and passively excreted.
- There is no development or multiplication of the infectious agent on or within the vector.

- **Biological transmission:**

Type	Explanation	Agent	Vector
Propagative	Only agent multiplication in vector	Plague bacilli	Rat flea
		Yellow fever	Aedes
Cyclo-propagative	Both multiplication and change in the form of agent	Malarial parasite	Anopheles mosquitoes
Cyclodevelopmental	Only change in the form of agents	Filarial parasite	Culex mosquito
		Guinea worm	Cyclops

- When the infectious agent is transmitted vertically from the infected female to her progeny in the vector, it is known as ***transovarial transmission*** (e.g., dengue virus in aedes mosquito).
- Transmission of the disease agent from one stage of the life cycle to another as for example nymph to adult is known as ***transstadial transmission*** (e.g., lyme disease in tick).

3. Air-borne

Droplet nuclei
- Droplet nuclei are dried residue of less than 5 microns in size. In contrast to droplets that fall to the ground within a few feet, droplet nuclei may remain suspended in the air for long periods of time and may be blown over great distances.
- Formed by evaporation of droplets coughed or sneezed into the air.
- Also be formed accidentally in microbiological laboratories, in abattoirs, rendering plants or autopsy rooms.
- Particles in the 1–5-micron range are liable to be easily drawn into the alveoli of the lungs and may be retained there.
- Example: Measles, tuberculosis, influenza, chickenpox, measles, Q fever

Dust
- Some of the larger droplets which are expelled during talking, coughing or sneezing, settle down by their sheer weight on the floor, carpets, furniture, clothes, bedding, linen and other objects in the immediate environment and become part of the dust.
- During the act of sweeping, dusting and bed-making, the dust is released into the air and becomes once again airborne.
- Dust particles may also, be blown from the soil by wind; this may include fungal spores.
- Airborne dust is primarily inhaled, but may settle on uncovered food and milk.
- Most-common in hospital-acquired (nosocomial) infection.
- Example: Streptococcal and staphylococcal infection, pneumonia, tuberculosis, Q fever, Coccidioidomycosis and psittacosis.

4. Fomite-borne
- Fomites-inanimate articles or substances other than water or food contaminated by the infectious discharges from a patient and capable of harbouring and transferring the infectious agent to a healthy person.
- Include soiled clothes, towels, linen, handkerchiefs, cups, spoons, pencils, books, toys, drinking glasses, door handles, taps, lavatory chains, syringes, instruments and surgical dressings.

- Example: Diphtheria, typhoid fever, bacillary dysentery, hepatitis A, eye and skin infections.

5. Unclean Hands and Fingers
- Hands—most common medium by which pathogenic agents are transferred to food from the skin, nose, bowel, etc. as well as from other foods.
- Both directly (hand-to-mouth) and indirectly.
- Imply lack of personal hygiene.
- Example: Staphylococcal and streptococcal infections, typhoid fever, dysentery, hepatitis A and intestinal parasites.

BIBLIOGRAPHY

1. Centers for Disease Control and Prevention. Principles of epidemiology, 2nd ed. Atlanta: US Department of Health and Human Services; 1992.

8.6 GLIMPSE ABOUT IMPORTANT CONCEPTS OF EPIDEMIOLOGY

8.6.1 IMPORTANT DEFINITIONS

Sanitation	Hygiene
• It is defined as the way in which human protects health by preventing human contact with wastes which contains disease causing microorganisms. • It is related to human waste, environmental waste. • It is keeping watch over external environment • Example: Management of human excreta	• It is defined as group of practices that is perceived by people to be a way towards healthy living or good health. • It is mainly associated with human body. • It is keeping watch over internal environment. • Example: Brushing of teeth

Source	Reservoir
• The source of infection is defined as "the person, animal, object or substance from which an infectious agent is acquired to the host". • Example: Feces in typhoid	• A **reservoir** is defined as "any person, animal, arthropod, plant, soil or substance (or combination of these) in which an infectious agent lives and multiplies, and depends primarily on it for survival, and where it reproduces itself in such a manner that it can be transmitted to a susceptible host". • Reservoir may or may be not the source • Example: Carrier in typhoid

Incubation period: It is defined as "the time interval between invasion by an infectious agent and appearance of the first sign or symptom of the disease."

Serial interval: The gap in time between the onset of the primary case and the secondary case is called the "serial interval".

Generation time: It is defined as "the interval of time between receipt of infection by a host and achieving maximal infectivity".

Period of communicability: It is defined as "the time during which an infectious agent may be transferred directly or indirectly from an infected person to another person, from an infected animal to man, or from an infected person to an animal, including arthropods".

Latent period: The interval between exposure to a carcinogen, toxin, or disease-causing organism and development of a consequent disease. It is mainly used for noncommunicable diseases and it has resemblance with incubation period.

Prepatent period: It is the interval between the entrance of the parasite (infective larvae of the *Wuchereria bancrofti*) and the first appearance of the microfilariae in the blood as in filariasis.

Window period: It is the period between the entry of the pathogen and the production of the antibodies.

Preclinical:
- Is the early stage of disease progression
- Disease is not clinically detected
- It is destined to become disease

Subclinical cases :
- They are also known as "**inapparent, covert, missed or abortive cases**".
- They are also important sources of infection.
- They are not destined to be cases.
- The disease agent may multiply in the host but does not manifest any signs and symptoms and it shows antibody response.
- The disease agent can contaminate the environment just like clinical cases.
- Subclinical cases maintain the chain of infection (endemicity) in the community.

Latent infection:
- Agent lies dormant within the host.
- The host does not shed the infectious agent.
- There are no symptoms.
- It's presence demonstration in blood, tissues or bodily secretions is mostly not possible.
- For example, latent infection occurs in herpes simplex, Brill-Zinsser disease in epidemic typhus, etc.
- The role of latent infection in the perpetuation of certain infectious agents appears to be great.

Primary case refers to the first case of a communicable disease introduced into the population unit being studied.

The term **Index case** refers to the first case to come to the attention of the investigator; it is not always the primary case.

Secondary cases are those developing from contact with primary case within same incubation period

A **Carrier** is defined as "an infected person or animal that harbours a specific infectious agent in the absence of discernible clinical disease and serves as a potential source of infection for others".

Communicable disease	Infectious disease
- An illness due to a specific infectious agent or its toxic products capable of being directly or indirectly transmitted from man to man, animal to animal, or from the environment (through air, dust, soil, water, food, etc.) to man or animal. - All communicable diseases are infectious	- A clinically manifest disease of man or animals resulting from an infection. - All infectious diseases are not communicable - Example: Tetanus

Isolation	Quarantine
• Isolation is defined as "separation, for the period of communicability of infected persons or animals from others in such places and under such conditions, as to prevent or limit the direct or indirect transmission of the infectious agent from those infected to those who are susceptible". • Isolation is done for the cases themselves. • It is secondary (treatment) level of prevention. • Duration for the isolation depends on period of communicability of the given disease.	• Quarantine has been defined as "the limitation of freedom of movement of such well persons or domestic animals exposed to communicable disease for a period of time not longer than the longest usual incubation period of the disease". • Healthy contacts of cases are quarantined. • It is primary (specific protection) level of prevention. • Duration of quarantine is the maximum incubation period of the given disease.

Endemic	It refers to the constant presence of disease or infectious agents within a given geographic area or population group
Epidemic	It refers to sudden occurrence of disease or specific health related behavior or events in community or region, clearly in excess of expected occurrence.
Outbreak	It is similar condition like epidemic but confined to small geographical region and can be managed locally available resources.
Pandemic	An epidemic usually affecting a large proportion of the population occurring over a wide geographic area such as a section of a nation, the entire nation, a continent or the world, e.g., influenza pandemics of 1918 and 1958 and 2009, cholera El Tor in 1962, COVID-19.
Sporadic	Cases are scattered and widely separated in space and time and little or no connection between cases.

Pasteurization	Sterilization	Disinfection
Pasteurization may be defined as the heating of milk to such temperatures and for such periods of time as are required to destroy any pathogens that may be present while causing minimal changes in the composition, flavor and nutritive value.	**Sterilization** is the process of destroying all life including spores. This is widely used in medical practice.	**Disinfection** is the killing of infectious agents outside the body by direct exposure to chemical or physical agents. It can refer to the action of antiseptics as well as disinfectants.

Disease control: Is reducing the transmission of disease agent to such a low level that it ceases to be a public health problem.

Elimination: Is complete interruption of transmission of disease in a defined geographical area, but the causative organism may be persisting in environment. The process of documenting elimination of transmission is called **verification** and declaring as elimination of public health problem is called **validation**.

Eradication: Termination of all transmission of infection by extermination of the infectious agent through surveillance and containment. The process of documenting eradication is called **certification.**

Vaccination	Immunization
• It means to inject a suspension of attenuated or killed microorganisms for the generation of immunity. • It is a process. • It does not guarantee immunity. • It is one of the ways for the immunization.	• It means make someone immune to particular disease. • It is a result. • It is guaranteed. • Immunization can be done with methods other than vaccination, like by breastfeeding (maternal antibodies) or exposure to natural infection.
Monitoring	**Surveillance**
• Performance and analysis of routine measurements aimed at detecting changes in environment or health status of a population. • One time linear activity. • No feedback present. • No inbuilt action component present. • Stops once disease is eliminated/eradicated. • Smaller concept.	• Continuous scrutiny of the factors that determine the occurrence and distribution of disease and other conditions of ill-health. • Continuous cycle. • Feedback present. • Inbuilt action component present • Continues even after disease is eliminated/eradicated. • Broader concept.
Antigenic shift	**Antigenic drift**
Sudden complete or major antigenic change	Antigenic change is gradual over a period of time
It is result from genetic recombination/rearrangements of human with animal or avian virus	It results from point mutation in the gene owing to selection pressure by immunity in the host population
It leads to epidemic or pandemic change	Sporadic cases

8.6.2 NATURAL HISTORY OF DISEASE

- Natural history of disease refers to the progress of a disease process in an individual over time, in the absence of intervention **(Fig. 8.6)**.
- Without medical intervention, the process ends with:
  - Recovery (influenza)
  - Disability (diabetes)
  - Death (cancer)
- The natural history of disease is best established by cohort studies.
- Knowledge of the natural history of disease ranks alongside causal understanding in importance for disease prevention and control.
- **Prepathogenesis phase:**
  - The disease agent has not yet entered man, but the factors which favor its interaction with the human host are already existing in the "environment"
  - This situation is frequently referred to as "man exposed to risk of disease"
- **Pathogenesis phase:**
  - This phase begins with entry of the disease "agent" in the susceptible "human host"
  - After the entry, agent multiplies and induces tissue and physiological changes the disease progresses through the period of incubation.
  - Pathogenesis phase usually divided into early and late pathogenesis.
  - The final outcome of the disease may be recovery, disability or death.

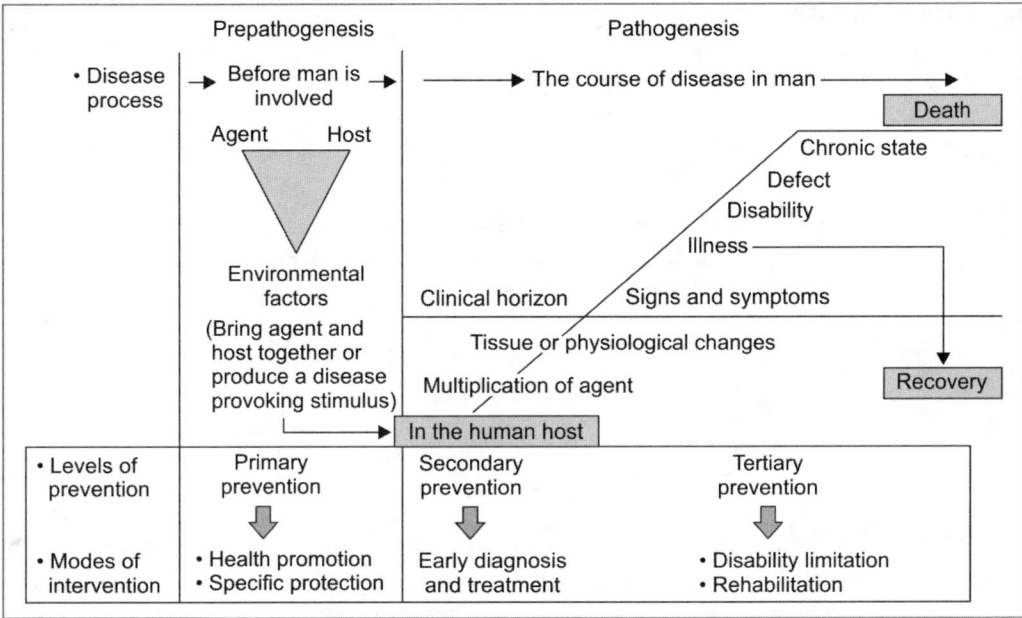

Fig. 8.6: Natural history of disease.

8.6.3 ICEBERG PHENOMENON

- Iceberg phenomenon of disease gives a picture of the spectrum of diseases in a community.
- The visible part of the iceberg denotes the clinically apparent cases of disease in the community.
- The part of the iceberg below the water level denoted the latent, subclinical, undiagnosed and carrier states in the community, which forms the major part.
- Screening test helps us to reduced the submerged portion of iceberg by finding the hidden cases.
- Iceberg phenomenon is commonly seen in the diseases where long latent or incubation period, more subclinical or carrier.
- But exceptionally following four diseases not showing iceberg phenomenon
  - Rabies
  - Rubella
  - Measles
  - Tetanus

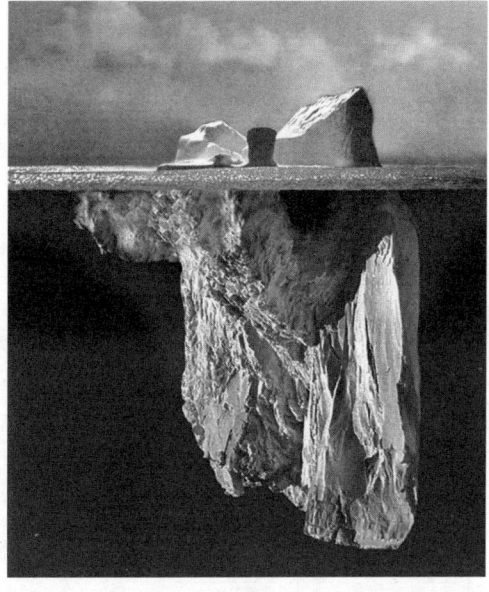

Spectrum of Health

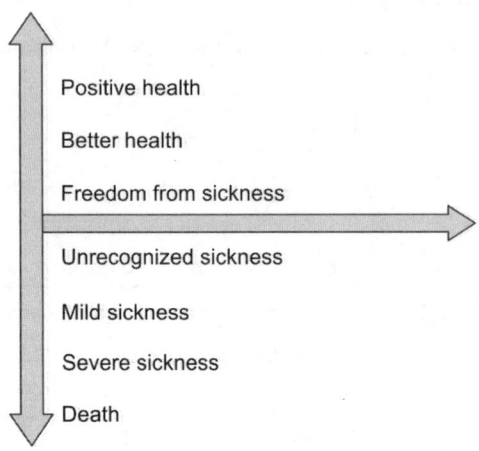

BIBLIOGRAPHY

1. https://ksumsc.com/download_center/Archive/3rd/436/Teams%20work/Community%20Medicine/1st%20semester/4.%20natural%20history%20of%20disease%20%28Final%20Draft%29.pdf
2. https://edisciplinas.usp.br/pluginfile.php/445608/mod_resource/content/1/Basic_epidemiology_2nd_edition.pdf

8.7 CLASSIFICATION OF DIFFERENT EPIDEMIOLOGICAL STUDY DESIGNS

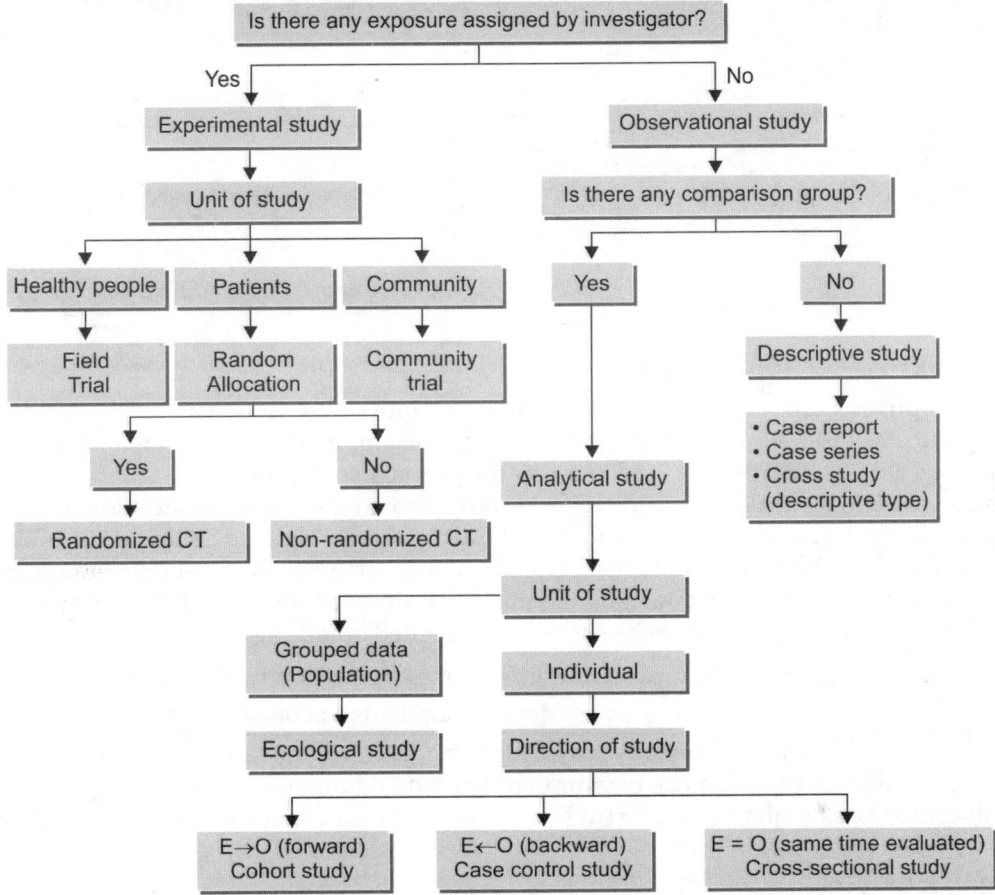

8.8 CROSS-SECTIONAL STUDY: DESIGN, STEPS, ANALYSIS AND INTERPRETATION

- Cross-sectional studies are carried out to examine the presence or absence of disease and the exposure at same and at particular time.
- The end result of this study design is prevalence of given disease or condition that's why it is also known **as prevalence study**.
- It gives the burden of given condition which in turn helps for better planning and allocating health resources.
- A cross-sectional study should be done among representative of the population for generalizations of the findings of the study.
- These studies provide **a snapshot** of the health of the populations at a particular time.
- Less expensive and lost to follow-up is not a problem in this study design.
- It gives relatively quick results and easy to conduct.
- Multiple outcomes and exposures can be studied.
- **Example** of cross-sectional study: NFHS, DLHS, CENUS.

Design

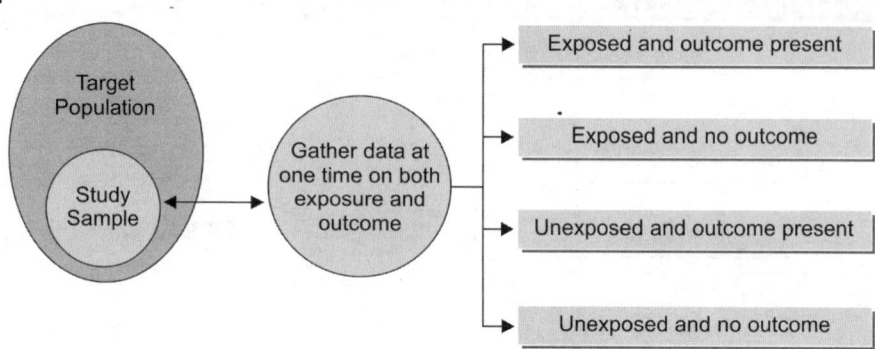

Type of Cross-sectional Study

- **Descriptive:** A cross-sectional study usually descriptive and used to assess the burden of a particular disease in a defined population. For example a random sample of pregnant women across city X may be used to assess the prevalence of anemia.
- **Analytical:** Analytical cross-sectional study is used to investigate the association between a putative risk factor and a health outcome. However, this type of study is limited in its ability to draw valid conclusions as to the association between a risk factor and health outcome because the risk factors and outcome are measured simultaneously, and therefore it may be difficult to determine whether the exposure proceeded or followed the disease.

Analysis: The main outcome measured from a cross-sectional study is prevalence:

$$\text{Prevalence} = \frac{\text{Number of cases in a defined population at one point in time}}{\text{Number of persons in a defined population at the same point in time}}$$

And in some cases we do calculation to obtain odds ratio and also we can apply test of significance like Chi square test, z test or t test based on types of data collected and sample size.

Disadvantages

- One of the weakest observational designs.
- It measures prevalence only and not the incidence of disease.
- The temporality (hills criteria) of exposure and effect may be difficult or impossible to determine because both outcome and exposure are ascertained at the same time.
- Not suitable for highly fatal or disease with shorter duration.
- Usually require bigger sample size.

BIBLIOGRAPHY

1. Grimes DA and Schulz KF. Descriptive studies: What they can and cannot do. Lancet 2002; 359:145--9.
2. https://journal.chestnet.org/article/S0012-3692(20)30462-1/fulltext
3. https://www.healthknowledge.org.uk/e-learning/epidemiology/practitioners/introduction-study-design-css

8.9 CASE CONTROL STUDY: DESIGN, STEPS, ANALYSIS AND INTERPRETATION

- It is analytical observational study used to know the strength of association between exposure and the outcome.
- Here two groups are recruited, one group of people who have the outcome are called as cases and the another group of people who do not have the outcome is called as controls.
- **Study design:**

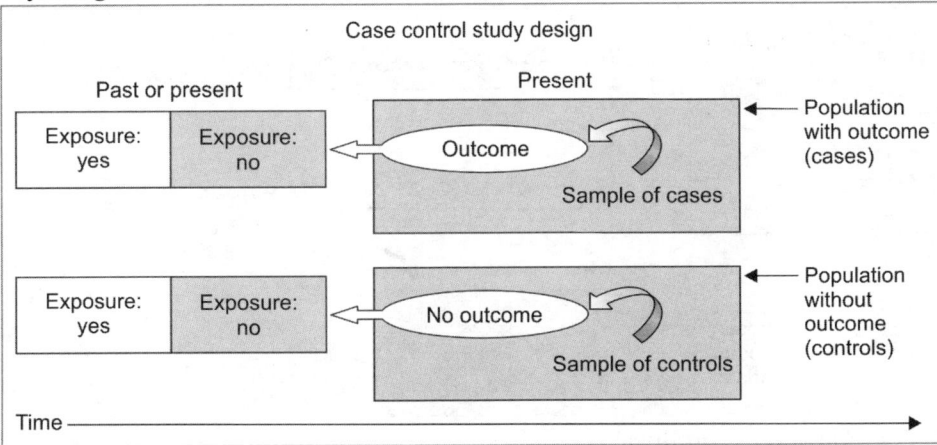

- **Synonyms of case control study:**
  - Retrospective study
  - Backward looking study
  - Effect to cause study
  - Outcome to exposure study
  - Disease to risk factor study
- There are four important components of case control study:
  - **Selection of cases and controls:**
    - Case definition and sources of cases and controls need to be clearly defined.
  - **Sources of cases:**
    - Hospital
    - General population (population based case control studies are generally more expensive and difficult to conduct)
  - **Sources of controls:** It depends on the source of cases.
    - Hospital
    - Neighbor
    - Relatives
    - Population
    - Peer or best friend
  - Control must be similar as much as possible to case except disease under study.
  - Generally, case to control ratio is taken as 1:1 in large studies but when the number of cases are less then control can be increased and **maximum** rewarding documented **ratio is 1:4 (cases: controls)**

- **Matching:** Cases and controls should be matched for at least known confounding factors (e.g., age, gender) to avoid biases.
- **Measuring exposure status:** It is very vital step to minimise recall and observer bias. Tools like standardized questionnaires, biological samples, interviews with the subject or spouse or other family members, records like medical, employment and pharmacy records. The approach used for the measuring exposure status should be the same for cases and controls.
- **Analysis:**
    - Example:

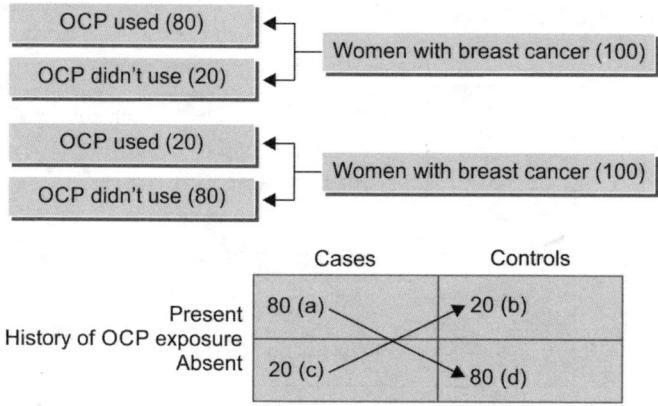

    - Odd's ratio or cross product ratio = ad/bc
    - Odd's ratio = (80 × 80)/(20 × 20)
              = 16
- **Interpretation of odd's ratio:**
    - OR >1: It means, that many times cases have more chances to have history of exposure as compared to controls. This indicates **positive** association. E.g., OCP and breast cancer.
    - OR = 1: It means that chances of history of exposure are same among cases and controls. It indicates **NO** association. E.g., Milk consumption and brain cancer.
    - OR <1: It means that many times cases have lesser chances to have history of exposure as compared to controls. This indicates **negative** association. E.g., Measles vaccine and measles.
- **Advantages of case control study:**
    - Multiple exposures for a single outcome can be studied.
    - Inexpensive and quick to carry out.
    - No attrition problem (no follow-up is required)
    - Case control study is very much useful for rare diseases and diseases with long incubation period.
    - It is preferred method for outbreak investigation to test the preliminary hypothesis.
- **Disadvantages of case control study:**
    - Recall bias
    - Selection bias: Berkesonian bias is a bias introduced in hospital based case-control studies, due to varying rates of hospital admissions
    - Observer bias or interviewer bias
    - The temporal sequence between exposure and disease may be difficult to determine.

BIBLIOGRAPHY

1. https://www.healthknowledge.org.uk/e-learning/epidemiology/practitioners/introduction-study-design-ccs
2. https://www.thelancet.com/journals/lancet/article/PIIS0140-6736%2802%2907605-5/fulltext
3. Schulz KF and Grimes DA. Case control Studies- Research in Reverse. Lancet 2002, 359:43-434.

8.10 COHORT STUDY: DESIGN, STEPS, ANALYSIS AND INTERPRETATION

- Cohort means a group of people sharing common characteristics, e.g., all those who are exposed to smoking will be called as cohort of smokers while who are not exposed will be called as cohort of nonsmokers.
- Here two groups are selected on the basis of their exposure status as exposed group (smokers) and nonexposed groups (nonsmokers).
- These two groups will be followed for a certain period of time to observe the outcome of interest (e.g., lung cancer)
- Cohort studies are preferred studies because we can calculate the incidence and we can determine the associated risk factors.

Cohort Study Design Overview

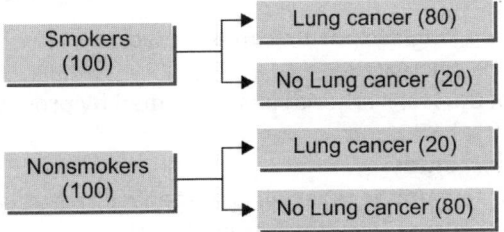

- **Synonyms of cohort study:**
  - Prospective study
  - Cause to effect study
  - Exposure to outcome study
  - Risk factor to disease study
  - Forward-looking study
  - Incidence study
  - Follow-up study
- There are five important steps of cohort study:
  1. **Selection of study population:** All study participants must be free of the outcome under investigation and have the potential to develop the outcome under investigation.
  2. **Obtain the baseline information:** Levels of exposure are measured for each individual at baseline and at intervals during the period of follow-up.
  3. **Selecting comparison group**
  4. **Follow-up:** The follow-up of study participants is a major challenge. A big amount of cost and time is required to ensure follow-up. The failure to collect outcome data for all members of the cohort may affect the validity of study findings.

5. **Analysis:**
   - Relative risk (RR)
   - Attributable risk (AR)
   - Population Attributable risk (PAR)
- There are three types of cohort studies:
  1. **Prospective or concurrent cohort study:**
     - Here two groups, one exposed and another nonexposed are recruited and followed for certain period of time to record the development of an outcome of interest.
     - **Example:** Framingham heart study.
  2. **Retrospective or historical cohort study:**
     - When there is long incubation period then retrospective cohort study seems more feasible.
     - It is time and money saving method.
     - Here we first we go back in time and take into account only exposure details (we obtain exposure details from school or college, hospital or industries records).
     - And at present we look for development of the outcome of interest in both groups.
     - **Example:** PVC exposure and angiosarcoma of liver.
  3. **Combined cohort study:**
     - Just like retrospective method we take the details of exposure and then like prospective method we follow both exposed and nonexposed groups to look for outcome.
     - **Example:** Court brown and Doll study on effects of radiation therapy.
- **Advantages of cohort study:**
  - Multiple outcome of a single exposure can be detected.
  - Incidence rate can be calculated.
  - Temporality (one of the Hill's criteria) is best studied by prospective cohort study.
  - We can calculate RR ad AR.
- **Disadvantages of cohort study:**
  - Expensive and time consuming (specially prospective cohort study)
  - Selection Bias in the form of "Healthy Worker Effect"
  - Attrition Bias (lost to follow up due to migration or death of the participants). Maximum Attrition allowable is 5%.
  - Cohort studies are not suitable for rare diseases.
  - Ethical problems (we are letting someone to keep exposing to risk factor is unethical)
- **Example of analysis of cohort study:**

	Lung cancer	No lung cancer
Smokers	80 (a)	20 (b)
Nonsmokers	20 (c)	80 (d)

- **Relative risk:**
  - RR= incidence among exposed/incidence among nonexposed
  - RR = (80/100)/(20/100)
  - RR = 4
  - Interpretation: Incidence of lung cancer among smokers is 4 times higher as compared to those nonsmokers.

- We need to understand two formulas here:
  1. Formula when RR is more than 1; RR (%) = (RR − 1) × 100
     For example RR is 3, RR (%) = (3 − 1) × 100 = 200%
  2. Formula when RR is less than 1; RR (%) = (1 − RR) × 100
     For example, RR is 0.70, RR (%) = (1 − 0.70) × 100 = 30%

RR	Interpretation
RR = 1	No association between exposure and disease (analytical study) or treatment and disease (experimental study)
RR = 2	100% more disease was observed among a population with exposure than among a population without exposure
RR = 3	200% more disease was observed
RR = 0.70	30% less disease was observed among a population with exposure than among a population without exposure
RR = 0.50	50% less disease was observed

- **Attributable Risk (AR):**
  - AR = {(incidence among exposed − incidence among nonexposed)/incidence among exposed} * 100
  - AR = {(0.8 − 0.2)/0.8}*100
  - AR = 75%
  - Interpretation: 75% of lung cancer patients can be attributed to smoking.
- **Population Attributable Risk:**
  - PAR = {(incidence among Total − incidence among nonexposed)/incidence among Total} * 100
  - PAR = {(100/200 − 20/100)/(100/200)} * 100
  - PAR = {(1.0 − 0.2)/1.0}*100
  - PAR = 60%
  - Interpretation: If we eliminate or reduce the level of smoking level then there will be 60% annual reduction in incidence of lung cancer in the given population.

BIBLIOGRAPHY

1. Grimes DA and Schulz KF. Cohort Studies: Marching Towards Outcomes. Lancet 2002;359:341-45.
2. https://www.healthknowledge.org.uk/e-learning/epidemiology/practitioners/introduction-study-design-cs

8.11 RANDOMIZED CONTROL TRIAL (RCT) STUDY: DESIGN, STEPS, ANALYSIS AND INTERPRETATION

- It is the experimental or interventional study.
- Basic study design is just like cohort study but the difference is that the level of exposure will be under control of investigator in RCT while in cohort study it will be natural phenomenon. It means the intervention (the preventative or therapeutic measure) being tested is allocated by the investigator to a group of two or more study subjects (individuals, households, communities).

- RCT also known as trials. Basically, there are broadly two types of trials: Therapeutic (ex. drug trial) and preventive trail (ex. vaccine trial).
- Randomization is the heart of any clinical trial as each participant has equal chance of being either in experiment group or control (reference group).

Design of RCT

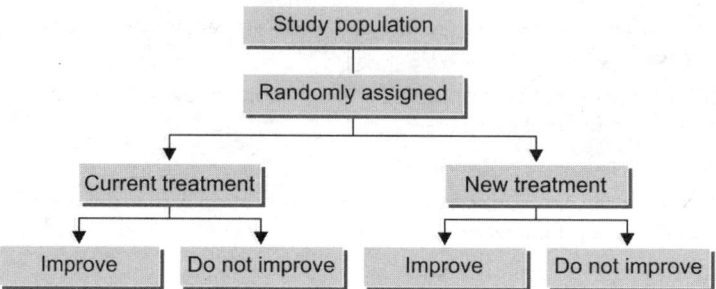

- **Steps of cohort study:**
  - **Drawing up a protocol:** Detailed planning in written and if necessary do the pilot study.
  - **Select experiment and reference group:** Experiment group who will get the new drug or any new intervention while reference group is control group who will receive old or existing intervention.
  - **Randomization:** Random allocation of selected participants into experiment and reference groups.
  - **Manipulation:** It is the phase of actually giving new drug or implementing new intervention.
  - **Follow-up:** Do the follow-up of both groups with equal intensity and similar circumstances at defined intervals.
  - **Assessment:** Assess the outcome in both groups. Apply test of significance either chi square test or Z test to decide the significance of the results.
- There are two types of RCT: 1. Concurrent rct and 2. Cross over design.
  1. **Concurrent design** is just like prospective cohort study.
  2. **Cross over design:** It is one in which the subjects are first assigned to the treatment group and, after a brief interval for cessation of residual effect of the drug, are shifted into the placebo/alternative group. Thus, the subjects act as their own control at the end of the study. However, such studies are not feasible if there is mortality, or if the disease is easily cured by one of the interventions.
- **Blinding:** "Blinding is a process where the critical information on allocation of treatment is hidden either from the patients, or from observer or the evaluator in the study". There are three types of blinding:
  1. **Single blinding:** Study participants don't know whether they are in control group or experiment group.
  2. **Double blinding:** Here neither the participants nor the investigator knows about the control group and experiment group. It is the most commonly used type of blinding.
  3. **Triple blinding:** Here participants, investigator and analyzer all are unaware about the group allocation. It is the ideal type of blinding.

Advantages of Randomized Controlled Trial
- It provides the strongest evidence of safety and efficacy of the given intervention.
- It is one of the best types of epidemiological study to draw conclusions on causality.
- Helps in establishing temporality-exposure clearly precedes outcome.
- It controls both known and unknown confounding factors.
- Enables blinding and therefore minimizes bias.
- Can measure disease incidence and multiple outcomes.

Disadvantages of Randomized Controlled Trial
- Ethical constraints.
- Expensive and time consuming.
- Inefficient for rare diseases or diseases with a delayed outcome.
- Internal validity of RCT is excellent but external validity is always questionable as standardized and controlled study conditions do not adequately reflect clinical reality.

BIBLIOGRAPHY
1. Hennekens CH, Buring JE. Epidemiology in Medicine, Lippincott Williams & Wilkins, 1987.
2. https://www.atlas101.ca/pm/concepts/randomized-controlled-trial-rtc/
3. https://www.healthknowledge.org.uk/e-learning/epidemiology/practitioners/introduction-study-design-is-rct
4. Kendall JM. Designing a research project: Randomised Controlled trials and their principles, Emerg Med J. 2003;20(2)164-8.

8.12 LEVELS OF PREVENTION: PRIMORDIAL, PRIMARY, SECONDARY AND TERTIARY

Definition of Prevention
- "Actions aimed at eradicating, eliminating, or minimizing the impact of disease and disability. The concept of prevention is best defined in the context of levels, traditionally called primary, secondary, and tertiary prevention". (John M Last)
- Leavel and Clark explained levels of prevention for the first time.

Primordial Prevention
- Primordial prevention consists of actions and measures that inhibit the emergence of risk factors in the form of environmental, economic, social, and behavioral conditions and cultural patterns of living, etc.
- It is the prevention of the emergence or development of risk factors in countries or population groups in which they have not yet appeared.
- For example, many adult health problems (e.g., obesity, hypertension) have their early origins in childhood, because this is the time when lifestyles are formed (e.g., smoking, eating patterns, physical exercise).
- In primordial prevention, efforts are directed towards discouraging children from adopting harmful lifestyles.
- The main intervention in primordial prevention is through individual and mass education.

Primary Prevention

- Primary prevention can be defined as the action taken prior to the onset of disease, which removes the possibility that the disease will ever occur.
- It signifies intervention in the prepathogenesis phase of a disease or health problem.
- Primary prevention may be accomplished by measures of "health promotion" and "specific protection".

Health promotion	Specific protection
• Health education • Environmental modifications • Nutritional interventions • Lifestyle modifications	• Immunization and seroprophylaxis • Chemoprophylaxis • Use of specific nutrients or supplementations • Protection against occupational hazards • Safety of drugs and foods • Control of environmental hazards, e.g. air pollution

- The WHO has recommended the following approaches for the primary prevention:
  - Population (mass) strategy
  - High-risk strategy

Population (Mass) Strategy

- "Population strategy" is directed at the whole population irrespective of individual risk levels.
- For example, studies have shown that even a small reduction in the average salt intake of a population would produce a large reduction in the incidence of cardiovascular disease.
- The population approach is directed towards socio-economic, behavioral and lifestyle changes.

High-risk Strategy

- The high-risk strategy aims to bring preventive care to individuals at special risk.
- This requires detection of individuals at high risk by the optimum use of clinical methods.

Secondary Prevention

- It is defined as "action which halts the progress of a disease at its incipient stage and prevents complications."
- The specific interventions are: early diagnosis (e.g., screening tests, and case finding programs) and adequate treatment.
- It acts at early pathogenesis phase of disease.
- Secondary prevention attempts to arrest the disease process, restore health by seeking out unrecognized disease and treating it before irreversible pathological changes take place, and reverse communicability of infectious diseases.
- It thus protects others from in the community from acquiring the infection and thus provide at once secondary prevention for the infected ones and primary prevention for their potential contacts.
- The earlier the disease is diagnosed, and treated the better it is for prognosis of the case and for the prevention of the occurrence of other secondary cases.

Tertiary Prevention

- It is used when the disease process has advanced beyond its early stages and usually has become permanent and irreversible.
- It is defined as "all the measures available to reduce or limit impairments and disabilities, and to promote the patients' adjustment to irremediable conditions."
- Intervention of tertiary prevention are disability limitation, and rehabilitation.

Summary

Levels of prevention	Stage	Target	Modes of intervention
Primordial	Underlying Condition leading to Causation	Target Population/ Selected Groups	Health education (at individual and mass level)
Primary	Specific Causal Factors	Target Population/ Selected Groups/ Individual	• Health Promotion • Specific Protection
Secondary	Early Stage of Disease	Patients	Early Diagnosis and Prompt Treatment
Tertiary	Late Stage of Disease	Patients	Disability Limitation and Rehabilitation

BIBLIOGRAPHY

1. https://www.ump.edu.pl/files/8_483_epidemiology_and_prevention.pdf
2. Leavell, H. R., & Clark, E. G. (1965). Preventive medicine for the doctor in his community (3rd ed.). New York: McGraw-Hill.

8.13 OUTBREAK INVESTIGATION

Epidemic: It refers to sudden occurrence of disease or specific health related behavior or events in community or region, clearly in excess of expected occurrence.

Outbreak: It is similar condition like epidemic but confined to small geographical region and can be managed locally available resources.

Warning Signs of an Outbreak

- Clustering of cases or deaths
- Increases in cases or deaths
- Single case of disease of epidemic potential
- Acute febrile illness of an unknown etiology
- Occurrence of two or more epidemiologically linked cases of a disease of outbreak potential (e.g., measles, cholera, dengue, JE, AFP or plague).
- Unusual isolate
- Shifting in age distribution of cases
- High vector density
- Natural disasters

The balance between investigation and control while responding to an outbreak: At time of outbreak how should we proceed depends on our knowledge about the causative agent and its mode of transmission which shown in details in the following table:

		Source / transmission	
		Known	Unknown
Causative agent	Known	Control +++ Investigate +	Control + Investigate +++
	Unknown	Control +++ Investigate +++	Control + Investigate ++[+]

Trigger level-1	Suspected/limited outbreak	Local response by health worker and MO
Trigger level-2	Outbreak	Local and district response by DSO and DEIT
Trigger level-3	Confirmed outbreak	Local, district and state level response
Trigger level-4	Wide spread epidemic	State level responce to an epidemic
Trigger level-5	Disaster response	Local, district, state, center and partners

Objectives of Outbreak Investigation
- To define the magnitude of the outbreak in terms of time, place and person.
- To determine the particular conditions and factors responsible for the occurrence of an outbreak or an epidemic.
- To identify the etiology of outbreak
- Determine the measures of control, and suggest recommendations to prevent future outbreaks.

Epidemiologic Steps of an Outbreak Investigation
- Preparation for the field work
- Verification of the diagnosis
- Establish the existence of an outbreak
- Develop working definition
- Find cases systematically and record the information
- Descriptive epidemiology
- Hypothesis generation
- Hypothesis testing by epidemiological methods
- Reconsider, refine and reevaluate hypothesis
- Comparison with environmental and/or laboratory studies
- Prevention and control
- Initiation or maintenance of the surveillance
- Reporting of the findings

First three steps are highly variable in sequence as we often verify the diagnosis and also confirms the existence of an outbreak before proceeding for the investigation of an outbreak.

Preparation for the Field Work
- Preparation can be divided in two groups: 1. Preparation for scientific and investigative issues and 2. Preparation for management and operational issues.
- We need to review of literature about the suspected etiological agents and get the lab staff ready with the required equipments.
- Personal protective equipment must be worn by every team member.
- Make plan of action before going for the field work.
- Make team including specialist of different area and distribute roles and responsibilities. Team may have following members:
  - Team Leader
  - Epidemiologist
  - Clinical Officer (Physician or Pediatrician)
  - Laboratory technician/scientist
  - Veterinarian or Animal Health Specialist
  - Social Mobilization Specialist

Verification of the Diagnosis
- Verification of diagnosis and verification of the existence of an outbreak are generally addressed at the same time.
- Verification of the diagnosis made by either expert lab person or expert clinician on the basis of distribution of presenting signs and symptoms.

Establish the Existence of an Outbreak
- As we know that to declare outbreak or epidemic the number of cases must be in excess of normal expectancy.
- The expected number is usually the number from the previous few weeks or months, or from a comparable period during the previous few years.
- If locally data are not available then we can use the state or national data.
- Clearly in excess of normal expectancy is decided when the number of cases is more than average number of cases (previous 3 years) + 2SE or 2 cases with epidemiologic linkage in short time or 1 case of a new emerging disease or even 1 case if endemicity is 0.
- Sometimes due to following reasons **false or pseudoepidemic** is declared:
  - Increasing of reporting
  - Change in the case definition
  - Improvement in diagnostic procedures
  - Increase of awareness among people so more people come for testing so more hidden case will be revealed.
  - Misdiagnosis or lab error
  - In-migration of people increase

Develop Working Definition
- Case definition: It is standard set of criteria for deciding whether an individual has that particular disease or not.
- Case definition should be restricted by time, place and person.
- It must be based on clinical criteria.
- Clinical definition must not include the risk factor which is under study.

- Types of case:
  - **Possible cases**: Events that can possibly be considered as cases following investigation
  - **Probable cases**: Events that are compatible upon clinical assessment
  - **Confirmed cases**: Events that are confirmed by laboratory assessment.

Find Cases Systematically and Record the Information
- Enhanced passive surveillance will help to find out the cases. (all treating facilities either private or public will be asked to report details about each case of the disease under study.)
- Active surveillance also makes contribution in finding of cases.
- Mass media helps to make people aware about the suspicious signs and symptoms of disease and people come forward for testing and at the same time they take precaution to control the spread of the disease.
- Just like snowball effect patient to patient information also helps to find out cases.

Descriptive Epidemiology
- Disease is described by time, place and person and this is called as descriptive epidemiology.
- Descriptive epidemiology helps to identify the population at risk, gives clue about the etiology and possible modes of transmission of disease.

Time Distribution
- Time distribution generally is shown by special type of histogram called as epidemic curve or epicurve.
- Epicurve shows the magnitude of disease over period of time and helps to distinguish epidemic from endemic.
- Its shape tells us that whether it is point or intermittent or propagated type of epidemic.
- Position of the curve tells about the future status of the outbreak; for example if we are at upswing slope of the curve then it means more case are yet about to occur while if we are at the down slope of the curve then it means only few cases are likely to occur.
- Epidemic curve is also used to decide the efficacy of the intervention.
- Most importantly it helps to know probable time of exposure.
- Types of the epidemic on the basis of epidemic curve:
  - **Point source epidemic:**
    - Epidemic curve has steep upslope and more gradual downslope.
    - Sudden rise in the number of the cases.
    - All cases occurred within one incubation period.
    - Example:

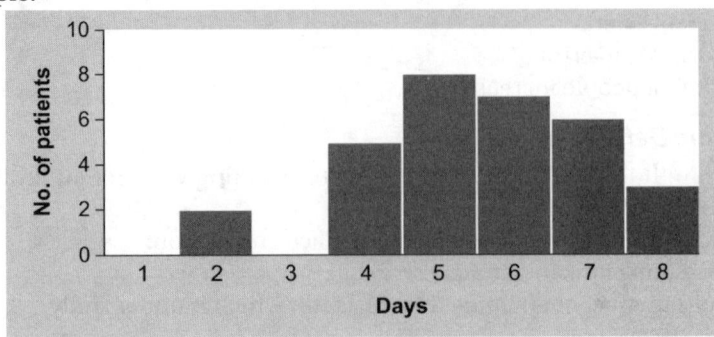

- **Continuous common source epidemic:**
  - The duration of exposure is prolonged.
  - Epidemic curve has plateau instead of peak.

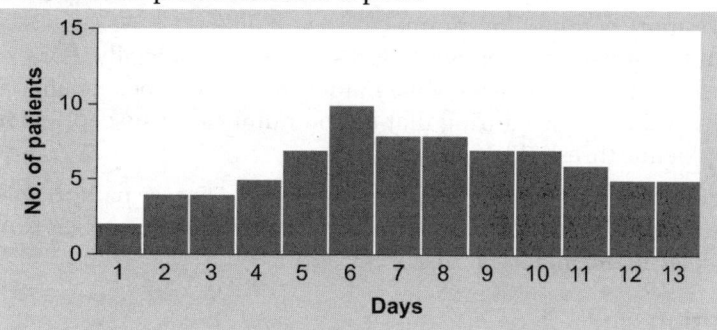

- **Intermittent common source epidemic:**
  - Exposure to causative agent is sporadic over time.
  - It usually produces an irregularly jagged epidemic curve.

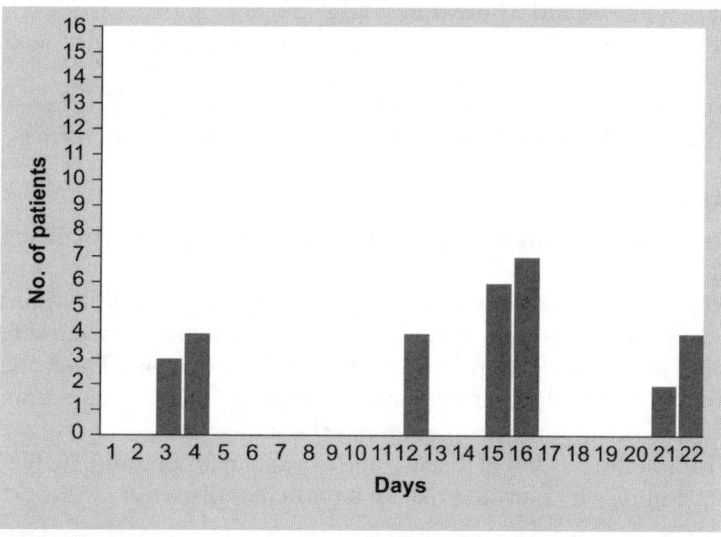

- **Propagated epidemic:**
  - It is generally seen when spread of disease takes place from person to person.
  - It shows progressively taller peaks and one incubation period apart.

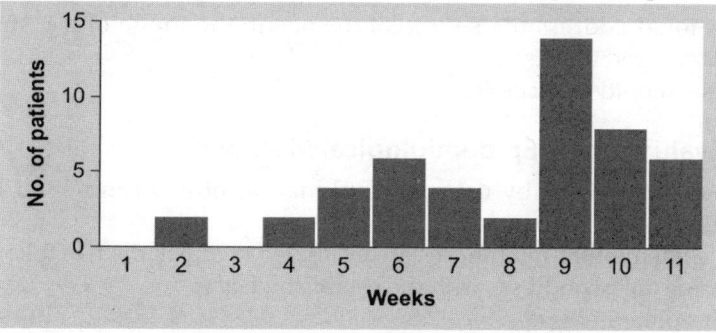

Periodic fluctuation: There are two patterns of periodic fluctuation:
- **Seasonal trend:** Some diseases prefer particular season because of favorable environmental factors. For example, respiratory diseases are more common during winter while diarrhea like diseases is more common in summer.
- **Cyclical trend:** It means tendency of disease to occur cyclically. For example, measles epidemic occurs once in 2–3 years while influenza epidemic occurs after a cycle of 7 to 10 years. It takes cycle because during that period numbers of susceptible individuals have reached to epidemic threshold.

Long-term fluctuations: It is also called as **secular trend**. Disease pattern takes long period of time even decades to change. For example, in the most developed countries Noncommunicable diseases have replaced the infectious diseases.

Place Distribution
- Assessment of an outbreak by place not only provides information on the geographic extent of a problem but may provide important etiologic clues.
- A spot map is a simple and useful technique for illustrating where cases may have been exposed, where they live and where they work.
- **Spot map** is useful for showing distribution of cases within a particular geographic area, but they do not take into account the size of the underlying population.
- While **an incidence map** or **area map** is preferable to show comparison between incidence of particular disease for different areas with different population densities.

Person Distribution
- Characterization of the outbreak by person provides a description of the case-patients and who is at risk.
- Host characteristics like age, sex, race, medical status and other possible exposures (occupation, use of medications, tobacco and drugs) influence susceptibility to disease.
- **Age and sex** are the two most important and commonly described host characteristics.
- Depending on the outbreak other personal characteristics like occupation, race which are specific to the disease under investigation may be important.
- Numbers tell about the burden of disease and are useful for planning while Rates are useful for identifying groups with elevated risk for a particular disease.

Hypotheses Generation
- Count, divide and compare (CDC) and time, place and person distribution help to generate hypotheses.
- Hypothesis should address the source of the agent, the mode of transmission and the exposures that caused the disease.
- The hypothesis should be testable.

Hypotheses Evaluation by Epidemiological Methods
- Hypotheses are evaluated by using a combination of environmental laboratory and epidemiological methods.
- Generally in epidemiology hypotheses are evaluated in one of the two following ways:
  - By comparing the hypotheses with the established facts
  - By analytic epidemiology

- The **first method** is used when the clinical, laboratory, environmental, and/or epidemiologic evidence so obviously supports the formal hypotheses then testing of formal hypothesis is unnecessary.
- When the circumstances are not as straightforward, and information from the investigation is not convincing then epidemiologists use **second method of analytic epidemiology** to test their hypotheses.
- Epidemiologists use analytic epidemiology to quantify relationships between exposures and disease and to test hypotheses about causal relationships.
- The two most common types of analytic epidemiology studies used are: 1. **retrospective cohort studies** and 2. **case-control studies**.
- A retrospective cohort study is the study of choice for an outbreak in a small, well-defined population and when it is possible to follow the population over a period of time.
- However, in many outbreak settings the population is not well defined and investigation's results are needed urgently then in such settings, the case-control study becomes the study design of choice.
- The most common statistical test for used during outbreak is the chi-square test.

Reconsider, Refine, and Re-evaluate Hypotheses

- Sometimes analytic studies are failed to give expected results when hypotheses are not well formed during initial phase.
- If you are not able to generate good hypotheses then conducting analytic epidemiology (such as a case-control study) is likely to be a waste of time it means when analytic epidemiology is unrevealing, rethink of your hypotheses.

Comparison with Laboratory and Environmental Studies

Laboratory evidence helps in confirming the epidemiologic findings.

Control and Prevention Measures

- The primary goal of investigation of an outbreak is to control of the ongoing outbreak and prevention of occurrence of new cases.
- If appropriate control measures are known and available, they should be implemented even before an epidemiologic investigation is started.

Initiation or Maintenance of the Surveillance

- Control and prevention measures must be monitored.
- If surveillance is not started yet for that particular disease, then it should be initiated now.
- If active surveillance has already initiated then it should be continued.

Reporting of the Findings

- Higher authorities and media should be informed orally as well through a detailed written report which includes introduction/background, methods, results, discussion, and recommendations.
- Declaring the outbreak to be over when there have been no new cases for a period of 2 incubation periods since the onset of the last case (after rigorous active case search).

Control Measures for Different Types of Outbreaks

Water-borne Disease Outbreak
- Identify and maintain a line list of cases
- Access to safe drinking water: Communicate to the people not to use any of the local sources and to supply safe water in sachets or through water tankers for the duration of the epidemic.
- Well (in the area)-cleaned or emptying out of water by portable pump sets and then chlorinated.
- Identification and surveillance of high risk cases—pregnant females in case of hepatitis E
- Sanitary disposal of human waste
- Adopting safe practices in food handling.
- If the source of an outbreak is a broken pipeline, it has to be repaired.
- Intersectoral coordination with public health engineering department (PHED) and local bodies.
- IEC—handwashing, sanitation and personal hygiene, safe drinking water, food handling and at household.

Vector-borne Disease Outbreak
- Fever survey and maintain a line list of cases
- Symptomatic management of cases
- Monitoring vector indices (e.g., breteau index, house index)
- Vector control: Integrated vector control measures as per NVBDCP guidelines
- Regular monitoring of vulnerable population (e.g., pregnant women in case of Zika)
- Intersectoral coordination with VBD Officer, PHED and Local bodies.
- IEC for
  - Prevent breeding of mosquitoes
  - Personal protective measures (mosquito nets, repellent, full clothes, wear light coloured clothes)
  - Better health seeking behavior.

Vaccine Preventable Disease Outbreak
- Enhanced case based surveillance and active case search
- Isolation and symptomatic management of cases
- Contact tracing
- Adequate supply of vaccines, syringes and needles
- Adequate staff those are able to administer the vaccines.
- Ring immunization where applicable.
- Supportive treatment, for example vitamin A prophylaxis in case of measles
- Prevention of complications.
  - Monitoring of vulnerable population
  - Intersectoral coordination (immunization officer, ICDS, public relation officer, etc.)
  - IEC

Zoonotic Disease Outbreaks
- Intersectoral coordination with animal husbandry department, wild-life and local bodies
- Safe disposal of dead body including animals
- Universal precautions to prevent exposure to blood and body fluids
- Reporting to higher authorities.

- Vaccination of vulnerable animal and human
- Adequate supply and usage of PPE
- Chemoprophylaxis (e.g., Doxycycline/Azithromycin prophylaxis for leptospirosis)
- Establishment and implementation of isolation facility as per guidelines
- Control the movement of animals
- IEC to avoid panic

Air-born Disease Outbreak
- Disease specific surveillance
- Isolation
- PPE for health worker/contacts
- Chemoprophylaxis and vaccination of vulnerable population
- IEC for:
  - Handwashing
  - Personal hygiene
  - Health seeking behavior
  - Cough etiquettes
- Vaccination as per GoI guidelines

BIBLIOGRAPHY

1. https://idsp.nic.in/WriteReadData/OldSite/2WkDSOSept08/Resources_files/DistrictSurvMan/Module8.pdf
2. https://www.cdc.gov/csels/dsepd/ss1978/lesson6/section2.html

8.14 EVIDENCE-BASED PUBLIC HEALTH

Definition
- Jenicek defined EBPH as the "conscientious, explicit, and judicious use of current best evidence in making decisions about the care of communities and populations in the domain of health protection, disease prevention, health maintenance and improvement (health promotion)."
- "Evidence-based public health is the process of integrating science-based interventions with community preferences to improve the health of populations".

Characteristics of Evidence-Based Public Health (EBPH)
- Decisions are based on best peer-reviewed evidence (both quantitative and qualitative research)
- Systematic use of data and information systems
- Application of program-planning frameworks
- Involvement of community in assessment and decision-making
- Conducting sound evaluation
- Dissemination of the findings to key stakeholders and decision makers.

Steps of EBPH

- Develop problem statement
- Review the scientific literature related to the problem under study and collect all relevant information
- Quantification of the problem under study by using existing data
- Develop and prioritize program options
- Implementation of the interventions
- Evaluation of the program or policy.

Level of Evidence

- Level I: Evidence from well-designed randomized controlled trial (at least one).
- Level II-1: Evidence from well-designed controlled trials without randomization.
- Level II-2: Evidence from well-designed cohort or case-control analytic studies (at least from more than one research center).
- Level II-3: Evidence from multiple times series with or without intervention or dramatic results in uncontrolled experiments
- Level III: Opinions of experienced and well known authorities, based on clinical findings, descriptive studies and case reports, or expert committee's reports.

Hierarchy of Evidence-based Medicine/Public Health

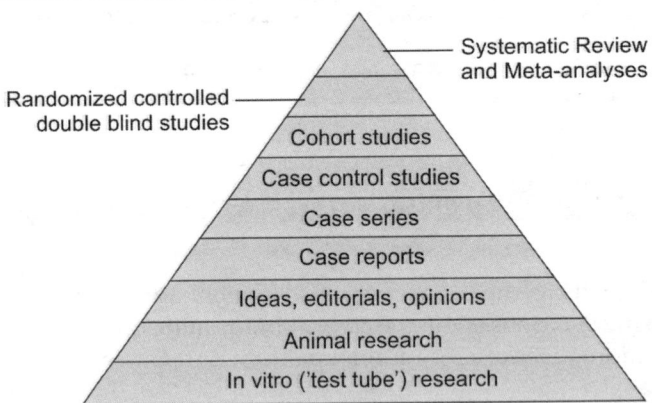

BIBLIOGRAPHY

1. Evidence-Based Public Health: A Fundamental Concept for Public Health Practice, Ross C. Brownson, Jonathan E. Fielding, Christopher M. Maylahn Annual Review of Public Health; 30(1):175–201.
2. https://www.downstate.edu/education-training/medical-research-library/evidence-based-practice.html

8.15 SCREENING

It is used to search for an unrecognized diseases or defect, in apparently healthy individuals, by means of rapidly applied test, examinations or other procedures.

Wilson and Jungner Criteria for Screening

- The disease or condition should be an important health problem
- The natural history of the disease/condition should be understood
- There should be a recognizable latent or early symptomatic stage
- There should be a test that is easy to perform and interpret, acceptable, accurate, reliable, sensitive and specific
- There should be an accepted treatment for the disease
- Treatment should be more effective if started early
- There should be a policy on who should be treated
- Diagnosis and treatment should be cost-effective
- Case-finding should be a continuous process.

Example of commonly done screening tests:

Screening test	Disease or condition
Visual inspection with acetic acid (VIA)	Cervical cancer
Pap smear	Cervical dysplasia or cervical cancer
Oral visual examination	Oral cancer
Clinical breast examination	Breast cancer
Mammography	Breast cancer
PSA test	Prostate cancer
Fecal occult blood	Colon cancer
Fasting blood sugar	Diabetes
Blood pressure	Hypertension
Rapid antigen test	COVID-19
Ocular pressure	Glaucoma
PKU test	Phenolketonuria in newborns
TSH	Hypothyroid and hyperthyroid

- Validity is the ability of a test to identify who have the disease and who do not have.
- Validity has main two characteristics: 1. Sensitivity and 2. Specificity.
- **2 × 2 contingency table:**

		Disease	
		Present	Absent
Screening test	Positive	True Positive (a)	False Positive (b)
	Negative	False Negative (c)	True Negative (d)

- Sensitivity is the ability of the test to identify correctly those who have the disease (a) from all individuals with the disease (a + c).
- Sensitivity = a/a + c.
- Specificity is the ability of the test to identify correctly those who do not have the disease (d) from all individuals free from the disease (b + d).
- Specificity = d/b + d.

Positive predictive value (PPV): It is ability of a screening test to identify correctly those who have the disease, out of all those tested as positive.

$$PPV = \frac{TP(a)}{TP(a) + FP(b)} \times 100$$

Negative predictive value: It is ability of a screening test to identify correctly those who do not have the disease, out of all those tested as negative.

$$NPV = \frac{TN(d)}{FN(c) + TN(d)} \times 100$$

Example of a Screening Test

- In population of 1,000 people, 100 have a disease X and 900 do not have the disease X.
- Result of the screening appears in this table:

Screening test results	Disease X status		Total
	Disease present	Disease absent	
Positive	80 (a)	100 (b)	180
Negative	20 (c)	800 (d)	820
Total	100	900	1000

- Sensitivity $= \frac{a}{a+c} \times 100$
  = 80/100 = 80%
- Specificity $= \frac{d}{b+d} \times 100$
  = 800/900 = 89%
- PPV $= \frac{a}{a+b} \times 100$
  = 80/180 = 44.44%
- NPV $= \frac{d}{c+d} \times 100$
  = 800/820 = 97.56%

BIBLIOGRAPHY

1. Andermann A, Blancquaert I, Beauchamp S, Déry V. Revisiting Wilson and Jungner in the genomic age: a review of screening criteria over the past 40 years. Bull World Health Organ. 2008;86(4):317-19. doi: 10.2471/blt.07.050112. PMID: 18438522; PMCID: PMC2647421.
2. https://sphweb.bumc.bu.edu/otlt/mph modules/ep/ep713_screening/EP713_Screening_print.html

CHAPTER 9

Communicable Diseases and Relevant National Health Programs

CHAPTER OUTLINE

- 9.1 Respiratory infections
- 9.2 Intestinal infections
- 9.3 Arthropod infections
- 9.4 Zoonotic infections/diseases
- 9.5 Other important diseases
- 9.6 Universal Immunization Program (UIP)
- 9.7 National Leprosy Eradication Program (NLEP)
- 9.8 The National Tuberculosis Elimination Program (NTEP)
- 9.9 Integrated Disease Surveillance Program (IDSP)
- 9.10 National AIDS Control Program (NACP)
- 9.11 National Vector Borne Disease Control Program (NVBDCP)
- 9.12 National Action Plan for Dog Mediated Rabies Elimination from India by 2030
- 9.13 National Viral Hepatitis Control Program (NVHCP)

9.1 RESPIRATORY INFECTIONS

SMALLPOX

Causative agent	Variola virus (major and minor)
Source of infection	Cases
Period of communicability	3 weeks from onset of rash (most infectious in first week of illness)
Secondary attack rate	30–40%
Host factor	All age groups and both genders are affected
Environmental factor	Overcrowding

Mode of transmission	Air droplet (direct, indirect, via contaminated items)
Incubation period (IP)	12 days (7–17 days)

Clinical Features
Fever, backache, headache followed by centrifugal, non-pleomorphic rash which is deep multilocular and affecting external surfaces of the body.
CFR: Up to 30%

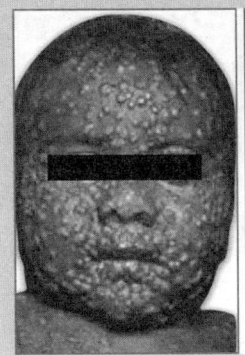
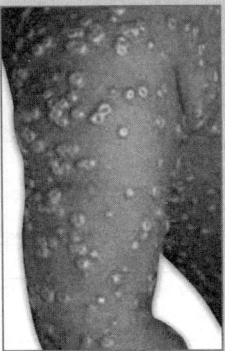
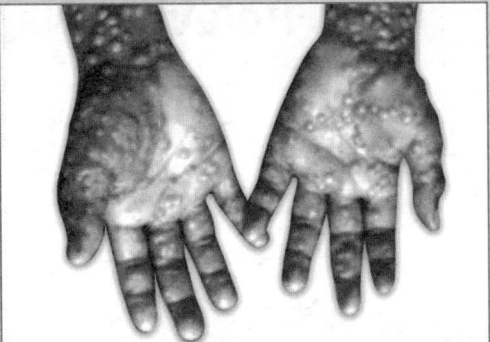

Complication	Scar, blindness, osteomyelitis
Diagnosis	Clinically, PCR
Prevention and treatment	• Live vaccine (Vaccinia virus) (given by bifurcated needle) • Isolate infected case • Nonspecific, symptomatic treatment • Antiviral drug cidofovir may be helpful
Remarks	• Smallpox vaccine invented by Edward Jenner in 1796 • Smallpox eliminated from India in 1977 • Smallpox eradicated from the world on 8th may, 1980

CHICKENPOX

Causative agent	Varicella-Zoster Virus [Human Herpes Virus-3 (Alpha)]
Source of infection	Cases
Period of communicability	1–2 days before the appearance of rash and 4–5 days the rash. Patient becomes noninfectious once the crusts have formed.
Secondary attack rate	90%
Host factors	*Age:* <10 years more commonly affected *Immunity:* durable and maternal antibody protects infant for few months *Pregnancy:* affects only when infection occurred during first 20 weeks of gestation.
Environmental factor	It shows seasonal variation as it peaks during winter and spring. Overcrowding facilitates transmission.
Mode of transmission	Droplet infection and droplet nuclei, direct contact with rash, Vertical transmission
Incubation period (IP)	14–16 days

Clinical Features
- In prodromal phase, fever, malaise and anorexia and these symptoms precede the rash by several days.
- Centripetal, unilocular, superficial, pleomorphic rash, dew drops like rash usually affect the flexor surfaces.
- Large outbreak occurs every 2-5 years.

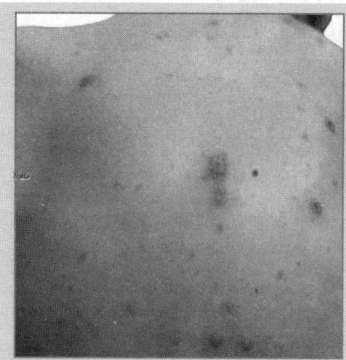

Complications	- Generally, no complications but in rare cases pneumonia, encephalitis and bacterial superinfection may occur. - Herpes zoster or shingles which is reactivation of latent varicella zoster virus infection. - High risk groups for complication are pregnant, people with HIV-AIDS, people with organ transplant or on long-term steroid therapy.
Diagnosis	- PCR or cell culture - IgM antibody (generally done when rashes present) - Four-fold rise in serum IgG antibody titer between acute and convalescent sera
Prevention and treatment	- Isolation of case for 6 days - Antipyretic, antihistaminic, acyclovir, ganciclovir or foscarnet drugs can be used - VZIG (can be used only in first 72 hours and only required for immunocompromised individuals) - Vaccine: live vaccine (OKA strain) for 12-18 months old child - Quarantine the exposed susceptible people - Calamine lotion for soothing effects for rash - Aspirin is not to be given as risk of Reye's syndrome high among children.

MEASLES (RUBEOLA)

Causative agent	Single stranded RNA virus with only one serotype Genus *Morbillivirus* and family paramyxovirus
Source of infection	Cases
Period of communicability	4 days before and 5 days after the appearance of rash
Secondary attack rate	80%
Host factors	Human are the only natural host *Age:* 6 months–3 years in developing countries while >5 years of age in developed countries *Immunity:* Maternal antibody protects infant for six months while natural infection or vaccine provides almost lifelong immunity. Malnourished child has more chances of mortality than normal child.

Environmental factor	It occurs mainly in winter and early spring
Mode of transmission	Droplet infection and droplet nuclei, direct contact with respiratory secretion
Incubation period (IP)	10–14 days but it is shortened to 7 days in vaccine induced measles
Clinical features • Fever, cough, coryza, conjunctivitis and cold • Koplik's spots (small bluish white spot with red background on the inner side of the cheek at upper 2nd molar tooth) • Maculopapular rash (begins behind the ear)	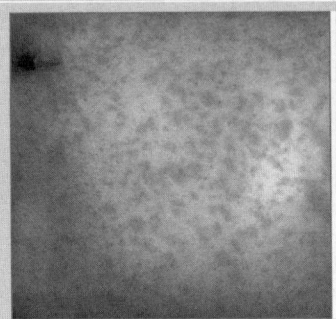 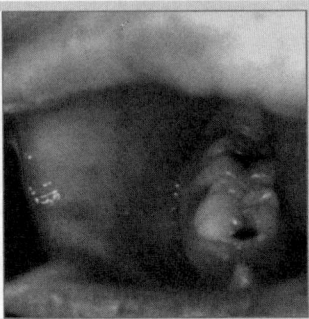
Complications	Otitis media, diarrhea, blindness Pneumonia (most common complication) SSPE (subacute sclerosing panencephalitis: rarest and most dangerous)
Diagnosis	Clinically, cell culture Samples like serum, throat swab and urine sample tested, IgM ELISA
Prevention and treatment	• Isolation of case for 7 days after rash • Measles vaccine and measles-rubella vaccine (Edmonston-Zagreb, Schwarz, Moraten strain) and passive immunization by measles immunoglobulin • Catch up, keep up and follow-up campaign • Accelerated measles mortality reduction strategy • Measles-Rubella campaign • Global measles and rubella strategic plan 2012-2020 • Vitamin A supplementation to all cases of measles (50,000 IU for infants aged less than 6 months, 1,00,000 IU for infants aged 6-11 months, and 2,00,000 IU for children aged 12 months. If the child has clinical signs of vitamin A deficiency (such as Bitot spots) a third dose should be given 4-6 weeks later • Antibiotic for prevention of secondary bacterial infection

MUMPS (ALSO KNOWN AS RUBULA)

Causative agent	RNA *Myxovirus parotitis* (only one serotype)
Source of infection	Cases and subclinical cases
Period of communicability	4–6 days before and 7 days after onset of symptoms
Secondary attack rate	86%
Host factors	Human is the only host *Age:* 5-9 years *Immunity:* maternal antibody protects infant for six months while natural infection or vaccine provides almost lifelong immunity

Environmental factor	It occurs mainly in winter and spring. Overcrowding may lead to epidemic.
Mode of transmission	Droplet infection and direct contact
Incubation period (IP)	14–18 days
Clinical features	Initially nonspecific symptoms like myalgia, headache and low grade fever followed by unilateral or bilateral salivary gland enlargement (m/c parotid gland) which cause pain during swallowing
Complications	Orchitis and oophoritis are most common complications among adolescents while overall most common complication is aseptic meningitis
Diagnosis	Usually clinically diagnosed but tests like blood, CSF and urine can be helpful
Prevention and treatment	• Isolation of cases till the disappearance of the symptoms. • Vaccine (Live-Jeryl Lynn strain) • Handwashing, mouth cover, cleaning of used material • Nonspecific, symptomatic treatment includes plenty of fluids and cold compression over the swollen gland

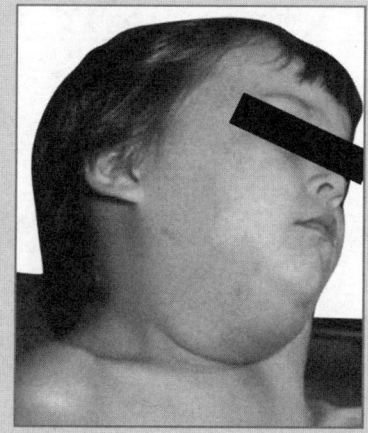

RUBELLA (also known as GERMAN MEASLES AND THREE DAYS MEASLES)

Causative agent	RNA virus from togavirus family (only one antigenic type)
Source of infection	Case and subclinical case
Period of communicability	A week before onset of symptoms to one week after appearance of rash
Host factors	*Age:* 3–10 years in developing country while >15 years in developed country *Immunity:* maternal antibody protects infant for 4–6 months while natural infection or vaccine provides almost lifelong immunity. 40% of women of childbearing age are susceptible.
Environmental factor	• Late winter and spring • Rubella shows cyclical trend every 4–9 years
Mode of transmission	Droplet infection and vertical transmission

Incubation period (IP)	18 days (2–3 weeks)
Clinical features	Fever, weakness, cough, cold, inflamed joint, conjunctivitis along with very peculiar feature as postauricular and posterior cervical lymphadenopathy 
Complications	Congenital rubella syndrome (if transmitted in the first trimester) (CRS: Cataract, sensorineural deafness and patent ductus arteriosus). And if rubella gets transmitted beyond the first trimester, then may lead to only sensorineural deafness while no abnormality reported if infection transmitted vertically in the third trimester. *Other complications:* Joint problems and thrombocytopenic purpura
Diagnosis	Hemagglutination inhibition test, RT-PCR
Prevention and treatment	• *Prevention:* RA 27/3 live vaccine 0.5 mL subcutaneously in a single dose, first priority will be women of reproductive age group. • Rubella vaccine is given as a MR vaccine at 9 month and 16–24 months under UIP. • *Treatment:* Nonspecific, symptomatic treatment

INFLUENZA

Causative agent	Influenza viruses—types A, B, C from the Orthomyxoviridae family. Pandemics are usually caused by Influenza A strain, Epidemic usually occurs every 2–3 years in case of Influenza A and every 3–6 years in Influenza B. There are 18 subtypes for hemagglutinin (H) viral protein and 11 subtypes for neuraminidase (N) viral protein
Source of infection	Case and subclinical case
Period of communicability	1–2 days before onset of symptoms to 1–2 days thereafter
Secondary attack rate	5–15% (H1N1-22–33%)
Host factors	All age and both sex are affected but highest mortality in <18 months and >65 years of age. Immunity lasts for 6–12 months only
Environmental factor	Jan to March and post-monsoon season (in India) overcrowding, poor ventilation Aquatics birds are the main reservoir of Influenza type A while humans are type B and C
Mode of transmission	Person to person by droplet infection and droplet nuclei, fomite-borne
Incubation period (IP)	18–72 hours

Clinical features	Fever, chills, cough, bodyache, headache, GIT illness
Complications	• Acute sinusitis, bronchitis, pneumonia and otitis media • Reye's syndrome can be seen with influenza B infection
Diagnosis	• ELISA for seasonal flu while RT-PCR for H_1N_1 • Viral culture from nasopharyngeal swab or throat swab
Prevention and treatment	• Personal hygiene and cough etiquette for Prevention. • Nonspecific symptomatic treatment: antipyretic, plenty of fluid and antiviral drugs (oseltamivir-Tamiflu 75 mg BD for 5 days for treatment and OD for 10 days for prophylaxis) • Other antiviral drug is zanamivir to be taken by inhaler (10 mg BD for treatment and OD for prophylaxis) • Vaccine [killed and live (nasal route)]
Remarks	**Antigenic shift**: Sudden major genetic reassortment, cause pandemic and epidemic **Antigenic drift**: Point mutation, Gradual changes over a period of time

DIPHTHERIA

Causative agent	*Corynebacterium diphtheria* (gram positive, non-motile bacteria, chinese letter appearance in slide) There are 4 types—gravis, mitis, belfanti and Intermedius
Source of infection	Case, subclinical case, carrier (ratio is 95 carriers to 5 cases) Diphtheria can have all types of carriers like Incubatory, convalescent and healthy carrier
Period of communicability	14–28 days after onset of symptoms
Host factors	1–5 years of age children, no bar for gender Maternal antibody protects for few weeks to few months of infancy
Environmental factor	All seasons but more in winter
Mode of transmission	Mainly person to person by droplet infection and through fomites also possible
Incubation period (IP)	2–6 days

Clinical features
Pseudomembrane (formation of grayish yellow membrane over the tonsil), sore throat, **bull necked** appearance due to edema and lymphadenopathy in the neck area, fever with chills, difficulty in swallowing
Types: Cutaneous, nasal, pharyngotonsillar and laryngotracheal diphtheria

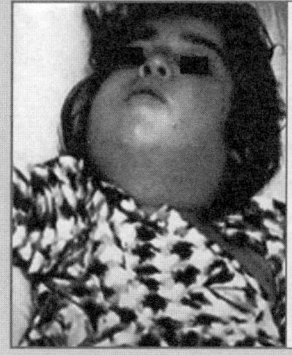
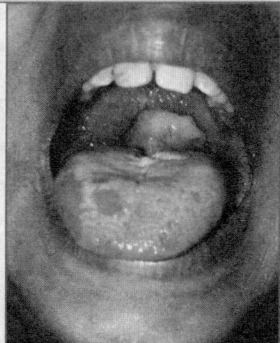

Complications	Airway blockage, myocarditis, kidney damage, nerve damage CFR: 10% (in untreated) and 5% (in treated)
Diagnosis	Culture
Prevention and treatment	• Isolation of case, penicillin or erythromycin for the treatment while DPT or pentavalent or Td vaccine for the prevention • Diphtheria antitoxin (20,000 to 1,00,000 U IM or IV) may be useful
Remarks	• Schick test—to decide susceptibility to infection and can be confirmed by HI test • Shake test—used to test that whether pentavalent or DPT vaccine is frozen or not.

PERTUSSIS (WHOOPING COUGH OR 100 DAYS COUGH)

Causative agent	95% of cases by *Bordetella pertussis* and 5% cases are by *Bordetella parapertussis*
Source of infection	Only cases
Period of communicability	A week after exposure to 3 weeks after onset of paroxysmal stage
Secondary attack rate	90%
Host factor	• Less than 5 years, incidence and fatality high in female • Maternal antibody provides no protection that's why children less than 6 months have highest mortality
Environmental factor	• All seasons but more in winter and during spring • Overcrowding favors the transmission
Mode of transmission	Mainly person to person by Droplet infection (direct contact)
Incubation period (IP)	7–14 days (max 3 weeks)

Clinical features

Paroxysmal of cough which is followed by an inspiratory, high pitch whoop, mild fever, runny nose

- *Catarrhal stage:* In the early stage, pertussis is highly contagious, with a secondary attack rate of up to 90% among non-immune household contacts. Untreated patients may transmit the infection for three weeks or more following the onset of typical coughing attacks. Lasts for 1–2 weeks.
- *Paroxysmal stage:* It is characterized by more frequent and spasmodic coughing, and followed by classic whoop with post-tussive emesis (vomiting). Lasts for 1–6 weeks.
- *Convalescent stage:* This stage is marked by less frequent and less severe coughing. Lasts for 2–3 weeks.

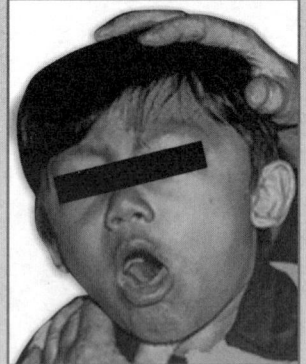

Complications	Bronchitis and bronchopneumonia, epistaxis, subconjunctival hemorrhage, encephalitis, convulsions and coma
Diagnosis	Culture and serological methods
Prevention and treatment	Nonspecific, symptomatic treatment. More fluids, antibiotics, oxygen treatment if necessary Erythromycin for the treatment and DPT or pentavalent vaccine for the prevention.

TUBERCULOSIS

Agent	Mycobacterium tuberculosis
Source of infection	Human source: smear +ve case Bovine source: infected milk One case of pulmonary tuberculosis can infect 10–15 persons per year
Period of communicability	Smear +ve case as long as remain untreated
Host factors	All ages are affected and males are more affected. Conditions like PLHIV, immunocompromised, diabetes and consumption of tobacco increase the risk
Environmental factors	Lower socio-economic condition, overcrowding, undernutrition, poor hygiene, lack of education.
Mode of transmission	Droplet infection and droplet nuclei
Incubation period (IP)	From receipt of infection to positive tuberculin test (3–6 weeks), thereafter disease development may take weeks/months/years
Clinical features	Fever with evening rise, cough more than two weeks, weight loss, night sweat
Complications	Hemoptysis, pleural effusion, fibrosis, generalized tuberculosis, death
Diagnosis	Sputum smear microscopy (ZN stain/fluorescent stain) Culture, LPA, CBNAAT, X-ray
Prevention and treatment	• For drug sensitive TB, treatment is given daily for 6 months (Four drugs: HRZE for 2 months and then HRE for next 4 months). • BCG vaccine at birth.
Remarks	• Mantoux test: 1 TU of PPD in 0.1 mL id and then read induration after 72 huors > 9 mm positive.

MENINGITIS

Agent	Neisseria meningitidis
Source of infection	Carrier more than case (nasopharyngeal discharge)
Host factors	Children and young adults
Environmental factors	Peak season between December to June. Overcrowding, as occurs in schools, barracks, refugee and other camps, is an important predisposing factor. Low socioeconomic groups living under poor housing conditions, with exposure to tobacco smoke, asplenia, HIV infection and travel to endemic areas
Mode of transmission	Droplet infection
Incubation period (IP)	2–10 days
Clinical features	Intense headache, fever, vomiting and stiff neck, photophobia and progresses to coma within a few hours. The meningitis is part of a septicemic process. The fatality of typical untreated cases is about 50 percent. With early diagnosis and treatment, case fatality rates can be less than 8–15 percent
Complication	Meningococcal septicemia

Diagnosis	CSF, culture
Prevention and treatment	Penicillin is the drug of choice, other useful drugs are rifampicin, ceftriaxone meningococcal vaccine (killed, sc)

COVID-19

Agent	SARS-CoV-2
Source of infection	Droplet, aerosol generating procedure
Period of communicability	In COVID-19 two days before and ten days after the initiation of symptoms
Host factors	All age groups and both the gender
Environmental factors	Humidity, temperature
Mode of transmission	Direct or indirect contact of mucous membranes of eyes, nose, or mouth with respiratory droplets or fomites. The use of aerosol-generating procedures (endotracheal intubation, bronchoscopy, nebulization treatments) in hospitals
Incubation period (IP)	2–14 days
Clinical features	Fever, cough, fatigue, shortness of breath, myalgia, sore throat, rhinorrhea, diarrhea, loss of smell (anosmia), loss of taste (ageusia)
Complications	ARDS, pulmonary decompensation, cardiac and renal complication
Diagnosis	Rapid antigen test, RT-PCR, X-ray/CT-scan, markers like CRP, LDH, ferritin
Prevention and treatment	<ul><li>Strict implementation of isolation and quarantine guideline</li><li>Government of India currently approved the vaccine like Covishield and Covaxin for routine use and only for emergency situation Sputnik-V, Moderna, Janssen, ZyCov-D, Corbevax, Covovax, Sputnik light vaccine</li><li>Hygienic measures such as handwashing after touching patients, use of appropriate and well-fitted masks, and infection control measures</li><li>Screening of international travelers</li><li>Timely and accurate reporting and sharing of information with other authorities and/or governments</li><li>Antivirals, interferon type 1, intravenous immunoglobulin, and systemic corticosteroids</li></ul>
Remarks	<ul><li>Coronavirus outbreak declared as Public Health Emergency of International Concern (30th January, 2020)</li><li>Coronavirus named as COVID-19 on 11th February, 2020</li><li>COVID-19 declared as Pandemic by WHO (11th March, 2020)</li></ul>

MONKEYPOX

Causative agent	Double-stranded DNA virus of *Orthopoxvirus* genus, Poxviridae family
Reservoirs	Natural reservoir is yet unknown. Certain rodents (including rope squirrels, tree squirrels, Gambian pouched rats, dormice) and non-human primates are known to be naturally susceptible to monkeypox virus.
Host factors	Monkeypox chiefly occurs in communities where there is often a high background prevalence of malnutrition, parasitic infections, and other significant health-compromising conditions.
Mode of transmission	• Respiratory droplets (after prolonged close contact) • Direct contact with body fluids or lesion material • Indirect contact through contaminated clothing or linens • Animal-to-human transmission: may occur by bite or scratch of infected animals like small mammals including rodents (rats, squirrels) and non-human primates (monkeys, apes) or through bush meat preparation.
Incubation period	6–13 days but may range 5–21 days
Period of Communicability	1–2 days before the rash to until all the scabs fall off/gets subsided

Clinical features	• Fever
	• Lymphadenopathy: occurs with fever onset usually in periauricular, axillary, cervical or inguinal region
	• Headache, muscle aches, exhaustion
	• Chills and/or sweats
	• Sore throat and cough
	• Skin involvement (rash):
	  ▪ Usually begins within 1–3 days of fever onset, lasting for around 2–4 weeks.
	  ▪ Deep-seated, well-circumscribed and often develop umbilication.
	  ▪ Painful until the healing phase when they become itchy (in the crust stage)
	  ▪ Stages of rash (slow evolution): Enanthem—first lesions on tongue and mouth—macules starting from face spreading to arms, legs, palms, and soles (centrifugal distribution), within 24 hours—the rash goes through a macular, papular, vesicular and pustular phase.
	  ▪ Classic lesion is vesicopustular: involvement by area—face (98%), palms and soles (95%), oral mucous membranes (70%), genitalia (28%), conjunctiva (20%).
	  ▪ Generally skin rashes are more apparent on the limbs and face than on the trunk.
	  ▪ A notable predilection for palm and soles is characteristic of monkeypox

Complications	• Secondary infections • Pneumonia, sepsis, encephalitis • Corneal involvement (may lead to loss of vision) • Hyperpigmented or hypopigmented atrophic scars • Patchy alopecia • Hypertrophic skin scarring and contracture/deformity of facial muscles

Case fatality rate	0 to 11% in the general population and has been higher among young children. In recent times, it has been around 3–6%.
Diagnosis	Polymerase chain reaction (PCR)
Differential diagnosis	Varicella (chickenpox), disseminated herpes zoster, disseminated herpes simplex, measles, chancroid, secondary syphilis, hand-foot-mouth disease, infectious mononucleosis, molluscum contagiosum
Treatment	Monkeypox is usually a self-limited disease with the symptoms lasting from 2–4 weeks • Patient isolation (until all lesions have resolved and scabs have completely fallen off) • Protection of compromised skin and mucous membranes • Rehydration therapy and nutritional support • Symptom alleviation • Monitoring and treatment of complications
Prevention	• Isolate cases to prevent further transmission • Provide optimal clinical care • Identify and manage contacts • Protect frontline health workers • Effective control and preventive measures • Vaccines
Remarks	WHO declared monkeypox as a public health emergency of international concern on 23rd July, 2022

9.2 INTESTINAL INFECTIONS

CHOLERA

Causative agent	It is gram-negative bacteria There are main two serogroups of *Vibrio cholerae*: O1 and O139 O1 is classified into two biotypes—classical and El tor Serotypes of El Tor are Ogawa, Inaba and Hikojima
Source of infection	Carrier and case. All 4 types of carriers found in cholera (incubatory, convalescent, healthy and chronic)
Period of communicability	Case remains infectious for 7–10 days while convalescent carriers remain infectious for 2–3 weeks and chronic carrier lasts from months to years.
Host factors	All age and both sexes but in endemic area highest cases are seen in children. Immunity—unknown as even post vaccination immunity lasts just for 3–6 months. Person with type O blood group and lowered gastric acidity are at higher risk.
Environmental factor	Poor environmental sanitation and nuisance of flies, poor personal hygiene and illiteracy. "5F" fingers, food, fomites, flies, fluids explain the interaction of environmental factors.
Mode of transmission	Contaminated water and food, direct contact

Communicable Diseases and Relevant National Health Programs

Incubation period (IP)	Hours to 5 days (more commonly 1–2 days)
Clinical features	Profuse and painless watery (rice watery) diarrhea followed by vomiting, dehydration, abdominal pain, leg cramp, less urine output in severe condition
Complications	Severe dehydration, renal failure, shock may lead to death
Diagnosis	Rectal swab or stool sample and Staining (darting motility) and culture, examination of contaminated food and water
Prevention and treatment	• Hygiene and sanitation • Proper food handling technique • Oral rehydration solution (ORS) • Rehydration therapy and doxycycline for the cases. Other: Azithromycin or ciprofloxacin, ampicillin and trimethoprim (TMP), sulfamethoxazole (SMX) • While for the prevention health education (most effective), proper excreta disposal, chemoprophylaxis (DOC: Tetracycline) for close contacts and vaccination (oral vaccines are Dukoral, Sanchol and Euvichol) • Zinc supplementation is an important adjunctive therapy for children less than 5 years, which also reduces the duration of diarrhea and may prevent recurrent episodes of diarrhea
Remarks	Notifiable disease under International Health Regulations Cholera is also known as father of public health

TYPHOID (ENTERIC FEVER)

Causative agent	*Salmonella typhi* (three main antigens O, H, Vi) and *S. paratyphi* A, B
Source of infection	Urine and feces of the carriers and cases, also contaminated food and water
Period of communicability	Till bacilli disappear from stool or urine
Host factors	Can occur at any age but highest incidence seen in 5–19 years of age. Cases are more in male while carrier rate is more in female *Immunity*: No solid immunity after natural infection
Environmental factor	Peaks in rainy season (July to Sept), poor sanitation and hygiene, open defecation
Mode of transmission	Feco-oral and urine-oral route—direct transmission through contaminated hand and indirect transmission from contaminated food and water, flies
Incubation period (IP)	10–14 days
Clinical features	Fever (stepladder pattern), pea soup diarrhea, bodyache, headache, abdominal pain, loss of appetite, constipation, bradycardia dicrotic pulse, splenomegaly and rose spots (occurs in 2nd week)
Complication	Rare; intestinal perforation (occurs in 3rd week), cholecysititis, urinary retention, pneumonia, nephritis, psychosis, osteomyelitis are rare complication

Diagnosis	Blood culture (best) and Widal test [Mnemonic **BASU**: Blood culture, Agglutination test/Widal test, Stool test, Urine test] Newer tests are: Typhidot, Typhidot-M, IDL Tubex test
Prevention and treatment	Fluoroquinolones like ciprofloxacin/ofloxacin 15 mg/kg for 7 days (drug of choice), cephalosporin like cefixime 20 mg/kg for 7 days antibiotics for cases while ampicillin + probenecid for carriers. Three types of vaccine: oral vaccine given >5 years of age, injectable vaccine >2 years of age • Typhoral (Ty21a strain-1 capsule to be taken on days 1, 3, and 5 every 3 years) • Typhim Vi (subcutaneous or IM) and • TAB vaccine Other measures like proper sanitation and hygiene, safe drinking water, pasteurization of milk are also important.
Remarks	Mary Mallon was the first known carrier of typhoid and thus formally known as "Typhoid Mary".

FOOD POISONING

	Staph Food poisoning	*Salmonella food poisoning*	*Bacillus cereus (emetic form) food poisoning*	*Bacillus cereus (diarrheal form) food poisoning*
Agent	*Staphylococcus aureus–enterotoxins* (preformed toxin)	*Salmonella typhimurium, Salmonella choleraesuis, S. enteritidis*	*Bacillus cereus-enterotoxins* (preformed toxin)	*Bacillus cereus*
Source of infection	Milk and its products	Meat, milk, eggs and its product, urine and feces of rat, mice, human carrier	Raw foods, processed food, fried rice, mashed potato, pasta	Soup, sauce, meat, gravy, custard
Incubation period (IP)	1–6 hours	12–24 hours	1–6 hours	12–24 hours
Clinical features	Vomiting, nausea, stomach cramps, diarrhea	Nausea, low grade fever, headache, vomiting, diarrhea, reactive arthritis in some cases	Upper gastro-intestinal tract symptom	Lower gastro-intestinal tract symptom
Prevention and treatment	Symptomatic treatment like fluid therapy, antiemetic Food safety measure: prevent contamination of food with specific health education to food handlers Personal hygiene and sanitary improvement			

Communicable Diseases and Relevant National Health Programs

	Botulism food poisoning	Clostridium perfringens food poisoning
Agent	Clostridium botulinum type-A, B or E exotoxin (preformed)	Clostridium perfringens (C. welchii)
Source of infection	Home preserved foods such as canned vegetables, smoked fish	Ingestion of meat, poultry (reheated)
Incubation period (IP)	18–36 hours	6–24 hours (peak 10–14 hours)
Clinical features	Dysphagia, diplopia, ptosis, dysarthria, blurring of vision, muscle weakness, quadriplegia	Diarrhea, abdominal cramp
Complication	Death due to respiratory/cardiac failure	Dehydration
Prevention and treatment	Antitoxin useful in prophylaxis and to reverse neuromuscular block, guanidine hydrochloride is useful.	Symptomatic treatment Food safety measure

POLIOMYELITIS

Agent	Poliovirus (RNA) type 1, 2, 3
Source of infection	Contaminated water, food and flies
Period of communicability	7–10 days before onset of symptoms to 3–4 weeks there after (max 3–4 months)
Host factor	Man is the only reservoir. Age group: 6 months to 3 years Male: Female (3:1)
Environmental factors	Rainy season (June to Sept), overcrowding, poor sanitation
Mode of transmission	Feco-oral route and rarely droplet infection
Incubation period (IP)	7–14 days (3–35 days)

Clinical features
- Subclinical, (inapparent) infection—asymptomatic
- Abortive polio: mild infection
- Non-paralytic illness: pain and stiffness in back and neck
- Paralytic illness: Asymmetrical flaccid paralysis, fever, malaise, nausea, vomiting, anorexia, headache, constipation

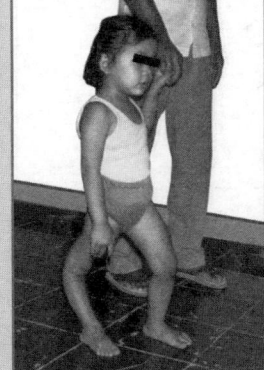

Complication	Deformity, post-polio syndrome
Diagnosis	Stool culture (stool sample is transported in the reversed cold chain)

Prevention and treatment	Vaccine: OPV (oral at 6, 10, 14 weeks), FIPV (at 6 and 14 weeks and 9 months)
Remarks	• Last case of polio in India is reported on 13th Jan, 2011 and India declared Polio free on 27th march, 2014 • Only two countries are endemic for polio: Pakistan, Afghanistan • AFP(acute flaccid paralysis) surveillance • Environmental surveillance • Pulse Polio Immunization Prgram

VIRAL HEPATITIS

	Hepatitis A/ infectious hepatitis/ epidemic jaundice	Hepatitis B/serum hepatitis	Hepatitis C/ Post-transfusion hepatitis	Hepatitis E/ non-A, non-B hepatitis
Agent	Hepatitis A virus (enterovirus type 72-picornaviridae family)	Hepatitis B virus (hepadnavirus) DNA virus also called as "Dane particle" Blumberg antigen/ Australian antigen	Hepatitis C virus (hepacivirus, flavivirus)	Hepatitis E virus (calcivirus, alphavirus)
Source of infection	Case	Carrier and case	Case	Contaminated drinking water
Period of communicability	2 weeks before and 1 week after the onset of jaundice	Several months or until disappearance of HBsAg	Indeterminate	Unknown
Host factors	Children are more affected than adult. Severity increase with age	Adult Surgeon, laboratory person, homosexual are high-risk group	Adult Dialysis and hemophilic patients are high-risk group	15–40 years
Environmental factors	Heavy rain fall, poor sanitation, over crowding	—	—	Hot climate, inadequate sewage disposal, unsafe drinking water
Transmission				
Feco-oral	+++			+++
Parenteral	+ (rare)	+++	+++	
Sexual	+ (oral or anal sex)	+++	+	
Perinatal (vertical)		+++	+	

Diagnosis	Abnormal liver function test, viral antigen, anti-HAV Acute: IgM anti-HAV	Liver function test which includes serum bilirubin, liver enzyme (SGPT, SGOT) and following markers HbsAg: first detected (acute and chronic) IgMAg: high infectivity (acute), IgGAg: (chronic), HbeAg: marker of infectivity and virus replication Anti-HbsAg; immunity/after vaccination Anti-Hbe; indicate stopping of viral infection	HCV, anti-HCV	Detection of IgM/IgG RT-PCR
Prevention and treatment	a. Vaccine: 1. Formaldehyde inactivated vaccine 2. Live attenuated vaccine b. Human immunoglobulin c. Personal and community hygiene safe and portable water education of food handler	• Hepatitis B vaccine (98–100% efficacy) is given at birth and also as pentavalent vaccine (6, 10, 14 weeks) • Adult hepatitis B vaccination at 0, 1 and 6 months • Hepatitis B immunoglobulin, • Tenofovir/Entecavir to suppress the virus • Screening of the blood donor and hygiene and strict sterilization protocol helps us to prevent hepatitis B infection	Interferon/ribavirin, antiviral agent Strict adherence to guidelines of blood safety policy	It is usually self-limiting, maintain hygiene, safe water and food, no specific treatment, no specific immunoglobulin and recently vaccine developed in china
Phases	*Phase I* (viral replication phase): Patients usually asymptomatic during this phase and serological and enzyme markers of hepatitis will be favoring presence of infection. *Phase II* (prodromal phase): Anorexia, nausea, vomiting, change in taste, joint pain, malaise, fatigue, urticarial, and pruritus. *Phase III* (icteric phase): Dark urine, followed by pale-colored stools, icteric (yellow discoloration) and right upper quadrant pain with hepatomegaly. *Phase IV* (convalescent phase): Symptoms and icterus resolve and liver enzymes return to normal			

| Risk of transmission after needle stick injury | HBV (HBsAg+, HBeAg−) 1–6%
HBV (HBsAg+, HBeAg+) 30%
HCV 3–10%
HIV 0.2–0.5% |

Remark: Timeline of Ag and Ab related to hepatitis B

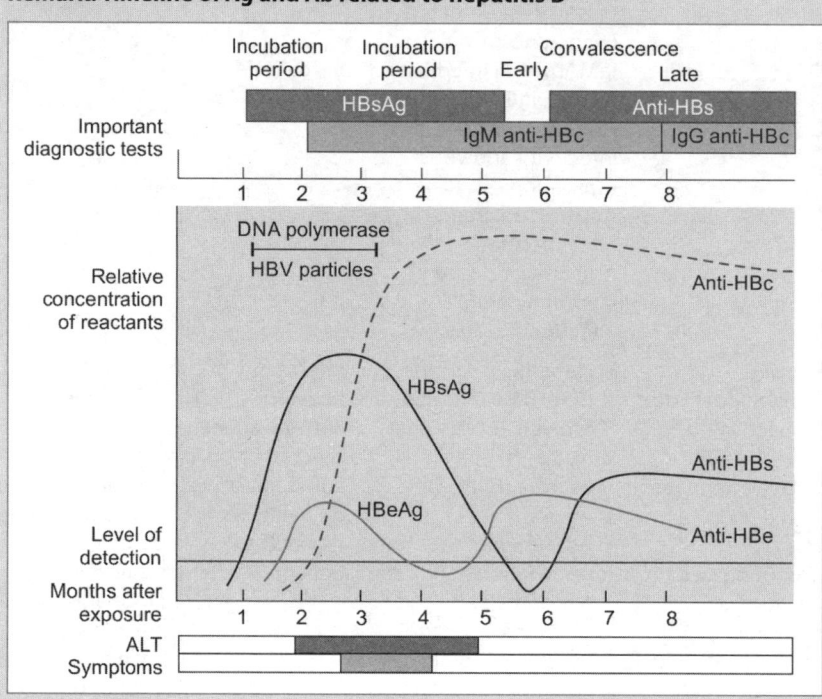

AMEBIASIS

Causative agent	*Entamoeba histolytica* There are two forms: vegetative and cystic (infective forms)
Source of infection	Ingestion of mature cyst through contaminated food, water or hands
Host factor	All age group can be affected and it almost affects whole family
Environmental factor	Poor sanitation, monsoon season, low socioeconomic group
Mode of transmission	Feco-oral route, vector-borne as flies, cockroach and rodents may carry cyst and contaminate food and water. In rare cases sexual transmission is seen among homosexuals
Incubation period (IP)	2–4 weeks or more

Communicable Diseases and Relevant National Health Programs

Life cycle

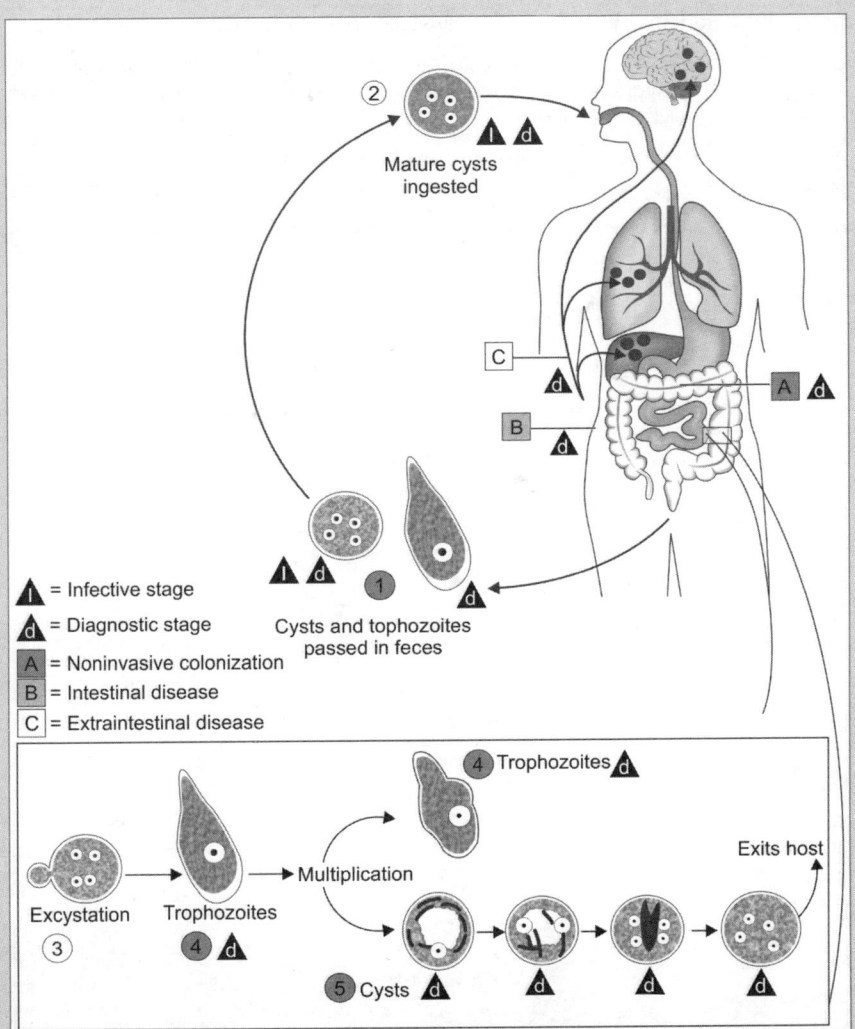

Clinical features	Stomachache, dysentery and in severe condition liver abscess
Diagnosis	Serological, ELISA, indirect hemagglutination test
Prevention and treatment	Proper hygiene and sanitation, boiling of water before use, health education, periodic examination of food handlers. Proper and safe disposal of human excreta. Metronidazole (30 mg/kg/day for 8 days): drug of choice. Other: Tinidazole

SOIL TRANSMITTED HELMINTHS

Hookworm (also known as **Ancylostomiasis/Tunnel disease/Egyptian chlorosis/Miner's disease/Brickmaker's anemia**)

Communicable Diseases and Relevant National Health Programs

Causative agent	*Ancylostoma duodenale, Necator americanus* (more common)
Host factor	Agriculture workers with bare feet are at higher risk.
Environmental factor	Higher contain of moisture in damp sandy soil necessary for survival of larva. Poor hygiene and sanitation, open air defecation, bare feet walking increasing the risk of infection.
Mode of transmission	Direct from skin of foot or sole (soil transmitted), oral
Incubation period (IP)	5 weeks – 9 months (*Ancylostoma duodenale*) 7 weeks (*N. americanus*)
Life cycle	

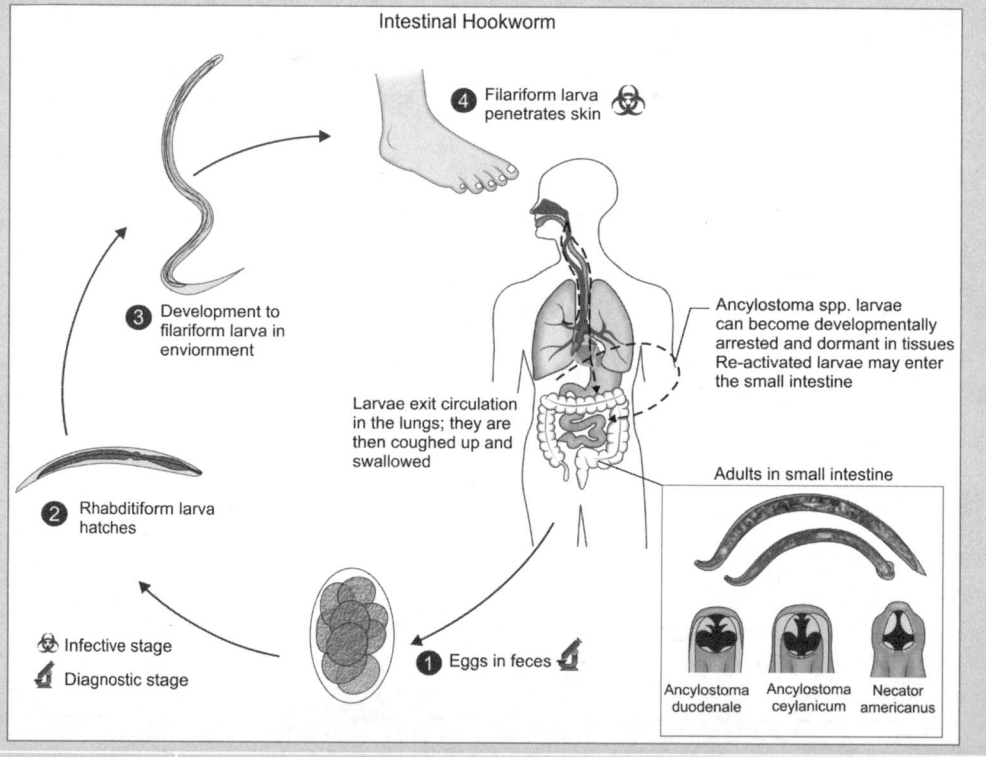

Clinical features	• Diarrhea, abdominal pain, weakness, weight loss, intestinal blood loss, itching, rash on skin site where contaminated soil coming in contact • Associated with iron deficiency anemia. • Average blood loss: 0.03–0.2 mL/worm/day
Complication	Anemia and malnutrition
Diagnosis	Clinical and sometimes identification of hookworm egg in feces.
Prevention and treatment	• Proper sanitation measure, use the vegetables and fruits after thoroughly washing, prevent barefoot walking, wear shoes, prevent open defecation, iron supplementation and iron-rich food • Albendazole (400 mg single dose), mebendazole (100 mg twice a day for 3 days)

Remark	**Chandler index**: Index to assess the level of endemicity of hookworm
	• <200 eggs per gram of stool: Not significant
	• 200–250 eggs per gram of stool: Potential danger
	• 250–300 eggs per gram of stool: Minor public health problem
	• >300 eggs per gram of stool: Severe or important public health problem

ASCARIASIS (ROUNDWORM)

Causative agent	Ascaris lumbricoides
Source of infection	Ingestion of infective eggs of worm
Host factor	Man is the only reservoir of infection
Environmental factor	Open air defecation, soil transmitted
Mode of transmission	Feco-oral (ingestion of fertilized eggs)
Incubation period (IP)	2 months

Life cycle

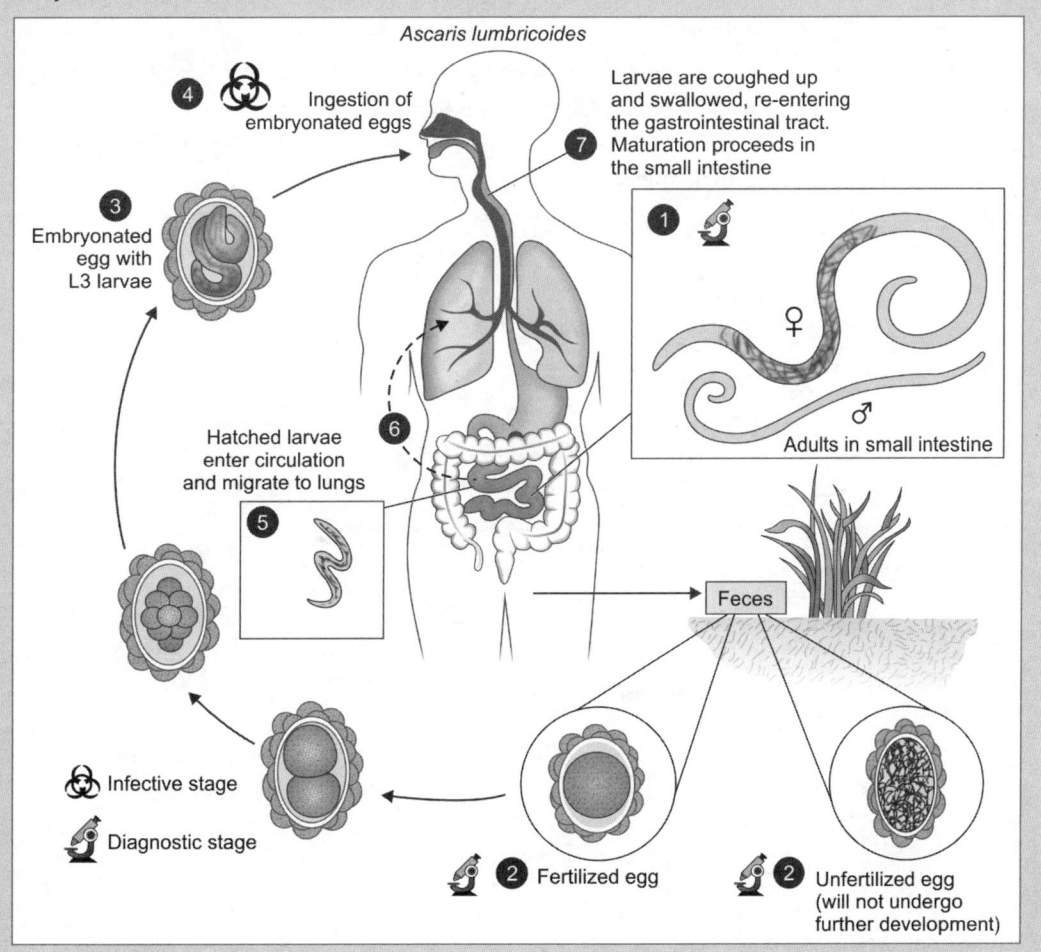

Clinical features	Usually, adults do not have symptoms but in case of high burden of worms they may present as nausea, vomiting, abdominal pain and intestinal obstructions, stunting among children due to malnutrition
Prevention and treatment	Thoroughly wash vegetable and fruits before cook, sanitation and hygiene, prevent open defecation Treatment: Mebendazole (100 mg twice a day for 3 days), other drugs, such as albendazole, pyrantel, piperazine
Remarks	Most common Helminthic infection per day 2 lacs egg excreted in stool

DRACUNCULIASIS (also known as GUINEA WORM)

Causative agent	*Dracunculus medinensis* (nematode)
Source of infection	Water
Host factor	Poor communities, males are more affected because of higher frequency of exposure
Environmental factor	Step well and surface water users are at higher risk, dry season
Mode of transmission	Inhabits through subcutaneous tissue (usually leg and foot), infection by cyclops infected drinking water, consumption of uncooked aquatic animal
Incubation period (IP)	10–14 months

Life cycle

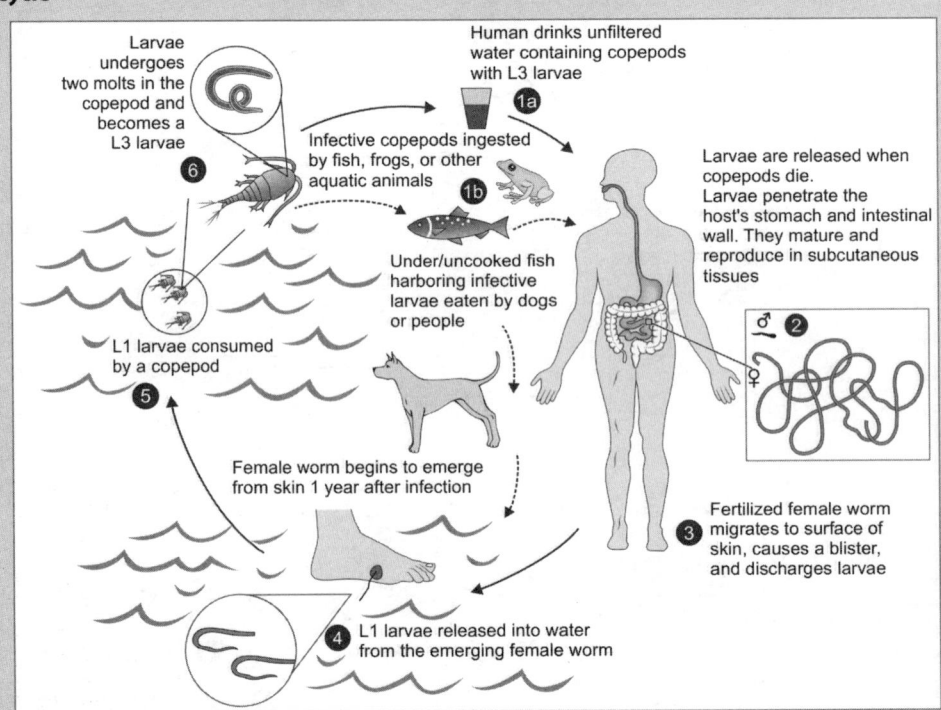

Clinical features Initially no any symptoms; fever, swelling, and pain is developed when worms come out of the skin mainly legs and feet	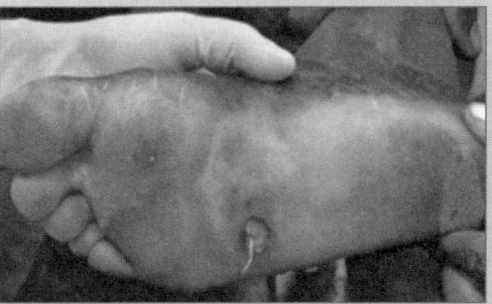
Complications	Cellulitis, abscess, arthritis, sepsis
Diagnosis	Clinically
Prevention and treatment	• Making drinking water safe, not allowing villagers, especially those with blisters and ulcers, to enter any source of drinking water, filtering water in endemic areas through fine mesh (size 100 micrometers) to remove cyclops, converting step wells to draw wells, controlling of cyclops by use of temephos, and increasing awareness among endemic communities about the disease and its control. • Symptomatic treatment like anti-inflammatory drugs, wet compression relieves discomfort and pain and worm removal by small stick or by surgery • Actual there is no effective drug or vaccine available but drug like metronidazole and mebendazole help to some extent to relieve inflammation and facilitate worm removal.
Remarks	• Multiple repeated infection may occur in same person. • It is a water-based disease. • In 1996, last case reported in India. • Eliminated from India in February, 2000

9.3 ARTHROPOD INFECTIONS

MALARIA

Causative agent	*Plasmodium vivax, Plasmodium falciparum, Plasmodium malariae* and *Plasmodium ovale*
Host factor	Man: Intermediate host Mosquito: Definite host Individuals with AS hemoglobin (sickle cell trait) have a milder illness with falciparum infection whereas persons whose red blood cells are "duffy negative" (a genetic trait) are resistant to *P. vivax* infection
Environmental factor	July-November Optimum temp. is 20–30°C, 60% to 65% humidity ill-ventilated and ill-lighted houses, burrow pits, garden pools, irrigation channels, etc.

Communicable Diseases and Relevant National Health Programs

Mode of transmission	• Vector transmission: *An. culicifacies* in rural and *An. stephensi* in urban • Direct transmission through blood transfusion, malaria in drug addicts • Congenital malaria: It is rare
Incubation period (IP)	Intrinsic incubation period (In human) • *P. falciparum*: 12 (9–14 days) • *P. vivax*: 14 (8–17 days) • Quartan malaria: 28 (18–40 days) • Ovale malaria: 17 (16–18 days) Extrinsic incubation period (in mosquito) • 10–12 days at 27°C • 25–30 days at 18°C

Life cycle
- **Asexual cycle (human cycle)**
  - Hepatic phase
  - Erythrocytic phase
  - Gametogony phase
- **Sexual cycle (mosquito cycle)**

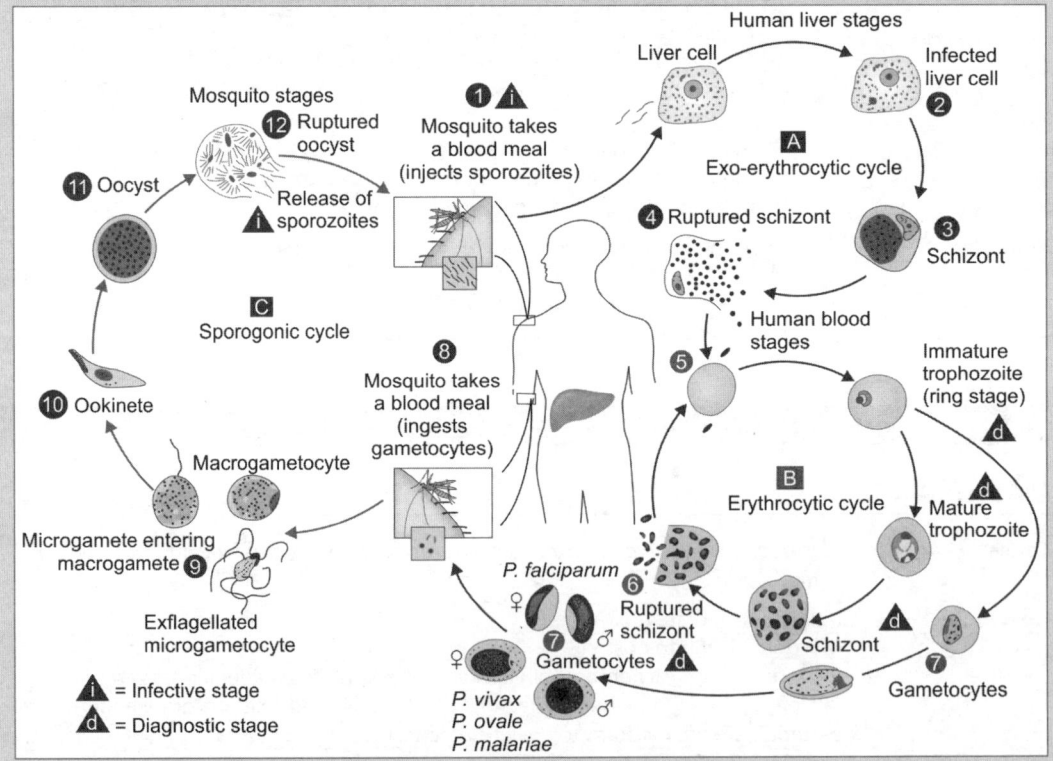

Clinical features	Fever, headache, vomiting and other flu-like symptoms. Due to destruction of red blood cells resulting in fatigue due to anemia, fits/convulsions and loss of consciousness may occur in cerebral malaria.

Diagnosis	**Microscopy**
	• Microscopy of stained thick and thin blood smears remains the gold standard for confirmation of diagnosis of malaria. It has high sensitivity.
	• Thick smear shows whether the slide is positive for malarial parasite or not
	• Thin smear shows the species of the MP and the stages of development in red cells
	Rapid diagnostic tests (RDTs)
	• RDTs are based on the detection of circulating parasite antigens. RDTs are available in the form of cassettes, cards or dipsticks
	• Some of them can only detect *P. falciparum*, while others can detect other parasite species also
	• The NVBDCP rolled out bivalent RDTs (for detecting *P. falciparum* and *P. vivax*) for use in the public health sector.
	Types of RDT kits:
	• Histidine rich protein 2 (HRP2)
	  ▪ Water soluble protein produced only by *P. falciparum*
	• *Plasmodium* lactate dehydrogenase (pLDH)
	  ▪ Currently used in products that include *P. falciparum* specific and *P. vivax* specific
	• Aldolase (for all species)

Prevention and treatment	**Malaria control strategies**
	1. Early case detection and prompt treatment
	  ▪ Chloroquine is the main anti-malaria drug for uncomplicated malaria.
	  ▪ Drug distribution centres (DDCs) and fever treatment depots (FTDs) have been established in the rural areas for providing easy access to anti-malarial drugs to the community.
	  ▪ Details of treatment given below.
	2. Vector control
	i. Chemical control
	  ▪ Use of indoor residual spray (IRS) with insecticides recommended under the program
	  ▪ Use of chemical larvicides like Abate in potable water
	  ▪ Aerosol space spray during day time
	  ▪ Malathion fogging during outbreaks
	ii. Biological control
	  ▪ Use of larvivorous fish such as *Gambusia, Lebister*
	  ▪ Use of biocides.
	iii. Personal protective measures
	  ▪ Use of mosquito repellent creams, liquids, coils, mats, etc.
	  ▪ Screening of the houses with wire mesh
	  ▪ Use of bednets treated with insecticide
	  ▪ Wearing clothes that cover maximum surface area of the body
	4. Community participation: Sensitizing and involving the community for detection of *Anopheles* breeding places and their elimination
	5. Environmental: Management and source reduction methods
	  ▪ Source reduction, i.e. filling of the breeding places
	  ▪ Proper covering of stored water
	  ▪ Channelization of breeding source
	6. Monitoring and evaluation of the program

Communicable Diseases and Relevant National Health Programs

	Treatment details: *P. vivax:* T. chloroquine 25 mg/kg divided over three days and T. primaquine 0.25 mg/kg daily for 14 days. *P. falciparum:* Artemisinin Combination Therapy (ACT), T. artesunate for 3 days + sulphadoxine-pyrimethamine on 1 day and single dose of primaquine (0.75 mg/kg) on day 2. In north eastern states Artemether–lumefantrine for 3 days and single dose of primaquine (0.75 mg/kg) on day 2.
Remarks	**Relapse:** • Some of the sporozoites invade liver cells and do not multiply rather go to sleep and called as hypnozoites. [hypno = sleep (dormant)] • In future (after days to months) they can start multiplying and bring an episode of malaria and this is called as relapse. • Its renewed clinical activity seen around 30th–40th week following primary attack (long-term relapse) • It is reactivation. • Seen only in *Plasmodium vivax* and *ovale*. **Recrudescence** • The occurrence of clinical symptoms in a malaria patient, because plasmodium is not eliminated completely either due to poor immune system or due to treatment failure, this is known as recrudescence. • It is revival. • Its renewed clinical activity seen during first 8-10 weeks after primary attack. (short-term relapse) • Seen in all species of *Plasmodium*. **Malariometric indices in Eradicaton era** • Annual parasite incidence (API): It is a measure of malaria incidence in a community. Areas with API ≥ 2 per 1,000 population per year have been classified as high risk areas in India. It is most sophisticated index. • Annual blood examination rate (ABER): It is an index of operational efficiency. • Annual falciparum incidence (AFI) • Slide positivity rate (SPR): It is the percentage of slides found positive for malarial parasite, irrespective of the type of species. • Slide falciparum rate (SFR): It provides trend of transmission. **Malaria vaccine:** Mosquirix (RTS,S/AS01) is recombinant protein based vaccine. World Malaria day: 25th April Anti-Malaria Week: 1st–7th May Anti-Malaria Month: June Target: Malaria free India by 2027 and elimination by 2030

DENGUE

Causative agent	Belongs to arboviruses-flavivirus Dengue virus four serotype (DEN-1, DEN-2, DEN-3 and DEN-4)
Host factor	All age group
Environmental factor	16°–30°C and a relative humidity of 60–80%. It breeds in the containers in and around the houses

Reservoir of infection	Viruses are maintained in human-mosquito cycle
Period of communicability	Infected person with Dengue becomes infective to mosquitoes 6–12 hours before the onset of the disease and remains so up to 3–5 days.
Mode of transmission	Vector: Aedes aegypti and Aedes albopictus usually day biter mosquito
Incubation period (IP)	3–10 days
Clinical features	**Dengue fever:**<ul><li>Abrupt onset of high fever</li><li>Severe frontal headache</li><li>Pain behind the eyes which worsens with eye movement</li><li>Muscle and joint pains</li><li>Loss of sense of taste and appetite</li><li>Measles-like rash over chest and upper limbs</li><li>Nausea and vomiting</li></ul>**Dengue hemorrhagic fever:** Symptoms similar to dengue fever with additional symptoms like:<ul><li>Severe continuous stomach pain</li><li>Skin becomes pale, cold or clammy</li><li>Bleeding from nose, mouth and gums and skin rashes</li><li>Frequent vomiting with or without blood</li><li>Sleepiness and restlessness</li><li>Patient feels thirsty and mouth becomes dry</li><li>Rapid weak pulse</li><li>Difficulty in breathing</li><li>Sometimes may worsen and results in Dengue shock Syndrome</li></ul>
Diagnosis	Viral antigen detection test: NS-1 (useful for early diagnosis) RT PCR, ELISA, Virus isolation from plasma, serum, etc. can be useful. Rapid diagnostic test: IgG and IgM Hematocrit and platelet count for monitoring
Prevention and treatment	<ul><li>No specific treatment. Symptomatic treatment is given. Aspirin should be avoided since they can increase the risk of bleeding.</li><li>Dengue vaccine: Dengvaxia under field trial</li><li>Integrated vector control measure is the main preventive measure.</li></ul>
Remarks	**Indices**<ul><li>**Container index:** Percentage of water holding containers infected with larvae or pupae</li><li>**House index:** Percentage of houses infected with larvae and/or pupae</li><li>**Breteau index:** Number of positive containers per 100 houses inspected</li><li>**Pupae index:** Number of pupae per 100 houses</li></ul>

CHIKUNGUNYA

Causative agent	Group A Alphavirus, belongs to the Togaviridae family of arboviruses
Host factor	Human particularly in Asia
Environmental factor	Climate: mainly rainy season. Aedes Mosquito is found predominantly in artificial water collection places.
Mode of transmission	Vector: infected female *Aedes aegypti* and *Aedes albopictus* (sometimes *Mansonia* mosquito)
Incubation period (IP)	3–7 days
Clinical features	Sudden onset with fever, severe headache, chills, nausea, vomitting, morbilliform rash, anorexia, conjunctivitis and adenopathy. Arthropathy is manifested by pain, swelling and stiffness, especially of the metacarpophalangeal, wrist, elbow, shoulder, knee, ankle and metatarsal joints. It can persist for many months and years.
Diagnosis	ELISA test
Prevention and treatment	There is no specific treatment and it is usually self-limiting. Symptomatic treatment for pain and fever with anti-inflammatory drugs Analgesics, antipyretics along with fluid supplementation. Drugs like aspirin and steroids should be avoided. No vaccine is available. Integrated vector control measure is the main preventive measure.
Remarks	In African language, Chikungunya word means "that which bends up" that reflects in disease presentation. It is reemerging disease.

FILARIASIS

Causative agent	Nematode worms— Bancroftian filariasis: *Wuchereria bancrofti* Brugian filariasis: *Brugia malayi* and *Brugia timori*
Host factor	Man: Definitive host Mosquito: Intermediate Host All age group
Environmental factor	The temperature between 22–38°C and humidity 70% favorable condition. Bad drainage and polluted water collection, poor sanitaion The common breeding places are septic tanks, cesspools, burrow pits, soakage pits, ill-maintained drains, etc.
Mode of transmission	Vector: *Culex quinquefasciatus* and *Mansonia annulifera/M. uniformis*
Incubation period (IP)	8–6 months

Communicable Diseases and Relevant National Health Programs

Life cycle

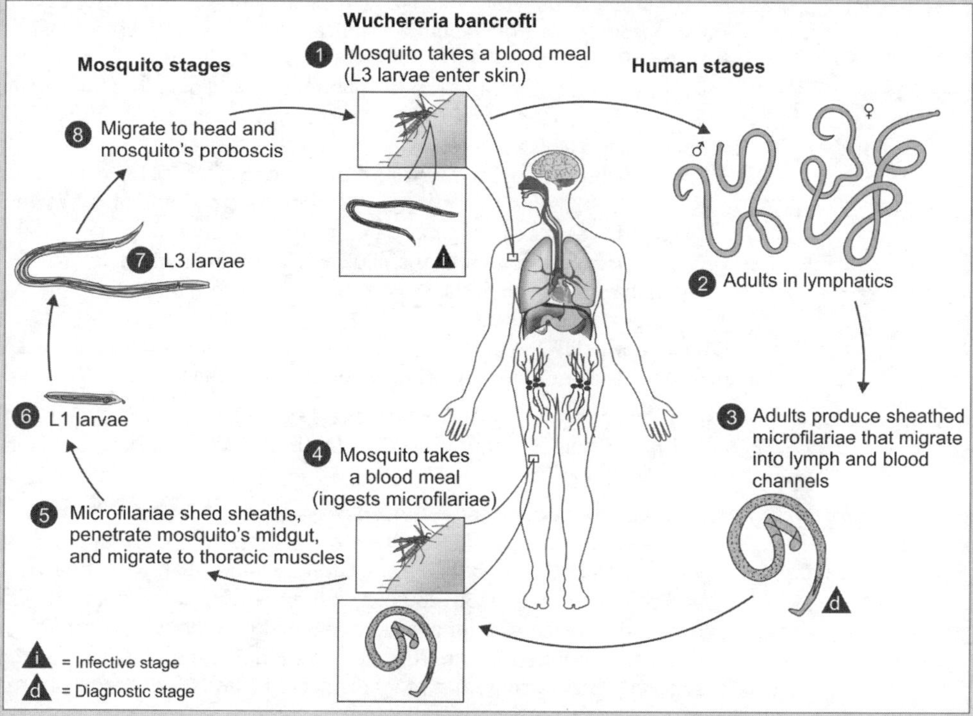

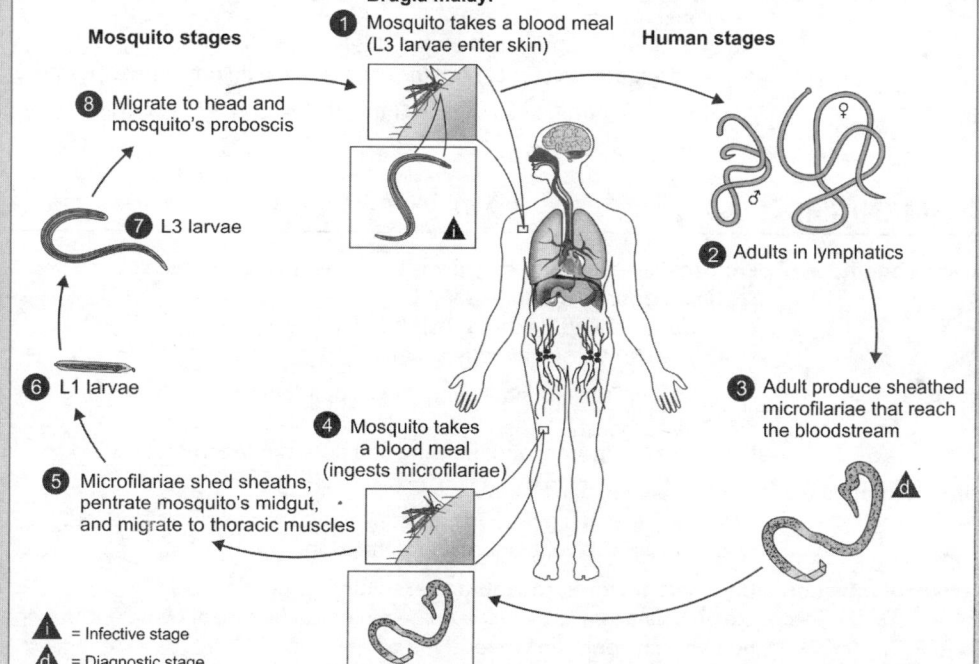

Clinical features	**Lymphatic filariasis:** Caused by the parasite in the lymphatic system • *Asymptomatic amicrofilaraemia:* no clinical symptom and absence of Mf • *Asymptomatic microfilaremia:* no clinical symptom but presence of Mf • Stage of acute manifestations: like fever, lymphadenitis, lymphangitis, lymphedema of the various parts of the body and of epididymo-orchitis in the male. Recurrent episodes of acute inflammation in lymph glands and vessels can be occurred. • Stage of chronic obstructive lesion: developed after 10-15 years from the onset of the first acute attack. It is due to fibrosis and obstruction of lymphatic vessels causing permanent structural changes. • In chronic bancroftian filariasis, clinical features are hydrocele, elephantiasis and chyluria. Elephantiasis may affect the legs, scrotum, arms, penis and vulva. **Occult filariasis:** Due to immune hypersensitivity reaction (e.g., tropical pulmonary eosinophilia). Also known as cryptic filariasis
Diagnosis	Mass Blood Survey: The Thick Film (collect between 8 pm to 12 midnight) Membrane Filter Concentration (MFC) Methods DEC Provocation Test

Prevention and treatment	**Twin pillar strategy for elimination of lymphatic filariasis**
	1. Annual Mass Drug Administration (MDA) of single dose of triple drugs includes DEC (Diethylcarbamazine citrate, 6 mg/kg) and Albendazole (400 mg) and Ivermectin (150–200 mcg/kg) for 5 years or more to the eligible population (except pregnant women, children below 2 years of age and seriously ill persons) to interrupt transmission of the disease (triple drugs in selected districts only while other districts DEC and Albendazole given).
	2. Home-based management of lymphoedema cases and up-scaling of hydrocele operations in identified CHCs/District hospitals/medical colleges.
	  ▪ DEC medicated salt (1–4 gm DEC/kg salt)
	  ▪ Integrated vector control measure is the main preventive measure.

Remarks	India is committed to eliminate lymphatic filariasis by 2027 (Global target 2030)

LEISHMANIASIS

Causative agent	Protozoa diseases caused by parasites of the genus *Leishmania* *Leishmania donovani:* Kala-azar (VL); *L. tropica:* cutaneous leishmaniasis (oriental sore); *L. braziliensis:* mucocutaneous leishmaniasis
Host factor	All age group, male is more affected. Occupation like farming, mining, forestry and fishing. Poverty, malnutrition, poor housing and poor sanitation
Environmental factor	November and March-April Sandflies breed in cracks and crevices in buildings, tree holes, soil etc. Overcrowding, ill-ventilation, poor sanitation
Reservoir of infection	Dogs, jackals, foxes, rodents are reservoir outside the India. Indian Kala-azar has a unique epidemiological feature of being anthroponotic; human is the only known reservoir of infection.

Mode of transmission	Bite of female phlebotomine sandfly and species of sandfly as below: *Phlebotomus argentipes* transmits kala-azar while *Phlebotomus sergenti* and *Phlebotomus papatasi* transmit cutaneous leishmaniasis
Incubation period (IP)	1–4 months
	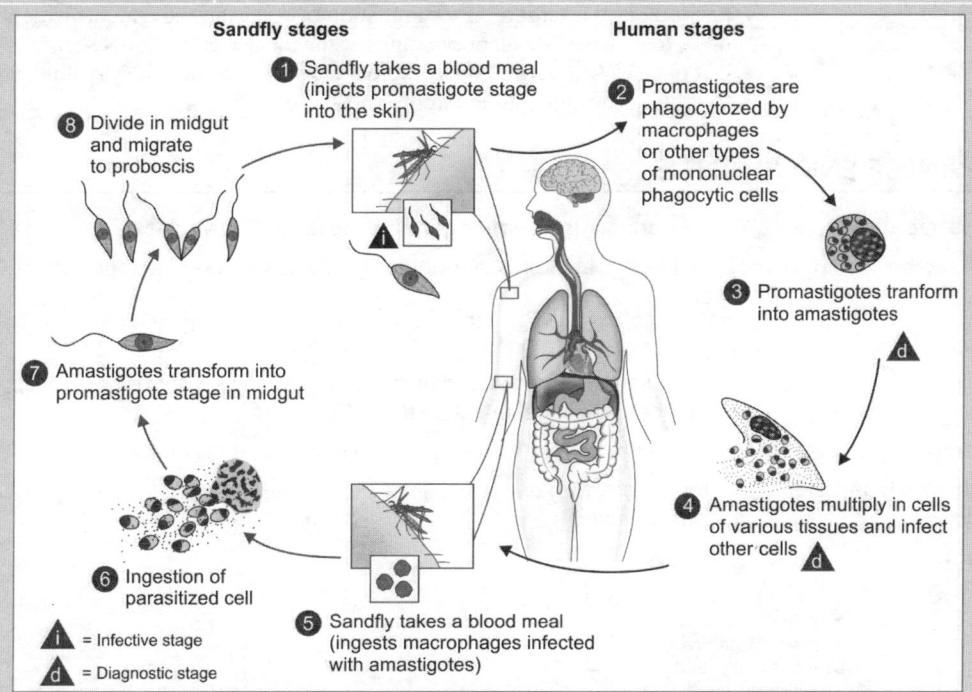
Clinical features	**Kala-azar or visceral leishmaniasis (VL):** (Kala-azar means black sickness) characterized by fever (recurrent intermittent), weight loss, hepatomegaly, splenomegaly and, anemia and darkening of the skin of the face, hands, feet and abdomen is common in India. **PKDL: Post-kala-azar dermal leishmaniasis,** caused by *L.donovani*, is common in India. It appears few years after apparent cure of kala-azar. The lesions (with numerous parasite) consist of multiple nodular infiltrations of the skin, usually without ulceration. **Cutaneous leishmaniasis (CL):** characterized by painful ulcers in the parts of the body exposed to sandfly bites (e.g., legs, arms or face) reducing the victim's ability to work. Other forms are anthroponotic cutaneous leishmaniasis (ACL) and zoonotic cutaneous leishmaniasis (ZCL). **Mucocutaneous leishmaniasis (MCL):** Ulcers appear around the margins of mouth and nose.
Diagnosis	• Rk39 dipstick test • Aldehyde test • Leishmanin (Montenegro) test • ELISA, direct agglutination test and indirect fluorescent antibody test • Parasite demonstration in bone marrow aspiration or culture is a confirmatory diagnosis.

Prevention and treatment	• Sodium stibogluconate, liposomal amphotericin B (LAMB), amphotericin B deoxycholate, paramomycin and miltefosine • Personal prophylaxis • Sandfly control measure (Highly sensitive to DDT)
Remarks	• Kala-azar (KA) is targeted for elimination by reducing the annual incidence of KA to <1 case/10,000 populations at the block level. • Out of 633 KA endemic blocks, 8 blocks (6 in Jharkhand and 2 in Bihar) yet to achieve the elimination target.

JAPANESE ENCEPHALITIS

Causative agent	Group B arbovirus, *Flavivirus* genus in the family Flaviviridae.
Host factor	Natural host: Water birds of Ardeidae family (mainly pond herons and cattle egrets) Pig: Amplifier host (they allow manifold virus multiplication without suffering from disease) Man: accidental and dead end host (due to low and short-lived viraemia, mosquitoes do not get infection from JE patient)
Environmental factor	Area with rice production and flooding irrigation are at higher risk
Mode of transmission	Vector: *Culex tritaeniorhynchus* and *Culex vishnui* groups, *Culex gelidus* Culicine mosquitoes
Incubation period (IP)	5–15 days
Life cycle	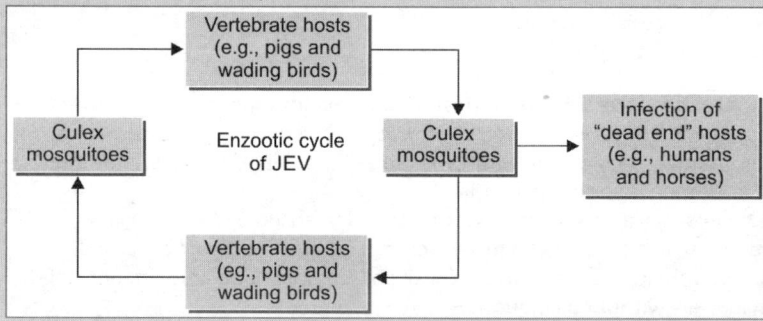
Clinical features	Clinical manifestation described in three stages: • **Prodromal stage:** fever, headache, lethargy and gastrointestinal disturbances. It is usually for 1-6 days. • **Acute encephalitic stage:** high grade fever, nuchal rigidity, focal CNS signs, convulsions sign of raised intracranial pressure, difficulty of speech, ocular palsies, dystonia, hemiplegia, quadriplegia, extrapyramidal signs like coarse tremors and altered sensorium progressing to coma. • **Late Stage:** Neurological sign starts to improve convalescence may be prolonged. The case fatality rate is around 20–40 %.
Diagnosis	• Antibody detection: Hemagglutination Inhibition Test (HI), Compliment Fixation test (CF), ELISA for IgG (paired) and IgM (MAC) antibodies, etc. • Antigen detection: RPHA, IFA, Immunoperoxidase, etc. • Genome detection: RTPCR • Isolation: Tissue culture, infant mice, etc.

Prevention and treatment	No specific treatment but supportive treatment like, analgesic, anticonvulsant and care can significantly reduce the number of deaths. Vaccination: cell culture-derived, live attenuated vaccine based on the SA 14-14-2 strain (JE-1 at 9 months and JE-2 at 16–24 months s.c.). Two other killed vaccines are available like JEEV and JENVAC. Integrated vector control measure is the main preventive measure.
Remarks	JE vaccine is only provided in endemic districts.

9.4 ZOONOTIC INFECTIONS/DISEASES

CLASSIFICATION OF ZOONOSIS

According to the lifecycle of infective organism.

Direct Zoonoses

These are transmitted from an infected vertebrate host to a susceptible host (man) by direct contact, by contact with a fomite or by a mechanical vector. The agent itself undergoes little or no propagative or developmental changes during transmission, e.g., rabies, anthrax, brucellosis, leptospirosis, toxoplasmosis.

Cyclozoonoses

These require more than one vertebrate host species, but no invertebrate host for the completion of the life-cycle of the agent, e.g., echinococcosis, taeniasis.

Metazoonoses

These are transmitted biologically by invertebrate vectors, in which the agent multiplies and/or develops and there is always an extrinsic incubation (prepatent) period before transmission to another vertebrate host, e.g., plague, arbovirus infections, schistosomiasis, leishmaniasis.

Saprozoonoses

These require a vertebrate host and a non-animal developmental site like soil, plant material, pigeon dropping, etc., for the development of the infectious agent, e.g., aspergillosis, coccidioidomycosis, cryptococosis, histoplasmosis, zygomycosis.

According to the direction of transmission

Anthropozoonoses

Infections transmitted to man from lower vertebrate animals e.g. rabies, leptospirosis, plague, arboviral infections, brucellosis and Q-fever.

Zooanthroponoses

Infections transmitted from man to lower vertebrate animals, e.g., human tuberculosis in cattle, streptococci, staphylococci, diphtheria, enterobacteriaceae.

Amphixenoses

Infections maintained in both man and lower vertebrate animals and transmitted in either direction, e.g., *Trypanosoma cruzi*, *Schistosoma japonicum*.

Factors Influencing Prevalence of Zoonoses

- **Ecological changes in man's environment:** With the expansion of human population, man is forced to exploit the virgin territories and natural resources like harnessing the power of rivers, constructing roads and pipelines through virgin or thinly populated areas, clearing, irrigating and cultivating new land, deforestation. Large scale expansion of agricultural and engineering resources, construction of dams, artificial lakes, irrigation schemes, clearing of forests—all these lead to changing of the biting habits of the blood sucking vectors and alteration in the population of reservoir animals which has led to the spread of leptospira, tuleraemia, helminthic infections etc.
- **Handling animal byproducts and wastes (occupational hazards):**
  - Anthrax in carpet weavers, **livestock** raisers and workers with animal hair in the textile industry
  - Leptospirosis in rice field workers
  - Listeriosis in agricultural workers
  - Erysipeloid in butchers and fish merchants
  - Tularemia and trypanosomiasis in hunters
  - Creeping eruptions in plumbers, trench diggers, etc.
  - Q-fever in abattoir and rendering plant workers
  - Jungle yellow fever and tickborne diseases in woodcutters
  - Salmonellosis in food processors
  - Bovine tuberculosis in farmers, etc.
- **Increased movements of man:** Land development, engineering project work, pilgrimages, tourism, etc. expose the people to contaminated food and water leading to diseases like amoebiasis, colibacilliosis, giardiasis, salmonellosis, shigellosis, etc.
- **Increased trade in animal products:** Countries which import hides, wool, bone meal, meat, etc. from an area where some of the zoonoses are endemic, are likely to introduce the disease into their territories, e.g., salmonellosis, foot and mouth disease, anthrax, newcastle disease etc.
- **Increased density of animal population:** Animals may carry potential risk of increased frequency of zoonotic agents in man, e.g., dermatophytosis, tuberculosis, brucellosis etc.
- **Transportation of virus infected mosquitoes:** Aircraft, ship, train, motor and other vehicles bring the viruses into a new area, e.g., yellow fever, chikungunya fever, dengue fever etc.
- **Cultural anthropological norms:** In Kenya, people allow the dogs and hyenas to eat human dead bodies infected with hydatidosis. This helps to perpetuate the transmission cycle of the disease.

RABIES

Causative agent
- Family: Rhabdoviridae
- Genus: Lyssavirus type 1
- Structure: Bullet shaped RNA virus
- Types: Street virus and Fixed virus

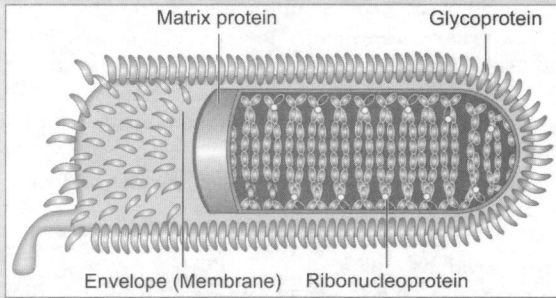

Source of infection	The source of infection to man is the saliva of rabid animals. In dogs and cats, the virus may be present in the saliva for 3–4 days (occasionally 5–6 days) before the onset of clinical symptoms and during the course of illness till death
Host factors	• All warm blooded animals including man are susceptible to rabies. Rabies in man is a dead-end infection • Approximately 40% of the cases are children less than 15 years of age. • Dog handlers, veterinary doctors and hunters are increased risk.
Environmental factor	• 80% of human cases occur in rural areas • Rabies is present in all continent except Antarctica. Rabies is present in India except Andaman Nicobar and Lakshadweep
Mode of transmission	• Animal bites particularly 99% cases in world and 95% cases in India are due to dog bite • Corneal grafts and organ transplantation • Licking or contamination, aerosol

Incubation period (IP)	30–90 days
	• Factors which may influence the length of the incubation period:
	  ▪ Site of bite
	  ▪ The amount of virus in saliva of the biting animal
	  ▪ Strain of the virus
	  ▪ Age of the victim
	  ▪ Immune status of the victim
	• Incubation period is shorter in case the bite is closer to brain and massive dose of virus has been inoculated

Clinical features	• The first symptom to appear may be pain and tingling in the affected limb, especially around the site of bite. This is seen in 35–65% cases. • Hydrophobia is the best-known symptom and pathognomonic feature for rabies. • Hydrophobia is usually the only neurologic abnormality found in patient presenting with furious rabies. It is due to a violent jerky contraction of the diaphragm and accessory muscles of inspiration that is triggered by the patient's attempts to swallow liquid and by a variety of other stimuli such as strong current of air, loud noise and bright light. As disease advances patient may become irritable, confused, angry, depressed and ultimately develop convulsion, paralysis and coma

Complication	Paralysis, Coma, CFR: 100%
Diagnosis	• Clinical diagnosis based on patient's presentation and history of exposure to a suspected rabid animal. • Laboratory confirmation of human rabies can be performed antemortem or post-mortem on saliva, spinal fluid or tissue biopsies to detect intact virions, viral genomic RNA and antibody or antigen

Prevention and treatment	• No specific treatment, isolated in a quiet room and symptomatic treatment.
	• Post-exposure prophylaxis: thorough wound washing, rabies immunoglobulin in severe cases, and a series of human rabies vaccines, is highly effective in preventing death.
	• Vaccinating dogs is the most cost-effective strategy for preventing rabies in people.
	Management of animal bite wound
	• Thoroughly wound toileting (at least for 15 minutes) with soap and water as soap has very good effect against rabies virus as it contains lipid layer.
	• Nothing should be applied over wound like cow dung or chilly.
	• Apply antiseptic solution, such as povidone iodine.
	• There should be no suture of wound, and if it is too much large wound and suturing is required then it should be loose suturing and should be delayed as much as possible.
	• TT/Td must be given to every patient.
	Rabies immunoglobin (RIG)
	• RIG can be given up to 7 days of animal bite because later on it may interfere with anti-rabies vaccine (ARV) and can create problem with the generation of the immunity.
	• RIG is given to the persons with category 3 wound only, exception is HIV patient, RIG is given in category 2 wound also.
	• Dosage of RIG; if it is equine origin then 40 IU/kg and if human origin then 20 IU/kg.
	Regime of ARV
	• **Updated Thai Red Cross regime: 2–2–2–0–2**
	  ▪ It consists of two injections of 0.1 mL tissue culture rabies vaccine, given intradermally at two sites on days 0, 3, 7, and 28 days.
	  ▪ It skips the day 14.
	  ▪ Intradermal route reduces the dose of the vaccine and thus cost of active immunization against rabies.
	  ▪ It gives prompt and effective immune response as from the subcutaneous fat the antigens will be taken directly by the lymphatic cells.
	• **Essen regime: 1–1–1–1-1**
	  ▪ It consists of one injection of 0.5 mL tissue culture rabies vaccine, given intramuscularly at deltoid muscles on days 0, 3, 7, 14 followed by one injection on days 28.
	  ▪ Subsequent exposure requires only two doses of ARV and that on day 0 and day 3 (subsequent exposure does not require RIG in cat 3 wound).
	  ▪ Pre-exposure prophylaxis requires three doses of ARV and that on day 0, day 7 and day 21. Last dose can be taken on day 28 also.

Remarks	• Negri bodies: intracytoplasmic eosinophilic inclusion bodies with basophilic granules in neurons. • National action plan for dog mediated Rabies elimination from India by 2030 is launched with vision to reduce human deaths to dog mediated rabies to zero by 2030. • Rabies can be prevented with vaccination coverage of 70% of dog population for consecutive 3 years.

PLAGUE (also known as MAHAMARI/BLACK DEATH)

Causative agent	*Yersinia pestis*
Source of infection	Infected rodents and fleas and case of pneumonic plague
Host factor	All ages and both sexes
Environmental factor	Heavy rainfall, especially in the flat fields tend to flood the rat burrows
Mode of transmission	• Infected flea bites to humans living: species of fleas are *Xenopsylla cheopis* (principal vector), *X astia* and *X brasiliensis*. • Direct contact with tissues of infected animal • Droplet infection for pneumonic plague
Incubation period (IP)	1–3 days for pneumonic plague 2–7 days for bubonic plague, septicemic plague

Clinical features: Initially patient present with flu like syndrome.
There are three types of plague:
1. **Bubonic plague:** It present as inflamed lymphnode (Bubo) which may turn into open ulcer. It is a most common type.
2. **Septicemic plague:** It happen without formation of bubo.
3. **Pneumonic plague:** It is usually extension of bubonic plague. It is least common type.
4. **CFR** ranges from 30–60% in case of bubonic plague while almost 100% in case of Pneumonic plague in left untreated.

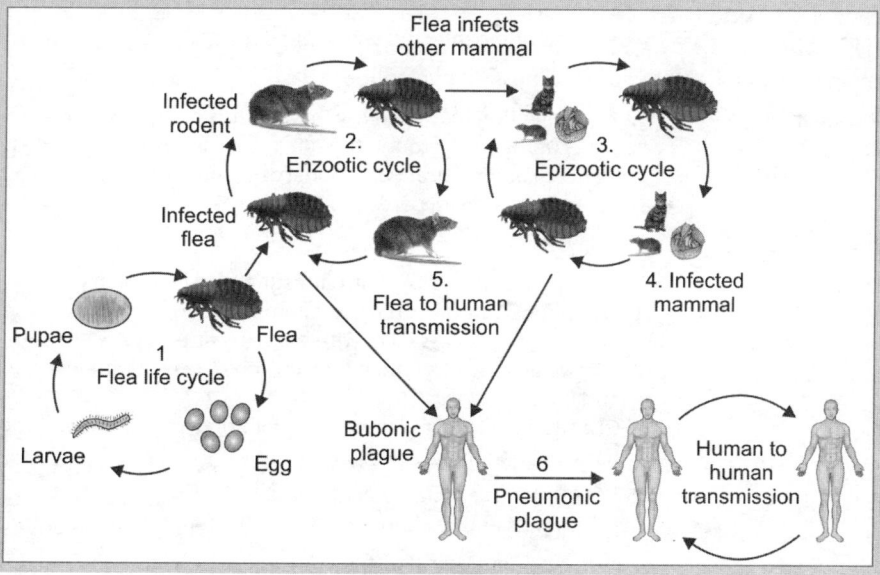

Diagnosis	Microscopic examination Sputum/throat swabs Wayson stain Direct fluorescent antibody (DFA) test
Prevention and treatment	• Surveillance • Vector control (10% DDT and 3% BHC for Flea control) • Rodent control always to be done after the vector control measure have been initiated which helps us to avoid jump of fleas to other hosts including human. • Chemoprophylaxis (Tetracycline 500 mg 6 hrly for 5 days) Drug of choice: Streptomycin (30 mg/kg/day IM for 7 to 10 days) Other drugs: Tetracycline (30–40 mg/kg/day orally), Chloramphenicol, Co-trimoxazole, Sulphonamide
Remarks	Notifiable disease under IHR Outbreak of Plague occurred in south central and western India from 26th August to 18th October, 1994.

ANTHRAX (also known as MALIGNANT PUSTULE, MALIGNANT EDEMA, WOOL SORTER'S DISEASE)

Causative agent	*Bacillus Anthracis* (Gram positive road shaped bacteria) spore forming bacteria
Host factor	Human handling infected animal tissues
Environmental factor	Poor hygiene at slaughter house
Mode of transmission	Human infection may occur by three routes of exposure to anthrax spores: cutaneous (through the skin), gastrointestinal (by ingestion of raw uncooked meat), and pulmonary (inhalation) Not transmitted from person to person
Incubation period (IP)	1–7 days
Clinical features	Three types: Cutaneous, Gastrointestinal and Pulmonary 1. Cutaneous anthrax is the most common anthrax (95% of cases). It presents as painless ulcer with black in center 2. Pulmonary anthrax (Inhalation anthrax) present with fever, chest pain and breathlessness. 3. GI anthrax presents with nausea, vomiting, diarrhea and abdominal pain or sometime as a dysentery.
CFR (%)	CFR: Cutaneous anthrax: 20% if untreated. 25-75% for GI anthrax and more than 80% for pulmonary anthrax
Diagnosis	Culture and serological test-ELISA, molecular testing-PCR

Prevention and treatment	- Disinfection, decontamination and proper disposal.
- Do not handle dead animals without protective measure
- Antibiotics like ciprofloxacin, doxycycline or amoxicillin, penicillin to be taken for two months.
- Vaccination of exposed susceptible humans (anthrax vaccine adsorbed)
- Animal immunization with anthrax vaccine
Remark	Risk of use in bioterrorism

LEPTOSPIROSIS (also known as WEIL'S DISEASE, MUD FEVER", "PEA PICKERS DISEASE", "CANICOLA FEVER", "HEMORRHAGIC JAUNDICE", "INFECTIOUS JAUNDICE", "SWINEHERD'S DISEASE", "SWAMP FEVER")

Causative agent	Bacteria *Leptospira interrogans* and *L.biflexa*
Source of infection	Urine of infected animals
Host factors	Major reservoir hosts of leptospira include: rodents, foxes, wild cats and rabbits. More common among male and in the age group of 20–45 years, occupations like agricultural and livestock farmers, rice fields and sugarcane field workers and underground sewers, veterinarians, abattoir workers, meat and animal handlers, etc.
Environmental factor	Poor living condition, inadequate water supply, inadequate method of waste disposal, Soil salinity and water logging are also favorable environment for leptospire.
Mode of transmission	There is a three R concept which includes rain, rice and rat; this concept explains the mechanism of modes of transmission.
Contact with urine or tissues from infected animals, usually rodents or contaminated water, soil or plants from the urine of infected animals.
Skin abrasions or exposed mucous membrane are the most common point of entry for infection.
Incubation period (IP)	4–20 days usually 10 days
Clinical features	Spectrum of the disease ranges from flu-like symptoms to headache, muscle pain and conjunctival suffusion can develop with progression to severe jaundice, anuria, kidney failure and even death.
Anicteric leptospirosis: Fever, headache, myalgia, conjunctival hemorrhage, renal manifestation, pulmonary manifestation.
Icteric leptospirosis: Jaundice, fever, headache, myalgia, acute renal failure, pulmonary insufficiency, circulatory collapse.
Complications	Pneumonia, bleeding from lungs and multiple organ dysfunction syndromes 5–10% but if lungs are involved than 50–70%.

| Diagnosis | - MAT (microscopic agglutination test)
- Immunofluorescent antibody test
- Seroconversion
- PCR test
- ELISA |
|---|---|
| Prevention and treatment | - Reduction of animal reservoir populations, such as rats
- Removal of rubbish and ensuring areas in and around homes are clean
- Avoid contact with animal urine, infected animals or an infected environment
- Wear protective clothing and cover wounds with waterproof dressings to reduce the chance of infection
- Prophylactic use of antibiotics during flooding times
- Penicillin (6 million unit/day IV) is the drug of choice and other antibiotics, such as tetracycline, amoxicillin, ampicillin and doxycycline are also effective
- Vaccination of animal
- Program for prevention and control of leptospirosis |

BRUCELLOSIS (also known as UNDULANT FEVER, MALTA FEVER, MEDITERRANEAN FEVER, BANG'S DISEASE)

Causative agent	Types of the *Brucella* species *B. abortus*, *B. melitensis* (most common), *B. suis*, *B. canis*
Source of infection	Raw dairy product, infected animal's birth product
Host factors	Occupation like farmer, veterinarians, livestock handlers and slaughter house workers are at higher risk
Reservoir:
- Cattle and buffalo: *B. abortus*
- Sheep and goats: *B. melitensis*
- Swine: *B. suis*
- Dogs: *B. canis*
Environmental factor	Poor hygiene and sanitation
Mode of transmission	**Contact infection:** Most commonly, infection occurs by direct contact with infected tissues, blood, urine, vaginal discharge, aborted fetuses and especially placenta.
Food-borne infection: Indirectly by the ingestion of raw milk or dairy products (cheese) from infected animals. Water contaminated with the excreta of infected animals may also serve as a source of infection.
Air-borne infection: Inhaled in aerosol form in slaughter houses and laboratories.

Incubation period (IP)	One week to several months (usually 1–3 weeks)
Clinical features	Gradual onset of persistent fever, chills, sweating, headache, muscle pain, backache, joint pain, fatigue, weakness and weight loss. Human brucellosis can cause chronic debilitating illness
Complication	Complications may affect any of the organ systems Rarely fatal <2% CFR
Diagnosis	ELISA, PCR, culture
Prevention and treatment	• Consume only pasteurized or boiled milk and dairy products and eat thoroughly cooked meat. • Use protective measure during disposal of animal waste and handling reproductive tissue of animal. • Animal: Vaccine of *B. abortus* strain 19 is commonly used for young animals. A compulsory vaccination program for all heifers in a given community on a yearly basis. • Human: Live vaccine of *B. abortus* strain 19-BA is available • Doxycycline 100 mg BD for 45 days and Inj Streptomycin 1 gm (IM) daily for 15 days. • Alternative regimen is doxycycline at 100 mg, twice a day for 45 days, plus rifampicin at 15 mg/kg/day (600–900 mg) for 45 days

KYASANUR FOREST DISEASE (KFD) (also known as MONKEY DISEASE)

Causative agent	Group B togavirus/flavivirus
Host factors	Man is the incidental dead end host Amplifier host: monkeys
Environmental factor	More cases are reported during dry season November to June Occupation like hunters, herders, farmers and forest workers particularly working in state of Karnataka are at increases risk for infection KFD is now also being reported from three neighboring states namely Kerala, Goa, Maharashtra
Mode of transmission	Vector: Hard tick-Haemaphysalis spinigera (India) Soft tick (outside India) Ticks remain infected for life Transmission to human after tick bite or contact with infected animals Animal like cattle, goats, sheep may be infected but less role in transmission of disease to human No person to person transmission Transovarial and transstadial transmission occur

Incubation period (IP)	3–8 days
Pathogenesis	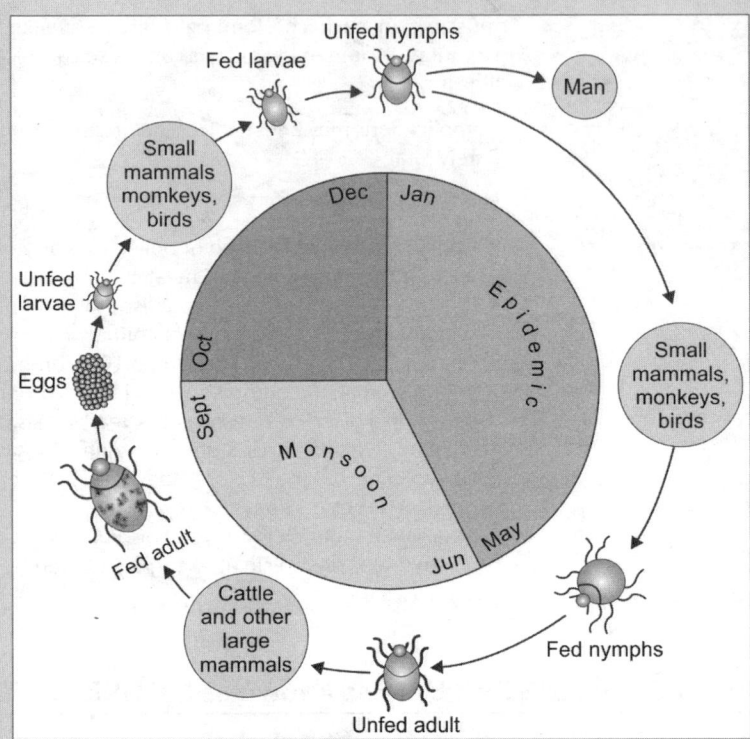
Clinical features	Fever with chills, headache, vomiting, muscle pain and sometimes bleeding after 3–4 days of initial symptoms
Complication	10–20% of cases may have serious complication like neurological problem and vision deficits CFR: 2–10%
Diagnosis	RT-PCR, IgM ELISA
Prevention and treatment	<ul><li>Personal protection, use of repellent</li><li>Tick control measure like spraying of insecticides with the help of aircraft</li><li>Regularly de-tick animal and apply insect repellents on animals</li><li>No specific treatment only supportive therapy and maintenance of hydration</li><li>Vaccine (inactivate cheek embryo vaccine)</li></ul>

RICKETTSIAL DISEASES

	Scrub typhus /Tsutsugamushi disease	Murine typhus/ Endemic typhus/ Flea borne typhus/Urban typhus	Epidemic typhus/ Louse borne typhus	Indian tick typhus	Rickettsial pox	Rocky mountain spotted fever/ Tick typhus	Q fever	Trench fever/Five day fever/ Quintan fever
Causative agent	Orientia tsutsugamushi (R. tsutsugamushi)	R. typhi (R. mooseri)	R. prowazekii	R. conorii	R. akari	R. rickettsii	C. burnetti	Bartonella quintana
Vector	Trombiculid mite	Flea	Louse	Tick	Mite	Tick (Ixodid ticks)	Nil	Louse
Reservoir	Rodents	Rodents	Human	Rodents and dogs	Mice	Rodents and dogs	Cattle, sheep and goat	Human
Mode of transmission	Bite of infected larval mite	Feces inoculation on skin or inhalation of dried infective feces	Inoculation/ inhalation of infected louse feces, crushing infected louse feces	Bite of infected tick	Bite of infected mite	Bite of infected tick	Inhalation of infected dust, aerosol transmission, direct contact. Contaminated food like milk, meat	Louse feces
Incubation period	10–12 days	1–2 weeks	1–2 weeks	3–7 days	7–9 days	5–7 days	2–3 weeks	2 weeks
Clinical features	Fever with chills, headache, malaise, Rash: Centrifugal. Eschar (punched out ulcer covered with blackened scab)	Fever, headache, gangrene Rash: Centrifugal	Rash: Centrifugal, prolong fever, vasculitis	Fever, malaise, headache, eschar, Rash: All over body (confused with atypical measles)	Rash: All over body (confused with chicken pox)	Fever, chills, Rash: Centripetal, and sometimes swollen lymph nodes, vasculitis, ulcer	Acute: No rash, fever with chills, headache, bodyache, Pneumonia Chronic Q fever present with endocarditis and meningoencephalitis	Fever, headache, muscle pain, rash
Diagnosis	Clinically, serological Weil-Felix reaction, indirect immunofluorescence test	Blood culture, Weil-Felix reaction positive in 2nd week	Serological test	Serological test	Serological test	Serological test and indirect immunofluores- cence assay (IFA)	Serological test	Serological test
Prevention and treatment	Vector control and personal protection, Doxycycline 100 mg twice daily for orally or intrave- nously for 7 days, other drug chloramphenicol, Rifampicin, Azithromycin	Rodent control, insecticide spraying, Tetracycline (DOC)	Anti louse measure, per- sonal hygiene, Tetracycline (include in IHR in the group of sur- veillance disease)	Personal protection, Tetracycline/ doxy	Habitat control and personal protection, doxycycline	Habitat control and personal protection, Doxycycline	Pasteurization of milk, sanitary cattel sheds, disinfection and coxiella vaccine, Doxycycline, Tetracycline	Doxycycline

TAENIASIS

Causative agent	Tape worm: Taenia Solium, Taenia Saginata
Source of infection	Undercooked beef or pork
Host factor	Man is a definitive host while cattle (C. bovis) and pig (C. cellulosae) are the intermediate host for the *T. saginata* and *T. solium* respectively.
Environmental factor	Poor sanitation
Mode of transmission	Ingestion of infective vegetable or any other food, water contaminated with eggs Ingestion of infective beef or pork
Incubation period (IP)	8–14 weeks
Life cycle	

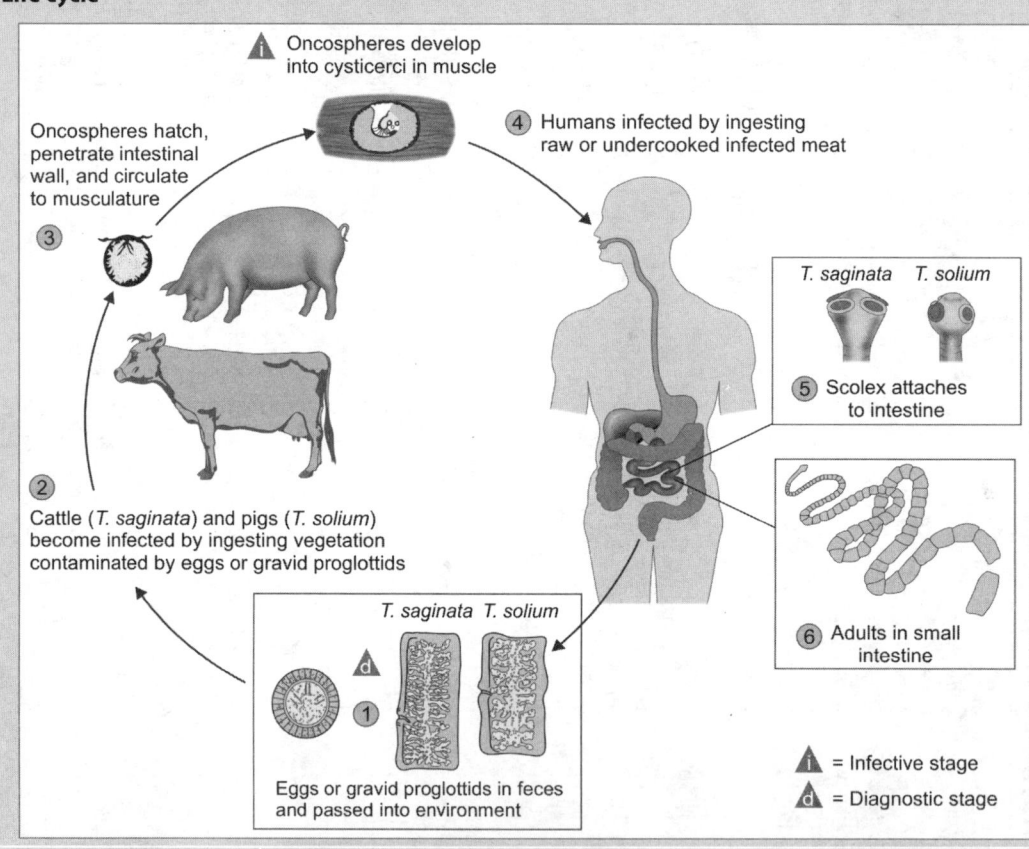

Clinical features	• Abdominal pain, loss of appetite, weight loss and indigestion. • When Cysticerci developed in central nervous system (Neurocysticercosis) is a serious condition which leads to epilepsy, hydrocephalus, intracranial hypertensive syndromes and death
Complication	• Cysticercosis due to *T. solium*
Diagnosis	• Stool sample • MRI/CT scan usually for neurocysticercosis

Prevention and treatment	- Hygiene and adequate sewage treatment - Meat inspection and thorough cooking - Handwashing - Single doses of Praziquantel (10 mg/kg) or Niclosamide (adults and children over 6 years: 2 g, children aged 2–6 years: 1 g). Albendazole at 400 g for 3 consecutive days has also been used. - For Neurocysticercosis steroid and antiepileptic drug may be required along with above mention drugs

HYDATID DISEASE

Causative agent	*Echinococcus granulosus, E. multilocularis*
Source of infection	Contaminated food and water
Host factors	Occupation like shepherds, shoe makers and workers of slaughter house Definitive host: carnivors (dog), Intermediate host: sheep, goat, cattle and sometimes human as incidental host
Environmental factor	Poor hygiene and sanitation
Mode of transmission	- Ingestion of the eggs of Echinococcus with food, unwashed vegetables or water contaminated with feces from infected dogs. - Infection can also take place while handling or playing with infected dogs, e.g., hand to mouth transfer of eggs, or by inhalation of dust contaminated with infected eggs. - Disease is not transmitted from person to person
Incubation period (IP)	Months to years
Life cycle	

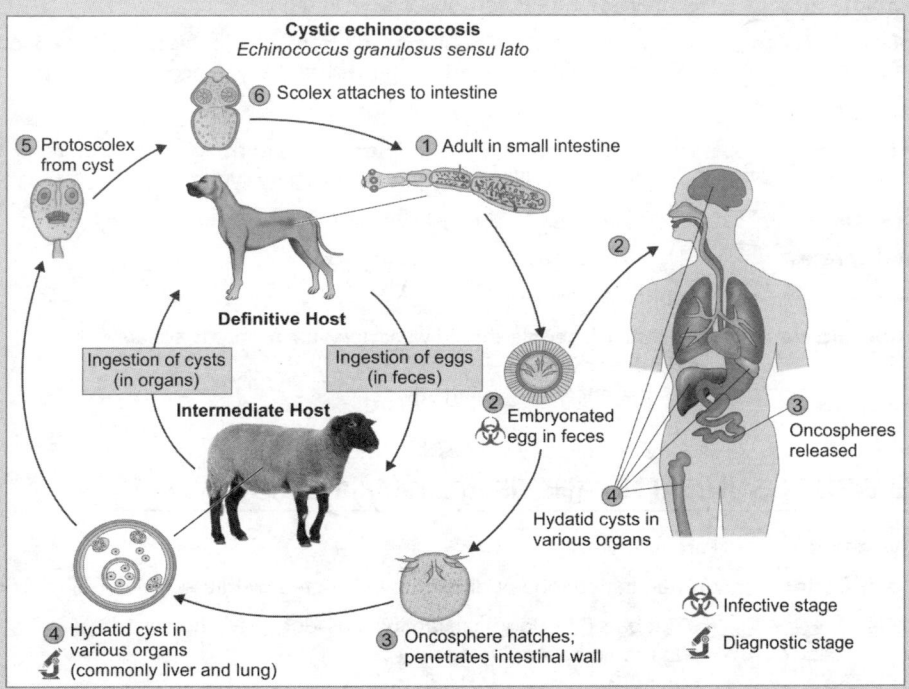

Clinical features	• After several years of exposure symptoms develop. • Majority of cyst develop in right lobe of liver, and lung, long bones, brain, peritoneum, kidney. If cyst size is small then asymptomatic and if enlarge then depending upon site of lodgments symptoms are developed.
Complication	Complications based on involved organ (e.g., Jaundice if liver is involved) and sometimes may lead to death
Diagnosis	Clinically, X-ray, Ultrasound, MRI, CT scan, Serological test, ELISA, Intradermal Casoni test

Prevention and treatment	• Hygiene and sanitation, thoroughly washing of vegetables and fruits,
	• Handwashing,
	• Stop defecation of dog near children playing area or vegetable farm,
	• There are four options for the treatment of cystic echinococcosis:
	  1. Percutaneous treatment of the hydatid cysts with the PAIR (Puncture, Aspiration, Injection, Re-aspiration) technique
	  2. Surgery
	  3. Anti-infective drug treatment (Albendazole/Mebendazole)
	  4. "Watch and Wait approach"

HANTA VIRUS

Causative agent	Belongs to Bunyaviridae family. Hantaan, Seoul and Thailand hanta virus types are mainly responsible for outbreaks in Asia
Source of infection	Urine or feces of infected rodents
Reservoirs	Wild rodents
Host factors	Farmers, sweepers and laborers are at high risk
Mode of transmission	• Inhalation of the virus in aerosols from urine or feces of infected rodents • Human-to-human transmission is less likely to occur
Incubation period	Usually 2–3 weeks
Clinical features	There are two types: HFRS (Hanta virus hemorrhagic fever with renal syndrome) and HPS (Hanta virus pulmonary syndrome)
Complication	Respiratory failure, kidney failure and profuse bleeding
Case fatality rate	CFR of HFRS is about 15% and in HPS 50%
Treatment	Supportive
Prevention and control	• High risk people should wear personal protective gears • Rodent control • Adherence to traveling advice

NIPAH VIRUS ("SUNGAI NIPAH" Village in Malaysia)

Causative agent	Paramyxovirus
Source of infection	Contaminated food or drink that in infected by bat secretion (saliva, urine).
Reservoirs	• Fruit bats (Pteropodidae family) pigs, dogs, cats, horses, etc. • Pigs could be amplifying host

Host factors	People involved with pigs and fruit bats and healthcare worker are higher risk
Mode of transmission	Transmitted to humans either from consumption of fruits or fruit products (such as raw date palm juice) contaminated with urine or saliva from infected fruit bats or animals (contact with urine, saliva or contaminated materials) or from other humans
Incubation period	4–14 days
Life cycle	

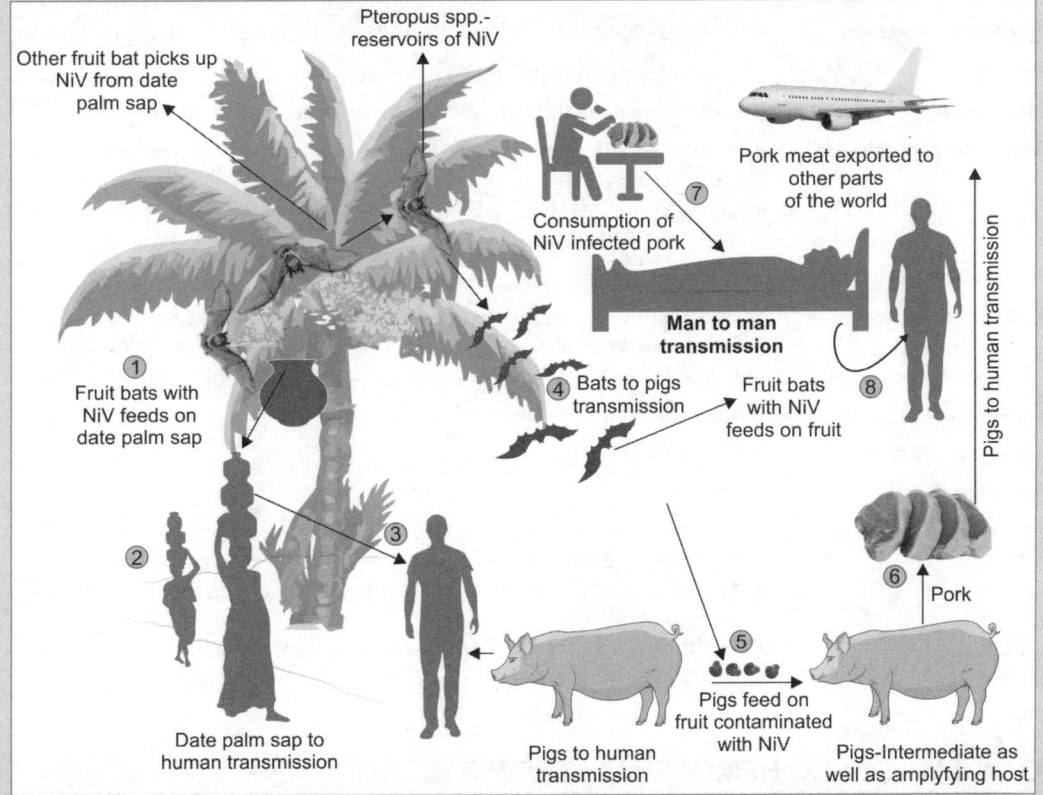

Clinical features	Clinical spectrum ranging from asymptomatic—flu like syndrome—fatal encephalitis.
Complication	Neurological complication
Case fatality rate	CFR in symptomatic cases is 40–75%
Treatment	Supportive
Prevention and control	• Avoid contact with bats and fruit potentially contaminated with bat urine, such as date palm sap. • Healthcare workers should implement standard precautions including PPE when treating patients with suspected or confirmed NiV infection • At present no vaccine available

EBOLAVIRUS DISEASE (name adopted from EBOLA RIVER)

Causative agent	Belongs to the Filoviridae family (filovirus). Ebolavirus comprises five different species: 1. Bundibugyo ebolavirus (BDBV) 2. Zaire ebolavirus (EBOV): most lethal 3. Sudan ebolavirus (SUDV) 4. Reston ebolavirus (RESTV) 5. Taï forest (formerly Côte d'Ivoire ebolavirus) ebolavirus (TAFV)
Source of infection	Infected raw meat of fruit bat, infected blood and body fluids of the patients
Reservoirs	Fruit bats (Pteropodidae family)
Host factors	Healthcare worker and laboratory personnel are at higher risk
Mode of transmission	• Human get infected through direct or close contact with patients, and particularly with blood and body fluids of patient. • Contact with infected fruit bats or monkeys and the consumption of their raw meat leads to infection.
Incubation period	2–21 days
Clinical features	Severe acute viral illness often characterized by the sudden onset of fever, rash, intense weakness, muscle pain, headache and sore throat can be followed by diarrhea, vomiting, internal and external bleeding
Complication	Hypovolemic hemorrhagic shock
Case fatality rate	25% to 90% (average 50%)
Treatment	Supportive
Prevention and control	• Raising awareness about the preventive measure measures (e.g., safe burial of dead person) • All animal products (blood, meat and milk) should be thoroughly cooked before eating. • Healthcare workers should follow standard precautions including PPE • Trial ongoing for vaccine (rVSV-ZEBOV)

CRIMEAN-CONGO HEMORRHAGIC FEVER (CCHF)

Causative agent	Nairovirus (Bunyaviridae family)
Reservoirs	Domestic and wild animals
Mode of transmission	• Vector: Transmitted by ticks (*Hyalomma* genus) • Transmission is mainly through direct contact with the blood or tissues of livestock, such as sheep, goats or cattle, but also from tick bites. • Human-to-human transmission may occur by exposure to blood and excreta from affected people. • Mode of transmission suggest that agricultural workers, slaughterhouse workers and veterinarians are at higher risk.
Incubation period	1–3 days following a tick bite, or 5–6 days following contact with infected blood or tissues.

Clinical features	• High grade fever and chills, headache, dizziness, and muscle pain. Gastrointestinal signs include abdominal pain, nausea, vomiting and diarrhea. • Conjunctival congestion and flushing of the face can be observed. Bleeding from the nose, gums, kidneys, and gastric mucosa are frequent manifestations.
Complication	Hemorrhage
Case fatality rate	10–40%
Treatment	Supportive care and Ribavirin (Antiviral Drug)
Prevention and control	• Insect repellents • Wearing gloves and other protective clothing by animal handlers. • Individuals should avoid contact with the blood and body fluids of sick livestock or patients. • Strict adherence to infection-control precautions is very important in healthcare settings. • Healthcare workers who have had contact with tissue or blood from suspected or confirmed CCHF patients, should do temperature and symptom monitoring for at least 14 days after exposure. • No vaccine for human or animal use is available. • Community awareness about the hazards of tick bites and personal protection is essential.

9.5 OTHER IMPORTANT DISEASES

HIV/AIDS (ACQUIRED IMMUNODEFICIENCY SYNDROME/SLIM DISEASE)

Causative agent	• Retrovirus: Human immunodeficiency virus (HIV) • There are two types of HIV—HIV-1 and HIV-2. HIV-1 is further divided into three main groups—major (M), outliers (O) and new groups (N). • Group M is further classified into subtypes A-K (except I) based on phylogenetic relatedness. 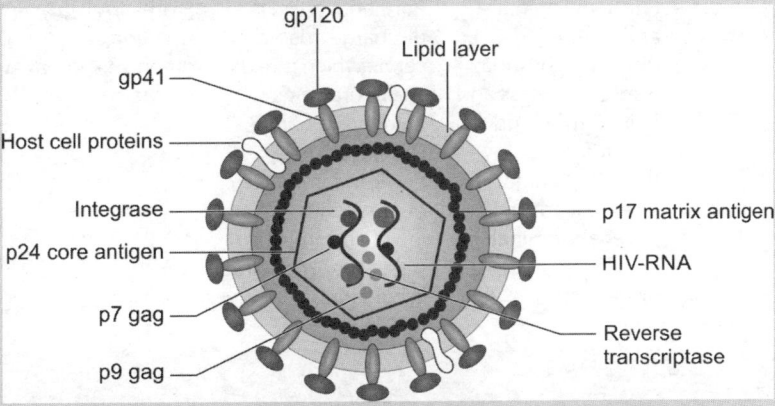
Host factor	20–49 age group, commercial sex worker, migrant worker, injectable drug abuser, truck driver, transgender, male homosexuals, unemployed, under employed, mobile and migrant youth, and street children vulnerable population

Mode of transmission	Sexual, mother to child, contaminated blood contact, needles
Incubation period (IP)	Few months to 10 years
Clinical features	a. **Initial infection with the virus and development of antibodies:** No symptom or mild fever, rash, sore throat b. **Asymptomatic carrier state:** Enlargement of lymph nodes c. **AIDS-related complex (ARC):** Diarrhea more than one month, weight loss more than 10% of body weight, fever, opportunistic infection d. **AIDS:** End stage of HIV: Chronic diarrhea and severe weight loss, opportunistic infection, candidiasis, pneumocystosis carini pneumonia, AIDS encephalopathy, generalized lymphadenopathy, Kaposi sarcoma, cryptococcal meningitis, etc.
Diagnosis	Clinically, ELISA, Western Blot
Prevention and treatment	• Preferred first-line ART regimen for all PLHIV with age >10 years and weight >30 kg is as follows: Tenofovir (TDF 300 mg) + Lamivudine (3TC 300 mg) + DOLUTEGRAVIR (DTG 50 mg) regimen (TLD) as FDC in a single pill once a day (at a fixed time every day as per patient's convenience). • Vaccines are under trials.
Remarks	• HIV progresses to AIDS when CD4 count < 200. • **Window period:** There is a period of time between HIV infection and the appearance of anti-HIV antibodies that can be measured. • For more details read Chapter 9.10 NACP

SEXUALLY TRANSMITTED DISEASES (STD)

High risk among single, divorced people, commercial sexual worker, poverty, urbanization and migration.

	Gonorrhea	Chlamydia	Trichomoniasis	Candidiasis	Bacterial vaginosis
Agent	Neisseria gonorrhoeae	Chlamydia trachomatis	Trichomonas vaginalis	Candida albicans	Gardnerella vaginalis
Clinical features	Purulent vaginal and urethral discharge, dysuria, urethral abscess and Epididymitis and Orchitis, Pelvic inflammatory disease leads to lower abdominal pain, fever, menstrual irregularities	Purulent cervical discharge, friable cervix which bleeds easily, urethritis Epididymitis and Orchitis in male, Pelvic inflammatory disease leads to lower abdominal pain, fever, menstrual irregularities	Frothy foul-smelling, greenish vaginal discharge	Whitish Curd-like vaginal discharge, vaginal itching, balanitis in male	Fishy odor grayish vaginal discharge

	Syphilis	Chancroid (Soft chancre)	Lymphogranuloma venereum (LGV)	Genital herpes	Granuloma inguinale (Donovanosis)
Agent	Treponema pallidum	Haemophilus ducreyi	Chlamydia trachomatis (L1, L2, L3)	Herpes simplex virus	Calymmato-bacterium granulomatis

Communicable Diseases and Relevant National Health Programs

Clinical features	Primary syphilis: Painless ulcer (chancre)—in women on the external genitalia and in men on the penis. Enlarged rubbery lymph node. Secondary syphilis: Rash, muscle pain, headache, low grade fever if untreated then involvement of heart and blood vessels which can be fatal	Painful ulcers on the external genitalia, painful enlarged lymph nodes (bubo) in the groin	Painless papule on vulva and penis, bubos in groin with fistulae, if untreated then develop swelling of genitals due to blockage of lymphatic system	Multiple painful vesicles and ulcer	Initially lumps below the skin then develop painless ulcers

	Molluscum contagiosum	*Genital warts (Condyloma acuminate)*	*Scabies*	*Pediculosis pubis*
Agent	Poxvirus	Human papillomavirus	Sarcoptes scabiei	Pthirus pubis
Clinical features	Multiple globular papules over the body	"Cauliflower" growth which appear around the anus, vulvovaginal area, penis, urethra and perineum, painless	Burrow on the skin, severe itching worsen at night	Small red papules and urticaria

Prevention and treatment
- Syndromic management
- Health education and counseling
- Safer sex practices
- Treatment adherence for both patients and their partners

Syndromic management

Kit number	Syndrome	Kit color	Drugs
Kit 1	Urethral discharge (UD), Cervical discharge (CD), Anorectal discharge (ARD), Painful scrotal swelling (PSS)	Gray	Tab. Azithromycin 1 g and Tab. Cefixime 400 mg
Kit 2	Vaginal discharge (VD)	Green	Tab. Secnidazole 2 g and Tab. Fluconazole 150 mg
Kit 3	Genital Ulcer Disease-Non-herpetic (GUD-NH)	White	Inj. Benzathine penicillin 2.4 MU and Tab. Azithromycin 1 g and Disposable syringe 10 mL with 21 gauge needle and Sterile water 10 mL
Kit 4	Genital Ulcer Disease-Non-Herpetic (GUD-NH)—for patients allergic to penicillin	Blue	Tab. Doxycycline 100 mg and Tab. Azithromycin 1 g
Kit 5	Genital Ulcer Disease-Herpetic (GUD-H)	Red	Tab. Acyclovir 400 mg
Kit 6	Lower abdominal pain (LAP/PID)	Yellow	Tab. Cefixime 400 mg and Tab. Metronidazole 400 mg and Cap. Doxycycline 100 mg
Kit 7	Inguinal bubo (IB)	Black	Tab. Doxycycline 100 mg and Tab. Azithromycin 1 g

TRACHOMA

Causative agent	• *Chlamydia trachomatis* endemic trachoma of developing countries is caused by *C. trachomatis* of immune types A, B or C. • The sexually-transmitted *C. trachomatis* (serotypes D, E, F, G, H, I, J or K)
Source of infection	• Infected ocular discharge
Host factor	• Children mainly 2–5 year of age group • Increased the risk if direct exposure of sunlight, irritants such as kajal, dust and smoke
Environmental factor	• April-May and July-September • poor personal hygiene, illiteracy, poverty, crowded households and poor housing
Mode of transmission	• Direct or indirect contact with ocular discharges of infected persons or fomites, e.g., infected fingers, towels, bedding, kajal
Incubation period (IP)	• 5–12 days
Period of communicability	• Low infectivity. It is infective as long as active lesions are present in the conjunctiva
Clinical features	It is a chronic infectious disease of conjunctiva and cornea. "Blinding trachoma" – characterized by: • Corneal blindness • Trachomatous trichiasis (inward deviation of eyelashes) and entropion (inward deviation of lid margin) • Moderate and severe trachomatous inflammation
Complication	Blindness
Diagnosis	Diagnostic criteria • Follicles on the upper tarsal conjunctiva • Herbert's pits, limbal follicles • Conjunctival scarring (trichiasis, entropion) • Vascular pannus
Prevention and treatment	**Mass or blanket treatment** (if prevalence >5% in <10-year age group): Application twice daily of tetracycline 1% ointment to all children, for 5 consecutive days each month or once daily for 10 days each month for 6 consecutive months Selective treatment Surgical correction of eye lid deformities Personal and environmental hygiene

Remarks	• **SAFE strategy** for eliminate Trachoma under GET (Global Elimination of Trachoma) 2020:
	  ▪ Surgery for advanced disease,
	  ▪ Antibiotics to clear *C. trachomatis* infection,
	  ▪ Facial cleanliness and
	  ▪ Environmental improvement to reduce transmission.
	• Trachoma is eliminated from India in 2017, as its prevalence is only 0.7% (WHO elimination target is <5% in less than 10 years of age)

TETANUS

Causative agent	*Clostridium tetani*
Source of infection	Soil and dust containing spores of bacilli
Host factor	5–40 years age group, more in male
Environmental factor	Presence of soil, agriculture and animal husbandry, unhygienic customs and delivery practices, lack of primary healthcare services, ignorance, crush injuries and wound
Mode of transmission	Contamination of wound with tetanus spores
Incubation period (IP)	6–10 days (1 day to several months)
Reservoir of infection	Soil and dust
clinical features	Characterized by muscular rigidity and painful paroxysmal spasms of the voluntary muscles like Trismus (lock jaw), facial muscle (Risus sardonicus), back and neck muscle (Opisthotonus)
	Types: • **Traumatic:** Trauma and wound • **Puerperal:** Tetanus during delivery or abortion • **Tetanus neonatorum:** Newborn delivered in non-aseptic condition; infection of the umbilical stump also known as "8th day disease". • **Otogenic:** Rare due to infected beads, pencils, etc. • **Idiopathic:** No definite history
Complication	Laryngospasm, fracture due to violent and strong contraction by muscle, asphyxia
Diagnosis	Clinically
Prevention and treatment	• **Active immunization:** Pentavalent, DPT, Td • **Passive immunization:** Human tetanus hyperimmunoglobulin (TIG), antitetanus serum (ATS) • Active and passive immunization usually required in unimmunized severe crush injury • Surgical toilet requires in all the wound • **Antibiotics:** Penicillin

Management of clean, nonpenetrating wound and less than 6 hours old wound

Category	Treatment
Category A: H/o complete course or Toxoid or booster dose within 5 years	Nothing required
Category B: H/o complete course or Toxoid or booster dose more than 5 years but less than 10 years	Toxoid 1 dose
Category C: H/o complete course or Toxoid or booster dose more than 10 years	Toxoid 1 dose
Category D: No H/o complete course or Toxoid or unknown immunity status	Toxoid complete course

Management of other wounds

Category	Treatment
Category A: H/o complete course of Toxoid or booster dose within 5 years	Nothing required
Category B: H/o complete course of Toxoid or booster dose more than 5 years but less than 10 years	Toxoid 1 dose
Category C: H/o complete course of Toxoid or booster dose more than 10 years	Toxoid 1 dose + Human Tetanus Ig
Category D: No H/o complete course of Toxoid or unknown immunity status	Toxoid complete course + Human Tetanus Ig

Remarks	• Lethal exotoxin produced by tetanus bacilli • Source and reservoir both are same • India was declared free of maternal and neonatal tetanus on 15th May, 2015

LEPROSY/HANSEN'S DISEASE

Causative agent	*Mycobacterium leprae* It is obligate intracellular bacteria It is acid fast bacillus It does not grow in artificial media
Source of infection	Multibacillary case (main)
Host factor	All age but in endemic area highest case in 10–20 years, cases are more in adult male
Environmental factor	Humidity, overcrowding, lack of ventilation, social beliefs
Mode of transmission	Droplet infection, contact transmission
Incubation period (IP)	3–5 years
Period of communicability	Highly infectious but low pathogenicity
Clinical features	Loss of sensation in hypopigmented patch thickening of nerve, nodule, loss of eyebrow, dry skin
Complication	Deformity
Diagnosis	Clinical examination, bacteriological examination, foot pad culture, histamine test biopsy, immunological test
Prevention and treatment	Read treatment Chapter 9.7 NLEP Rehabilitation **Post-exposure prophylaxis:** Single dose of Rifampicin **Leprosy vaccine:** Mycobacterium indicus pranii vaccine (under research)
Remarks	**Lepromin test:** To detect the cell mediated immunity Read classification Chapter 9.7 NLEP

YAWS (ENDEMIC TREPONEMATOSES)

Causative agent	*Treponema pertenue*
Host factor	More common in less than 15 years. Males are more affected than females.
Environmental factor	High humidity region and overcrowding, poor sanitation and hygiene
Mode of transmission	Direct contact with secretions from infectious lesions and infected fomites
Incubation period (IP)	9–90 days (average 21 days)
Reservoir of Infection	Case
Clinical features	Chronic skin infection **Early yaws:** Primary lesion or "mother yaw" appears at the site of inoculation. The lesion founds on exposed parts of the body like arms legs, face. Enlargement of lymph node **Late yaws:** After 5 years destructive lesion appear **Crab yaws:** Lesions on sole and palms **Gangos:** Lesions of soft palate, hard palate, and nose **Goundu:** Swelling around nose due to osteoperiostites of the superior maxillary bone

Complication	Destructive lesion and deformity
Diagnosis	Microscopic examination of skin lesion and serological test (RPR and TPPA), PCR is usually confirmatory test
Prevention and treatment	Single dose of Azithromycin (30 mg/kg) oral or a single injection of long-acting penicillin Benzathine penicillin (0.6 to 1.2 million units) Personal hygiene, environmental sanitation The WHO has recommended three treatment policies: 1. **Total mass treatment:** For hyperendemic area (>10% prevalence of clinically active yaws) treatment is given to the all 2. **Juvenile mass treatment:** In meso-endemic communities (5 to 10% prevalence) treatment is given to all cases and to all children under 15 years of age and other obvious contacts 3. **Selective mass treatment:** In hypoendemic areas (<5% prevalence) treatment to the cases and their household
Remarks	Yaws eliminated from India in 2006 and Yaws free declared on 5th May, 2016.

SCABIES

Causative agent	Sarcoptes scabiei or Acarus scabiei
Source of infection	Close contact
Host factor	Children are more affected
Environmental factor	Poor hygiene, overcrowding, poor
Mode of transmission	Close contact with affected patient and sharing of contaminated linen and clothes
Incubation period (IP)	3–4 weeks
Clinical features	Intense itching worse at night, affects the hands and wrist (63%), the extensor aspect of elbows being next (10.9%). The axillae, buttocks, lower abdomen, feet and ankles, palms in infants are all common sites of infestation. Irregular burrow tracks, the disease also affects the breasts in women and the genitals in men. Similar complains among family members and close contact is very common.
Complication	Secondary bacterial infection over skin lesion like impetigo
Diagnosis	Clinical history like night itching at night, follicular lesion, pustules, microscopic examination
Prevention and treatment	• 5% permethrin cream (most effective): only one application required • Benzyl Benzoate (12.5% for children and 25% for adults): Usually require three application 12 hours apart. • Ivermectin—as a single oral dose (200 mcg/kg) • Symptomatic treatment for itching • All close contact must be treated at the same time • Scabicidal lotion applied at bedtime all over the body from head to toes and washed off in next morning
Remarks	Norwegian scabies is a rare form, occurs in immunocompromised patients and presents as hyperkeratotic and crusted lesion

PEDICULOSIS

Causative agent	• Head louse (Pediculus humanus capitis) • Body louse (Pediculus humanus corporis) • Pubic louse (Pthirus pubis)
Host factor	All age group
Environmental factor	Poor hygiene and overcrowding
Mode of transmission	Contact with a person who is already infested, wearing clothing transmission via fomites like towel, bed linens Pediculus humanus capitis caused by hair contact and fomites while Pthirus pubis transmitted by sexually and fomites
Clinical features	Itching is the main presenting complain. Sometimes may be presented as a papule and secondary bacterial infection.
Diagnosis	Clinically
Prevention and treatment	• **Pediculus capitis:** Topical application of Permethrin (1%), gamma benzene hexachloride (1%). Ivermectin can be used. • **Pediculus corporis:** Proper hygiene and washing clothes with gamma benzene hexachloride (10%) • **Pubic louse:** Removal of hair is effective
Remarks	Louse is an important vector for following diseases: 1. **Epidemic typhus:** Rickettsia prowazekii 2. **Trench fever:** Bartonella quintana 3. **Louse-borne relapsing fever:** Borrelia recurrentis Chronic body louse infestation is also known as Vagabond disease.

BIBLIOGRAPHY

1. http://naco.gov.in/sites/default/files/India%20HIV%20Estimates%202020__Web_Version_0.pdf
2. http://ncdc.gov.in/linkimages/YAWS_Elimination%20in%20India%20a%20step%20towards%20eradication3178866818.pdf
3. http://nhp.gov.in/disease/communicable-disease/kyasanur-forest-disease
4. http://nhp.gov.in/disease/whooping-cough-pertu
5. http://www.who.int/topics/infectious_diseases/factsheets/en/
6. https://apps.who.int/iris/rest/bitstreams/909329/retrieve
7. https://cltri.gov.in/TrainingMaterial/Epid_lep_dr_vmb_Apr.2022.pdf
8. https://main.mohfw.gov.in/sites/default/files/195431585071489665073.pdf
9. https://main.mohfw.gov.in/sites/default/files/Guidelines%20for%20Management%20of%20Monkeypox%20Disease.pdf
10. https://ncdc.gov.in/index1.php?lang=1andlevel=1andsublinkid=142andlid=73
11. https://ncdc.gov.in/showfile.php?lid=360
12. https://ncdc.gov.in/WriteReadData/l892s/File618.pdf
13. https://ncdc.gov.in/WriteReadData/linkimages/May%20June-20098604739980.pdf
14. https://ncdc.gov.in/WriteReadData/linkimages/OCT-NOV_098132922884.pdf
15. https://nhm.assam.gov.in/sites/default/files/swf_utility_folder/departments/nhm_lipl_in_oid_6/portlet/level_2/epidemiology.pdf

16. https://nhm.gov.in/images/pdf/guidelines/nrhm-guidelines/rtis-stis/chapter-2.pdf
17. https://nhm.gov.in/New_Updates_2018/NHM_Components/Immunization/Guildelines_for_immunization/Td_vaccine_operational_guidelines.pdf
18. https://nvbdcp.gov.in/index1.php?lang=1andlevel=1andsublinkid=5784andlid=368
19. https://pib.gov.in/newsite/PrintRelease.aspx?relid=174210
20. https://tbcindia.gov.in/WriteReadData/NTEPTrainingModules1to4.pdf
21. https://www.cdc.gov/anthrax/basics/index.html
22. https://www.cdc.gov/brucellosis/index.html
23. https://www.cdc.gov/chickenpox/about/index.html
24. https://www.cdc.gov/chikungunya/index.html
25. https://www.cdc.gov/dengue/index.html
26. https://www.cdc.gov/dpdx/amebiasis/
27. https://www.cdc.gov/dpdx/pediculosis/index.html
28. https://www.cdc.gov/foodsafety/food-poisoning.html
29. https://www.cdc.gov/japaneseencephalitis/index.html
30. https://www.cdc.gov/leptospirosis/index.html
31. https://www.cdc.gov/mumps/index.html
32. https://www.cdc.gov/parasites/ascariasis/index.html
33. https://www.cdc.gov/parasites/hookworm/gen_info/faqs.html
34. https://www.cdc.gov/parasites/leishmaniasis/gen_info/faqs.html
35. https://www.cdc.gov/parasites/lymphaticfilariasis/
36. https://www.cdc.gov/parasites/scabies/epi.html
37. https://www.cdc.gov/rubella/index.html
38. https://www.nhp.gov.in/disease/communicable-disease/plague
39. https://www.nhp.gov.in/national-viral-hepatitis-control-program-(nvhcp)_pg
40. https://www.who.int/health-topics/smallpox#tab=tab_1
41. https://www.who.int/news-room/fact-sheets/detail/cholera
42. https://www.who.int/news-room/fact-sheets/detail/measles
43. https://www.who.int/news-room/fact-sheets/detail/poliomyelitis
44. https://www.who.int/news-room/fact-sheets/detail/trachoma
45. https://www.who.int/news-room/fact-sheets/detail/typhoid
46. https://www.who.int/news-room/questions-and-answers/item/diphtheria
47. K Park. Park's Textbook of Preventive and Social Medicine, 24th ed. Jabalpur: Bhanot Publishers; 2017.

9.6 UNIVERSAL IMMUNIZATION PROGRAM (UIP)

- Expanded Program on Immunization was launched in 1978. It was renamed as Universal Immunization Program in 1985 when its reach was expanded beyond urban areas.
- In 1992, it was included in Child Survival and Safe Motherhood Program and in 1997, it became part of Reproductive and Child Health Program.
- UIP is one of the largest immunization programs in the world on the basis of quantities of vaccine used, number of beneficiaries (2.76 crore newborns and almost 3 crore pregnant women), number of immunization sessions organized, geographical spread and diversity of areas covered.
- It is one of the most cost-effective public health interventions and largely responsible for reduction of vaccine preventable disease.
- Under UIP 12 vaccines are being provided free of cost. These are—BCG, bOPV, Hepatitis B, Pentavalent, Rotavirus, PCV, fIPV, Measles/MR, JE, DPT, and Td.

Communicable Diseases and Relevant National Health Programs

Table 9.1: Milestones.

Year	Milestone
1978	Expanded program of immunization BCG, DPT, OPV, typhoid (urban areas)
1983	TT vaccine for pregnant women
1985	Universal immunization program—measles added, typhoid removed, focus on children less than 1 year of age
1990	Vitamin-A supplementation
1995	Polio national immunization days
1997	VVM introduced on vaccines in UIP
2002	Hep B introduced as pilot in 33 districts and cities of 10 states
2005	• National rural health mission launched • Auto Disable (AD) syringes introduced into UIP
2006	JE vaccine introduced after campaigns in endemic districts
2007–8	Hep B expanded to all districts in 10 states and schedule revised to 4 doses from 3 doses
2010	Measles 2nd dose introduced in RI and MCUP (14 states)
2011	• Hepatitis B universalized and *Haemophilus influenzae* type b introduced as pentavalent in 2 states • Open vial policy for vaccines in UIP
2013	• Pentavalent expanded to 9 states • Second dose of JE vaccine
2014	India and south east asia region certified POLIO-FREE
2015	• India validated for maternal and neonatal tetanus elimination • Pentavalent expanded to all states • IPV introduced
2016	• Rotavirus vaccine introduced in 4 states in phase 1 • tOPV to bOPV switch • Switch to fractional IPV (phased) • Rotavirus vaccine introduced (phased launch)
2017	• MR vaccine introduced • PCV (phased launch) • Use of adrenaline IM by ANM in AEFI
2019	• Tetanus and adult Diphtheria (Td) introduced • RVV expanded to all states
2021	PCV expanded to all states
2022	IMI 4.0 was conducted
2023	Third dose of fIPV introduced

The objectives of UIP:
- Rapidly increase immunization coverage
- Improve the quality of services
- Establish a reliable cold chain system up to the health facility level
- Introduce a district-wise system for monitoring of performance
- Achieve self-sufficiency in vaccine production

Table 9.2: National immunization schedule.

Vaccine	Type	Schedule	Dose	Route	Site	Strain and VVM	Remarks
TT-1 or Td 1	Toxoid	As early as possible in pregnancy	0.5 mL	Intra-muscular	Upper arm	VVM 30	• Currently TT is replaced by Td • **Td**- Tetanus and adult diphtheria • **Td Booster** if pregnancy occurs within 3 years of last pregnancy and two Td dose were received.
TT-2 or Td 2	Toxoid	4 weeks after TT-1/Td-1	0.5 mL	Intra-muscular	Upper arm		
For infant							
BCG	Live	At birth	0.1 mL (0.05 until 1 month age- because neonatal skin is too thin)	Intra-dermal	Left upper arm	• DANISH 1331 Strain • **VVM 2** (VVM 2 means vaccine remain stable for 2 days at 37°C)	• **Diluent:** 1 mL sodium chloride • **Discard** 4 hour after reconstitution • Reconstituted vaccine is light sensitive and it should be protected from sunlight – hence vial is amber color • **Maximum age limit:** Till one year of age • If scar does not appear after vaccination, there is no need for revaccination.

Communicable Diseases and Relevant National Health Programs

Vaccine	Type	Schedule	Dose	Route	Site	Strain and VVM	Remarks	Images
Hepatitis B-0 (Birth dose)	Recombinant	At birth (within 24 hours)	0.5 mL	Intramuscular	Anterolateral aspect of mid-thigh-left	VVM 30	• It is freeze sensitive vaccine and never to be frozen • Give within 24 hours of birth	
OPV-0 (zero dose)	Live	At birth	2 drops	Oral	Oral	• Bivalent strain (Type 1 and 3) • VVM 2	**Maximum age limit:** Within 15 days of birth	
OPV-1,2,3	Live	At 6 weeks, 10 weeks, 14 weeks	2 drops	Oral	Oral	• Bivalent strain (Type 1 and 3) • VVM 2	**Maximum age limit:** Till five years of age	
PENTA 1,2,3	DPT: Diphtheria and Tetanus are toxoid, Pertussis killed, Hepatitis B recombinant	At 6 weeks, 10 weeks, 14 weeks	0.5 mL	Intramuscular	Anterolateral side of mid-thigh Left	VVM 30	• It contains DPT, Hepatitis B, H. Influenza type B • **Maximum age limit:** till one year of age	

Communicable Diseases and Relevant National Health Programs

Vaccine	Type	Schedule	Dose	Route	Site	Strain and VVM	Remarks	Images
fIPV (Fractional inactivated polio vaccine)	Killed	At 6 weeks, 14 weeks and 9 months	0.1 mL	Intra-dermal	Anterolateral side of mid thigh-right	Strains of IPV are Mahoney (type 1 poliovirus), MEF-1 (type 2 poliovirus), and Saukett (type 3 poliovirus)	**Maximum age limit:** Till one year of age	
Rota-virus-1,2,3 (Rotasiil)	Live attenuated freeze dried vaccine	At 6 weeks, 10 weeks, 14 weeks	2.5 mL	Orals	Oral	• **Rotasiil** (RV5) vaccine containing five viruses (Human and Bovine reassortant strains) of serotype G1, G2, G3, G4 and G9. • **VVM 30**	• **Procedure:** 2.5 mL Orally, administer slowly with the nozzle of the 6 mL oral syringe pointed toward the inner cheek (buccal cavity) of the infant. • **Diluent:** (citrate bicarbonate) • It can be used up to maximum of 4 hours after reconstitution • **Maximum age limit:** Till one year of age	

Communicable Diseases and Relevant National Health Programs

Vaccine	Type	Schedule	Dose	Route	Site	Strain and VVM	Remarks	Images
Rotavirus-1,2,3 Rotavac	Live (liquid formulation)	At 6 weeks, 10 weeks, 14 weeks	5 drops	Orals	Oral	• **Rotavac** (ORV116E), a live vaccine containing suspension of Rotavirus 116E • **VVM 2**	• Rotavirus vaccine vial can be used up to a maximum of 4 hours after opening. • **Maximum age limit:** Till one year of age	
PCV-1, PCV-2, PCV B (Pneumococcal conjugate vaccine)	Conjugate vaccine	**Two primary doses:** At 6 weeks, 14 weeks **Booster dose:** 9 months	0.5 mL	Intramuscular	Anterolateral side of mid thigh-right	• PCV13 • **VVM 30**	• **Maximum age limit:** Till one year of age	
Measles	Live	9 month completed	0.5 mL	Subcutaneous	Right upper arm	Edmonston-Zagreb strain (Most common), Schwartz strain, Moraten strain	• **Diluent:** 2.5 mL double distilled water • Reconstitution vaccine should be used within 4 hours • Reconstituted vaccine looses potency on exposure to light and is very heat labile and needs to be protected, from light. Hence the vaccine vial is available in amber color	

Communicable Diseases and Relevant National Health Programs

Vaccine	Type	Schedule	Dose	Route	Site	Strain and VVM	Remarks	Images
MR-1 (Measles, Rubella)	Live	First dose at-9 month completed	0.5 mL	Sub-cutaneous	Right upper arm	Rubella: RA 27/3 Measles strain as above	• Diluent should be kept at 2–8°C at least 24 h before use, • **Maximum age limit:** Till five years of age • Currently MR vaccine has replaced the current two doses of measles vaccine in the national immunization schedule • Diluent: Sterile water • **Maximum age limit:** Till five years of age *All other remarks same as Measles	
JE* 1st dose (Japanese Encephalitis)	Live	9–12 months	0.5 mL	Sub-cutaneous	Left supper arm	• SA 14-14-2 strain • VVM 14	• **Diluent:** Phosphate buffer solution • **Maximum age limit:** Till fifteen years of age • **JenVac** vaccine to be launched which is to be given IM and will be under open vial policy	

Communicable Diseases and Relevant National Health Programs

Vaccine	Type	Schedule	Dose	Route	Site	Strain and VVM	Remarks	Images
Vitamin A	First dose at 9 months with measles		1 mL (1 lakh IU)	Oral	Oral		• Second dose at 16th months (with 2nd dose of measles). Then after every 6 months 2 lakh IU/2 mL up to 5 years of age • Administer 2,00,000 IU of vitamin A to child >1 year of age immediately after diagnosis To be followed by 2,00,000 IU of vitamin A 1-4 weeks later • Vitamin A syrup should be discarded after 8 weeks of opening	
For Children								
DPT Booster-1	Formalin-inactivated diphtheria toxin (killed), with whole cell Pertussis and tetanus toxoid	16–24 months	0.5 mL	Intra-muscular	Anterolateral side of mid thigh-left		• Freeze sensitive and need to be protected from freezing • **Maximum age limit:** Till seven years of age	

Communicable Diseases and Relevant National Health Programs

Vaccine	Type	Schedule	Dose	Route	Site	Strain and VVM	Remarks
OPV Booster	Live	16–24 months	2 drops	Oral	Oral		**Maximum age limit:** Till five years of age
MEASLES 2nd dose Or MR-2	Live	16–24 months	0.5 mL	Sub-cutaneous	Right upper arm		**Maximum age limit:** Till five years of age
JE 2nd dose	Live	16–24 months	0.5 mL	Sub-cutaneous	Left upper arm		**Maximum age limit:** Till fifteen years of age
5–6 years							
DPT Booster-2	As same as DPT Booster 1	5–6 years	0.5 mL	Intra-muscular	Left upper arm		**Maximum age limit:** Till seven years of age
For 10–16 years							
Td-1, Td-2	Toxoid	10 years, 16 years	0.5 mL	Intra-muscular	Upper arms	VVM 30	• Td: Tetanus and adult diphtheria • **Maximum age limit:** Till sixteen years of age • If schedule started with TT then also Td vaccine can be given in subsequent dose.

*JE wherever introduced

*Multiple injections can be given in the same thigh but the distance between the two injections should be at least 2.5 cm (1 inch)

*Pentavalent, IPV, PCV and Rotavirus vaccines, if at least one dose is given before one year of age, then remaining doses can be administered and schedule must be completed irrespective of the age of child. If the first dose is not administered before one year of age, then these vaccines cannot be administered to the child under UIP.

Note: If 1st dose of MR vaccine delayed beyond 12 months, then ensure minimum 1 month gap between two MR doses while JE vaccine delayed beyond 12 months then ensure minimum 3 months gap between two JE doses.

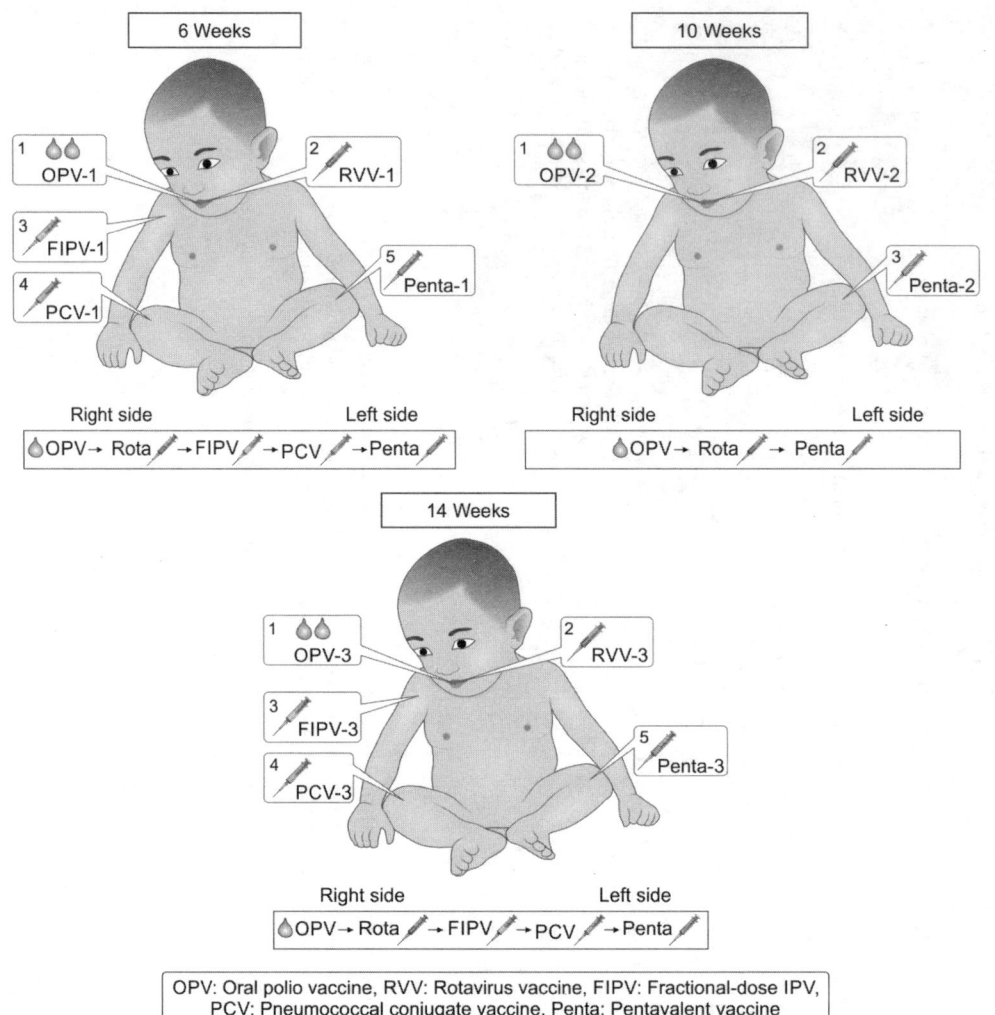

Fig. 9.1: Ideal sequence of administration of vaccines.

Some Important FAQs Regarding Due Vaccines as per Different Age Group

- What vaccines should be given to a 7-month old child who has not been vaccinated?
  Answer: BCG, OPV-1, RVV-1, Penta-1, fIPV-1, PCV-1
- What vaccines should be given to a 9-month old child who has received BCG, OPV-2, RVV-1, Penta-2, fIPV-1, PCV-1 only?
  Answer: Give OPV-3, RVV-2, fIPV-2, Penta-3, PCV-2, MR-1, JE-1
- What vaccines should be given to 16-month old child who has never been vaccinated?
  Answer: OPV-1, DPT-1, MR-1, JE-1
- What vaccines should be given to 18-month old child who has received BCG, OPV-2, RVV-2, fIPV-1 Penta-2, PCV-1 only?
  Answer: OPV-3, RVV-3, fIPV-2, Penta-3, PCV-2, MR-1, JE-1

Definition of Full and Complete Immunization

- **Full immunization:** Before age of 1 year: one dose of BCG, 3 doses of OPV, 3 doses of Rotavirus, 3 doses of Pentavalent, 3 doses of fractional IPV, 3 doses of PCV, MR vacccine 1st dose, JE 1st dose (where applicable)
- **Complete immunization:** Before the age of 2 years received 2nd dose of Measles/MR, DPT booster, Polio booster, 2nd dose of JE (where applicable)
- **Common vaccine reaction:**
  - *BCG:* Local reaction (swelling, pain, redness)
  - *DPT, Pentavalent:* Local reaction (swelling, pain, redness), fever
  - *HEPATITIS B:* Local reaction (swelling, pain, redness), fever
  - *OPV:* None
  - *IPV:* None
  - *TETANUS:* Local reaction (swelling, pain, redness), malaise and nonspecific symptoms

Rare Serious Adverse Events

Vaccine	Reaction
BCG	Suppurative lymphadenitis, BCG Osteitis, Disseminated BCG infection
Hepatitis B	Guillain-Barre Syndrome (plasma derived), Anaphylaxis
Measles	Febrile seizures, Anaphylaxis, Thrombocytopenia
OPV	Vaccine-associated paralytic polio, Vaccine derived polio virus
Tetanus	Brachial neuritis, Thrombocytopenia
DPT	Persistent (>3 hours) inconsolable screaming, Seizures Hypotonic hyporesponsive episode (HHE), Anaphylaxis/shock encephalopathy

Contraindication of Vaccine

- **Live vaccine:** Pregnancy, radiation therapy
- **BCG:** Symptomatic HIV infection
- **Pertussis:** Neurological disease, anaphylactic reaction to previous dose
- **All other vaccines:** Any current serious illness, anaphylactic reaction to previous dose

Responsibilities of ANM for Routine Immunization Session

ANM can take help from ASHA and AWW.
a. Map of area under SC with names of villages, urban areas including all hamlets (tola), sub-villages, sub-wards, sector, mohalla, hard to reach areas, etc.
b. Demarcation map—allocate areas for each ANM if more than 2 ANMs are present in a SC. It can also show the exact boundaries and areas for ASHAs and AWWs
c. Master list of the area—this list includes all villages/tolas/HRAs/wards/mohalls
d. An estimation of beneficiaries
e. An estimation of vaccines and logistics
f. ANM work plan including mobilization plan

Types of Routine Immunization Session
- **Fixed:** These sessions are held where vaccine storage is possible because of availability of ILR and deep freezer (DF), i.e., the sessions conducted at PHC/CHC.
- **Outreach:** All sessions conducted where vaccine has to be taken by vaccine carrier.
- **Mobile:** Sessions conducted using a vehicle which moves from site to site along with the immunization team and vaccine.
- **Tagged:** Site/area which does not have a session but is linked to the nearest session site.

Give these Four Key Messages to the Caregiver after Vaccination
1. What vaccine was given and what disease it prevents (e.g. BCG for preventing TB)
2. When to come for the next visit.
3. What are the minor side-effects and how to deal with them.
4. To keep the vaccination card safe and to bring it along for the next visit.

BIBLIOGRAPHY
1. https://nhm.gov.in/New_Updates_2018/NHM_Components/Immunization/Guildelines_for_immunization/Immunization_Handbook_for_Medical_Officers%202017.pdf

9.7 NATIONAL LEPROSY ERADICATION PROGRAM (NLEP)

In 1955, launched as National Leprosy Control Program and renamed as National Leprosy Eradication Program (NLEP) in 1983.
- National Leprosy Eradication Program (NLEP) is a Centrally Sponsored public health program under the umbrella of National Health Mission (NHM).
- In December 2005, India has achieved the elimination of leprosy as a public health problem, i.e., defined as less than 1 case per 10,000 populations, at the National level.
- The NLEP aims at eliminating leprosy in each of the districts by 2030.
- Leprosy related statistics:
  - ANCDR (annual case detection rate)—5.52 per 100,000 population
  - Prevalence rate (PR)—0.45 per 10,000 population
  - Child proportion—6.87%
  - Grade 2 Disability proportion—2.41%
  - Grade 2 Disability rate—1.96/million population

Vision: Leprosy-Free India

Mission: "To provide quality leprosy services free of cost to all sections of the population, with easy accessibility, through the integrated healthcare system, including care for disability after cure of the disease".

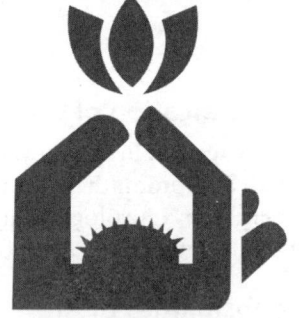

Symbolizes beauty and purity in lotus

1. Symbolizes beauty and purity in lotus
2. Leprosy can be cured and a leprosy patient can be a useful member of the society in the form of a partially affected thumb; a normal fore-finger and the shape of house
3. The symbol of hope and optimism in a rising sun

Objectives

1. To reduce the prevalence rate to less than 1/10,000 population at sub-national and district level.
2. To reduce Grade II disability % to <1 among new cases at national level.
nNational level.
4. Zero disabilities among new child cases.
5. Zero stigma and discrimination against persons affected by leprosy.

NLEP Strategies

1. Decentralized integrated leprosy services through general healthcare system.
2. Early detection and complete treatment of all new leprosy cases.
3. Carrying out household contact survey for early detection of cases.
4. Capacity building of all general health services functionaries.
5. Involvement of ASHAs in the detection and completion of treatment of leprosy cases on time.
6. Strengthening of Disability Prevention and Medical Rehabilitation (DPMR) services.
7. IEC activities in the community to improve self-reporting to PHC and reduction of stigma.
8. Intensive monitoring and supervision at Health and Wellness centers and at PHC/CHC.

Domains of NLEP

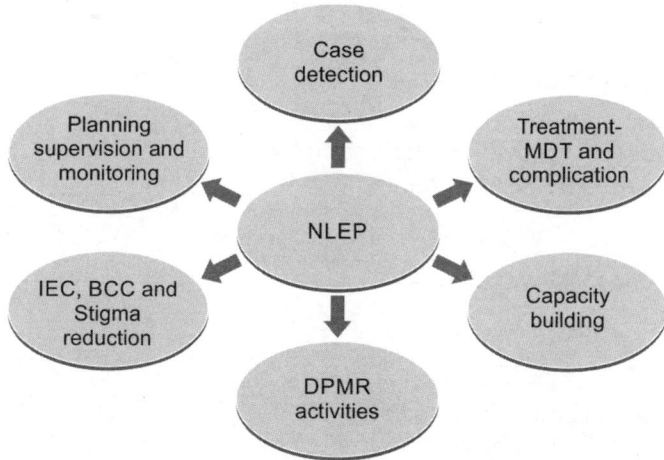

Classification of Leprosy

Characteristics	Paucibacillary (PB)	Multibacillary (MB)
Skin lesions	1–5 lesions	6 and above
Peripheral nerve involvement	No nerve/only one nerve involvement	>1 nerve irrespective of no. of skin lesion
Skin smear	Negative at all sites	Positive at any site

Treatment of Leprosy

Type of leprosy	Drugs used	Frequency of administration adults	Dosage (adult) 15 years and above	Dosage (children 10–14 years)#	Dosage children below 10 years*	Criteria for RFT
MB leprosy	Rifampicin	Once monthly	600 mg	450 mg	300 mg	Completion of 12 monthly pulses in 18 consecutive months **(12 BCP/18 months)**
	Clofazimine	Monthly	300 mg	150 mg	100 mg	
	Dapsone	Daily once	100 mg	50 mg	25 mg	
	Clofazimine	Daily for adults (every other day for children)	50 mg	50 mg (alternate days)	50 mg (weekly twice)	
PB leprosy	Rifampicin	Once monthly	600 mg	450 mg	300 mg	Completion of 6 monthly pulses in 9 consecutive months **(6 BCP/9 months)**
	Dapsone	Daily	100 mg	50 mg	25 mg daily or 50 mg alternate days	

#For children 10–14 years with body weight > 35 kg, adult BCP should be given
*For children <10 years doses (as per body weight) should be provided loose after opening appropriate BCP (Blister calender pack)

Role of Multipurpose Health Worker

- Suspect identification
- Availability of MDT and providing MDT, compliance
- Record Maintenance and Report Preparation
- IEC activities
- DPMR activities
- Supervision of ASHA/AWW/Volunteer
- Assist MO

Role of ASHA

- Suspect identification and referral to PHC
- Timely completion of treatment
- Counseling and IEC
- Contact screening, support for active case detection campaigns

ASHA's incentive as below:
i. At confirmation of diagnosis ₹ 250/-
   - Finding a case before the occurrence of any visible deformity ₹ 250/-
   - A new case with visible deformity in hand, feet or eye ₹ 200/-
ii. On completion of full course of treatment in time:
   - Paucibacillary (PB)—additional ₹ 400/-
   - Multibacillary (MB)—additional ₹ 600/-

Major Initiatives under NLEP are as Follows:
- Leprosy Case Detection Campaigns (LCDC) for 14 days in high endemic districts.
- ASHA Based Surveillance for Leprosy Suspects (ABSULS).
- LCDC and ABSULS have now been clubbed together as "Active Case Detection and Regular Surveillance" (ACDRS) both in rural and urban areas in order to ensure detection of leprosy cases on regular basis and at an early stage in order to prevent Grade II disabilities.
- Focused Leprosy Campaign (FLC) in low endemic districts for case detection.
- Special plans for Hard-to-Reach areas for early case detection and treatment on time.
- Sparsh Leprosy Awareness Campaigns on 30th January.
- Convergence of leprosy screening under Rashtriya Bal Swasthya Karyakram (RBSK) for screening of children (0–18 years) and under Ayushman Bharat for screening of people above 30 years of age.
- NIKUSTH—A real time leprosy reporting software implemented across India.
- For encouraging the district heath functionaries, provision of certification and award to the districts for achieving leprosy elimination. Under two categories: (1) Gold category and (2) Silver category.
- Contact tracing is done and Post-exposure Prophylaxis (PEP) with Single dose of Rifampicin (SDR) is administered to the eligible contacts of index case in order to interrupt the chain of transmission.
- Immunoprophylaxis—Mycobacterium indicus pranii (MIP) vaccine.
- Various services are provided under the program for Disability Prevention and Medical Rehabilitation (DPMR), i.e., reaction management, provision of Microcellular Rubber (MCR) footwear, Aids and Appliances, self-care kits, etc.
- Reconstructive Surgeries are conducted at District Hospitals/Medical Colleges/Central Leprosy Institutes, and welfare allowance @ ₹ 8,000 is paid to each patients undergoing RCS.

BIBLIOGRAPHY
1. https://cltri.gov.in/AboutLeprosy/NLEP_Program%20Management_DLO.pdf

9.8 THE NATIONAL TUBERCULOSIS ELIMINATION PROGRAM (NTEP)

CHRONOLOGY OF NTEP

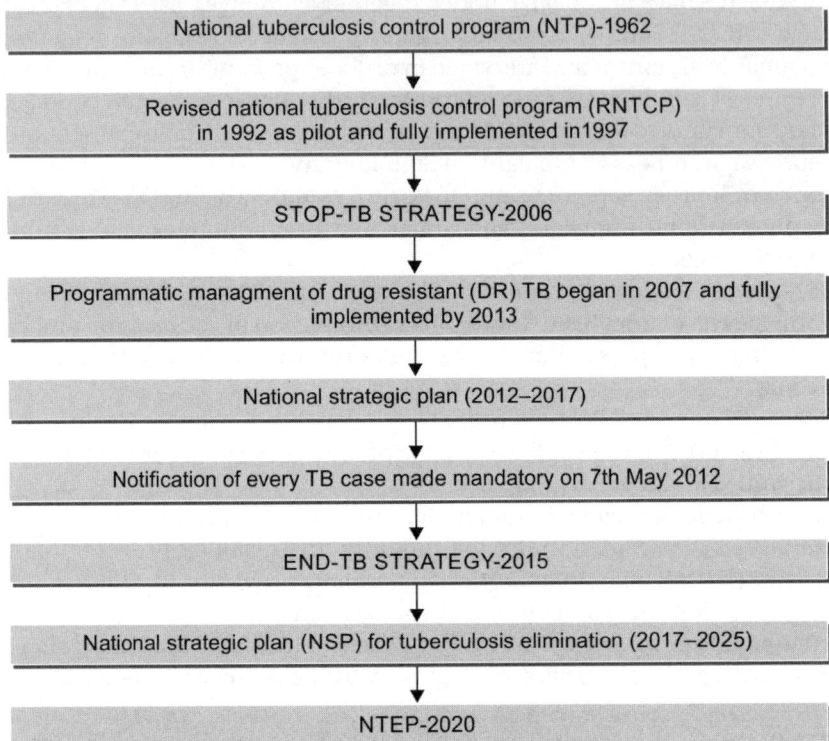

- Tuberculosis (TB) represents one of the world's public health greatest challenges. Along with disease burden, TB also leads to socioeconomic burden.
- Current statistics of TB in INDIA as per GLOBAL TB report 2022:

Indicator	(Rate per 1,00,000 population)
Total TB incidence	210
HIV-positive TB incidence	3.9
HIV-negative TB mortality	35
HIV-positive TB mortality	0.81
Microbiologically confirmed TB prevalence (2019–21) among more than 15 years of age	316

Treatment Success Rate and Cohort Size

Type of TB	Success
New and relapse cases registered in 2020	85%
Previously treated cases, excluding relapse, registered in 2020	80%
HIV-positive TB cases registered in 2019	71%
MDR/RR-TB cases started on second-line treatment in 2019	57%
XDR-TB cases started on second-line treatment in 2018	48%

- TB kills an estimated 5,25,600 Indians every year and more than 1,440 every day.
- Sustainable Development Goals envisage achieving a 90% reduction in TB deaths and an 80% decrease in TB incidence by 2030 compared to 2015. The National Tuberculosis Elimination Program (NTEP) also aims to eliminate TB by 2025.
- **National TB Elimination Program** is a Centrally Sponsored Scheme being implemented under the aegis of National Health Mission with resource sharing between the State Governments and the Central Government.

NTEP ORGANOGRAM

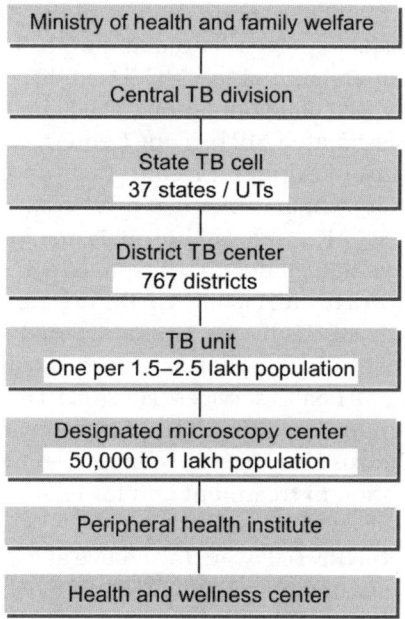

NTEP STRUCTURE COMPRISES OF FIVE LEVELS

1. **National:** Central TB Division (CTD) manages the National TB Control Program for the entire country at the central level under AS and DG (RNTCP and NACO) through a National Program manager, Deputy Director General TB (DDG TB).
2. **State:** State Health Society or its equivalent under National Health Mission of the state manages the TB Control Program. A full-time State Tuberculosis Officer (STO) is responsible for planning, training, supervising and monitoring the program in all the districts of their respective states. State TB cell is being supported by State TB Training and Demonstration Center (STDC) in many states through its three units—a training unit, supervision and monitoring unit and an Intermediate Reference Laboratory (IRL). Operational Research is also a component of STDC. Each state also has one fully operational State Drug Store (SDS) for each 5 crore of population.
3. **District:** The Chief District Health Officer (CDHO)/Chief District Medical Officer (CDMO)/Civil Surgeon in the district is responsible for all activities for control of TB. The District Tuberculosis Center (DTC) is the nodal point for TB control activities in the district. A full-time District Tuberculosis Officer (DTO) is responsible for planning, training, supervising and monitoring the program in the district.

4. **Subdistrict (Tuberculosis unit level):** The TU is the nodal point for TB control activities in the subdistrict. TUs have been created based on a population of 1 per 2,00,000 (range 1.5-2.5 lakh) for rural and urban population and 1 per 1,00,000 (0.75-1.25 lakh) population in hilly/tribal/difficult areas. The Tuberculosis unit (TU) consists of a designated Medical Officer-Tuberculosis Control (MO-TC), as well as one full-time supervisory staff - Senior Treatment Supervisor (STS). However, One Senior TB Laboratory Supervisor (STLS) will continue to be in 5 lakh population (one per 2.5 lakh population for tribal/hilly/difficult areas). The Block Medical Officer also functions as a Medical Officer TB Control (MO-TC). For the urban TB units, a medical officer from the health facility where TU is located should be designated, in coordination with CM and HO/DHO to function as a MO-TC. MO-TC has the overall responsibility of management of TB Control Program at the TU and is expected to undertake supervisory visits for seven days in a month. The team of STS and STLS are under the administrative supervision of the MO-TC and the DTO. The TU will have one Microscopy Center for every 1,00,000 population (50,000 in tribal, desert, remote and hilly regions) referred to as the Designated Microscopy Center.
5. **Peripheral health institution:** Peripheral Health Institutions (PHIs) for the purpose of NTEP, a PHI is a health facility which is manned by at least a medical officer. At this level, there are dispensaries, PHCs, CHCs, referral hospitals, major hospitals, specialty clinics or hospitals (including other health facilities), TB hospitals, ART Centers and Medical colleges within the respective district. All health facilities in the private and NGO sectors participating in NTEP are also considered as PHIs by the program. Some of these PHIs also function as DMCs. Peripheral health institutions undertake tuberculosis case-finding and treatment activities as a part of the general health services. There is 1 TB Health Visitor (TBHV) per one lakh urban population to support the urban TB control activities.

For the treatment of tuberculosis Health and Wellness Centers will serve as the last level of healthcare facility for continuation of treatment and for receiving ancillary drugs to support TB treatment.

Previously the objectives of the RNTCP were to achieve at least 85 percent cure rate among the new smear positive cases initiated on treatment, and thereafter a case detection rate of at least 70 percent of such cases.

The objectives of the national strategic plan are:
- To achieve 90% notification rate for all cases
- To achieve 90% success rate for all new and 85% for retreatment cases
- To significantly improve the successful outcomes of treatment of DR-TB cases
- To achieve decreased morbidity and mortality of HIV associated TB
- To improve outcomes of TB care in the private sector

National TB Elimination Program (NTEP) Government of India has committed to end TB by 2025, five years ahead of the global target under Sustainable Development Goals.

NATIONAL STRATEGIC PLAN FOR TB (2017–2025)

Vision: TB-Free India with zero deaths, disease and poverty due to TB

Goal: To achieve a rapid decline in burden of TB, morbidity and mortality to achieve the Sustainable Development Goals of 80% reduction in incidence and 90% reduction in deaths by 2025; five years earlier of the global targets.
- The NSP objectives are translated into four pillars: BUILD-PREVENT-DETECT-TREAT (BDPT) that is required to achieve the goals of the NSP.

Communicable Diseases and Relevant National Health Programs

- TB elimination requires the country to BUILD strong foundations for PREVENT-DETECT-TREAT components of the program.
- These cut across all areas of NTEP activities and is critical in building an enabling environment that enhances the performance of the program, ensuring quality, equity, efficiency, accountability, resilience, and sustainability in the delivery of TB care services.
- The schematic diagram below represents the foundational pillar of BUILD with its cross cutting components at the bottom on which rest the core TB care activities represented by the pillars of PREVENT, DETECT and TREAT.

PILLARS AND STRATEGIES OF THE NSP (2017-25)

While the pillars remain the same, it must be noted that the pillars in NSP 2017–25 has been reconfigured in **BUILD–PREVENT–DETECT-TREAT** sequence.

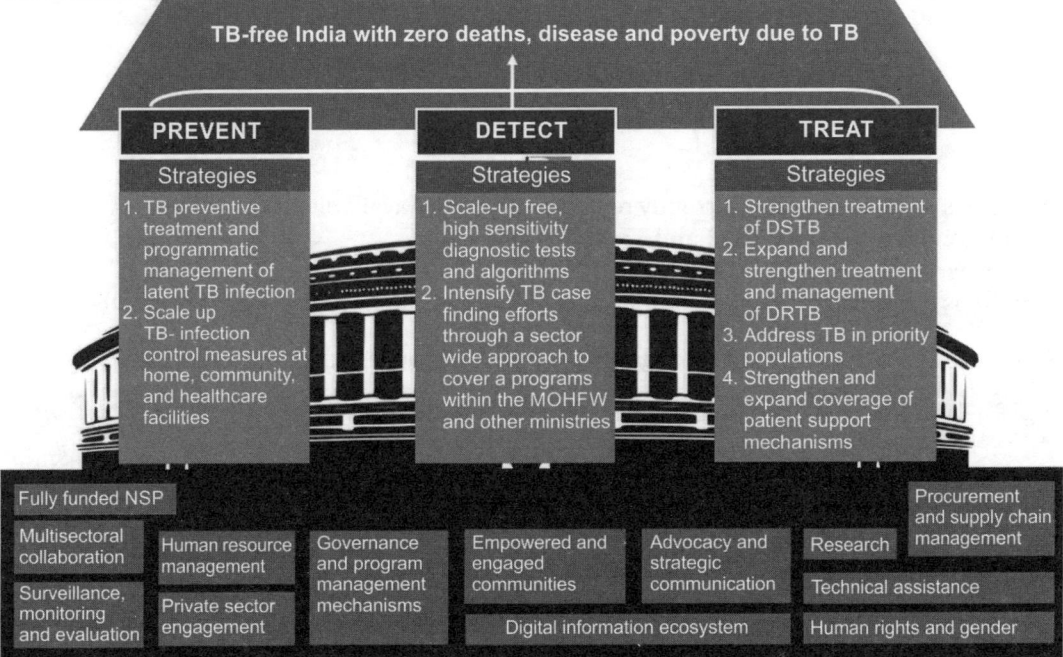

PREVENT

Tuberculosis Preventive Treatment (TPT)

Overview of TB Infection

- India has the highest estimated burden of tuberculosis infection (TBI) globally, with nearly 35–40 crore Indian population having TBI, of which 26 lakh (18–36 lakh) are estimated to develop tuberculosis (TB) disease annually.
- 5–10% of those infected will develop TB disease over the course of their lives, usually within the first 2 years after initial infection.
- Risk of developing TB disease after TPT decreases by approximately 60% and the reduction can be up to 90% among people living with HIV (PLHIV).

Cascade of TB Case Finding and TPT

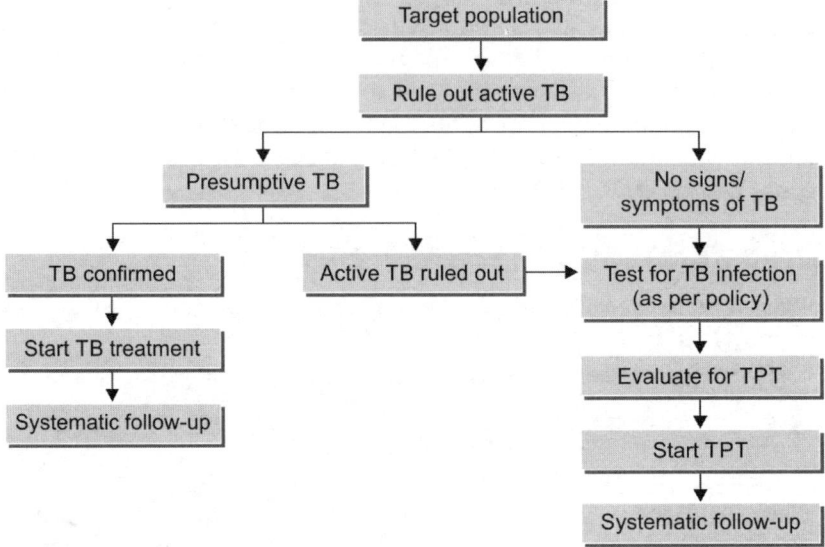

Diagnosis of TB infection: Currently recommended and available tests for TBI
1. Tuberculin Skin Test (TST) and
2. Interferon-Gamma Release Assay (IGRA)

IGRA is more specific test as compared to TST even in BCG vaccinated individuals.

TPT: Target Population, Strategy and Regimen (for Drug Sensitive TBI)

Target Population	Strategy	TPT Regimen

• People living with HIV (+ ART)
  ▪ Adults and children >12 months
  ▪ Infants <12 months with HIV in contact with active TB
• HHC below 5 years of pulmonary* TB patients
	TPT to all after ruling out active TB disease	• 6-month daily isoniazid (6H)
		• 3-month weekly isoniazid and Rifapentine (3HP) in persons older than 2 years

HHC 5 years and above of pulmonary* TB patients#	TPT among TBI positive# after ruling out TB disease	• 3-month weekly isoniazid and Rifapentine (3HP) • 6-month daily isoniazid (6H)
Individuals who are: • On immunosuppressive therapy • Having silicosis • On anti-TNF treatment • On dialysis • Preparing for organ or Hematologic transplantation	TPT after ruling out TB disease among TBI positive	• 3-month weekly isoniazid and Rifapentine (3HP) • 6-month daily isoniazid (6H)

*Bacteriologically confirmed pulmonary TB patients will be prioritized for enumeration of the target population for TPT
#Chest X-ray (CXR) and TBI testing would be offered wherever available, but TPT must not be deferred in their absence

TPT Regimen and Dosages for Contacts of DR-TB Index Patients

1. Six months of daily levofloxacin (6Lfx) for contacts of R resistant FQ sensitive patients
2. Four months of rifampicin daily (4R) for contacts of H resistant R sensitive patients

Communicable Diseases and Relevant National Health Programs

3. 6H can be considered as the TPT regimen option for contacts of index patients with RR-TB with FQ and H sensitive, after ruling out active TB in them.

Note: Regimen decision based on resistance and drug dosage to be adjusted based on age and weight.

DETECT

Drug-sensitive TB (DS TB)
- Patients with pulmonary TB are diagnosed using sputum smear microscopy/Chest X-ray and NAAT (Nucleic Acid Amplification Tests).
- Smear replacement by NAAT and offer of upfront NAAT for diagnosis of TB has been prioritized by the program.
- Response to DS TB treatment is monitored using sputum smear microscopy.

Drug-resistant TB (DR TB)
- Microbiologically confirmed TB patients are offered NAAT for determining resistance to Rifampicin.
- Line Probe Assay (LPA–First Line) is offered to patients with Rifampicin Sensitive (RS) TB.
- First and Second Line LPA is offered to Rifampicin-resistant (RR) and Isoniazid (H) resistant TB patients. Liquid Culture (LC) and DST is performed for determining amplification of resistance to drugs used for managing DR TB.
- LC is used for monitoring response to DR TB treatment.

New Diagnostic Algorithm for Pulmonary TB

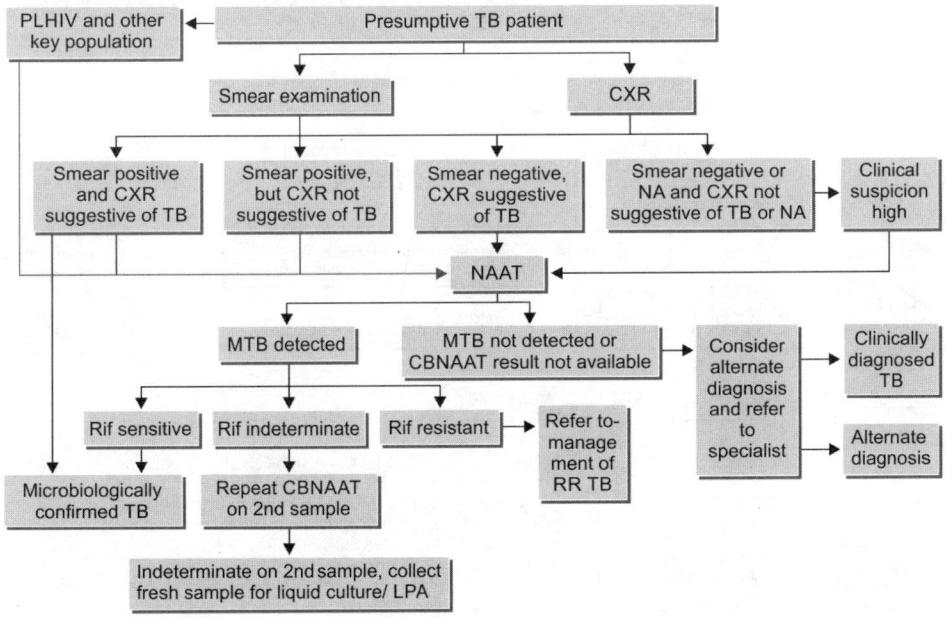

New Diagnostic Algorithm for Extrapulmonary TB

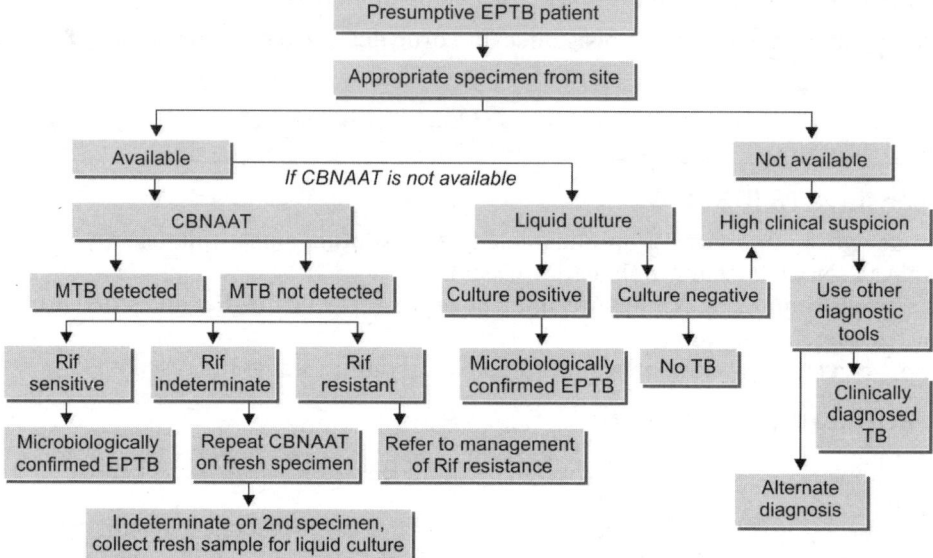

Algorithm for Pediatric Intrathoracic TB among Children with No Risk Factor for Drug Resistance

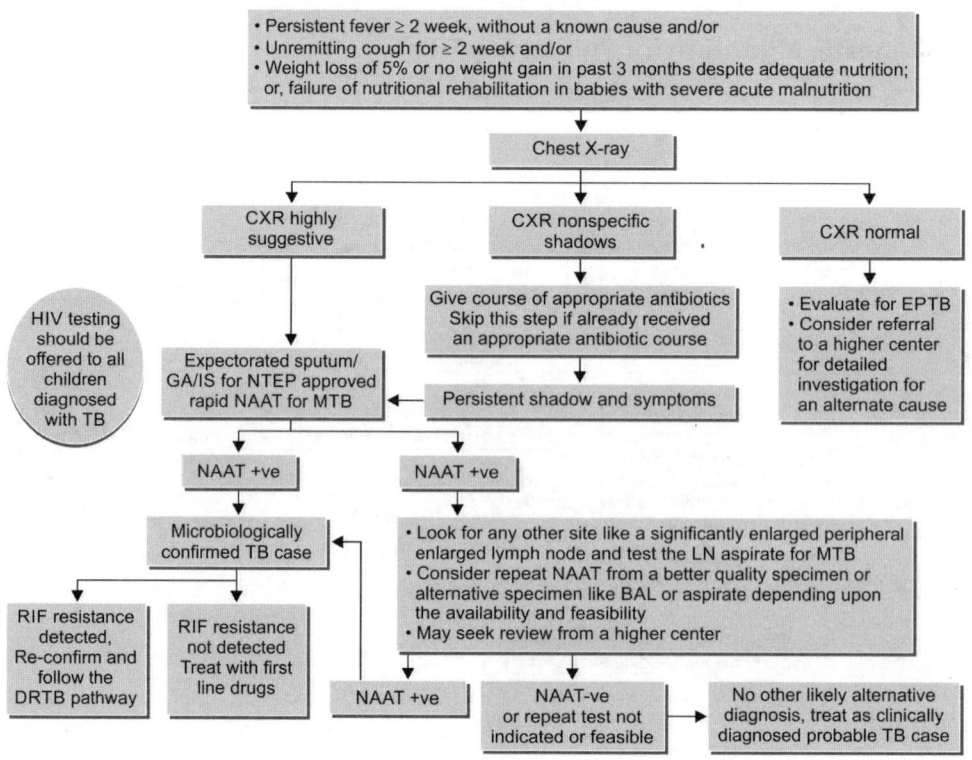

Diagnostic Algorithm for DR Tuberculosis

Integrated DR-TB diagnosis and treatment algorithm

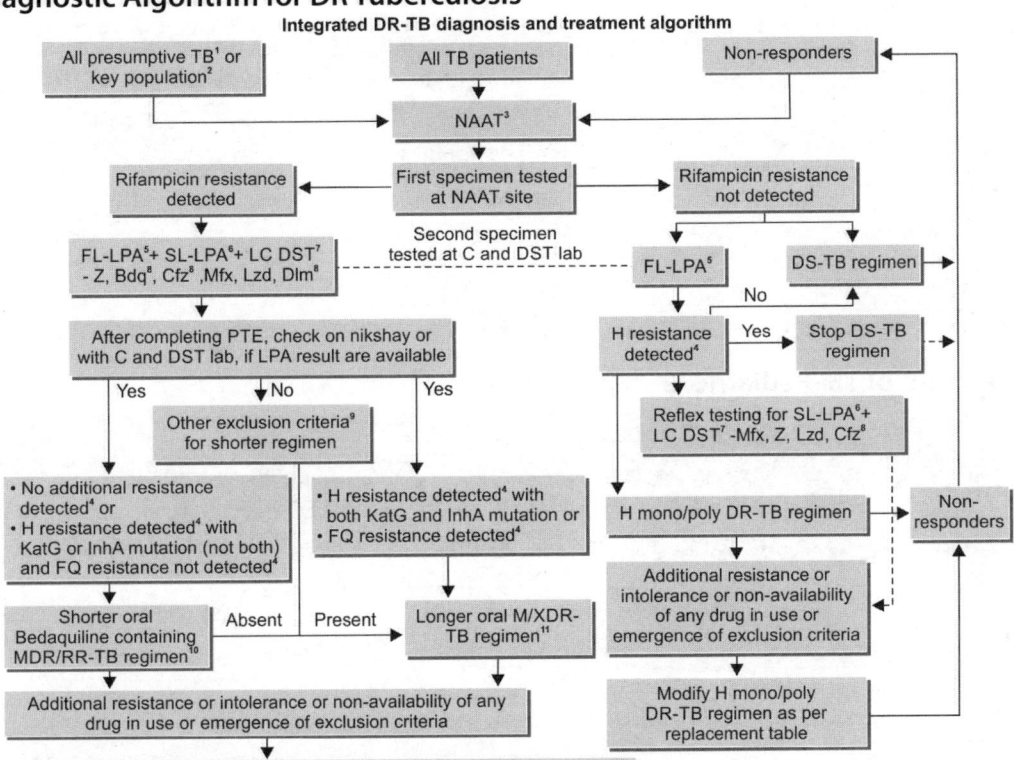

Approaches for Detection

- **Passive case finding:** When the Patient Voluntarily reports symptoms to the Medical Officer.
- **Intensified case findings:** When the Medical Officer searches for TB symptoms among the individual seeking care in the health facility, e.g., ART Center, Diabetic Clinics, NCD Clinics.
- **Active case finding:** When the community health workers seeks for TB symptoms among the vulnerable key population. The program encourages Active Case finding as an intervention for Ending TB.

TREAT

Regimen for Drug-sensitive TB (DSTB) cases:

Drug-sensitive TB	Intensive phase (IP)	Continuation phase (CP)
New or Previously Treated Cases (H and R sensitive/unknown)	2HRZE 56 Doses (8 Weeks)	4HRE 112 Doses (16 Weeks)

The CP may be extended by 12–24 weeks in certain forms of TB like CNS TB, Skeletal TB, Disseminated TB, etc. based on clinical decision of the treating physician on case to case basis. Extension beyond 12 weeks should only be on recommendation of specialists.

Treatment of TB for Adults

Weight category	Number of tablets (FDCs)	
	Intensive phase	Continuation phase
	HRZE	HRE
	75/150/400/275	75/150/275
25–34 kg	2	2
35–49 kg	3	3
50–64 kg	4	4
65–75 kg	5	5
≥75	6	6

Treatment of TB–Pediatric (0–18 years)

Weight category	Number of tablets (dispersible FDCs)			
	Intensive phase		Continuation phase	
	HRZ	E	HR	E
	50/75/150	100	50/75	100
4–7 kg	1	1	1	1
8–11 kg	2	2	2	2
12–15 kg	3	3	3	3
16–24 kg	4	4	4	4
25–29 kg	3 + 1A*	3	3 + 1A*	3
30–39 kg	2 + 2A*	2	2 + 2A*	2

A = Adult FDC (HRZE = 75/150/400/275; HRE = 75/150/275). It is added in higher weight band categories, i.e., >25 kg as these children may be able to swallow tablets.

Name	Resistance to drugs
Mono-resistant TB	One first-line anti-TB drug
Isoniazid-resistant TB	Isoniazid
Poly-drug resistant TB	More than one first-line anti-TB drug, other than both H and R
Rifampicin resistant TB	Resistant to R, with or without resistance to other anti-TB drugs. It includes any resistance to R, in the form of Mono-resistance, Poly-resistance, MDR or XDR
Multidrug-resistant TB	Both H and R with or without resistance to other first-line anti-TB drugs
Pre-extensively drug resistant TB	MDR/RR-TB fluoroquinolone
Extensively drug resistant TB	MDR/RR-TB fluoroquinolone (levofloxacin or moxifloxacin) One additional Group A drug (presently to either bedaquiline or linezolid [or both])

Regimes for DR TB

	H-mono regimen	Shorter oral regimen	Oral longer regimen
Duration	6 to 9 months	9 to 11 months	18 to 20 months
IP	–	4 to 6 months	–
CP	–	5 months	–
IP	Lfx, R, E, Z	BDq (6 M), Lfx, Cfz, Z, E, Hh, Eto	BDq (6 months or longer), Lfx, Lzd, Cfz, Cs
CP		Lfx, Cfz, Z, E	
Pre-treatment evaluation	Same as DSTB	Same as DSTB and ECG, TSH, LFT, Serum electrolytes (Na, K, Mg, Ca), UPT	

[Lfx (Levofloxacin), R (Rifampicin), E (Ethambutol), Z (Pyrazinamide), Bdq (Bedaquiline), Lzd (Linezolid), Cfz (Clofazimine), Cs (Cycloserine), Eto (Ethionamide), Hh (High dose isoniazid)]

Note: BPaL (Bedaquiline-Pretomanid-Linezolid) being tried for XDR TB as a shorter regimen for 6–9 months.

Direct Benefit Schemes

- **NIKSHAY Poshan Yojana** – Nutrition support can improve the overall nutritional status of people with TB which results in better adherence and treatment outcomes while at the same time it will increase notification rate and reduction in out of pocket expenses. All notified TB patients enrolled on or after 1st April 2018, are beneficiaries of the scheme. Under this scheme, ₹500/- per month is given to the person with TB till the completion of the treatment. This payment is given in installments. The payments will be made through DBT.

Here example is given for drug sensitive TB patient:

1st incentive	On notification	₹1,000/-
2nd incentive	At the end of IP	₹1,000/-
3rd incentive	At the end of treatment	₹1,000/-

- Private provider incentives – ₹500 for notification and ₹500 for reporting of treatment outcome have been initiated for private practitioners
- Informant incentives – To encourage referral from private sector and community volunteers, ₹500 are being provided for each referral of patient who is diagnosed as TB in public sector
- Incentive to treatment supporter is ₹1,000/- on completion of drug sensitive TB.
- Incentive to treatment supporter is ₹5,000/- on completion of drug resistant TB.
- Patient form tribal area is eligible to get ₹750/- as travel support.

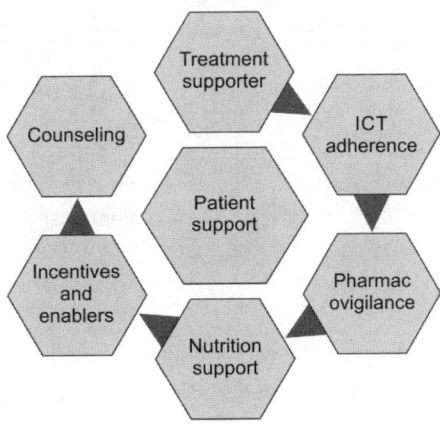

Treatment adherence interventions are grouped in categories that can be remembered as **SIMPLE:**
- **S**implifying regimen characteristic
- **I**mparting knowledge
- **M**odifying patient beliefs
- **P**atient communication
- **L**eaving the bias
- **E**valuating adherence

MONITORING ADHERENCE TO TB MEDICATIONS

- Direct Observation of Therapy (DOT) to monitor medication adherence.
- Cell phone-based adherence monitoring strategy known as **99DOTS** in which patients calling a phone number dispensed with each day's TB pills to report taking every dose.
- **Real-time medication event reminder-monitor device (RT-MERM)** is highly accurate, affordable, reusable, and suitable for TB medications, provides programmable visual and audible reminders of daily dosing and monthly refill, and compiles and transmits automatically detailed and patient-specific information regarding medication taking and medication adherence. Electronic pillboxes can record when the box containing TB drugs is opened and closed to indicate doses taken.
- The patient can also be remotely monitored with the help of Interactive Voice Response (**IVR**), **SMS** reminders. A call center has been established for care cascade and adherence monitoring.
- A mobile app for patients to report treatment compliance using video, audio or text message.

DOTS and STOP TB Strategies Overview

DOTS strategy (Directly observed treatment short course strategy)	STOP TB strategy
DOTS strategy adopted by revised national TB control program in 1997	2006
Components:	Components:
1. Political will and administrative commitment	1. Pursue high-quality DOTS expansion and enhancement
2. Diagnosis by quality assured sputum smear microscopy	2. Address TB/HIV and MDR-TB
3. Adequate supply of quality assured short course chemotherapy drugs	3. Contribute to health system strengthening
4. Directly observed treatment	4. Engage all care providers
5. Systematic monitoring and accountability	5. Empower people with TB and communities
	6. Enable and promote research (diagnosis, treatment, vaccine)

END TB STRATEGY

Vision: A world free of tuberculosis zero deaths; disease and suffering due to tuberculosis.

Goal: End the global tuberculosis epidemic.

Indicators	Milestones		Targets	
	2020	2025	SDG 2030	END TB 2035
Reduction in number of TB deaths compared with 2015 (%)	35%	75%	90%	95%
Reduction in number of TB incidence rate compared with 2015 (%)	20% (<85/10,0,000)	50% (<55/10,0,000)	80% (<20/1,00,000)	90% (<10/1,00,000)
TB affected families facing catastrophic costs due to TB (%)	Zero	Zero	Zero	Zero

Principles
- Government stewardship and accountability with monitoring and evaluation
- Strong coalition with civil society organization and communities
- Protection and promotion of human rights, ethics and equity
- Adoption of the strategy and targets at country level, with global collaboration.

Pillars and Components
- **Integrated, patient—centered care and prevention:**
  - Early diagnosis of tuberculosis of tuberculosis including drug—susceptibility testing and systematic screening of contacts and high risk groups
  - Treatment of all people with tuberculosis including drug-resistant tuberculosis and patient support
  - Collaborative tuberculosis/HIV activities and management of comorbidities
  - Preventive treatment of person at high risk, and vaccination against tuberculosis.
- **Bold policies and supportive systems:**
  - Political commitment with adequate resources for tuberculosis care and prevention.
  - Engagement of communities, civil society organizations, and public and private care providers.
  - Universal health coverage policy, and regulatory frameworks for case notification, vital registration, quality and rational use of medicines, and infection control.
  - Social protection, poverty alleviation and actions on other determinants of tuberculosis.
- **Intensified research and innovation:**
  - Discovery, development and rapid uptake of new tools, interventions and strategies.
  - Research to optimize implementation and impact and promote innovations. The Global Plan's targets are designed as 90-90- 90 targets reach at least 90% of all people with TB and place all of them on appropriate therapy first-line, second-line and preventive therapy as required as a part of this approach, reach at least 90% of the key populations the most vulnerable, underserved, at-risk populations. Achieve at least 90% treatment success for all people diagnosed with TB through affordable treatment services, adherence to complete and correct treatment, and social support.

Sub-national Disease Certification: At District Level

Award	Criteria Decline in incidence rate compared to 2015	Monetary award for district (in ₹)
Bronze	20%	2 lakhs
Silver	40%	3 lakhs
Gold	60%	5 lakhs
TB free status	80%	10 lakhs

Sub-national Disease Certification: At State Level

Award	State/UTs with population <50 lakh	State/UTs (population 50 lakh – 5 Cr)	State/UTs population >5 Cr
Bronze	10 lakhs	15 lakhs	25 lakhs
Silver	20 lakhs	35 lakhs	50 lakhs
Gold	40 lakhs	60 lakhs	75 lakhs
TB free status	60 lakhs	75 lakhs	1 Crore

Roles and Responsibilities MPW (Male)/ANM (MPW Female) at HWC-SHC

- Creating awareness through IEC and social behavior change communication (SBCC)
- Coordinate and participate in the outreach activities for patient support and regular active case finding
- Educate and screen pregnant women for TB and support pregnant women with TB to undergo TB treatment
- Mobilization of community members and leaders
- Refer patients for diagnosis and management
- Sample collection for transport to the nearest appropriate health facility/referral center
- Home visits of patients for public health action
- Monitoring patient adherence and facilitate follow-up and ADR management.
- Undertake minimum three visits to each DSTB patient and minimum six visits to DRTB patients during treatment
- Support in retrieval of TB patients who have stopped taking anti-TB drugs before prescribed period
- Supervision of treatment supporters in the area
- Work as treatment supporter
- Maintain of TB records
- Long-term follow-up of treated patients every six months for next two years
- Map vulnerable population for active case finding and screening and referral for LTBI
- Supply of drugs to treatment supporter.

Roles and Responsibilities of Community Health Officer (CHO) at HWC Sub-center

- Plan and monitor awareness and community mobilization activities
- Sensitize VHSNC members, Jan Arogya Samiti members, PRI members, etc. on TB and their potential role in eliminating TB
- Screen person for symptoms of TB and ensure periodic screening of patients with diabetes and those on immunosuppressants, and smokers.

- Refer the presumptive TB patient to AB-HWC-PHC to ensure complete diagnostic evaluation with microscopy radiology and molecular test
- Ensure follow-up testing of patients at regular frequency
- Clinically monitor patients identified as high-risk for complications/death and ensure that they undergo required investigations at suggested intervals
- Monitor treatment of patients through visits at least once a month and review treatment record on fortnightly basis. Support in retrieval of TB patients who have stopped taking anti-TB drugs before prescribed period
- Plan, organize and implement active case finding in their area
- Early identification of adverse drug reaction and prompt management
- Ensure comorbidity and drug susceptibility testing, linkages of comorbidity patients, and drug-resistant TB patients
- Ensure inventory of laboratory request form, specimen container and anti-TB drugs
- Coordinate with PHC for logistics, patient's management
- Ensure record maintenance, reporting on NIKSHAY
- Identify and engage community treatment supporters and train them on supporting and monitoring TB treatment
- Educate patients and family members on TB, treatment, etc.
- Ensure screening and testing of contacts of sputum positive TB patients for TB/LTBI
- Coordinate with RBSK team and PHC MO for ensuring screening for pediatric TB
- Facilitate for ruling out TB complete evaluation by microbiological and/or radiological examination and/or other investigations for contacts of TB patients and others vulnerable for LTBI
- Ensure that eligible person undergo TB treatment or TB preventive treatment as needed
- Identify potential TB champions among TB survivors and facilitate their participation in the program
- Coordinate, guide and monitor village level activities for TB control

JEET FOR TB

Joint effort for elimination of tuberculosis (JEET) is the largest private health sector engagement initiative for tuberculosis (TB) ever to be carried out in India. Under the project, private patients can receive free, quality-assured diagnostic and treatment services to minimize out-of-pocket expenses. The project provides patients with treatment adherence support by facilitating regular interaction between patients and providers; it also facilitates the provision of incentives by the national TB control program to patients for nutritional support, and to private providers for notification.

Nikshay Mitra

"Nikshay"–Elimination of TB and "Mitra"–Friend ; "Friend to help in elimination of TB"
Nikshay Mitra under the Pradhan Mantri TB Mukt Bharat Abhiyan would provide support to on treatment TB patients through the following ways:
a. Nutritional support
b. Additional investigations for the diagnosed TB patients
c. Vocational support
d. Additional nutritional supplements

It is expected to give such support for at least 1 year.
- **Nikshya sampark: (1800-11-6666):** It is toll free is operational in 14 languages for information, for patient support, for service linkage and grievance redressal.
- **Nikshya patrika:** Quarterly publication of TB central division.
- **Nutrition-TB App (N-TB App):** A mobile-based application to simplify nutritional assessment, counseling and care of patients with tuberculosis.
- **TB arogya sathi:** Citizens using the TB Aarogya Sathi App will have access to common FAQs regarding TB, information on the symptoms of TB and side effects of Anti-TB drugs. Using the app, any user will be able to find the closest health facilities that can assist in diagnosis of TB. Patients registered with Nikshay will have access to update their treatment adherence and bank details using the app along with viewing the DBT details, adherence details and treatment progress.

BIBLIOGRAPHY

1. http://tbcindia.gov.in/WriteReadData/l892s/090220211600NSP_2020_2025_Draft_V7_28th_Aug_20.docx
2. https://tbcindia.gov.in/WriteReadData/NTEPTrainingModules1to4.pdf
3. https://tbcindia.gov.in/WriteReadData/NTEPTrainingModules5to9.pdf
4. https://tbcindia.gov.in/WriteReadData/India%20TB%20Report%202019.pdf
5. https://tbcindia.gov.in/WriteReadData/NSP%20Draft%2020.02.2017%201.pdf
6. https://www.finddx.org/tb/jeet/
7. https://www.who.int/tb/post2015_TBstrategy. pdf?ua=1
8. The Guidelines on Programmatic Management of TB Preventive Treatment (PMTPT) in India (2021)
9. https://tbcindia.gov.in/index1.php?lang=1andlevel=1andsublinkid=5527andlid=3591
10. https://tbcindia.gov.in/showfile.php?lid=3327

9.9 INTEGRATED DISEASE SURVEILLANCE PROGRAM (IDSP)

Introduction
- Launched in 2004 as project with world bank assistance in selected states and later on with NHM fund it is now pan India implemented.
- **Integrated disease surveillance program:** Here integration means sharing of surveillance information of various disease control programs, developing effective partnership with health and non-health sectors in surveillance, including communicable and non-communicable diseases in the surveillance system, working with the private sector and nongovernmental organization and bringing academic institutions and medical colleges into disease surveillance.

Objectives
- Integration and decentralization of surveillance activities through establishment of surveillance units at Center, State and District level, so:
  - Districts would be able to detect **early warning signals** of impending outbreaks and timely, effective public health actions can be initiated
  - Disease **trends** can be traced over a period of time
  - Districts can provide essential data to **monitor progress of ongoing disease control programs** and control strategies can be periodically evaluated and suitably tailored
  - **Health resources can be allocated more efficiently**

- Human resource development—Training of State Surveillance Officers, District Surveillance Officers, Rapid Response Team and other Medical and Paramedical staff on principles of disease surveillance.
- Information communication technology—for collection, collation, compilation, analysis and dissemination of data.
- Strengthening of public health laboratories.
- To **involve all stakeholders** including private sectors and communities in surveillance activities.

Program Components

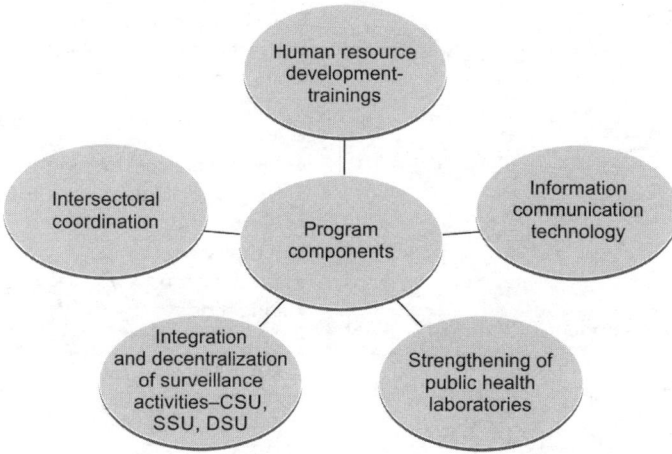

Strategies

Syndromic Surveillance

- **The paramedical health staff (MPHW/ASHA) will undertake disease surveillance (both active and passive)**
- The clinical syndromes under surveillance are:
  - Fever
    - Fever <7 days
      - Only fever
      - With rash
      - With bleeding
      - With daze/semi-consciousness/unconsciousness
      - Fever >7 days
    - Cough with or without fever
      - <2 weeks
      - >2 weeks
    - Loose watery stools of less than 2 weeks duration
      - With some/much dehydration
      - With no dehydration
      - With blood in stools
    - Jaundice cases of less than 4 weeks duration
    - Acute flaccid paralysis cases in <15 yrs of age
    - Unusual symptoms leading to death or hospitalization that do not fit into above.

Diseases under presumptive surveillance	Diseases under lab surveillance
• Acute diarrheal disease (including acute gastroenteritis) • Dysentery (with blood in stool) • Acute encephalitis syndrome • Acute hepatitis • Anthrax • Chickenpox • Chikungunya • Crimean congo hemorrhagic fever • Dengue • Diphtheria • Enteric fever/typhoid • Human rabies • ARI/ILI • Kyasanur-forest disease • Leptospirosis • Malaria • Measles • Meningitis • Mumps • Pertussis • SARI (including pneumonia) • Scrub Typhus • Any other state specific diseases (e.g., brucellosis/chandipura virus disease) • Unusual syndromes NOT captured above (undiagnosed hemorrhagic fevers)	• Anthrax • Chikungunya • Cholera • Crimean congo hemorrhagic fever • Dengue • Diphtheria • Typhoid • Hepatitis A • Hepatitis E • Influenza • Japanese encephalitis • Kyasanur-Forest disease • Leptospirosis • Malaria • Measles • Meningococcal meningitis • Non-typhoidal salmonellosis • Pertussis • Rubella • Scrub typhus • Shigellosis • Two state specific diseases (e.g., brucellosis/chandipura virus disease) • Any other

Regular Surveillance

Types of disease	Disease
Vector-borne diseases	Malaria
Water-borne diseases	Diarrhea, cholera, typhoid
Respiratory diseases	Tuberculosis
Vaccine preventable diseases	Measles
Disease under eradication	Polio
Other conditions	Road traffic accidents
International commitment	Plague, yellow fever
Unusual syndromes (Causing death/hospitalization)	Meningoencephalitis Respiratory distress Hemorrhagic fever, jaundice Other undiagnosed condition

Sentinel Surveillance

- ☐ HIV/HBV, HCV
- ☐ Water quality
- ☐ Outdoor air quality (large urban centers)

Regular Periodic Surveys

- **NCD risk factors:** Anthropometry, physical activity, blood pressure, tobacco
- Nutrition
- Blindness and any other unusual health condition

State Specific Diseases under Surveillance (Provisional): Up to 5 Diseases

Reporting Mechanism

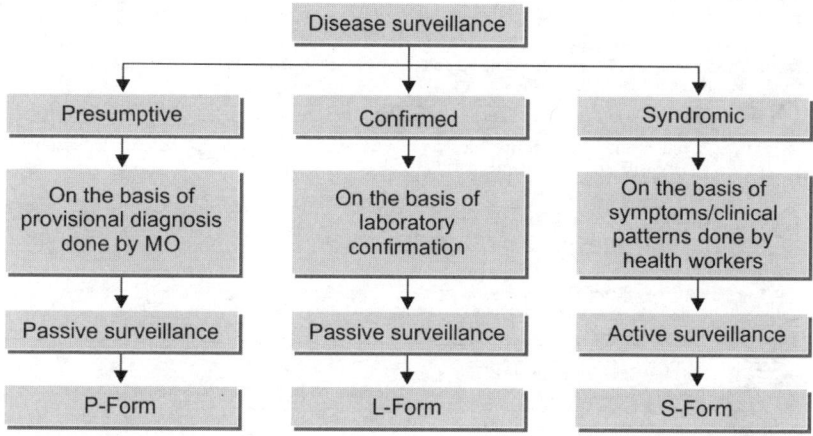

Organizational Structure of IDSP

Central surveillance unit (CSU): Integrated administratively and financially with National Centre for Disease Control (NCDC), Delhi.

State surveillance unit (SSU): One in each State/UT with a regular officer identified as State Surveillance Officer (SSO). Supported by 7 contractual staff.

District surveillance unit (DSU): One in each district with a regular officer as District Surveillance Officer (DSO). Supported by 3 contractual staff.

Differences between IDSP and IHIP

	IDSP portal	IHIP portal
1.	Capture aggregate data only	Capture disaggregate data of persons at all levels
2.	Paper-based data collection	Web-based data collection
3.	Manually links data from S, P and L forms	Electronically linked data of S, P, L forms
4.	Weekly surveillance	Capture real-time or daily surveillance data
5.	Monitoring 22 health conditions	Monitor more than 33+ health conditions
6.	Not being done	Integrate with ongoing surveillance programs Provide analysis on mobile and electronic devices

BIBLIOGRAPHY

1. https://idsp.nic.in/index.php

9.10 NATIONAL AIDS CONTROL PROGRAM (NACP)

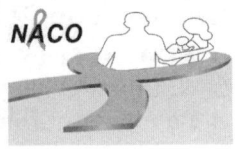

HIV (HIV estimation 2020 report): Adult (15–49 years) HIV prevalence was estimated at 0.22% (0.17%–0.29%); 0.23% (0.18%–0.31%) among males and 0.20% (0.15%–0.26%) among females.

Milestones of the NACP Program

- **1986**: Identification of first case of HIV in India
- **1992**: NACP-1 (1992–99)
  - Objective of slowing down the spread of HIV infections so as to reduce morbidity, mortality and impact of AIDS in the country
- **2000**: NACP-2 (2000–05)
  - To reduce the spread of HIV infection in India, and to increase India's capacity to respond to HIV/AIDS on a long-term basis
- **2006**: NACP-3 (2006–11)
  - Goal of halting and reversing the epidemic over its five-year period
- **2012**: NACP-4 (2012–17)
  - Aims to accelerate the process of reversal and further strengthen the epidemic response in India
- **2017**:
  - National Strategic Plan, 2017–2024
  - The HIV and acquired immune deficiency syndrome (prevention and control) Act, 2017
  - NACP-5 (2021–26): Focus is on ensuring PLHIV survive longer and lead productive lives

Objectives

- Reduce new infections by 50% (2007 Baseline of NACP III)
- Comprehensive care, support and treatment to all persons living with HIV/AIDS
- The objective of NACP IV is to consolidate the trend of reversal of the epidemic seen at the national level to all the key districts in India.

Note: Target 3.3 of SDG goal no. 3 states 'Ending of the AIDS epidemic as a public health threat' by 2030.

Components

Component 1

Intensifying and consolidating prevention services with a focus on high-risk group (HRG) and vulnerable populations.

Activities

- **Scaling up coverage of targeted interventions (TIs) among HRG:**
  - Behavior change interventions to increase safe practices, testing and counseling, and adherence to treatment, and demand for other services.
  - The promotion and provision of condoms to HRG to use in each sexual encounter.
  - Provision or referral for STI.
  - Needle and syringe exchange for IDUs as well as scaling up of opioid substitution therapy (OST) provision.

- **Scaling up of interventions among other vulnerable populations:**
  - Risk assessment and size estimation of migrant population and truckers at transit points and at workplaces.
  - Behavior change communications (BCC) for creating awareness about risk and vulnerability, prevention methods, availability of services, increase safe behavior and demand for services as well as reduce stigma.
  - Promotion and provisioning of condoms through different channels like social marketing.
  - For testing, counseling and STI treatment services, linkages will be developed with local institutions, both public and NGO owned.
  - Creation of "peer support groups" and "safe spaces" for migrants at destination.

Component 2: Expanding IEC Services
- Behavior change communication strategies for HRGs, vulnerable groups and hard to reach populations.
- Increasing awareness among general population, particularly women and youth.

Component 3: Comprehensive Care, Support and Treatment
- To provide high-quality treatment and follow-up services, Additional Centers of Excellence (CoEs) and upgraded ART Plus centers will be established.
- Provision of anti-retroviral treatment (ART) including second line.
- Management of opportunistic infections.
- Facilitating social protection through linkages with concerned Departments/Ministries.
- Public-private partnerships to avail better care, support and treatment services.
- Activities to reduce stigma and discrimination at all levels particularly at health care settings will be carried out.

Component 4: Strengthening Institutional Capacities
There will be integration of the HIV services with the routine public sector health delivery systems in phase manner for better execution.

Component 5: Strategic Information Management Systems (SIMS)
- The surveillance system will be further strengthened to track the epidemic, for the incidence analysis, identifying pockets of infection and estimating the burden of infection.
- Research will be priority to serve the emerging needs of the program.
- The relevant, measurable and verifiable indicators will be identified and used appropriately.

Treatment
Preferred first-line ART regimen for all PLHIV with age >10 years and weight >30kg is as follows: Tenofovir (TDF 300 mg) + Lamivudine (3TC 300 mg) + Dolutegravir (DTG 50 mg) regimen (TLD) as FDC in a single pill once a day (at a fixed time every day as per patient's convenience)

NATIONAL STRATEGIC PLAN FOR HIV/AIDS AND STI 2017–2024: "PAVING WAY FOR AN AIDS FREE INDIA"

Vision: An AIDS Free India

Mission: Attain universal coverage of HIV prevention, testing, treatment to care continuum that is effective, inclusive, equitable and adapted to population and local needs.

Goal: Achieving zero new infections, zero AIDS-related deaths and zero AIDS related stigma and discrimination.

Target	2020	2024
New HIV infections	75% reduction in new infections	80% reduction in new HIV infections
Diagnosis and treatment	90-90-90: 90% of those who are HIV positive in the country know their status, 90% of those who know their status are on treatment and 90% of those who are on treatment experience effective viral load suppression	95-95-95: 95% of those who are HIV positive in the country know their status, 95% of those who know their status are on treatment and 95% of those who are on treatment experience effective viral load suppression
Mother to child transmission	Elimination	NA
Stigma and discrimination	Elimination	NA

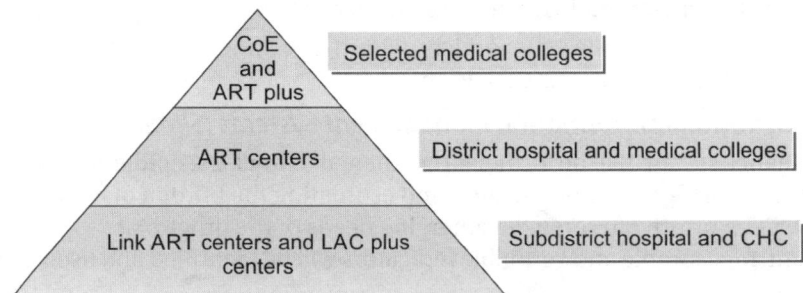

Fig. 9.2: HIV treatment services.

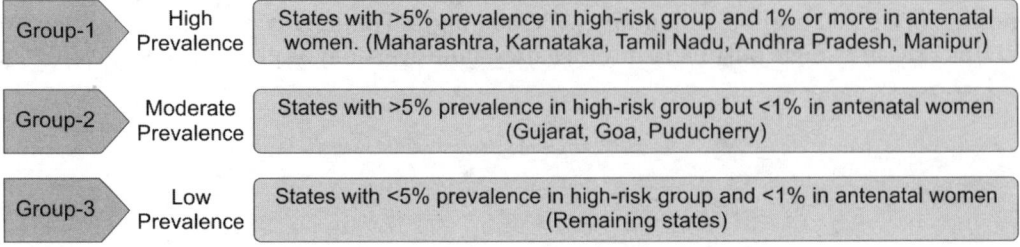

Communicable Diseases and Relevant National Health Programs

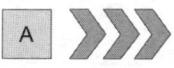 More than 1% ANC/Parents to child transmission prevalence in district at any time in any of the sites in the last 3 years

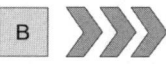 Less than 1% ANC/PTCT prevalence in all the sites in the last 3 years associated with >5% prevalence in any high-risk group

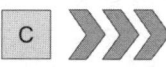 <1% ANC prevalence in all the sites in the last 3 years with <5% prevalence in all STD clinic attendees or any HRG with known hotspots

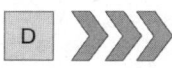 <1% ANC prevalence in all the sites in the last 3 years with <5% prevalence in all STD clinic attendees or any HRG or poor data with no known hotspots

NACP Phase-V (2021–2026)

Goal
1. Reduce annual new HIV infections by 80%
2. Reduce AIDS-related mortalities by 80%
3. Eliminate vertical transmission of HIV and syphilis
4. Promote universal access to quality STI/RTI services to at-risk and vulnerable populations
5. Eliminate HIV/AIDS related stigma and discrimination

The specific objectives:
- HIV/AIDS prevention and control
  - 95% of people who are most at risk of acquiring HIV infection use comprehensive prevention
  - 95% of HIV positive know their status, 95% of those who know their status are on treatment and 95% of those who are on treatment have suppressed viral load
  - 95% of pregnant and breastfeeding women living with HIV have suppressed viral load toward attainment of elimination of vertical transmission of HIV
  - Less than 10% of people living with HIV and key populations experience stigma and discrimination
- STI/RTI prevention and control
  - Universal access to quality STI/RTI services to at-risk and vulnerable populations
  - Attainment of elimination of vertical transmission of syphilis

Table 9.3: Risk of HIV transmission from mother to child with or without interventions.

ARV intervention	Risk of HIV transmission from mother to child
No ARV: no breastfeeding	30–45%
No ARV: breastfeeding	20–25%
Short course with one ARV: breastfeeding	15–25%
Short course with one ARV: no breastfeeding	5–15%
Short course with two ARVs: breastfeeding	5%
3 ARVs (ART) with breastfeeding	2%
3 ARVs (ART) with no breastfeeding	1%

ART regimen in pregnant and breastfeeding women with HIV

Group	Regime	Duration
Pregnant or breastfeeding women with HIV	Tenofovir + Lamivudine + Dolutegravir TDF + 3TC + DTG (TLD)	Once daily lifelong
Pregnant women presenting in active labor	**Intrapartum** Initiate TLD TDF (300 mg) + 3TC (300 mg) + DTG (50 mg) **Postpartum** Continue TLD TDF (300 mg) + 3TC (300 mg) + DTG (50 mg)	
Low-risk infants Infants born to mothers with suppressed viral load (<1000 copies/mL) done any time after 32 weeks of pregnancy up to delivery	1. Syrup Nevirapine (NVP) or 2. Syrup Zidovudine	From birth till 6 weeks of age
High-risk infants Mother not on ART or maternal viral load not done or not suppressed between 32 weeks of pregnancy till delivery or mother newly identified HIV positive within 6 weeks of delivery	Syrup NVP + Syrup Zidovudine	In case of Exclusive Replacement Feeding (ERF): From birth till 6 weeks of age In case of Exclusive breast-feeding (EBF): From birth till 12 weeks of age

BIBLIOGRAPHY

1. http://naco.gov.in/sites/default/files/Paving%20the%20Way%20for%20an%20AIDS%2015122017.pdf
2. Govt. of India, NACP IV components, NACO, Ministry of health and Family Welfare, New Delhi. Available at: http://naco.gov.in/nacp-iv-components
3. https://vikaspedia.in/health/nrhm/national-health-programmes-1/communicable-diseases/national-aids-control-programme

9.11 NATIONAL VECTOR BORNE DISEASE CONTROL PROGRAM (NVBDCP)

Evolution of NVBDCP

1947	75 million cases and 0.8 million deaths estimated to be due to malaria
1953	National Malaria Control Program (NMCP)
1958	National Malaria Eradication Program (NMEP)
1971	Urban Malaria Scheme
1977	Modified Plan of Operation
1995	Modified Action Program for Malaria Control
1997	Enhanced Malaria Control Project (World Bank Assisted)
1998	National Anti-malaria Program (NAMP)
2003	National Vector-borne Disease Control Program (NVBDCP)

Epidemiology of Malaria (According to the 2021 Data)

Year	Blood smears examined	Positive cases	Falciparum case (%)	ABER	API	SPR/TPR	Deaths
2021	114.2 million	161516	63.09	8.25	0.12	0.14	90

Hierarchy of Malaria Control Administrative Framework

Central Level
- There are 19 Regional Offices located in 19 States which are overall under the DGHS jurisdiction.
- These offices do the monitoring of the activities of NVBDCP in collaboration with the states.

State Level
- There is a vector-borne diseases (VBD) Control Division (under Health and Family Welfare) in every state which is headed by the State Programme Officer (SPO).
- State Program Officer is responsible for supervision, guidance and proper implementation of the program.
- Each state has **"State VBD Control Society"** which has civil society and sometimes private sector representation.

Divisional Level
There are **zonal officers** (under the overall supervision of Senior Divisional Officers) at the divisional level who have the technical and administrative responsibilities of the program in their respected areas.

District Level
- Chief Medical Officer (CMO)/District Health Officer (DHO) is the overall responsible person for the management the program at district level.
- District malaria office is the main planning and monitoring unit of the program.
- There is one DVBDC officer while an Assistant Malaria Officer (AMO) and Malaria Inspectors (MIs) to assist him.
- DVBDC officer under overall supervision of CMO conducts spray operations in the entire district.
- District VBD Control Societies now merged with District Health Societies to assist the management of funds, planning and monitoring of program activities.

PHC Level
- The MO-PHC is the overall in charge of the activities like malaria surveillance, laboratory services and supervision of the spray operations.
- MPWs, ASHAs and other community health volunteers do the case detection, management and other community outreach services.

GLOBAL TECHNICAL STRATEGY FOR MALARIA ELIMINATION (2015–2030)

Vision: A world free of Malaria

Goals

Goals	Milestones for 2020	Milestones for 2025	Targets for the year 2030
Reduce malaria mortality rates globally compared with 2015	At least 40%	At least 75%	At least 90%
Reduce malaria case incidence globally compared with 2015	At least 40%	At least 75%	At least 90%
Eliminate malaria from countries in which malaria was transmitted in 2015	At least 10 countries	At least 20 countries	At least 35 countries

Strategy Framework

In the strategy framework, there are **three pillars** and **two supporting elements** to guide the member nations to fight against malaria.

Pillar 1: Ensure Universal Access to Malaria Prevention, Diagnosis and Treatment

Pillar 1 is built of the following guiding principles:
- Integrated vector control
- Chemoprevention
- Diagnostic testing and treatment

Pillar 2: Accelerate Efforts Toward Elimination and Attainment of Malaria Free Status

Pillar 2 is built of the following guiding principles:
- Refocus the program target time to time
- Enact strict legislation (e.g., civic by law)
- Renew political commitment and deepen regional collaboration
- Reduce the number of undetected infections
- Implement targeted malaria vector control
- Prevent re-establishment of local malaria transmission
- Implement transmission blocking chemotherapy
- Detect all infections to attain elimination and prevent re-establishment

Pillar 3: Transform Malaria Surveillance into a Core Intervention

Pillar 3 is built of the following guiding principles:
- Surveillance in areas of high transmission, in areas of low transmission and even in the targeted areas for elimination of malaria
- Data collection is important for understanding disease trends and overall performance of the program
- Develop national strategic plans that take into account the epidemiology and heterogeneity of malaria in a country and monitor the progress of the national strategic plans

Supporting Element 1: Harnessing Innovation and Expanding Research

It can be summarized as follows:
- Basic research for the development of new and improved tools.
- Operational research should be conducted to know the impact and cost-effectiveness of existing tools and strategies
- Ensure rapid uptake of new tools, interventions and strategies

Supporting Element 2: Strengthening the Enabling Environment

This supporting element can be summarized as follows:
- Strong political and financial commitments
- Multisectoral approaches, and cross-border and regional collaborations
- Stewardship of entire heath system including the private sector, with strong regulatory support
- Capacity development for both effective program management and research

In the line of this global strategy government of India has launched:

NATIONAL FRAMEWORK FOR MALARIA ELIMINATION IN INDIA (2016–2030)

Vision
Eliminate malaria nationally and contribute to improved health, quality of life and alleviation of poverty.

Goals
- Eliminate malaria (zero indigenous cases) throughout the entire country by 2030; and
- Maintain malaria-free status in areas where malaria transmission has been interrupted and prevent re-introduction of malaria.

Objectives
- Eliminate malaria from all 26 low (Category 1) and moderate (Category 2) transmission states/union territories (UTs) by 2022.
- Reduce the incidence of malaria to less than 1 case per 1000 population per year in all states and UTs and their districts by 2024.
- Interrupt indigenous transmission of malaria throughout the entire country, including all high transmission states and union territories (UTs) (Category 3) by 2027.
- Prevent the re-establishment of local transmission of malaria in areas where it has been eliminated and maintain national malaria-free status by 2030 and beyond.

Classification of States/UTs Based on API as Primary Criteria

Category 0: Prevention of re-establishment phase
States/UTs with zero indigenous cases of malaria.

Category 1: Elimination phase
States/UTs (15) including their districts reporting an API of less than 1 case per 1000 population at risk.

Category 2: Pre-elimination phase
States/UTs (11) with an API of less than 1 case per 1000 population at risk, but some of their districts are reporting an API of 1 case per 1000 population at risk or above.

Category 3: Intensified control phase
States/UTs (10) with an API of 1 case per 1000 population at risk or above.

EXPECTED ROLE OF MPW (MALE)

- For early diagnosis and complete treatment, he should conduct a fortnightly house-to-house visit for collecting blood smears (thick and thin) or perform RDT from fever cases or cases with history of fever during domiciliary visits to households and keep the records in M-1.
- He transports slide collected along with M-1 to lab for examination.
- He provides treatment to confirmed malarias cases as per the treatment guidelines.
- He should advise seriously ill cases to visit PHC/referral center for immediate treatment after collection of blood smear and performing RDT.
- He should cross verify records of ASHA workers, replenish the stock of microslides, RDKs and drugs to them wherever necessary.
- MPW (Male) should give advance intimation to the residents a fortnight before the actual spray date and he should facilitated spraying activity. He also must ensure safety of spraymen and also water and food in the house.
- He will make a record of spray output showing insecticide consumed, squads utilized, human dwellings sprayed, missed, locked, refused and rooms sprayed/rooms missed in the proforma prescribed.
- In case of refusals or locked houses, he will contact persons concerned/panchayat personnel to get mopping up done to cover these houses.
- He will aware the community about signs and symptoms of malaria, its treatment, prevention and vector control.
- He will maintain record of fever cases diagnosed by blood slides/RDTs in M-1 and prepare a Subcenter report (M-2) for all cases in the area, including those of ASHAs and submit it to PHC by 5th of the following month.
- He should keep a record of supervisory visits in tour diary and submit to MO-PHC during monthly meetings for verification.

EXPECTED ROLE OF MPW (FEMALE)

- **MPW (FEMALE)** will be responsible for collecting blood smears from all antenatal, postnatal cases as well as from infants.
- If the pregnant woman has fever or history of fever, MPW (FEMALE) will collect thick and thin blood smears and perform RDT and keep records in M-1.
- She will give malaria treatment as per drug policy. (Note: Primaquine should not be administered to pregnant women and during postpartum period of 45 days and also to infants).
- Screening of households if any of them has fever or history of fever.
- She will ensue that all samples reached to the nearest Malaria Clinic/PHC laboratory on priority and obtain the results and give treatment within 24 hours of malaria positives.
- She should refer the seriously ill cases immediately to PHC/other nearest referral center for proper treatment but make sure that before referral collection of blood smear and RDT are done.
- She should take help of AWW/Community Volunteers/ASHAs of her area during the visit to the village and collect blood smears and M-2 forms for transmission to laboratory.
- If MPW-M post is vacant or MPW-M is on leave, the duties will be carried out by MPW (F).
- She will educate the community about malaria, its diagnosis and treatment.

Communicable Diseases and Relevant National Health Programs

- Helping in spraying activities like intimation of spraying schedule till the acceptance of the community and safe execution of spraying activity.
- Details of all tests conducted and diagnosed cases will be entered in M1 and provided to MPW-M.
- She should keep a record of supervisory visits in tour diary and submit to MO-PHC during monthly meetings for verification.

Case Detection and Management Forms—M-1, M-2, M-3 and M-4.
- M-1: Fortnightly Report of Fever Cases by ASHA/MPW/Health Facility
- M-2: Laboratory Request for Slide Examination
- M-3: Record of Slide Examination in PHC Laboratory
- M-4: Fortnightly Report of Cases from Subcenter/PHC/District/State.

Strategies for Prevention and Control of Dengue and Chikungunya

- **Surveillance:** Disease and entomological surveillance.
- **Case management:** Laboratory diagnosis and clinical management.
- **Vector management:** Environmental management for source reduction, chemical control, personal protection and legislation.
- **Outbreak response:** Epidemic preparedness and media management.
- **Capacity building:** Training, strengthening human resource and operational research.
- Behavioural change communication Social mobilization, and information, education and communication (IEC).
- **Intersectoral coordination:** With ministries of urban development, rural development, panchayati raj, surface transport and education sector.
- **Monitoring and supervision:** Analysis of reports, review, field visit and feedback.

Strategies for Elimination of Kala-azar

- **Parasite elimination and disease management**
  - Expansion of new tools through case introduction of rK39 rapid diagnostic kits and oral drug miltefosine for treatment of Kala-azar cases
  - Early case detection and complete treatment
  - Strengthening of referral
- **Integrated vector control**
  - Indoor Residual Spraying (IRS)
  - Environmental management by maintenance of sanitation and hygiene and provision of pucca houses in Kala-azar affected villages PMAY-G
- **Supportive interventions**
  - Behavior change communication for social mobilization
  - Intersectoral convergence
  - Capacity building by training and monitoring and evaluation

Elimination Strategies for Lymphatic Filariasis

Elimination is defined as "lymphatic filariasis ceases to be public health problem, when the number of microfilaria carriers is less than 1 percent and the children born after initiation of ELF are free from circulating antigenemia (presence of adult filaria worm in human body).

Twin pillar strategy adopted for elimination.

- **Annual mass drug administration:** Triple Drug Therapy (Ivermectin + DEC + Albendazole) (triple drugs in selected districts only while in other districts DEC and Albendazole are given)
- **Morbidity management and disability prevention (MMDP):** Home based management of lymphoedema cases and up-scaling of hydrocele operations in identified CHCs/district hospitals/medical colleges.

Implementation of vector control measure through anti-larval operations and source reduction.

Strategies for Prevention and Control of Japanese Encephalitis

- Strengthening of monitoring and surveillance activity
- Strengthening diagnostic facilities and referral facilities
- JE vaccination
- Case management
- Capacity building for proper case management at different health care facility
- BCC for hygiene and sanitation

BIBLIOGRAPHY

1. Govt. of India, Strategic action plan for malaria control in India 2012–2017, Scaling up malaria control interventions with high a focus on high burden areas, Directorate of national vector borne disease control programme, DGHS, ministry of health and family welfare, New Delhi.
2. Govt. of India, National Framework for Malaria Elimination in India (2016–2030), Directorate of national vector borne disease control programme, DGHS, ministry of health and family welfare, New Delhi.
3. https://wwwn.cdc.gov/nndss/conditions/malaria/case-definition/2010/
4. World Health Organization. Global Technical Strategy for Malaria 2016–2030 Geneva. WHO; 2015.

9.12 NATIONAL ACTION PLAN FOR DOG MEDIATED RABIES ELIMINATION FROM INDIA BY 2030

Introduction

- 97% of the rabies cases are due to dog bite.
- 2% due to cat bite and 1% due to jackals, mongoose and other animals bite.
- Rabies is 100% fatal yet 100% preventable disease.
- Around 20,000 estimated deaths are due to rabies.
- Rabies can be prevented with at least 70% of the dog population should be vaccinated for rabies.
- Four organizations namely World Health Organization (WHO), World Organization for Animal Health (OIE), Food and Agriculture Organization of the United Nations (FAO) and the Global Alliance for Rabies Control (GARC) have determined to reach the global target of "Zero human deaths due to dog-mediated Rabies by 2030".

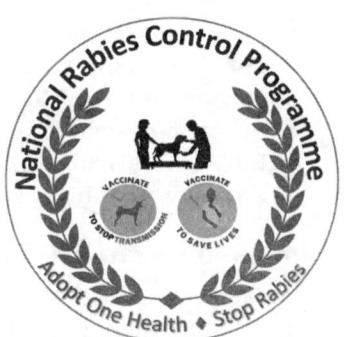

- Countries like Western Europe, Canada, the US, Mexico, Japan and Latin America have already eliminated dog-mediated Rabies through successful canine rabies vaccination and one health approach.
- In India, Rabies is endemic in all States/UTs except Andaman and Nicobar, and Lakshadweep Islands.
- WHO has also divided countries into five different stages of Rabies elimination:
  i. **Endemic stage**
  ii. **Control stage**—Indicates a steep decrease in Rabies incidence after mass interventions.
  iii. **Zero human rabies death**—Shows interruption of dog-human Rabies transmission and no human deaths.
  iv. **Elimination stage**—Shows interruption of Rabies transmission and no canine case.
  v. **Maintenance stage**—Refers to continuing freedom from disease, e.g., by preventing incursion and/or reemergence of canine or human Rabies.
- Validation of elimination of Rabies as a public health problem: zero human death from dog-mediated Rabies for at least 24 months in a country with adequate surveillance and an effective Rabies control program in human and animal populations.
- Verification of elimination of dog-mediated Rabies: Interrupting Rabies transmission, defined as the absence of dog-mediated Rabies cases for a period of at least 24 months in the presence of high-quality surveillance according to international standards.
- Be declared Rabies-free, which follows from verification, and recognizes countries or areas that are free of both dog Rabies and terrestrial Rabies.

Milestones for National Rabies Control Programme

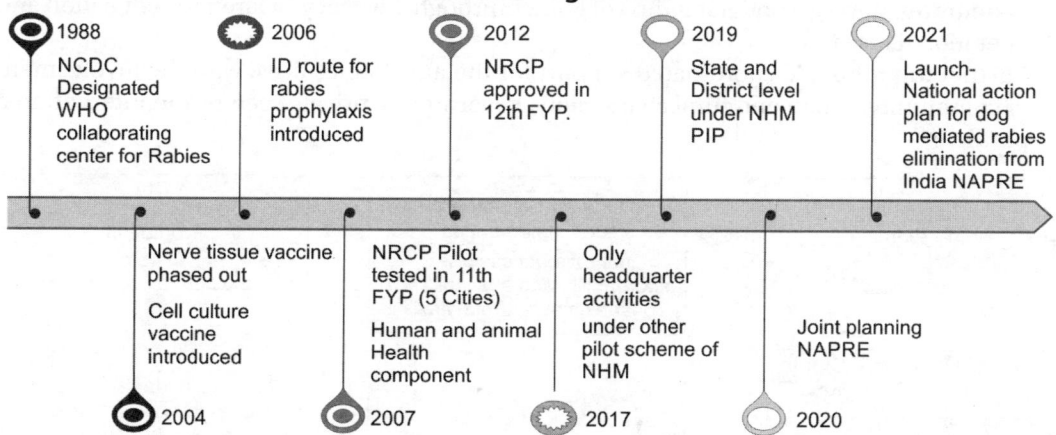

Fig. 9.3: Milestones for national rabies control program.

The National Action Plan for dog-mediated Rabies Elimination in India is based on recommendations of various international agencies such as WHO, OIE, and GARC.

The successful implementation of NAPRE is based on 5 major pillars.

Five Major Pillars of NAPRE

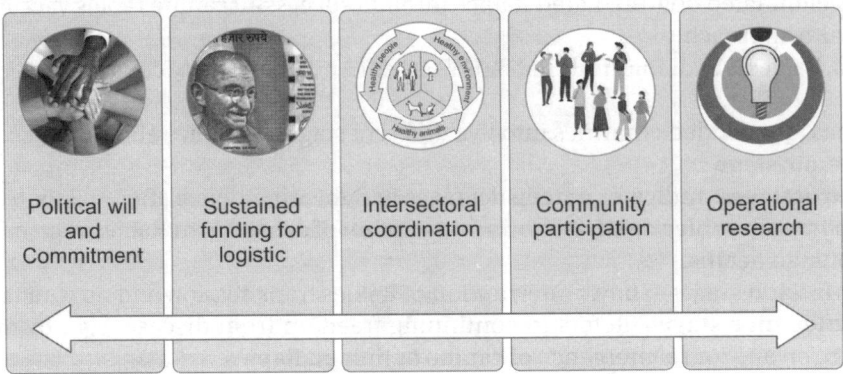

- Political will and Commitment
- Sustained funding for logistic
- Intersectoral coordination
- Community participation
- Operational research

Vision: To achieve zero human deaths due to dog-mediated Rabies by 2030.

Mission: To progressively reduce and ultimately eliminate human Rabies in India through sustained, mass dog vaccination and appropriate post-exposure treatment.

Key Principles

- **Prevention:** Introduce cost-effective public health intervention techniques to improve accessibility, affordability, and availability of post-exposure prophylaxis to all people in need.
- **Promotion:** Improve understanding of Rabies through advocacy, awareness, education and operational research.
- **Partnership:** Provide coordinated support for the anti-Rabies drive with the involvement of community, urban and rural civil society, government, private sectors and international partners.

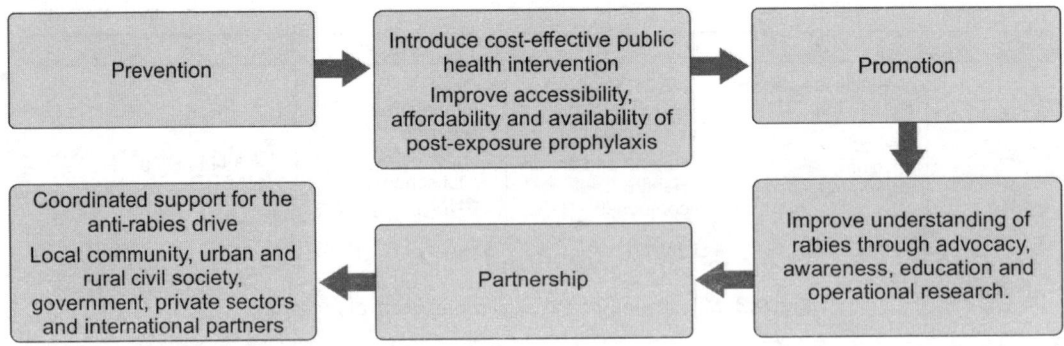

Core Components of NAPRE

There are two core components:

A. **Human health component:** To prevent human deaths due to Rabies by ensuring timely access for post-exposure prophylaxis for all animal bite victims and creating well responsive Public Health System.

B. **Animal health component:** To achieve at least 70% Anti-Rabies vaccination coverage among dogs in a defined geographical area annually for 3 consecutive years.

Strategies of Human Health Component of NAPRE

- To ensure availability of anti-rabies vaccine (ARV) and anti-rabies serum (ARS) to all animal bite victims at all levels of health facilities
- Capacity building of professionals in appropriate animal bite management
- To encourage pre-exposure prophylaxis for high-risk groups
- Strengthening surveillance of animal bites and rabies cases in human
- To strengthen diagnostics capacity on Rabies
- To promote operational research in the Rabies
- To strengthen intersectoral coordination mechanism between the veterinary and medical sectors
- Information education and communication (IEC)
- Public-private partnership through involvement of NGO and community organizations.

Strategies for Animal Health Components

- Estimation of canine population
- Identification of rabies risk zone
- Planning and implementing strategic mass dog vaccination program
  - To achieve anti-rabies vaccination in at least 70% of the dog population, annually for three consecutive years and maintain the 70% vaccination status in a defined geographic area.
- Assessment of post vaccination coverage
- Dog population management (DPM)
  - Animal birth control (ABC)
- To promote responsible dog ownership
- Solid waste management (SWM)
- Community involvement
- Confinement and containment
- Operational research

BIBLIOGRAPHY

1. http://www.awbi.in/awbi-pdf/NationalActiopPlan.pdf
2. https://dahd.nic.in/livestock-health/national-action-plan-dog-mediated-rabies-elimination-india-2030

9.13 NATIONAL VIRAL HEPATITIS CONTROL PROGRAM (NVHCP)

- It has been launched on 28th July 2018 (world hepatitis day) by MOHFW for the prevention and control of viral hepatitis in India as to achieve Sustainable Development Goal (SDG) 3.3 which targets "By 2030, end the epidemics of AIDS, tuberculosis, malaria and neglected tropical diseases and combat hepatitis, water-borne diseases and other communicable diseases".
- It covers all major viral hepatitis like A, B, C, D and E (these five types are responsible for 96% of overall viral hepatitis related mortality).

- HAV-is responsible for 10-30% of acute hepatitis and 5-15% of acute liver failure cases in India. It is further reported that HEV accounts for 10-40% of acute hepatitis and 15-45% of acute liver failure.
- Hepatitis B surface Antigen (HBsAg) positivity in the general population ranges from 1.1% to 12.2%, with an average prevalence of 3-4%.
- Endemicity of countries is based on prevalence of HBsAg carrier as follows:
  - <2%: Low Endemicity
  - 2-4%: Low Intermediate Endemicity
  - 5-7 %: High Intermediate Endemicity
  - ≥8 %: High Endemicity
- It is estimated that in India, approximately 40 million people are chronically infected with Hepatitis B and 6-12 million people with Hepatitis C.
- Hepatitis B prevalence is highest in the WHO Western Pacific Region (6.2%) while lowest in WHO Region of the Americas (0.7%) while in SEARO it is 2.0%.

Aims
- Combat hepatitis and achieve country wide elimination of Hepatitis C by 2030;
- Achieve significant reduction in the infected population, morbidity and mortality associated with Hepatitis B and C viz. Cirrhosis and Hepato-cellular carcinoma (liver cancer);
- Reduce the risk, morbidity and mortality due to Hepatitis A and E.

Key Objectives
- Enhance community awareness on hepatitis and lay stress on preventive measures among general population especially high-risk groups and in hotspots.
- Provide early diagnosis and management of viral hepatitis at all levels of healthcare.
- Develop standard diagnostic and treatment protocols for management of viral hepatitis and its complications.
- Strengthen the existing infrastructure facilities, build capacities of existing human resources and raise additional human resources, where required, for providing comprehensive services for management of viral hepatitis and its complications in all districts of the country.
- Develop linkages with the existing national programs toward awareness, prevention, diagnosis and treatment for viral hepatitis.
- Develop a web-based "Viral Hepatitis Information and Management System" to maintain a registry of persons affected with viral hepatitis and its sequelae.

Components

Preventive Component
This is the main component of the NVHCP.
- Awareness generation and behavior change communication
- Immunization of Hepatitis B (birth dose, high-risk groups, healthcare workers)
- Safety of blood and blood products
- Injection safety, safe sociocultural practices
- Safe drinking water, hygiene and sanitary toilets

Diagnosis and Treatment
- Screening of pregnant women for HBsAg to be done in areas where institutional deliveries are <80% to ensure their referral for institutional delivery for birth dose Hepatitis B vaccination.
- Free screening, diagnosis and treatment for both hepatitis B and C (approximately 5 crore patients will be benefited) would be made available at all levels of health care in a phased manner.
- Provision of linkages, including with private sector and not for profit institutions, for diagnosis and treatment.
- Engagement with community/peer support to enhance and ensure adherence to treatment and demand generation.

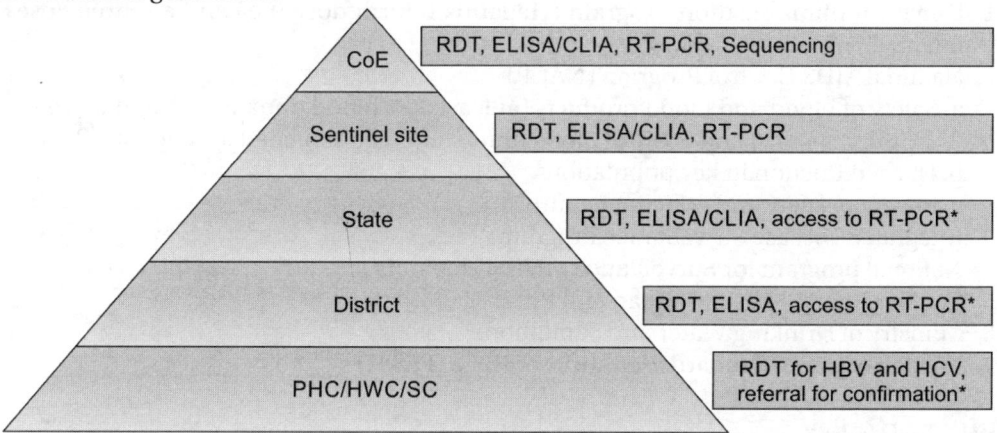

Monitoring and Evaluation, Surveillance and Research
- Effective linkages to the surveillance system would be established and operational research would be undertaken through Department of Health Research (DHR).
- Standardized monitoring and evaluation framework would be developed and an online web based system is established.

Training and Capacity Building
- The hepatitis induction and update programs for all level of healthcare workers would be made available using both, the traditional cascade model of training through master trainers and various platforms available for enabling electronic, e-learning and e-courses.
- This will be a continuous process and will be supported by NCDC (National Center for Disease Control), ILBS (Institute of Liver and Biliary Sciences) and state tertiary care institutes and coordinated by NVHCP.

National Viral Hepatitis Control Management Unit
The NVHCP will be coordinated by the units at the center and the states.

National Viral Hepatitis Management Unit (NVHMU)
- It is established at the center with in the NHM.
- It will be responsible for implementation of program in the country.
- Joint Secretary will be head of NVHMU and report to the Mission Director (NHM) will be submitted.

State Viral Hepatitis Management Unit (SVHMU)
The State Health Society with nodal officer and required essential manpower will coordinate the program at state level.

District Viral Hepatitis Management Unit (DVHMU)
- A program officer at the district level from available manpower would act as the nodal person to supervise the program and facilitate the logistics, supply chain, outreach, training at district level.

List of other ministries and programs which can have very important role in ending viral hepatitis as public health threat:
1. Universal Immunization Program (Hepatitis B birth dose 90% and all three doses for infant 95%)
2. National AIDS Control Program (NACP)
   a. Safety of blood and blood products (at least 80% blood donation should be voluntary by the year 2020 and 100% of blood units should be screened for hepatitis B and C)
   b. Harm reduction in key populations
   c. Injection safety and infection control
3. Integrated Disease Surveillance Program
4. National program for Surveillance of Viral Hepatitis
5. Swachh Bharat Mission-Urban and Rural
6. Ministry of Drinking Water and Sanitation
7. Food Safety and Standards Authority of India (FSSAI)

BIBLIOGRAPHY
1. https://www.nhp.gov.in/national-viral-hepatitis-control-program-(nvhcp)_pg
2. https://vikaspedia.in/health/nrhm/national-health-programmes-1/national-viral-hepatitis-control-program
3. https://www.who.int/news-room/fact-sheets/detail/hepatitis-b
4. https://www.inasl.org.in/national-viral-hepatitis-control-program.pdf

CHAPTER 10

Non-communicable Diseases and Relevant National Health Programs

CHAPTER OUTLINE

10.1 Basics of Non-communicable Diseases (NCDs)
10.2 Common Non-communicable Diseases
10.3 Common Cancers (Breast, Cervical and Oral)
10.4 National Program for Prevention and Control of Cancer, Diabetes, Cardiovascular Diseases and Stroke (NPCDCS) and National Program for Healthcare of the Elderly (NPHCE)
10.5 National Cancer Control Program
10.6 National Program for Palliative Care
10.7 National Program for Control of Blindness and Visual Impairment (NPCBVI)
10.8 National Program for Prevention and Control of Deafness (NPPCD)
10.9 National Iodine Deficiency Disorders Control Program (NIDDCP)
10.10 National Tobacco Control Program

10.1 BASICS OF NON-COMMUNICABLE DISEASES (NCDs)

- **Definition:** Non-communicable diseases (NCDs), also known as chronic diseases, are not passed from person-to-person. They are of long duration and generally slow progression. NCDs do not result from an (acute) infectious process and hence are not communicable. They have a prolonged course and does not resolve spontaneously.
- **Differences between CDs and NCDs:**

Communicable diseases (CDs)	Non-communicable diseases (NCDs)
Sudden onset	Gradual onset
Single cause	Multiple causes
Usually, short natural history	Generally long natural history
Short treatment in most of cases	Prolonged treatment

Non-communicable Diseases and Relevant National Health Programs

Communicable diseases (CDs)	Non-communicable diseases (NCDs)
Cure is achieved	Care predominates
Single discipline approach	Multidisciplinary approach
Short follow-up	Prolonged follow-up
Back to normalcy	Adjustment may require with quality of life

- Cardiovascular diseases, diabetes, cancers and chronic respiratory diseases are common NCDs.
- They are the leading cause of death even ahead of communicable diseases, maternal, perinatal, and nutritional conditions (WHO 2014). This shows a rapid epidemiological transition with a shift in disease burden to NCDs.
- NCDs are rapidly increasing largely due to globalization, industrialization, and rapid urbanization with demographic and lifestyle changes.
- Tobacco use, physical inactivity, the harmful use of alcohol and unhealthy diets all increase the risk of dying from an NCD.
- Non-communicable diseases (NCDs) kill 41 million people each year, equivalent to 74% of all deaths globally.
- Cardiovascular diseases account for most NCD deaths, or 17.9 million people annually, followed by cancers (9.3 million), chronic respiratory diseases (4.1 million), and diabetes (2.0 million including kidney disease deaths caused by diabetes).
- In India, non-communicable diseases (NCDs) contribute to 60–63% of all deaths. The four major causes of NCD deaths are:
  1. Coronary heart disease, stroke, and hypertension (45%)
  2. Chronic respiratory disease (22%)
  3. Cancers (12%)
  4. Diabetes (3%)
- 1 in 4 Indians has a risk of dying from an NCD before they reach the age of 70.
- At national level, prevalence of tobacco consumption among >15 years of age is 38% in males and 9% in females (NFHS5).
- Globally the prevalence of tobacco consumption is 22.3%, and 36.7% of all men and 7.8% of the women.
- Rapid increase in obesity and overweight is seen as prevalence of obesity increasing from 9.3% to 18.6% in males and from 12.6% to 20.7% in females.
- In India, 21.3% of women and 24% of men aged above 15 have hypertension.
- The level of physical inactivity among Indian adults is around 13%.

Major Risk Factors for NCDs

Non-modifiable Risk Factors

There are risk factors which cannot be modified or changed as they are inherent in nature.
- **Age:** As age increases the risk of NCDs increases.
- **Gender:** Both male and female are at risk of NCDs but male is slightly on higher side but after menopause among women the risk of NCDs increases multiple times.
- **Family history:** The chances of getting some NCDs are higher if a close family member-parents, siblings also have the disease.

Modifiable Risk Factors

These are the risk factors which can be modified by change in behavior.
- **Diet:** Poor in fruits and vegetables and rich in salt, sugar and fat are at high risk for NCDs.
- **Obesity:** BMI >30 kg/m² put person at higher risk.
- **Tobacco:** People start to consume tobacco for various reasons like:
  - Peer pressure, curiosity, media influence, enjoyment
  - Family history of tobacco use
  - To kill hunger
  - For toothache (toothpain) relief
  - As stress/tension reliever/relaxation
- **Dangerous impact of tobacco (Fig. 10.1):**

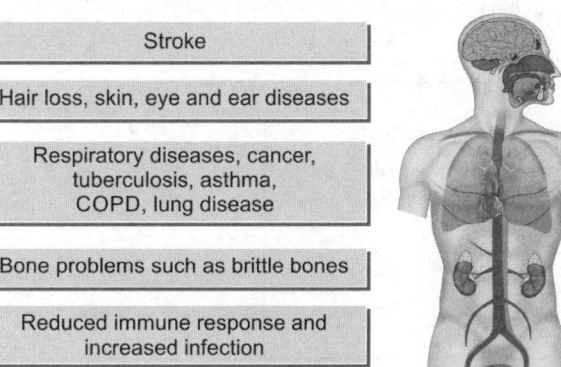

Fig. 10.1: Dangerous impact of tobacco.

- Second-hand smoke (SHS) is the inhalation of smoke breathed out by a smoker including smoke from the burning end of cigarettes, cigars, pipes and bidis. It is also called passive smoking or environmental tobacco smoke (ETS).
- **Children and second-hand smoke:**
  - One in three children in India aged 2 months to 5 years is exposed to SHS.
  - Nearly two out of six deaths due to SHS worldwide occurs in children under five
  - One in four children is exposed to SHS at home
  - Children exposed to SHS fall sick very often and have frequent attacks of asthma, pneumonia and bronchitis
- **Alcohol:** Harmful use of alcohol is linked with NCDs. WHO recently quoted that actually there is no safe limit of alcohol intake.
- **Physical activity:** Lack of physical activity not only the reason for overweight or obesity, but also increases risk of getting NCDs.
- **Stress:** Stress is linked with all modifiable risk factors responsible for NCDs. It influences the physical activity, diet and even consumption of tobacco and alcohol.

Classification of all risk factors for NCDs: Intermediate risk factors as result of above mentioned modifiable and non-modifiable risk factors explained here **(Fig. 10.2)**:

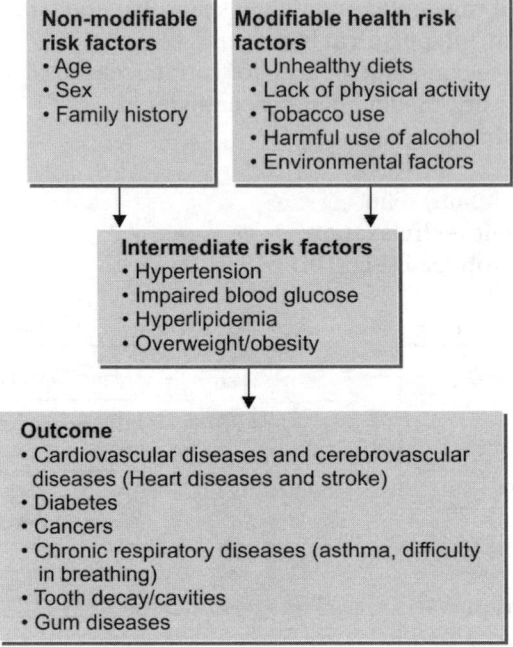

Fig. 10.2: NCD risk factors.

These risk factors also can be categorized as **Physiological** (obesity, high blood sugar, high blood pressure, high cholesterol), **Biological** (age, gender, family history), **Environmental** (pollution including air, water and food) and **Social** (poverty, culture and living/working conditions).

Prevention of NCDs

There are certain targets for these risk factors as shown in **Figure 10.3** to be achieved by the year 2025:

- **Those with an identified NCD:** This group will benefit from appropriate treatment of the NCD, an assessment of risk factors and guidance to modify the risk factors for better control of the NCD, preventing other NCDs and preventing complications from the NCD.
- **Those with risk factors and undiagnosed NCD:** This group will benefit from early detection and intervention for the NCD and guidance to modify the risk factors.
- **Those with risk factors but no NCD:** This group will benefit from guidance to modify the risk factors to lower risk for NCD and early warning signals.
- **Health persons without risk factors:** This group will benefit from encouragement to lead a healthy lifestyle with awareness on risk factors and ways of avoiding them.

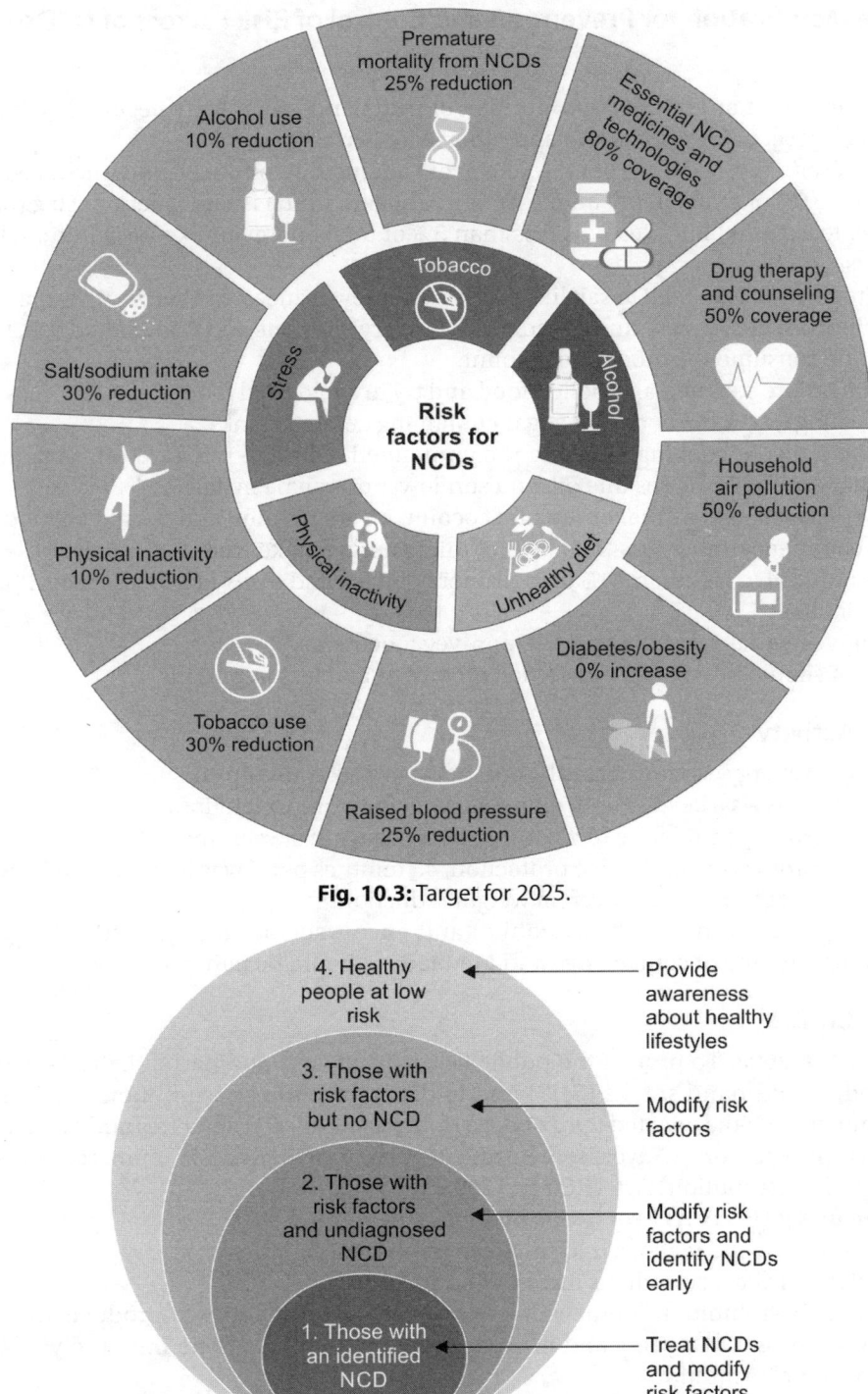

Fig. 10.3: Target for 2025.

Fig. 10.4: Relationship between extent of risk factor for NCD and modes of intervention.

Lifestyle Modification for Prevention and Control of Risk Factors of NCDs

Diet
- Consumption of at least 400 gm per day of fruits and green leafy vegetables excluding potatoes, sweet potatoes, cassava and other starchy roots.
- Intake of salt must be <5 gm per day and avoid adding salt to cooked and uncooked food.
- Less than 10% of total energy intake from free sugars which is equivalent to 50 g (or about 12 level teaspoons) but ideally is less than 5% of total energy intake for additional health benefits.
- Food items which are high in salt like pickles, chutneys, sauces and ketchups, papads, chips and salted biscuits, cheese and salted butter, bakery products and dried salted fish, these all should be consumed in moderate amount.
- Consume more steamed and boiled food and try to avoid fried food.
- Avoid eating fast/junk foods and sugar containing aerated drinks.
- Mixture of oils in cooking is highly recommended. Oils like mustard oil, soya bean oil, groundnut oil, olive oil, sesame oil, and sunflower oil can be mixed.
- Ghee, vanaspati, margarine, butter and coconut oil are harmful and should be moderated.
- It is recommended that less than 30% of total energy intake from fats, intake of saturated fats be reduced to less than 10% of total energy intake and *trans*-fats to less than 1% of total energy intake.
- For non-vegetarians, avoid frying the non-veg food items.
- Red meat should be consumed in small quantities and less frequently.

Physical Activity
- To increase energy expenditure, physical activity is a key determinant.
- Regular exercise is a key factor in either weight control or weight loss.
- Exercise regularly (moderate to vigorous) for 5–7 days in a week and at least 30 minutes per day gives cardiovascular disease protection, 45 minutes per day is good for fitness while 60 minutes per day has been proven in weight reduction.
- Discourage screen time (TV or mobile) and encourage outdoor activities like cycling, gardening, etc. and of course Yoga and Meditation should be part of life.

Tobacco Control
- **COTPA Act, 2003:** To protect the public from the adverse and harmful effects of tobacco use and second-hand smoke (SHS) and to discourage the consumption of tobacco, the Government of India enacted the Tobacco Control law titled "Cigarettes and other Tobacco Products (Prohibition of Advertisement and Regulation of Trade and Commerce, Production, Supply and Distribution) Act, (COTPA) 2003".
- **Section of Act (COTPA) Provisions of the Act:**
  - Section 4: No one is allowed to smoke in public places
  - Section 5: Tobacco products must not be advertised
  - Section 6: Prohibition on the sale of cigarettes or other tobacco products to a person below the age of 18 years and in an area within a radius of one hundred yards of any educational institution
  - Sections 7, 8 and 9: Tobacco packets should carry warnings about the risks of using tobacco.

Prevention, Screening and Management of Non-communicable Diseases at Different Level of Health facilities

At Community Level
- Population empanelment, support screening for universal screening for population—age 30 years and above for hypertension, diabetes, and three common cancers—Oral, Breast and Cervical Cancer
- Health promotion activities—to promote healthy lifestyle and address risk factors
- Early detection and referral for respiratory disorders—COPD, Epilepsy, Cancer, Diabetes, Hypertension and occupational diseases (pneumoconiosis, dermatitis, lead poisoning) and Fluorosis
- Mobilization activities at village level, schools and other community based institutions—for primary and secondary prevention
- Treatment compliance and follow-up for positive cases
- Counseling on steps to perform self-examination of breast
- Use of IEC material regarding prevention of NCDs in community

Care at the Health and Wellness Center-Sub-Health Centers
- Screening and treatment compliance for hypertension and diabetes, with referral if needed
- Screening and follow-up care for occupational diseases (pneumoconiosis, dermatitis, lead poisoning); fluorosis; respiratory disorders (COPD and asthma) and epilepsy
- Cancer—screening for oral, breast and cervical cancer and referral for suspected cases of other cancers
- Confirmation and referral for deaddiction—tobacco/alcohol/substance abuse
- Treatment compliance and follow-up for all diagnosed cases
- Linking with specialists and undertaking two-way referral for complications
- Sensitization of community to form patient support groups
- Conduct yoga sessions

Care at the Referral Site
- Diagnosis, treatment and management of complications of hypertension and diabetes
- Diagnosis, treatment and follow-up of cancers (esp. cervical, breast, oral)
- Diagnosis and management of occupational diseases such as silicosis, fluorosis and respiratory disorders (COPD and asthma) and epilepsy

BIBLIOGRAPHY

1. https://main.mohfw.gov.in/sites/default/files/Training%20Module%20for%20Medical%20Officers%20for%20Prevention%2C%20Control%20and%20Population%20Level%20Screening%20of%20NCDs_1.pdf
2. https://main.mohfw.gov.in/sites/default/files/Module%20for%20Multi-Purpose%20Workers%20-%20Prevention%2C%20Screening%20and%20Control%20of%20Common%20NCDS_2.pdf
3. https://www.who.int/news-room/fact-sheets/detail/healthy-diet

10.2 COMMON NON-COMMUNICABLE DISEASES

DIABETES MELLITUS

- Diabetes is a chronic disease that occurs either when the pancreas does not produce enough insulin or when the body cannot effectively use the insulin it produces. It results in hyperglycemia.
- As per the NFHS-5, blood sugar level-high or very high (>140 mg/dL) or taking medicine to control blood sugar level (%) among women and men is 13.5% and 15.6% respectively.

Risk Factors

- Overweight
- Physically inactivity (exercise less than 3 times a week)
- High blood pressure
- Impaired fasting glucose or impaired glucose tolerance
- Triglyceride and/or cholesterol levels are higher than normal
- Parents/siblings or grandparents have or had diabetes
- If she has had diabetes or even mild elevation of blood sugars during pregnancy
- If she delivered a baby whose birth weight was 4 kg or more

Presenting complaints where we need to suspect diabetes are:

- Polydipsia (excess thirst), polyuria (excess urination), polyphagia (excess hunger) with loss of weight
- Recurrent and frequent infections
- Non-healing wounds
- Unexplained lassitude (lack of energy) and fatigue

Etiological Classification of Diabetes Mellitus

- **Type 1 diabetes (absolute insulin deficiency):**
    - "Insulin-dependent diabetes mellitus" (IDDM)
    - It is mainly immune mediated or idiopathic.
    - This may be due to genetics, changes in environmental risk factors and/or viral infections.
    - Body does not produce insulin at all.
    - It can affect people of any age, but onset usually occurs in children, adolescents and younger age group.
    - Its management requires daily insulin injections in order to control the blood sugar.
- **Type 2 diabetes (relative insulin deficiency):**
    - "Non-insulin-dependent diabetes mellitus" (NIDDM)
    - It is the most common type of diabetes (95%).
    - The body produces some insulin, but not enough or the cells cannot use this insulin properly or efficiently.
    - It usually affects adults. People with family history, excess body weight, unhealthy lifestyle-poor dietary habits, lack/low of physical activity, tobacco and alcohol consumption, etc. are at higher risk for this type of diabetes.
    - Symptoms may be similar to those of type 1 diabetes but are often less marked. As a result, the disease may be diagnosed several years after onset, after complications have already arisen.

- People with type 2 diabetes usually treated with oral medication but may also require insulin injections.
- **Gestational diabetes mellitus:**
  - It occurs during pregnancy.
  - It is found in 10–15% of total pregnancy in various studies.
  - Screening of all pregnant women should be done in first antenatal visit. If first test is negative then blood sugar should be done again at 24–28 weeks of gestation.
  - GDM is associated with a risk of complications during pregnancy and delivery.
  - The children of women with GDM are at an increased risk of type 2 diabetes in the future.
- **Other specific types include:**
  - Genetic defect of beta cell function
  - Genetic defects in insulin action
  - Diseases of the exocrine pancreas
  - Endocrinopathies
  - Drug or chemical-mediated
  - Infections
  - Uncommon forms of immune-mediated diabetes
  - Other genetic syndromes associated with diabetes.

Diagnosis

Criteria based on Plasma Glucose Level

Test	Results	Interpretation
Fasting plasma glucose (no food intake for at least 8 hours)	≥126 mg/dL	Diabetes
	110–125 mg/dL	Impaired fasting glucose
	70–110 mg/dL	Normal
Postprandial blood sugar (PPBS) (2 hours after intake of food or 75 g glucose)	≥200 mg/dL	Diabetes
	140–199 mg/dL	Impaired glucose tolerance
	<140 mg/dL	Normal
Random blood sugar (RBS) or glucose + presence of symptoms of diabetes	≥200 mg/dL	Diabetes

Criteria Based on HbA1c

Test	Results	Interpretation
HbA1c	≥6.5%	Diabetes
	5.7–6.4%	Impaired fasting glucose
	≤5.6%	Normal

Criteria for Diagnosis of Prediabetes

Impaired fasting glucose	≥110 mg/dL to <126 mg/dL
Impaired glucose tolerance	≥140 mg/dL <200 mg/dL

Management of Diabetes

- **Modify lifestyle:** Diet and physical activity.
- Reduce insulin resistance through reduction in weight, specifically reduction of fat mass.
- **Pharmacological treatment:** Metformin/Sulfonylureas.

- A healthy diet, regular physical activity, maintaining a normal body weight and avoiding tobacco use are ways to prevent or delay the onset of type 2 diabetes.
- Diabetes can be treated and its consequences avoided or delayed with diet, physical activity, medication and regular screening and treatment for complications.

Foot Care Advice to the Patients
- Inspect your feet daily for cracks, blisters, infections, and injuries as we usually able to see a problem before we feel it.
- Cleanse your feet with using warm water (avoid hot water) and mild soap. Dry your feet with a soft towel and special attention for drying the area in between the toes.
- Apply oil to moisturize dry skin.
- Clip toenails straight across. Use a nail cutter; don't use a scissor and also smooth down the edges. If it is difficult for you to reach your feet you may have help from someone experienced trim your nails.
- Always wear something on your feet (socks, slippers, shoes) to protect from injury - even in your house.
- Choose soft good shoes. Let them be a size bigger that what you feel is appropriate. Wear socks made of cotton or wool (in winter).

Complications
- Cardiovascular disease (Angiopathy)
- Nerve damage (Neuropathy)
- Kidney damage (Nephropathy)
- Eye damage (Retinopathy)
- Diabetic foot ulcer
- Skin infections
- **Acute emergencies like** diabetic ketoacidosis, nonketotic hyperosmolar diabetic coma, hypoglycemia/hyperglycemia, diabetic coma and respiratory infections

BIBLIOGRAPHY
1. http://rchiips.org/nfhs/NFHS-5_FCTS/India.pdf
2. https://main.mohfw.gov.in/sites/default/files/Operational%20Guidelines%20on%20Prevention%2C%20Screening%20and%20Control%20of%20Common%20NCDs_1.pdf

HYPERTENSION
- Hypertension or 'High blood pressure' is a pathological condition which increases the work load on the heart, i.e., heart has to pump harder than normal for blood to get to all parts of the body.
- Hypertension is also called as "silent killer" as it exists without causing any warning signs or symptoms. So, it is very important to screen all individuals 30 years of age and above at least once in a year.
- As per NFHS-5 data, prevalence of elevated blood pressure (Systolic ≥140 mm of Hg and/or Diastolic ≥90 mm of Hg) or taking medicine to control blood pressure (%) among women and men are 21.3% and 24.0% respectively.

There are two types of hypertension:
- **Primary/Essential:** Primary or "essential" hypertension has no known cause, however many of the lifestyle factors are associated with this condition. It is the main type of hypertension as 90–95% of patients are having essential hypertension.
- **Secondary:** Secondary hypertension is caused by some other medical conditions/problem or the use of certain medications. Secondary hypertension is seen only in very few individuals in the community.

  The causes of secondary hypertension include:
  - **Kidney diseases (renovascular disease and chronic renal disease):** Most common cause
  - **Endocrine disorders:** Hyperthyroidism, Cushing's syndrome, pheochromocytoma, hyperaldosteronism, hyperparathyroidism
  - Coarctation of the aorta and non-specific aortoarteritis
  - Pregnancy
  - Contraceptive pills, etc.

Risk Factors for Hypertension
- Age
- Physical inactivity
- Smoking
- Excessive alcohol consumption
- Overweight or obese
- Salt take in excess (>5 g per day)
- Consumption of foods which are high in salt, fat and processed
- Stress
- Family history

Guide for Proper Measurement of Blood Pressure
- Ensure the patient is sitting comfortably with back supported, with their feet flat on the floor.
- The legs should not be crossed.
- Ensure the measurement is taken in a quiet room with comfortable temperature.
- Make sure if patient has not consumed tea or smoked cigarette/bidi within last 1 hour, had not done some heavy work or is not anxious or at discomfort.
- It is suggested to take a minimum of 2 readings at interval of 1 minute. The average of those readings should be used to represent the patient's blood pressure.
- Additional readings should be taken if the difference between the first two is greater than 5 mm Hg, and then the average of these multiple readings is used.

Classification of Hypertension

Category	Systolic blood pressure (mm Hg)	and/or	Diastolic blood pressure (mm Hg)
Normal	<120	And	<80
Elevated	120–129	And	<80
Hypertensive stage-1	130–139	or	80–89
Hypertensive stage-2	≥140	or	≥90
Hypertensive crisis	>180	And/or	>120

Common Symptoms of Hypertension
- Most people with hypertension have no warning signs or symptoms.
- Symptoms may occur, such as early morning headaches, nosebleeds, irregular heart rhythms, vision changes, and buzzing in the ears.
- Severe hypertension can cause fatigue, nausea, vomiting, confusion, anxiety, chest pain, and muscle tremors.
- **Complications** may occur like heart failure, kidney, eye problems. Some patients may develop acute severe emergencies as heart attack or stroke or sudden loss of vision.

Tracking of blood pressure: It has been seen that who were normotensive in childhood age they remain normotensive in adulthood as well while who were hypertensive in childhood they also become hypertensive in adulthood also.

Rule of Halves
- Only about half of hypertensive subjects in general population of most of the developed countries are aware of condition, only half of those aware of the problem were being treated and only half of those treated were considered adequately treated.
- It means only one in eight of the hypertensive population are receiving optimal treatment.
- But nowadays as result of improvement in screening and treatment these things are getting improved.

Prevention and Management
Prevention
- **Dietary approaches to stop hypertension (DASH Diet):** It advocates low in saturated fat, cholesterol and total fat while increase intake of fruits, vegetables along with consumption of Fat-free or low-fat milk and milk products. It recommends reducing salt intake (to less than 5 g daily)
- Being physically active on a regular basis
- Avoiding use of tobacco
- Reducing alcohol consumption
- Eliminating/reducing trans fats in diet

Management
- Reducing and managing stress
- Regularly checking blood pressure
- Treating high blood pressure
- Managing other medical conditions

BIBLIOGRAPHY
1. https://www.acc.org/latest-in-cardiology/articles/2017/11/08/11/47/mon-5pm-bp-guideline-aha-2017
2. https://main.mohfw.gov.in/sites/default/files/Module%20for%20Multi-Purpose%20Workers%20-%20Prevention%2C%20Screening%20and%20Control%20of%20Common%20NCDS_2.pdf

CARDIOVASCULAR DISEASES

Cardiovascular diseases (CVDs) are a group of disorders of the heart and blood vessels. They include:
- Coronary heart disease—a disease of the blood vessels supplying the heart muscle
- Cerebrovascular disease—a disease of the blood vessels supplying the brain
- Peripheral arterial disease—a disease of blood vessels supplying the arms and legs
- Rheumatic heart disease—damage to the heart muscle and heart valves from rheumatic fever, caused by streptococcal bacteria
- Congenital heart disease—birth defects that affect the normal development and functioning of the heart caused by malformations of the heart structure from birth
- Deep vein thrombosis and pulmonary embolism—blood clots in the leg veins, which can dislodge and move to the heart and lungs

The common risk factors are as follows:
- Advancing age
- Family history
- Gender—a man is at a greater risk of heart disease than a pre-menopausal woman. But once past the menopause, a woman's risk is similar to a mans.
- Unhealthy diet—high in fat, sugar, salt, animal fat and low in fruits, vegetables, whole grains and whole pulses
- Lack of physical activity/low physical activity
- Use of tobacco-smoking or chewing tobacco and passive smoking
- Excess intake of alcohol
- Hypertension
- High blood glucose level/diabetes
- Abnormal blood lipids (hyperlipidemia): High total cholesterol, LDL-cholesterol and triglyceride levels, and low levels of HDL cholesterol
- Being overweight/obese
- Stress, social isolation, anxiety and depression

Heart Attack

A heart attack (myocardial infarction) occurs when the heart's supply of blood is stopped due to deposition of fat, thus blockage in the blood vessel of the heart. It is defined as severe chest pain for more than 30 minutes, radiating to left arm, shoulder or jaw and not relieved by pain killers.

Warning Signs of Heart Attack

- Intense pain, pressure or constriction in the center of the chest that lasts more than a few minutes, or that goes away and comes back
- Discomfort in other areas of the upper body such as pain or discomfort in one or both arms, the back, neck, jaw or stomach
- Shortness of breath with or without chest discomfort
- Other signs like sweating, nausea or lightheadedness

Simple Ways of Preventing Heart Attack

- Lifestyle changes like eating a healthy diet, being physically active, avoiding the use of tobacco in any form/avoiding exposure to second-hand smoke, reducing the intake of

alcohol amongst heavy drinkers, managing stress, maintain healthy weight, people who are overweight/obese should lose weight, restriction of caffeinated beverages, etc.
- Ensure that all above 30 years of age are screened annually for hypertension and diabetes.
- Blood pressure and blood sugar should be monitored regularly in high-risk individuals including those with a family history of heart attack.
- Motivate those with high blood pressure and high blood sugar to change their lifestyle and regularly take their medicines to keep the BP or glucose under control.
- Create awareness among the community on the warning signs of heart attack and these are both preventable and treatable.
- Create awareness among the community on the services available for early management of heart diseases in health facilities.
- Emphasize that if there are any signs of heart attack, she/he should seek immediate medical attention by a qualified health professional at the higher facilities.
- WHO's initiative as **"HEARTS"** technical package (Healthy-lifestyle counseling, Evidence-based treatment protocols, Access to essential medicines and technology, Risk-based management, Team-based care, and Systems for monitoring) provide a strategic approach to improve cardiovascular health in countries across the world.

BIBLIOGRAPHY

1. https://www.who.int/news-room/fact-sheets/detail/cardiovascular-diseases-(cvds)

STROKE

- Stroke is the second leading cause of death worldwide and 4th leading cause of death and 5th leading cause of disability adjusted life years (DALY) in India.
- **Stroke:** 'Rapidly developed clinical signs of focal (or global) disturbance of cerebral function, lasting more than 24 hours or leading to death, with no apparent cause other than of vascular origin'. (WHO)
- **Transient ischemic attack (TIA):** "A transient episode of neurological dysfunction caused by focal brain, spinal cord, or retinal ischemia without acute infarction". [AHA/ASA (2009)]
- **Risk factors for stroke:**
  - Hypertension, diabetes, heart diseases (including rheumatic valvular diseases), dyslipidemia, atrial fibrillation
  - Positive family history
  - Unhealthy diet, obesity
  - Lack of physical activity, stress
  - Tobacco use and excessive alcohol consumption
  - Sickle cell disease.

Presenting Features of Stroke
- Sudden numbness or weakness in the face, arm, or leg, especially on one side of the body
- Sudden confusion, trouble speaking, or difficulty understanding speech
- Sudden trouble seeing in one or both eyes

- Sudden trouble walking, dizziness, loss of balance, or lack of coordination
- Impairment or loss of consciousness

Presenting Features of TIA
- Transient weakness, numbness or paralysis of face, arm or leg, typically on one side of your body
- Transient slurred or garbled speech or difficulty understanding others
- Transient blindness in one or both eyes or double vision
- Curtain like appearance in front of eye (amaurosis fugax)
- Transient dizziness or loss of balance or coordination

Prevention

Primary Prevention
- Primary stroke prevention aims at reducing the likelihood of having a stroke by either reducing the chances of developing risk factors or controlling various risk factors that increase the chance of having a stroke.
- Usually, there are two strategies for primary prevention: Population-based and high-risk strategy.
- Recommended steps for primary stroke prevention includes: Management of hypertension and diabetes as per the guidelines, tobacco cessation and reduction of alcohol consumption, treatment of existing heart diseases like atrial fibrillation and valvular diseases and antiplatelet among high risk people.
- Lifestyle modifications always important for prevention of stroke.

Role of Nurse
- Derive the score based on CBAC to highlight risk factors
- Undertake blood pressure and blood glucose measurement
- Refer cases with high BP and blood glucose to the appropriate facility for confirmation and initiation of treatment plan
- Provide follow-up management for patients (monthly drug supply, periodic BP/blood sugar measurement, referral for complications)
- Supportive supervision for ASHAs conducting NCD screening
- Referring those who are suspected of any of the risk factors to MO of PHC
- Identify warning signs of stroke and referral
- In case of suspicion of stroke, refer the patient to nearest stroke-ready healthcare facility
- Create awareness among the community on the warning signs of heart attack and stroke and including delivering the message that these are both preventable and treatable
- Imparting education to women, men, adolescents, on what is stroke, what are the risk factors for stroke and how can someone decrease one's risk of having a stroke
- To motivate the patient to comply with home exercise program as prescribed by physiotherapists
- Encourage caregivers to comply with safety instructions and prescribed home exercise program
- Advise the patient and caregivers to maintain a diary for daily exercise and report any adverse event. Motivate the patient to use the affected side in activities of daily living

❏ Acronym for stroke is **FAST** (F–Face drooping, A–Arm numb/weak, S–Speech slurred, T–Time) [Time not to be wasted, should act fast for the treatment].

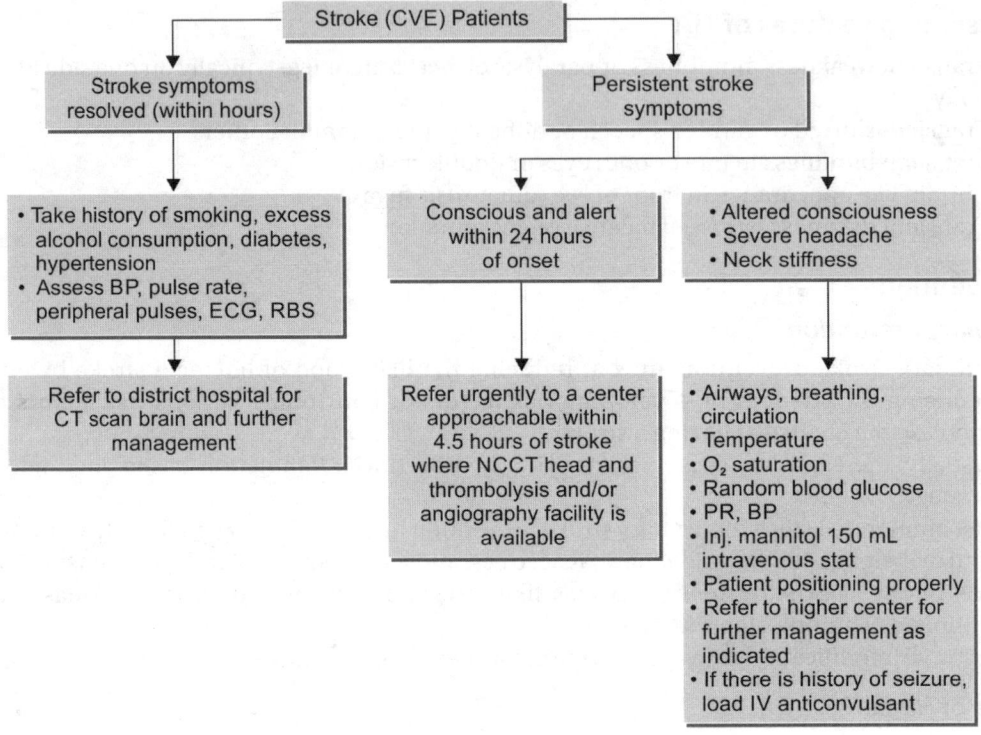

Fig. 10.5: Algorithm for stroke patients management at primary health center.

❏ **Secondary prevention:** This includes measures to reduce the risk of recurrence of stroke in patients who have had TIA or stroke.

BIBLIOGRAPHY

1. https://main.mohfw.gov.in/sites/default/files/Guidelines%20for%20Prevention%20and%20Managment%20of%20Stroke.pdf

OBESITY

❏ Obesity is usually the result of an imbalance between calories consumed and calories expended.
❏ Lifestyle changes like eating habits, increasing consumption of tobacco, alcohol and reduced physical activity affected the nutritional status which makes people overweight/obese.
❏ Obesity is now recognized as a chronic or non-communicable disease.

Non-communicable Diseases and Relevant National Health Programs

- "Double burden of malnutrition" many countries continue to deal with the problems undernutrition and experiencing a rapid upsurge in non-communicable disease risk factors such as obesity and overweight.
- It is not uncommon to find undernutrition and obesity co-existing within the same country, the same community and the same household.
- The common perception is that non-communicable diseases occur only in overweight or obese individuals. However, undernourished women are more likely to have low birth weight babies, who are at increased risk of developing non-communicable diseases when they grow into adults.
- In 2016, more than 1.9 billion adults, 18 years and older, were overweight. Of these over 650 million were obese. It means 39% of adults aged 18 years and over were overweight and 13% were obese.
- In India, as per NFHS-5, women who are overweight or obese (BMI ≥25.0 kg/m² and men who are overweight or obese (BMI ≥25.0 kg/m² are 24% and 22.95 respectively).

Causes of Overweight/Obese

- Family history
- Eating an unhealthy diet
- Lack of physical activity/low physical activity
- Depression, anxiety, stress, and low esteem can result in over eating
- Hormonal imbalance
- Over-feeding during infancy, childhood and adolescence predisposes to overweight/obesity during adulthood

Risks Associated with being Overweight/Obese

- Cardiovascular diseases and cerebrovascular diseases (stroke)
- Hyperlipidemia
- Hypertension
- Diabetes
- Musculoskeletal disorders (especially osteoarthritis)
- Sleep disorder
- Cancer—cancer of breast, cervix, ovary, liver, gallbladder, kidney, colon, rectum and prostrate
- Lung disorders
- Gallstones
- Psychological and social stigma that accompany being overweight and obese, those affected by these conditions are also vulnerable to discrimination in their personal and work lives, low self-esteem, and depression

Methods to diagnosis of obesity: The most accurate methods are underwater weighing, dual-energy X-ray absorptiometry (DEXA) scanning, computed tomography (CT), and magnetic resonance imaging (MRI) but are impractical for use in routine. Estimates of body fat by body mass index and waist provide relevant information and are easily implemented in a variety of practice settings.

- **BMI:**
  - BMI is body mass index.
  - It is the ratio of weight to height, calculated as weight (kg)/height (m²).

Table 10.1: Classification of weight status in adults as per BMI (WHO).

Classification	BMI (kilogram/m²)	Risk of comorbidities
Underweight	<18.5	Low (but risk of other clinical problems increased)
Normal weight	18.5–24.9	Average
Overweight:	≥25	
Pre-obese	≥25–29.9	Increased
Obesity Class 1	30–34.9	Moderate
Obesity Class 2	35–39.9	Severe
Extreme Obesity Class 3	≥40	Very severe

Table 10.2: Classification of weight status in Asian and Indian adults as per BMI.

Classification	BMI		
	Global population	Asian population	Indian population
Underweight	<18.5	<18.5	<18.5
Normal BMI	18.5–24.9	18.5–22.99	18.5–22.99
Overweight	≥25–29.9	23–26.99	23–24.99
Obesity	≥30.0	≥27.0	≥25.0

Other methods:
- *Ponderal index*:

$$PI = \frac{\text{Height (cm)}}{3\sqrt{\text{Body weight (kg)}}}$$

- *Broca index:*
Ideal weight = Height (cm) − 100
- *Lorentz formula:*

$$LF = Ht\,(cm) - 100 - \frac{Ht\,(cm) - 150}{2\,(\text{women})\,\text{or}\,4\,(\text{men})}$$

- *Corpulence index* (normal <1.2)

$$CI = \frac{\text{Actual weight}}{\text{Desirable weight}}$$

- **Skin fold thickness (SFT):** It is rapid and non-invasive method of fat assessment. Fat is measured at total 4 sites: Mid-triceps (most reliable), biceps, sub-scapular, supra-iliac with help of 'Harpenden skin fold calipers'. Cut off: Sum > 50 mm in girls and Sum > 40 mm in boys indicate obesity.
- **Waist hip ratio (WHR):** High WHR (>1.0 in men and >0.85 in women) indicates abdominal fat accumulation. Good predictor of risk of cardiovascular diseases. Women who have high risk waist-to-hip ratio (≥0.85) and men who have high-risk waist-to-hip ratio (≥0.90) as per NFHS-5 are 56.7% and 47.7% respectively.
- **Waist circumference:** It is measured at the midpoint between the lower border of the rib cage and the iliac crest. Globally, waist circumference ≥102 cm in men and ≥88 cm in females while in India ≥90 cm in men and ≥80 cm in females is associated with an increased risk of metabolic complications.

- **Waist height ratio (WHtR):** It is now more being used as WHO has declared WHtR as "best indicator" of cardiovascular risk. It is age and sex independent. Cut-off for WHtR: 0.5

Prevention of Obesity

- Limit energy intake from total fats and sugars
- Increase consumption of fruit and vegetables, as well as legumes, whole grains and nuts
- Engage in regular physical activity (60 minutes a day for children and 150 minutes spread through the week for adults)
- Exclusive breastfeeding reduces the risk of infants becoming overweight or obese

BIBLIOGRAPHY

1. https://www.maso.org.my/spom/chap3.pdf
2. https://www.who.int/news-room/fact-sheets/detail/obesity-and-overweight
3. http://rchiips.org/nfhs/NFHS-5_FCTS/India.pdf
4. Purnell JQ. Definitions, Classification, and Epidemiology of Obesity. [Updated 2018 Apr 12]. In: Feingold KR, Anawalt B, Boyce A, et al., editors. Endotext [Internet]. South Dartmouth (MA): MDText.com, Inc.; 2000-. Available from: https://www.ncbi.nlm.nih.gov/books/NBK279167/

BLINDNESS

- **Definitions of blindness and visual impairment:**

Blindness	Presenting visual acuity <3/60 in better eye with available correction
Severe visual impairment (SVI)	Presenting visual acuity <6/60–3/60 in better eye with available correction
Moderate visual impairment (MVI)	Presenting visual acuity <6/18–6/60 in better eye with available correction
Early visual impairment (EVI)	Presenting visual acuity <6/12–6/18 in better eye with available correction
Moderate severe visual impairment (MSVI)	Presenting visual acuity <6/18–3/60 in better eye with available correction
Visual impairment (VI)	Presenting visual acuity <6/18 in better eye with available correction
Functional low vision	A person with impairment of visual functioning even after treatment and/or standard refractive correction, and a visual acuity of less than 6/18 to light perception, or a visual field of less than 10 degree from the point of fixation, but who uses, or is potentially able to use, vision for planning and/or execution of a task
Blindness (BCVA/Pinhole <3/60)	Best corrected visual acuity <3/60 in better eye

- Prevalence of blindness in all age groups: 0.36%
- Prevalence of blindness in population aged ≥50 years: 1.99%
- Prevalence of severe visual impairment (SVI) in all age groups: 0.35%
- Prevalence of severe visual impairment (SVI) in population aged ≥50 years: 1.96%

- **Causes of blindness:**
  - Major cause of blindness in population aged ≥50 years is cataract (71.2%) followed by corneal opacity (8.2%) while major cause of blindness in population aged ≤50 years of age is corneal opacity (37.5%).
  - Major cause of visual impairment in population aged ≥50 years is cataract (71.2%) followed by refractive error (13.4%) while major cause of visual impairment population aged ≤50 years of age is refractive error (29.6%).
  - Overall cataract is the most common cause of blindness (66.2%).
  - Overall, the most common cause of early visual impairment is refractive error (70.6%) while cataract is the principal causes of severe visual impairment (80.7%), and moderate visual impairment (70.2%).
- **Vitamin A deficiency and blindness:**
  Classification of Xerophthalmia:
  - Night blindness (XN)
  - Conjunctival xerosis (X1A)
  - Bitot spots (X1B)
  - Corneal xerosis (X2)
  - Corneal ulceration/keratomalacia <⅓ corneal surface (X3A)
  - Corneal ulceration/keratomalacia ≥⅓ corneal surface (X3B)
  - Corneal scar (XS)
  - Xerophthalmic fundus (XF)

Prevalence criteria for determining the public health significance of xerophthalmia and vitamin A deficiency in children aged 6 months to 6 years:

Indicator	Minimum prevalence, %
Night blindness (XN)	>1
Bitot spots (X1B)	>0.5
Corneal xerosis/corneal ulceration/keratomalacia (X2/X3A/X3B)	>0.01
Corneal scar (XS)	>0.05

Prophylactic Vitamin A as per the following Dosage Schedule

- 1,00,000 IU at 9 months with measles immunization
- 2,00,000 IU every 6 months, up to the age of 5 years

SAFE strategy: This strategy was launched in 1996 by WHO to eliminate trachoma.
- **S: Surgery** for trichiasis and entropion
- **A: Antibiotic** (use of Azithromycin as mass treatment)
- **F: Facial hygiene** (facial cleanliness)
- **E: Environmental** (environmental improvement)

GET 2020: This campaign is launched in 1997 for the Global Elimination of Trachoma by the year 2020.

Vision 2020

- To eliminate avoidable blindness (preventable and curable) by 2020 **(Fig. 10.6).**

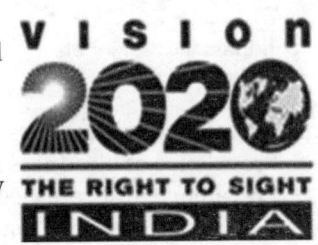

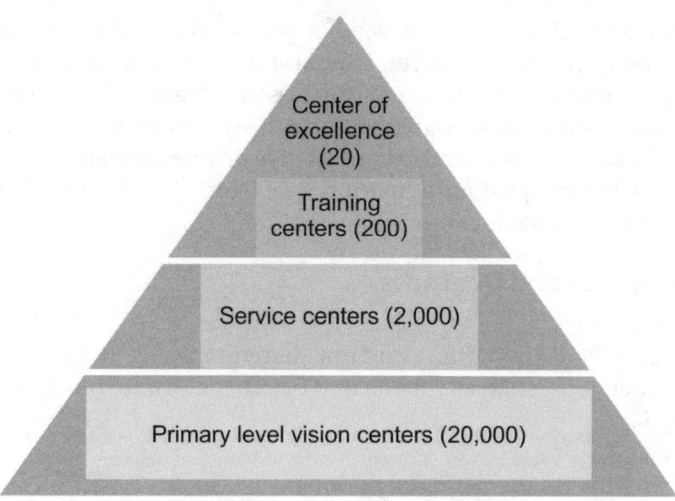

Fig. 10.6: Structure of vision 2020.

Global vision 2020 (5 diseases)	Indian vision 2020 (7 diseases)
Cataract	Cataract
Refractive errors and low vision	Refractive errors and low version
Childhood blindness	Childhood blindness
Trachoma	Trachoma (focal)
Onchocerciasis	Glaucoma Diabetic retinopathy Corneal blindness

BIBLIOGRAPHY

1. https://npcbvi.mohfw.gov.in/writeReadData/mainlinkFile/File341.pdf.

DEAFNESS

Hearing Loss and Deafness

- Human ear is sensitive to sound frequency: 20–20,000 Hz.
- Daily maximum tolerable sound level to human ear (without substantial damage to their hearing): 85–90 dB.
- Auditory fatigue appears in: 90 dB
- Usual noise level during whispering 20–30 dB, during routine conversation 60–70 dB while highest during Jet take off 150–160 dB which can lead to mechanical damage to eardrum.
- As per WHO, a person who is not able to hear as well as someone with normal hearing–hearing thresholds of 20 dB or better in both ears—is said to have hearing loss.
- 'Disabling' hearing loss refers to hearing loss greater than 35 decibels (dB) in the better hearing ear.

- Hearing loss may be mild, moderate, severe, or profound. It can affect one ear or both ears, and leads to difficulty in hearing conversational speech or loud sounds.
- 'Hard of hearing' refers to people with hearing loss ranging from mild to severe. People who are hard of hearing usually communicate through spoken language and can benefit from hearing aids, cochlear implants, and other assistive devices as well as captioning.
- 'Deaf' people mostly have profound hearing loss, which implies very little or no hearing. They often use sign language for communication.

Causes of Hearing Loss and Deafness

- **Prenatal period**
  - Genetic factors-include hereditary and non-hereditary
  - Intrauterine infections, such as rubella and cytomegalovirus infection
- **Perinatal period**
  - Birth asphyxia
  - Hyperbilirubinemia (in the neonatal period)
  - Low-birth weight
  - Other perinatal morbidities and their management
- **Childhood and adolescence**
  - Chronic ear infections (chronic suppurative otitis media)
  - Collection of fluid in the ear (chronic **nonsuppurative** otitis media)
  - Meningitis and other infections
- **Adulthood and older age**
  - Chronic diseases
  - Smoking
  - Otosclerosis
  - Age-related sensorineural degeneration
  - Sudden sensorineural hearing loss
- **Factors across the life span** (all age group)
  - Cerumen impaction (impacted ear wax)
  - Trauma to the ear or head
  - Loud noise/loud sounds
  - Ototoxic medicines
  - Work related ototoxic chemicals
  - Nutritional deficiencies
  - Viral infections and other ear conditions
  - Delayed onset or progressive genetic hearing loss

The Impact of Unaddressed Hearing Loss

- Communication and speech issues
- Cognition development suffers
- Children with hearing loss usually do not receive schooling and adults with hearing loss usually remains unemployed which indirectly affects overall economy
- Hearing loss or deafness brings social isolation, stigma and loneliness
- Hearing loss is one of the leading cause of DALYs (Disability adjusted life years)

Prevention

Effective strategies for reducing hearing loss at different stages of the life course include:
- Immunization (e.g., MR vaccine)
- Good maternal and childcare practices
- Genetic counseling
- Identification and management of common ear conditions
- Occupational hearing conservation programs for noise and chemical exposure
- Safe listening strategies for the reduction of exposure to loud sounds in recreational settings
- Rational use of medicines to prevent ototoxic hearing loss

More details are given in the Chapter 10.8.

BIBLIOGRAPHY

1. https://www.who.int/news-room/fact-sheets/detail/deafness-and-hearing-loss

THYROID DISEASES

- Diseases of thyroid gland are the second most common form of endocrine disorders.
- Diseases of thyroid gland may occur due to problems with thyroid gland itself (primary), pituitary gland (secondary) and hypothalamus (tertiary).
- Thyroid diseases are often serious and sometimes life threatening but usually manageable, curable and even preventable.
- Broadly, there are two types: hypothyroidism and hyperthyroidism.

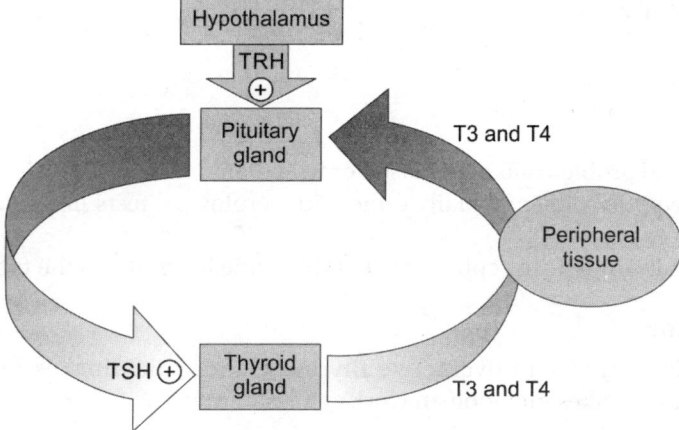

Fig. 10.7: Regulation of thyroid hormone.

Hypothyroidism

- Hypothyroidism is the most common type of thyroid disorder.
- Hypothyroidism can be overt (OH) or subclinical (SCH).

- In overt hypothyroidism, S.TSH levels are elevated and S.T4/Free T4 (FT4) levels are low. S.TSH ≥10 mIU/l is taken as OH irrespective of FT4 levels. In SCH, the TSH level is elevated (≤10 mIU/l) with normal serum T4/FT4.
- Women, family history, thyroid surgery or radiation, other metabolic problems like diabetes are common risk for hypothyroidism.
- Hypothyroidism during pregnancy may affect fetus development and may lead to neonatal hypothyroidism and even results in cretinism. So, screening of hypothyroidism during pregnancy is very important.
- **Causes** of hypothyroidism:
  - **Autoimmune (Hashimoto's Thyroiditis):** Most common cause
  - As consequence of treatment of overactive thyroid gland
  - **Pituitary gland dysfunction:** Secondary hypothyroidism
  - Iodine deficiency.

Presenting Signs and Symptoms of Hypothyroidism

- Dull facial expressions
- Tiredness (fatigue)
- Cold intolerance
- Hoarse voice
- Slow speech
- Puffy and swollen face
- Weight gain
- Constipation
- Sparse, coarse, and dry hair
- Coarse, dry, and thickened skin
- Carpal tunnel syndrome
- Bradycardia
- Muscle cramps
- Sides of eyebrows thin or fall out
- Confusion
- Menstrual related problems like increased or irregular
- Diagnosis of hypothyroidism usually done with serological tests like serum TSH, free T3 and T4 level.
- Treatment usually done with replacement of thyroxine hormone in the tablet form.

Hyperthyroidism

- Hyperthyroidism means an overactive thyroid gland which makes too much thyroid hormone and that makes metabolism work at a faster rate.
- **Causes:**
  - **Graves' disease: It is the most common cause:** It is an autoimmune disorder. Mostly affects young to middle-aged women and also tends to run in families.
  - **Toxic nodular goiter:** 1 or more nodules of the thyroid gland become too active.
  - **Thyroiditis:** It occurs when the thyroid becomes irritated. It temporarily causes the thyroid to be overactive. The thyroid then often becomes underactive.
  - Taking too much thyroid hormone medicine to treat an underactive thyroid
  - Having too much iodine in your diet

- Having a noncancer (benign) tumor in the pituitary gland that makes your thyroid overactive.

What are the Signs and Symptoms of Hyperthyroidism?
- Nervousness
- Irritability
- Sweating more than normal
- Thinning of the skin
- Fine, brittle hair
- Weak muscles, especially in the upper arms and thighs
- Tremor
- Palpitations
- High blood pressure
- More bowel movements than normal
- Weight loss
- Problems sleeping
- Prominent eyes (exophthalmos)
- Sensitivity to bright light
- Confusion
- Irregular menstrual cycle
- Tiredness
- Thyroid gland is larger than normal (goiter)

How is Hyperthyroidism Diagnosed?
- **Blood tests:** To measure the amount of thyroid hormone and thyroid stimulating hormone.
- **Thyroid ultrasound:** This test can see if it is there any nodules.
- **Thyroid scan:** This test uses a radioactive substance to make an image of the thyroid.

How is Hyperthyroidism Treated?
- **Medicine:** It can help lower the level of thyroid hormones in the blood. Usually carbimazole/methimazole is given to the general population and propylthiouracil is the drug of choice.
- **Radioactive iodine:** It comes in the form of a pill or liquid. It slowly destroys the cells of the thyroid gland so that less thyroid hormone is made.
- **Surgery**
- **Beta blockers:** These medicines block the action of the thyroid hormone on the body. That helps with rapid heart rate and palpitations.
- **Steroids:** These can be used to quiet the inflammation causing some forms of thyroiditis.

BIBLIOGRAPHY
1. https://www.hopkinsmedicine.org/health/conditions-and-diseases/hyperthyroidism
2. https://www.hopkinsmedicine.org/health/conditions-and-diseases/hypothyroidism
3. https://apps.who.int/iris/bitstream/handle/10665/66342/WHO_DIL_00.4_eng.pdf

10.3 COMMON CANCERS (BREAST, CERVICAL AND ORAL)

☐ **Current cancer statistics:**

		Number of new cases of common cancer			
Both genders		Male		Female	
Type	% of total cases	Type	% of total cases	Type	% of total cases
Breast	13.5	Lip, oral cavity	16.2	Breast	26
Lip, oral cavity	10.3	Lung	8	Cervix uteri	18.3
Cervix uteri	9.4	Stomach	6.3	Ovary	6.7
Lung	5.5	Colorectal	6.3	Lip, oral cavity	4.6
Colorectal	4.9	Esophagus	6.2	Colorectal	3.7
Other	56.5	Other	57	Other	40.4

Warning Signals for Cancers: "CAUTION"

☐ C: Change in bowel or bladder habits
☐ A: A wound that does not heal
☐ U: Unusual bleeding or discharge
☐ T: Thickening or lump in the breast or elsewhere
☐ I: Indigestion or difficulty in swallowing
☐ O: Obvious change in a wart or mole
☐ N: Nagging cough or hoarseness of voice

BREAST CANCER

Breast cancer is a group of cancer cells (malignant tumor) that develops from the cells of the breast. Women are more affected than men. Men can have breast cancer too, but this disease is about 100 times more common in women than in men.

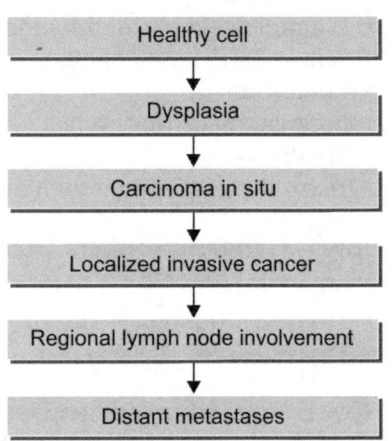

Fig. 10.8: Phases of cancer development.

Risk Factors for Breast Cancer

☐ Family history
☐ Early onset of menstrual period (before age 12 years) and late menopause (after age 55 years)
☐ Late age at first child birth (after age 30 years)
☐ No pregnancy-never having a full-term pregnancy
☐ Shorter duration or no breastfeeding
☐ Previous treatment using radiation therapy
☐ Being overweight/obese especially after menopause
☐ Smoking and second-hand smoke
☐ Lack of physical activity
☐ Consumption of alcohol
☐ Using combination hormone therapy after menopause

Common Warning Signs of Breast Cancer

- Lump in the breast or underarm area (armpit)
- Thickening or swelling of part of the breast
- Irritation or puckering/dimpling of breast skin
- Redness or flaky skin in the nipple area or the breast
- Pulling in of the nipple or change in position or shape and pain in the nipple area
- Nipple discharge other than breast milk, including blood
- Any change in the size or the shape of the breast
- Constant pain in any area of the breast or armpit

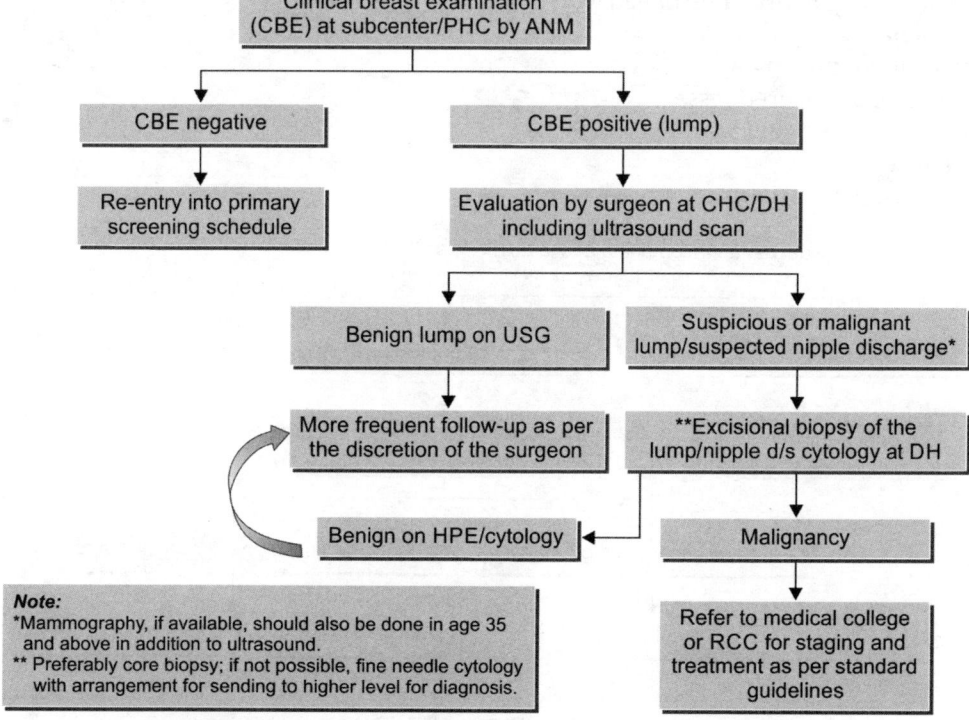

Fig. 10.9: Screening and management algorithm for breast cancer.

CERVICAL CANCER

The cervix is the lower, narrow end of the uterus in the female reproductive system. Cervical cancer occurs when abnormal cells develop and spread in the cervix.

Risk Factors for Cervical Cancer

- Human papillomavirus (HPV) infection (most common) particularly serotype 16 and 18
- Smoking
- Young age at first sexual activity
- Multiple sexual partners
- Unprotected sex or poor sexual hygiene
- Early marriage
- Early childbirth—in women younger than 17 years

- Frequent childbirth
- Weakened immune system such as HIV/AIDS

Common Signs and Symptoms of Cervical Cancer

- Vaginal bleeding between periods
- Menstrual periods that are longer or heavier than usual
- Postmenopausal bleeding
- Bleeding after sexual intercourse
- Pain during sexual intercourse
- Smelly vaginal discharge
- Unusual vaginal discharge tinged with blood
- Backache
- Lower abdominal pain
- Fatigue/extreme tiredness
- Unexplained weight loss
- Pain in legs
- Pain during urination

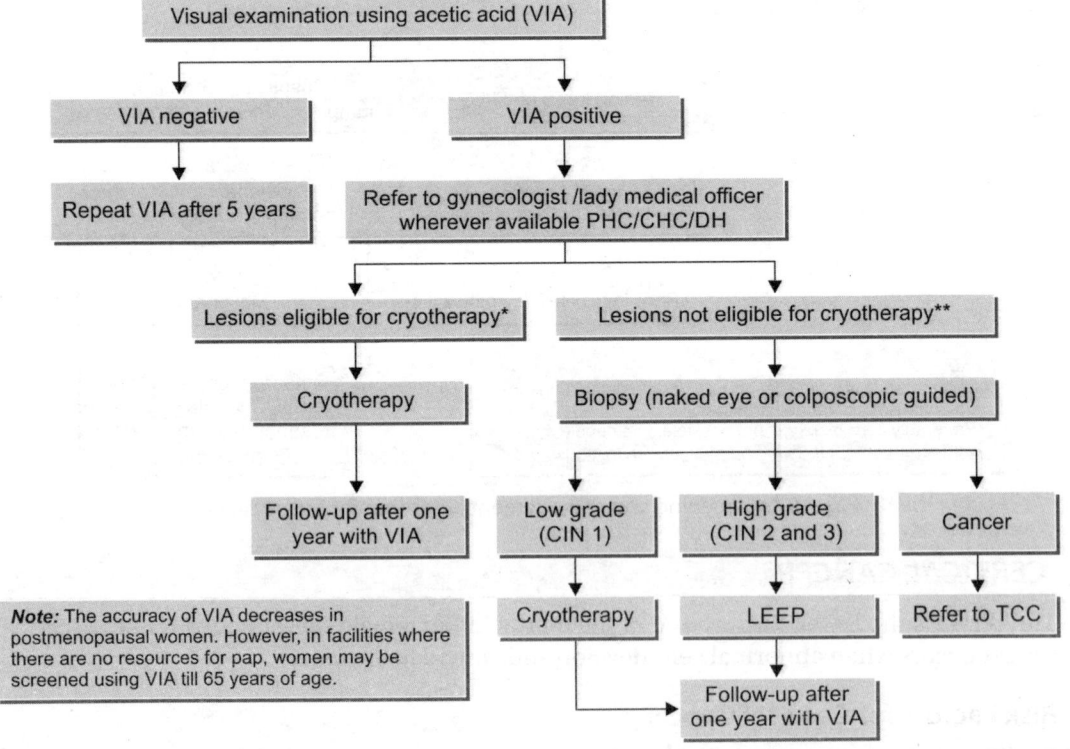

Fig. 10.10: Screening and management algorithm for cervical cancer.

Note

*Eligibility or cryotherapy: Fully visible lesion, only in ectocervix, not >2 quadrant involved.

**Cryotherapy not recommended if: Postcoital or postmenopausal bleeding, lesion bleeds on touch or with irregular surface and having overt cervical growth.

Prevention of Cervical Cancer

- Removal or modification of all possible risk factors as mentioned above.
- Currently, there are three licensed HPV vaccines: Cervarix, gardasil and CERVAVAC.
- Cervarix vaccine protects against infection with HPV-16 and HPV-18, the 2 serotypes that cause the majority of HPV-associated cancers.
- Gardasil protects against HPV 16, 18, 6 and 11.
- CERVAVAC is a first Indian origin quadrivalent vaccine (16, 18, 6 and 11) resulted from a partnership of DBT's biotechnology industry research assistance council (BIRAC) and the Bill and Melinda Gates Foundation that supported Serum Institute of India's development efforts.
- Government of India is in planning to include vaccine for prevention of cervical cancer in UIP.

ORAL CANCER

- It is the cancer that occurs in the oral cavity. The oral cavity includes the lips, the inner lining of the lips and cheeks (buccal mucosa), teeth, gums, front of the tongue, floor of the mouth below the tongue, and the bony roof of the mouth (hard palate).
- Oral cancer is both preventable and curable.
- It is the most common cancer among male in India because of the high prevalence of tobacco chewing.

Risk Factors for Oral Cancer

- Tobacco consumed in any form—smoking and chewing tobacco products
- Chewing betel quid (paan), which is made up of areca nut (supari) and lime (chuna) wrapped in a betel leaf, chewing gutka—a mixture of betel quid and tobacco
- Alcohol
- Weakened immune system
- Poor oral hygiene
- Sharp teeth and ill-fitting dentures

Common Signs and Symptoms of Oral Cancer

- Mouth ulcers that persist for more than three weeks
- Persistent pain in the mouth
- A lump or thickening in the cheek
- A white or red patch on the gums, tongue, tonsil, or lining of the mouth
- A sore throat or a feeling that something is stuck in the throat
- Difficulty in chewing or swallowing
- Difficulty in moving the jaw or tongue
- Difficulty in tolerating spicy foods
- Bleeding or numbness of the tongue or other area of the mouth
- Swelling of the jaw
- Loosening of the teeth or pain around the teeth or jaw
- Changes in voice or having speech problems
- A lump or mass in the neck
- Weight loss
- Constant bad breath
- Excessive salivation

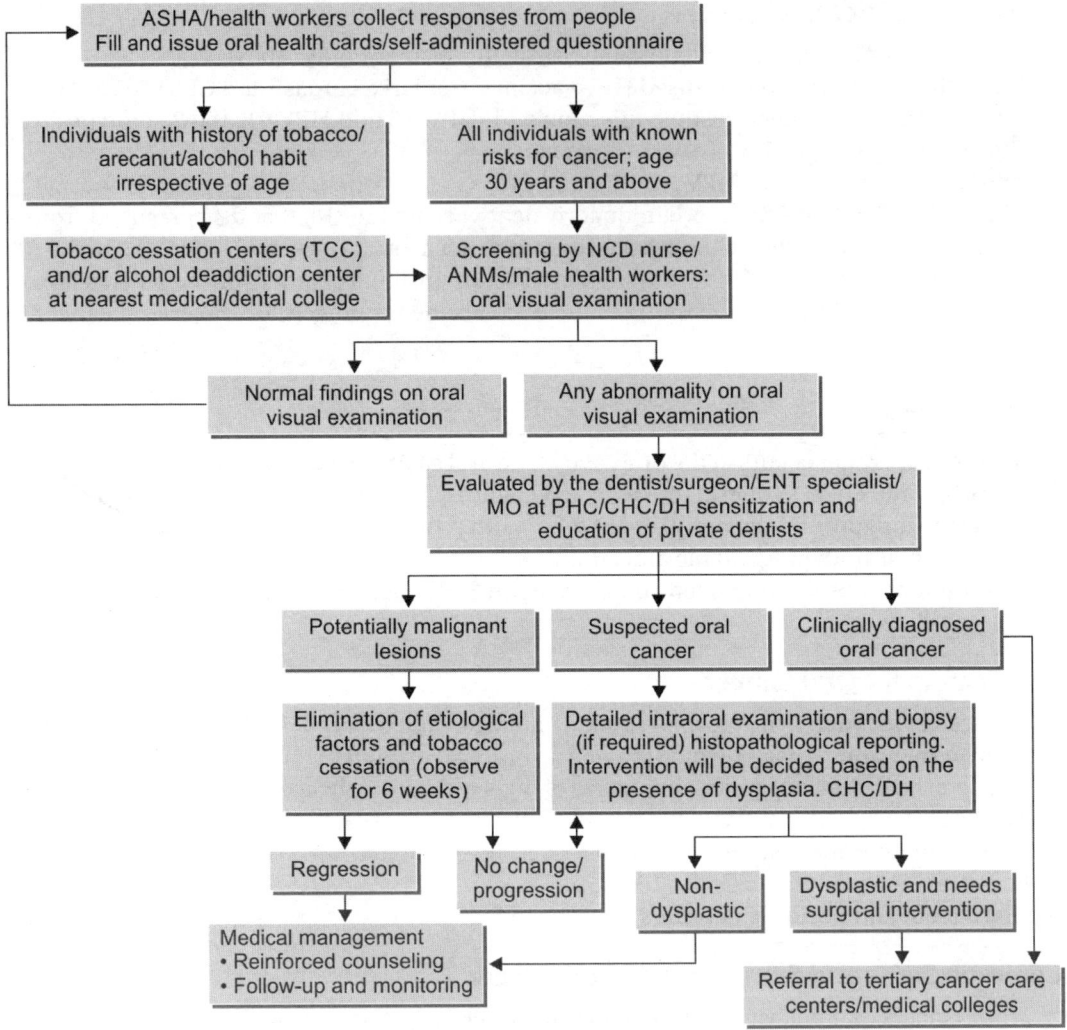

Fig. 10.11: Screening and management algorithm for oral cancer.

Overall Screening Framework for all Common NCDs

- ☐ **Population enumeration to cover the eligible population:** ASHA is the main person to conduct population enumeration of all those aged 30 years and above. She maintains this data in a specific register and updates it every 6 months. She fills Health Card for each eligible individual. MPHW is going to cross verify 10% of enumerated data.
- ☐ **Completing the community-based assessment checklist (CBAC) for NCD screening:** In CBAC form, details like tobacco and alcohol consumption, physical activity, waist circumference, family history of NCD like high blood pressure or diabetes, etc. are usually filled. Usually CBAC form is filled by ASHA. Person with score of 4 or more in CBAC form then he or she will be prioritized for further screening.

- **Community mobilization:** It is very important that high risk individuals found after CBAC form assessment, they should be mobilized for further screening at SC or PHC level. People like ASHA, PRI, AWC, VHSNC or MAS committee members could serve as mobilizer.
- **Screening for non-communicable diseases:** Screening to be done with be easy to apply, preferably noninvasive, acceptable tests. Once any person found suspect for having NCD in screening tests, he or she must be motivated to visit nearby PHC or CHC for further confirmation of the diagnosis and initiation of the treatment. It is estimated that approximately 37% of the population of given area is more than 30 years of age so that would be the screening load. It is expected that at least 30 individuals to be screened per day.

Frequency of Screening for different NCDs (for all who are >30 years of age)

NCD	Estimated beneficiaries	Methods of screening	Frequency of screening
Diabetes	370 people/1,000 population	Glucometer	Once in a year
Hypertension	370 people/1,000 population; (182 women and 188 men)	Digital or aneroid Sphygmomanometer	Once in a year
Breast cancer	182 women/1,000 population	Clinical breast examination (CBE)	Once in 5 years
Cervical cancer	182 women/1,000 population	Visual inspection with acetic acid (VIA)	Once in 5 years
Oral cancer	370 people/1,000 population	Oral visual examination (OVE)	Once in 5 years

- Screening for hypertension, diabetes, oral and breast cancer can be offered in the outreach session like at village level, while screening of cervical cancer to be done at least at the SHC/HWC. This process should be supportively supervised by a trained lady health visitor/staff nurse or even a medical officer.
- Awareness cum mobilization campaign should be conducted before conduction of screening days thus we can ensure high levels of participation.
- ANMs, LHVs, SNs, and midlevel providers should get trained in oral visual examination (OVE), clinical breast examination (CBE) and visual inspection using acetic acid (VIA). LHVs and SNs would serve as mentors and trainers to the subcenter staff and also assist when there are shortages/absences.

BIBLIOGRAPHY

1. https://nhsrcindia.org/sites/default/files/202103/Operational%20Framework%20Management%20of%20Common%20Cancers.pdf
2. https://main.mohfw.gov.in/sites/default/files/Module%20for%20Multi-Purpose%20Workers%20%20Prevention%2C%20Screening%20and%20Control%20of%20Common%20NCDS_2.pdf
3. http://www.nrhmorissa.gov.in/writereaddata/Upload/Documents/Cancer%20Screening%20Rationale%20Framework.pdf

10.4 NATIONAL PROGRAM FOR PREVENTION AND CONTROL OF CANCER, DIABETES, CARDIOVASCULAR DISEASES AND STROKE (NPCDCS) AND NATIONAL PROGRAM FOR HEALTHCARE OF THE ELDERLY (NPHCE)

National Program for Prevention and Control of Cancer, Diabetes, Cardiovascular Diseases and Stroke (NPCDCS)

Objectives of NPCDCS

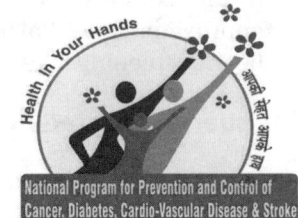

- Health promotion through behavior change with involvement of community, civil society, community-based organizations, media, etc.
- Opportunistic screening at all levels in the healthcare delivery system from subcenter and above for early detection of diabetes, hypertension and common cancers. Outreach camps are also envisaged.
- To prevent and control chronic non-communicable diseases, especially cancer, diabetes, CVDs and stroke.
- To build capacity at various levels of healthcare for prevention, early diagnosis, treatment, IEC/BCC, operational research and rehabilitation.
- To support for diagnosis and cost-effective treatment at primary, secondary and tertiary levels of healthcare.
- To support for development of database of NCDs through surveillance system and to monitor NCD morbidity and mortality and risk factors.

Strategy

- Health promotion, awareness generation and promotion of healthy lifestyle
- Screening and early detection
- Timely, affordable and accurate diagnosis
- Access to affordable treatment
- Rehabilitation

Activities under NPCDCS at PHC/Sub-center

- Health promotion activities for lifestyle changes
- **At community/sub-center:** Outreach activities
  - ***Population based screening of common NCDs***
  - *ASHA/ANM/Health workers to screen persons >30 years of age for NCD risk factors, DM, High BP and common cancers*
  - *Referral of suspected cases of DM/HTN/Cancer to PHC/CHC*
- **At PHC:** Confirmation of DM/HTN diagnosis and management, and follow-up of cases
- **Data recording and reporting:**
  - Filling up of family folder at community level
  - Maintain register at SC/PHC (details of suspected, referred or follow-up cases)
  - Monthly reporting of data
    - Form 1: From SC to PHC
    - Form 2: From PHC to CHC NCD Clinic

Activities under NPCDCS at CHC-NCD Clinic

- Opportunistic screening of persons (≥30 years)
- Promotion of healthy lifestyle through health education
- Diagnosis, management, counseling and rehabilitation services related to common NCDs (CVDs, DM, HTN, COPD, Stroke and common cancers)
- Referral of complicated cases to district hospital/empaneled referral hospital
- Data management:
  - Maintain records of diagnosis, treatment and referral
  - Monthly reports (Forms 3A and 3B) to District NCD Cell
  - **Contractual manpower**: Medical Officer, Nurse, Counselor, Lab Technician, Data Entry Operator.

Recent Initiatives

- Strategy for "Population-based screening (Universal NCD Screening)" for early detection of common NCDs in community, utilizing the services of frontline health workers.
- National urban health mission offers a platform for strengthening NCD services in urban areas through NPCDCS.
- Inclusion of guidelines for prevention and management of chronic obstructive pulmonary disease (COPD) and chronic kidney disease (CKD) under NPCDCS.
- National strategy for 'bi-directional screening', early detection and better management of Tuberculosis-Diabetes comorbidities, as a joint collaborative activity between NTEP and NPCDCS.
- Pilot intervention on rheumatic heart disease.
- Joint collaborative venture through platforms of NPCDCS and RBSK.
- Integration of alternative systems of medicine (AYUSH) with NPCDCS.
- National multisectoral action plan.
- Integration of non-alcoholic fatty liver disease (NAFLD) into NPCDCS.
- India hypertension control initiative (IHCI), a collaborative project of ICMR, MoHFW, State Governments and WHO has been rolled out to leverage and strengthen the ongoing efforts of hypertensive control interventions.
- Recently NPCDCS has been renamed as national programme for prevention and control of non-communicable diseases (NP-NCD).

National Programme for Health Care of Elderly (NPHCE)

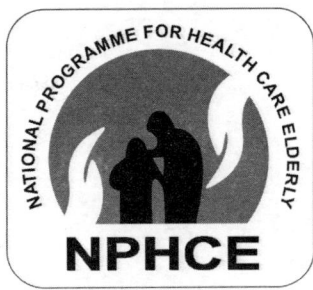

Vision of the NPHCE

- To provide accessible, affordable, and high-quality long-term, comprehensive and dedicated care services to an Aging population.
- Creating a new "architecture" for aging.
- To build a framework to create an enabling environment for "a Society for all Ages".
- To promote the concept of active and healthy aging.

Specific Objectives of NPHCE

- To provide an easy access to promotional, preventive, curative and rehabilitative services to the elderly through community-based primary healthcare approach.

- To identify health problems in the elderly and provide appropriate health interventions in the community with a strong referral backup support.
- To build capacity of the medical and paramedical professionals as well as the care-takers within the family for providing healthcare to the elderly.
- To provide referral services to the elderly patients through district hospitals, regional medical institutions.
- Convergence with national rural health mission, AYUSH and other line departments like Ministry of Social Justice and Empowerment.

Core Strategies

- Community-based primary healthcare approach including domiciliary visits by trained healthcare workers.
- Dedicated services at PHC/CHC level including provision of machinery, equipment, training, additional human resources (CHC), IEC, etc.
- Dedicated facilities at District Hospital with 10 bedded wards, additional human resources, machinery and equipment, consumables and drugs, training and IEC.
- Strengthening of 8 Regional Medical Institutes to provide dedicated tertiary level medical facilities for the Elderly, introducing PG courses in Geriatric Medicine, and in-service training of health personnel at all levels.
- Information, education and communication (IEC) using mass media, folk media and other communication channels to reach out to the target community.
- Continuous monitoring and independent evaluation of the program and research in geriatrics and implementation of NPHCE.

Supplementary Strategies

- Promotion of public private partnerships in Geriatric Healthcare.
- Mainstreaming AYUSH—revitalizing local health traditions, and convergence with programs of Ministry of Social Justice and empowerment in the field of geriatrics.
- Reorienting medical education to support geriatric issues.

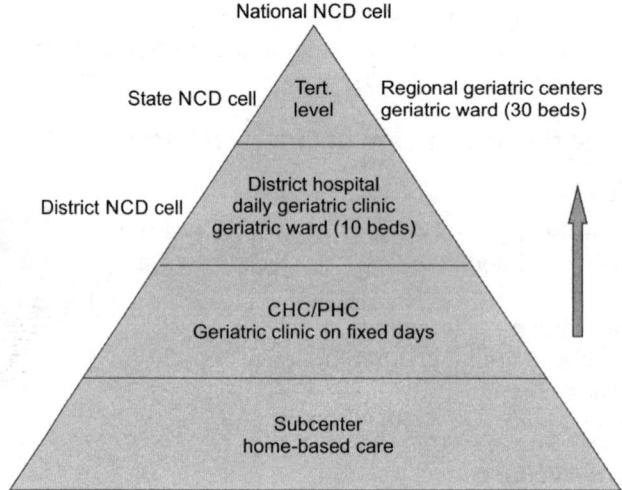

Fig. 10.12: Institutional framework of NPHCE along with NPCDCS.

Activities under NPHCE at Various Levels
Subcenter
- The ANM/male health workers will do domiciliary visits to the elderly persons in their areas and also give training to the family healthcare providers about care of bedridden elderly persons.
- The ANM/male health worker will provide information about:
  - Health education related to healthy aging
  - Environmental modifications
  - Nutritional requirements
  - Lifestyles and behavioral changes.
- They will arrange calipers and supportive devices for the elderly disabled persons.
- They arrange annual check-up of all the elderly at village level.

Primary Health Center
- **A weekly geriatric clinic** will be arranged at PHC level
- Simple clinical examination is carried out to assess vision, hearing, BP blood sugar, etc. and all the information will be recorded as baseline data.
- Proper advice on chronic diseases like chronic obstructive lung disease, diabetes, hypertension, etc. will be given.
- Provision of medicines to the elderly people.
- Referral for further investigations and treatment to higher level facility as per need.

Community Health Center
- **Geriatric clinic: Twice a week**
- **Rehabilitation services:** Physiotherapy and medical rehabilitation will be provided at CHC and for bed-ridden elderly patients it will be given at home by rehabilitation worker.
- Data received from all the PHCs in jurisdiction of CHCs on elderly will be compiled and forwarded to the district program officer (NCD).
- Referral is done to district hospitals/medical colleges as per need.

District Hospital
There will be special **Geriatric Unit** in District Hospitals with following services:
- OPD services to the elderly for examination and management of their illnesses
- Indoor services in Geriatric Ward (10-bedded); out of the 10 beds, 2 beds will be reserved for the bed ridden
- Facilities for lab. investigations and provision of medicines
- It will give training to the medical officers and paramedical staff of CHCs and PHCs
- Provide referral services to the elderly patients referred from the lower level
- Conducting camps in PHCs/CHCs and other sites
- Referral services for severe cases to the higher level

Note: There are 19 regional geriatric center in India and at every center there will be two seats of MD (Geriatric Medicine).

BIBLIOGRAPHY

1. Govt. of India (2011), Operational guidelines for national programme for health care of the elderly, DGHS, Ministry of Health and Family Welfare, New Delhi. Available at: http://www.mohfw.nic.in/showfile.php?lid=2171
2. https://main.mohfw.gov.in/sites/default/files/Operational%20Guidelines%20of%20NPCDCS%20%28Revised%20-%202013-17%29_1.pdf

10.5 NATIONAL CANCER CONTROL PROGRAM

INTRODUCTION

- The National Cancer Control Programme was launched in the year 1975 and then modified on 1983-84.
- During 12th FYP, it was modified to further augment the existing facilities.

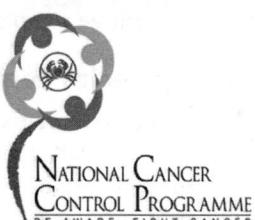

- **Cancer Statistics (GLOBOCAN 2020):**

Number of new cases of common cancer					
Both genders		Male		Female	
Type	% of total cases	Type	% of total cases	Type	% of total cases
Breast	13.5	Lip, oral cavity	16.2	Breast	26
Lip, oral cavity	10.3	Lung	8	Cervix uteri	18.3
Cervix uteri	9.4	Stomach	6.3	Ovary	6.7
Lung	5.5	Colorectal	6.3	Lip, oral cavity	4.6
Colorectal	4.9	Esophagus	6.2	Colorectal	3.7
Other	56.5	Other	57	Other	40.4

Goals and Objectives of NCCP

- Primary prevention of cancers by health education specially regarding hazards of tobacco consumption and necessity of genital hygiene for prevention of cervical cancer.
- Secondary prevention, i.e., early detection and diagnosis of cancers, for example, cancer of cervix, breast and of the oropharyngeal cancer by screening methods and patients' education on self-examination methods.
- Strengthening of existing cancer treatment facilities, which are woefully inadequate.
- Palliative care in terminal stage of the cancer.

Existing Schemes under National Cancer Control Programme (NCCP):
- **Recognition of new regional cancer centers (RCCs):** To enhance the cancer treatment facilities across the country and reduce the geographical gap in the country in the availability of cancer care facilities, New Regional Cancer centers are being recognized. A one-time grant of ₹5.00 crores is being provided for New RCCs.

- **Strengthening of existing Regional Cancer Centers:** A one-time grant of ₹3.00 crores is provided to the existing Regional Cancer Centers to further strengthen the cancer care services.
- **Development of Oncology Wing:** Government Hospitals and Government Medical Colleges are provided with a grant of ₹3.00 crores for the development of Oncology Wing.
- **District Cancer Control Program:** The DCCP will be implemented by a nodal agency, which may be a Regional Cancer Center or Government Medical College or Government Hospital with radiotherapy facility. A cluster of 2-3 districts are taken up for prevention, early detection, minimal treatment and provision of supportive cancer care at district levels. A grant-in-aid of ₹90.00 lakhs spread over a period of 5 years is provided per DCCP proposal.
- **Decentralized NGO Scheme:** A grant of ₹8,000/- per camp will be provided to the NGOs for IEC activities. The funds are released through a Nodal agency which could be a Regional Cancer Center or Government Medical College or Government hospital with radiotherapy facilities.

Note: Keeping in view that there are common preventable risk factors for Cancer, Diabetes, CVD and Stroke, Government of India initiated a National Programme for Prevention and Control of Cancers, Diabetes, Cardiovascular Diseases and Stroke (NPCDCS) during 2010-11 after integrating the National Cancer Control Programme (NCCP) with National Programme for Prevention and Control of Diabetes, Cardiovascular Diseases and Stroke.

BIBLIOGRAPHY

1. https://main.mohfw.gov.in/sites/default/files/4249985666nccp_0.pdf
2. http://www.nrhmhp.gov.in/sites/default/files/files/NCD_Guidelines.pdf

10.6 NATIONAL PROGRAM FOR PALLIATIVE CARE

Introduction

- 'Palliative care is an approach that improves the quality of life of patients and their families facing the problems associated with life-threatening illnesses, through the prevention and relief of suffering by means of early identification, impeccable assessment and treatment of pain and other problems, physical, psychosocial and spiritual'.
- Effective palliative care requires a broad multidisciplinary approach that includes the family and makes use of available community resources.
- It can be provided in tertiary care facilities, in community health centers and even in patients' homes.
- Palliative care is one of the 12 services to be provided at health and wellness centers.

◘ **"Continuum of care" approach:**

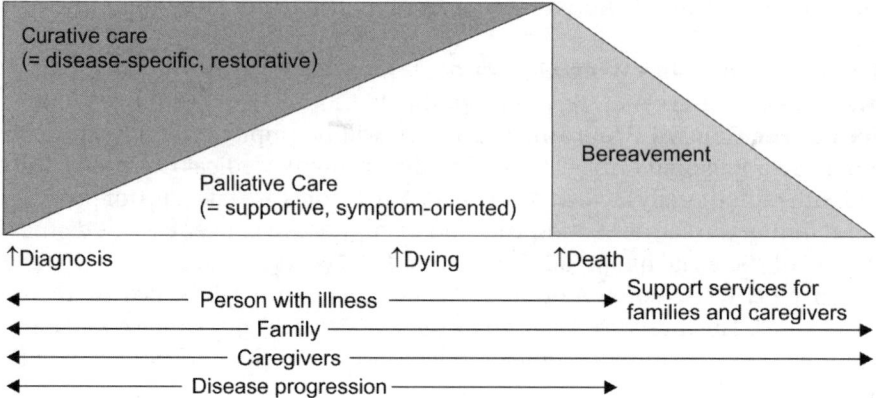

Fig. 10.13: Palliative care continuum.

Beneficiaries: Those with:
◘ Cancer
◘ HIV/AIDS
◘ Organ failures like heart failure, lung failure or kidney failure
◘ Chronic neurological diseases, e.g., Parkinson's disease
◘ Stroke or spinal cord injuries
◘ Old age conditions like Alzheimer's disease
◘ Children with cerebral palsy or birth defects

Goal: Availability and accessibility of rational, quality pain relief and palliative care to the needy, as an integral part of Healthcare at all levels, in alignment with the community requirements.

Objectives

◘ Improve the capacity to provide palliative care service delivery within government health programs such as the National Programme for Prevention and Control of Cancer, Cardiovascular Disease, Diabetes, and Stroke; National Programme for Healthcare of the Elderly; the National AIDS Control Programme; and the National Rural Health Mission.
◘ Refine the legal and regulatory systems and support implementation to ensure access and availability of opioids for medical and scientific use while maintaining measure for preventing diversion and misuse.
◘ Encourage attitudinal shifts amongst healthcare professionals by strengthening and incorporating principles of long-term care and palliative care into the educational curricula (of medical, nursing, pharmacy and social work courses).
◘ Promote behavior change in the community through increasing public awareness and improved skills and knowledge regarding pain relief and palliative care leading to community owned initiatives supporting healthcare system.
◘ Develop national standards for palliative care services and continuously evolve the design and implementation of the national program to ensure progress toward the vision of the program.

Implementation Mechanism
- Activities would be initiated through National Programme for Prevention and Control of Cancer, CVD, Diabetes and Stroke.
- The regulatory aspects for increasing morphine availability would be addressed.
- Cooperation of international and national agencies in the field of palliative care would be taken for successful implementation of the program.
- Provision of funds for establishing state palliative care cell and palliative care services at the district hospital.

BIBLIOGRAPHY
1. https://dghs.gov.in/WriteReadData/userfiles/file/a/5127_1558685685054(1).pdf
2. https://dghs.gov.in/content/1351_3_NationalProgramforPalliativeCare.aspx

10.7 NATIONAL PROGRAM FOR CONTROL OF BLINDNESS AND VISUAL IMPAIRMENT (NPCBVI)

- India was the first country in the world to launch a comprehensive nationwide programme for the prevention and control of blindness.
- National Programme for Control of Blindness was launched in the year 1976 as a 100% Centrally Sponsored scheme (now 60:40 in all states and 90:10 in NE States) with the goal to reduce the prevalence of blindness from 1.4% to 0.3% by 2020.
- It was renamed as National Programme for Control of Blindness and Visual Impairment (NPCB and VI) and is implemented all over the country uniformly, with a goal of reducing the prevalence of avoidable blindness to 0.25% by the year 2025.
- As per the National Blindness and Visual Impairment Survey 2015–2019, current prevalence of blindness is 0.36%.

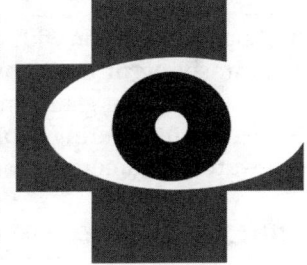

Goals and Objectives of NPCBVI
- To reduce the backlog of blindness through identification and treatment of blind at primary, secondary and tertiary levels based on assessment of the overall burden of visual impairment in the country.
- Develop and strengthen the strategy of NPCBVI for "Eye Health" and prevention of visual impairment; through provision of comprehensive eye care services and quality service delivery.
- Strengthening and upgradation of RIOs to become center of excellence in various sub-specialties of ophthalmology.
- Strengthening the existing and developing additional human resources and infrastructure facilities for providing high quality comprehensive Eye Care in all Districts of the country.
- To enhance community awareness on eye care and lay stress on preventive measures.
- Increase and expand research for prevention of blindness and visual impairment.
- To secure participation of Voluntary Organizations/Private Practitioners in eye care.

Role of ASHA Facilitators/MPW/ANM

- Supportive supervision and monitoring
- Creating awareness about personal hygiene and environmental cleanliness
- Enabling community for lifestyle modifications through various community-based platforms
- For low vision patients:
  - Community-based rehabilitation
  - Social acceptance
  - Vocational training
  - Inclusive education for low vision patients

Role of Community Heath Officer (CHO)

- Record maintenance (e.g., blind and visual impairment register)
- Data compilation and validation
- Monthly review meeting with ASHAs/ANM/MPW
- Screening of target population for near and distant vision
- Screening of target population for common eye conditions like cataract, presbyopia (poor near vision related to ageing), trachoma and corneal disease
- Providing treatment of common eye issues like conjunctivitis, dry eye, trachoma and follow-up medicines for chronic eye disease (e.g., Cataract, glaucoma and diabetes) treated at referral center
- Health promotion with main focus on eye care
- Counseling of the known patients for cataract surgery, wearing spectacles regularly, compliance for glaucoma, fundus examination for diabetics
- Regular monitoring of blood pressure and blood sugar
- Awareness generation on eye donation

BIBLIOGRAPHY

1. https://npcbvi.gov.in/Home
2. https://dghs.gov.in/content/1354_3_NationalProgrammeforControlofBlindnessVisual.aspx

10.8 NATIONAL PROGRAM FOR PREVENTION AND CONTROL OF DEAFNESS (NPPCD)

- The most common sensory deficit in human body is hearing loss.
- It is the second leading cause for *'Years lived with disability (YLD)'* (depression ranks first in terms of YLD).
- As per WHO estimates in India, estimated prevalence of significant auditory impairment is 6.3% which means approximately 63 million people are suffering from it.
- As per NSSO survey, currently there are 291 persons per one lakh population who are suffering from severe to profound hearing loss.

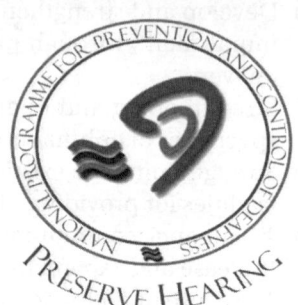

- A large percentage of children between the ages of 0 to 14 years are also suffering from significant auditory impairment. It may cause to a severe loss of productivity, both physical and economic in future.
- Hence, NPPCD was launched with a purpose of early identification, diagnosis and treatment of ear problems responsible for hearing loss and deafness in them.
- This program is being implemented by Ministry of Health and Family Welfare with the technical support of Directorate General of Health Services.
- State Nodal Officer preferably an ENT surgeon provides technical guidance and expertise to the State Health Society for the purpose of implementation of the program in the various districts of the state.
- National Programme for Prevention and Control of Deafness (NPPCD) was initiated on pilot basis in the year 2006–07 (January 2007) in 25 districts of 10 states and 1 UT and then it was expanded to 228 districts of 27 States/Union Territories.

Objectives of the Program

- To prevent avoidable hearing loss on account of disease or injury.
- Early identification, diagnosis and treatment of ear problems responsible for hearing loss and deafness.
- To medically rehabilitate persons of all age groups, suffering with deafness.
- To strengthen the existing intersectoral linkages for continuity of the rehabilitation program, for persons with deafness.
- To develop institutional capacity for ear care services by providing support for equipment, material and training personnel.

Long-term Objective

To prevent and control major causes of hearing impairment and deafness, so as to reduce the total disease burden by 25% of the existing burden by the end of 12th Five Year Plan (2012–2017).

Components of the Program

- **Manpower training and development:** For prevention, early identification and management of hearing impaired and deafness cases, training would be provided from medical college level specialists (ENT and audiology) to grass root level workers.
- **Capacity building:** For the district hospital, CHC and PHC in respect of ENT/Audiology infrastructure.
- **Service provision:** Early detection and management of hearing and speech impaired cases and rehabilitation, at different levels of healthcare delivery system.
- **Awareness generation through IEC/BCC activities:** For early identification of hearing impaired, especially children so that timely management of such cases is possible and to remove the stigma attached to deafness.
- **Program execution and expansion:** The program was an initially a 100% centrally sponsored scheme but later on, the center and the states have contribution in resources as per the financial norms of NRHM.

BIBLIOGRAPHY

1. https://dghs.gov.in/content/1362_3_NationalProgrammePreventionControl.aspx

10.9 NATIONAL IODINE DEFICIENCY DISORDERS CONTROL PROGRAM (NIDDCP)

- Iodine is an essential micronutrient required for the synthesis of the thyroid hormones, thyroxine (T4) and triiodothyronine (T3) and its daily requirement is 100–150 micrograms for normal human growth and development.
- During pregnancy requirement goes to 250 micrograms daily.
- It is also estimated that more than 71 million persons are suffering from Iodine Deficiency Disorders. These disorders include:
  - Goiter
  - Subnormal intelligence
  - Neuromuscular weakness
  - Endemic cretinism
  - Stillbirth
  - Hypothyroidism
  - Defect in vision, hearing, and speech
  - Spasticity
  - Intrauterine death
  - Mental retardation

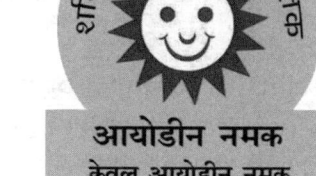

- Launched as National Goiter Control Programme (NGCP) in 1962 and in 1992, it was restructured and renamed as National Iodine Deficiency Disorders Control Programme (NIDDCP).
- Ministry of Health and Family Welfare is the nodal ministry for implementation of National Iodine Deficiency Disorders Control Programme (NIDDCP).

Goal

- To bring the prevalence of IDD to below 5% in the country
- To ensure 100% consumption of adequately iodated salt (15 ppm) at the household level.

Objectives and Components

- Surveys to assess the magnitude of the Iodine Deficiency Disorders.
- Supply of iodated salt in place of common salt.
- Resurvey after every 5 years to assess the extent of Iodine Deficiency Disorders and the impact of Iodated salt.
- Laboratory monitoring of iodated salt and urinary iodine excretion.
- Health education and publicity.

Structure

For example, Gujarat has a fulltime functional State IDD cell which is a part of the State Nutrition Cell. Gujarat's IDD cell consists of one Technical Officer, one Statistical Assistant, two Laboratory Technicians and one clerk.

BIBLIOGRAPHY

1. https://dghs.gov.in/content/1348_3_NationalIodineDeficiency.aspx
2. https://nhm.gov.in/images/pdf/programmes/ndcp/niddcp/revised_guidelines.pdf
3. http://www.nihfw.org/NationalHealthProgramme/NATIONAL IODINED EFICIENCY DISORDERS.html

10.10 NATIONAL TOBACCO CONTROL PROGRAM

- Tobacco is viewed as a crop by the Agriculture Ministry.
- Tobacco is viewed as a source of revenue by the Commerce Ministry.
- Tobacco is viewed as a livelihood issue by the Labour Ministry.
- Tobacco is viewed as a cause of major public health problems by Health Ministry.
- Tobacco kills up to half of its users.
- Tobacco users feel ten years older and die ten years younger than people who do not use tobacco.
- Tobacco kills more than 8 million people each year. More than 7 million of those deaths are the result of direct tobacco use while around 1 million are the result of non-smokers being exposed to second-hand smoke.
- 26.7 crores (28.6%) tobacco users among persons aged 15+ in India
- The use of smokeless tobacco is much more prevalent than smoking tobacco. The prevalence of smokeless tobacco use is almost twice of the prevalence of smoking.
- More than 75 percent of tobacco users, both smokers as well as users of the smokeless tobacco, are daily users of the tobacco.
- Khaini (tobacco lime mixture) is the most commonly used tobacco product in India. One in every eight adults chew Khaini (12%) and 8 percent and 6 percent adults use Gutkha and betel quid with tobacco (paan) respectively.
- Bidi is the most commonly used smoking product, followed by cigarette and hukkah.
- About 3500 deaths daily in India are attributable to tobacco use.

Levels of Prevention of Tobacco Use

- **Primordial prevention to prevent** initiation of tobacco use.
  - Health education to prevent initiation of tobacco use especially at school level and also to be provided in the community and the clinic.
  - Enforcing policies must be strictly implemented.
- **Primary prevention** to help tobacco users quit
  - Tobacco cessation services for tobacco users who haven't yet exhibited any tobacco related diseases and it is to be provided mainly at clinical set up.
- **Secondary prevention** for early diagnosis and treatment of diseases in tobacco users.
- **Tertiary prevention** to help heavy users quit, many of whom have tobacco related symptoms and diseases and this has to be done in special clinics or hospitals.
  - Treatment for heavy users and victims of tobacco related diseases (oral cancer, cardiovascular and lung diseases, etc.): disease treatment plus cessation services.

Some Tips that can be Helpful in Prevention Like

- **5As:** It is 5As intervention for supporting smoking cessation:
  - *Ask:* Ask all patients about current smoking status
  - *Assess:* Assess readiness or willingness to quit
  - *Advise:* Advise all smokers to quit and provide information on benefits of quitting smoking
  - *Assist:* Assist all smokers in quitting smoking
  - *Arrange:* Arrange follow-up

- **5Rs**: It is motivational tool specially used for those smokers who are not ready to quit:
  - *Relevance:* Show the relevance of smoking
  - *Risks:* Help the patients to identify the negative consequences of smoking
  - *Rewards:* Help the patient to know the benefits of stopping of smoking
  - *Roadblocks:* Ask the patients to know the barriers to quitting
  - *Repetition:* This motivational interaction should be repeated everytime

National Tobacco Control Programme (NTCP)

- Government of India launched the NTPC in the year 2007–08, during the 11th Five-Year Plan.
- It was up scaled in the 12th Five-Year Plan with a goal to reduce the prevalence of tobacco use by 5% by the end of the 12th FYP.

Objectives of NTCP

- Create awareness about the harmful effects of tobacco consumption
- Reduce the production and supply of tobacco products
- Ensure effective implementation of the provisions under "The Cigarettes and Other Tobacco Products (Prohibition of Advertisement and Regulation of Trade and Commerce, Production, Supply and Distribution) Act, 2003" (COTPA)
- Help the people quit tobacco use
- Facilitate implementation of strategies for prevention and control of tobacco advocated by WHO Framework Convention of Tobacco Control

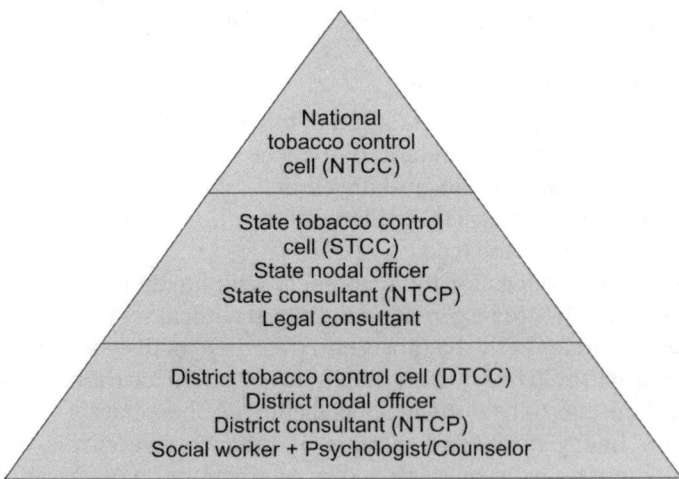

Fig. 10.14: Structure of NTCP.

NTCP Structure

- The National Tobacco Control Cell (NTCC) at the Ministry of Health and Family Welfare (MoHFW) is responsible for overall policy formulation, planning, implementation, monitoring and evaluation of the different activities envisaged under the National Tobacco Control Programme (NTCP).
- The technical assistance is provided by the identified officers in the Directorate General of Health Services.

- Currently, the program is being implemented in all 36 States/Union Territories covering around 612 districts across the country.

National Level
- Public awareness/mass media campaigns for awareness building and behavioral change
- Establishment of tobacco product testing laboratories at national level
- Mainstreaming research and training on alternative crops and livelihood with other nodal ministries
- Monitoring and evaluation including surveillance
- Integrating NTCP as a part of healthcare delivery mechanism under the National Health Mission framework.

State Level
Dedicated state tobacco control cells for effective implementation and monitoring of tobacco control initiatives. The key activities include:
- State level advocacy workshop
- Training of trainers program for staff appointed at DTCC under NTCP
- Refresher training of the DTCC staff
- Training on tobacco cessation for healthcare providers
- Law enforcers training/sensitization program

District Level
Dedicated district tobacco control cells for effective implementation and monitoring of tobacco control initiatives. The key activities include:
- **Training of key stakeholders:** Health and social workers, NGOs, school teachers, enforcement officers, etc.
- Information, education and communication (IEC) activities
- School programs monitoring tobacco control laws
- Setting-up and strengthening of cessation facilities including provision of pharmacological treatment facilities at the district level
- Coordination with Panchayat Raj Institutions for inculcating concept of tobacco control at the grassroots

WHO MPOWER Strategy
- To help countries fulfill the obligations under FCTC, WHO has established MPOWER, the policies of which are proven to reduce tobacco use.
- Following six policies are advocated to reverse the epidemic of tobacco:
    1. MONITOR tobacco use and prevention policies.
    2. PROTECT people from tobacco smoke.
    3. OFFER help to quit tobacco use.
    4. WARN about the dangers of tobacco.
    5. ENFORCE bans on tobacco advertising, promotion and sponsorship.
    6. RAISE taxes on tobacco products.

BIBLIOGRAPHY

1. https://www.who.int/news-room/fact-sheets/detail/tobacco
2. https://ntcp.nhp.gov.in/assets/document/Guideline-manuals/Training-Manual-for-Doctors-National-Tobacco-Control-Programme.pdf
3. http://nhm.gov.in/index1.php?lang=1andlevel=2andsublinkid=1052andlid=607

11 CHAPTER

School Health Program

CHAPTER OUTLINE

11.1 History of School Health
11.2 Objectives of School Health
11.3 Health Problems of School Children
11.4 Components of School Health Services
11.5 Initiation and Planning of School Health Services
11.6 Role of a School Health Nurse
11.7 RBSK/School Health Program

11.1 HISTORY OF SCHOOL HEALTH

- As per census 2011, 47.3 crore children (0–18 years) comprising 39 percent of the country's total population.
- And around 26 crore children from the age group of 6–18 years are attending schools.
- It is important to educate the children early in life, about their health and the right behaviors, so that they lead a healthy life and realize their full potential.
- Schools serve as an ideal platform to impart education on health issues and school health program offer high cost benefit ratio in terms of implementing health activities efficiently.
- Historically speaking, the introduction of medical inspection of school going children in the city of Baroda in 1909 was a landmark in the development of school health services in India.
- Between 1909 and 1937 Bengal, Bombay, Punjab, Uttar Pradesh, Bihar, Madras and Delhi also introduced the medical inspection of school children.
- In 1941, the Joint Committee of the Central Advisory Board of Health and Education emphasized the need for satisfactory medical inspection, treatment and school-feeding in any system of public education.

- In 1946, Bhore Committee put stress on the provision of the physical and nutritional program for school going children and stated that the functions of school health services should be under the Health Department and not that of Education Department. The Committee strongly recommended the inclusion of school health services as one of the important component of Primary Health Center for the school children of rural areas. The Committee had also recommended that the instruction of school children in hygiene should begin at the earliest possible stage.
- In 1953, Secondary Education Committee of the Government of India recommended comprehensive policy interventions dealing with school health and school feeding programs.
- In 1953, Secondary Education Committee reiterated the need for medical inspection of students and the introduction of School Feeding Program.
- In 1957, the Ministry of Education set up the Health Education—Nutrition Education Committee to initiate the preparation of syllabi on health education for schools and teacher training institutions. The Central Health Education Bureau set up the School Health Education Division in 1958 to serve as a technical resource agency to the Ministry of Health and the Ministry of Education and coordinated the preparation of syllabi and conducted national workshops and state-level joint workshops of health and educational personnel as an orientation for implementing the syllabus.
- The Ministry of Education appointed a School Health Committee under the Chairmanship of Smt. Renuka Ray in 1960 to assess the present standard of health and nutrition of school children and suggest ways and means of improving them. The Committee submitted its report in 1961 and considering the prevailing conditions and the available resources, made important recommendations for drawing up school health program and referred to other areas like school meal, pre-school child, school health education, training, studies, research, school environment and school health administration. The committee recommended that School Health Services should form part and parcel of the general health services for the community.
- It further said that with adequate training in health education and school health services, it should be possible for the teacher to undertake certain functions related to school health services such as:
  - Observation of students for defects and deviations from normal health,
  - Screening them for height, weight, vision and hearing,
  - Providing first aid,
  - Maintaining cumulative health cards and filling in relevant portions of the same,
  - Giving health education for prevention of preventable problems and development of healthful living practices among students.

The Links Between Health and Education
- School-based nutrition and health interventions can improve academic performance.
- Students' health and nutrition status affects their enrolment, retention, and absenteeism.
- Education benefits health.
- Education can reduce social and gender inequities.
- Health promotion for teachers benefits their health, morale, and quality of instruction.
- Health promotion and disease prevention programs are cost-effective.

- Treating youngsters in school can reduce disease in the community.
- Multiple coordinated strategies produce a greater effect than individual strategies, but multiple strategies for any one audience must be targeted carefully.
- Health education is most effective when it uses interactive methods in a skills-based approach.
- Trained teachers delivering health education produce more significant outcomes in student health knowledge and skills than untrained teachers.

11.2 OBJECTIVES OF SCHOOL HEALTH

School health team members include school principal, school teacher, medical officer, nurse, community member, parents and children.

Objectives of School Health Services

1. To include healthy practices and positive health among students
2. To develop knowledge and attitude for healthy behavior
3. To awake health consciousness in children
4. To ensure provision of healthy environment
5. To promote appropriate social and emotional behavior
    - In 2013, Government of India launched the Rashtriya Bal Swasthya Karyakram (RBSK) under the National Health Mission for early detection and timely management of illnesses among children (0–18 years) by periodic screening through the platform of Schools and Anganwadi centers.
    - In 2014, Government also launched another comprehensive program called, 'Rashtriya Kishor Swasthya Karyakram' (RKSK) to respond to the health and development requirements of adolescents in a holistic manner.
    - Recently, the School Health Program has been incorporated as a part of the Health and Wellness component of the Ayushman Bharat Program to strengthen the preventive and promotive aspects through health promotion activities. These health promotion activities will be a joint initiative of Ministry of Health and Family Welfare and Department of School Education and Literacy, Ministry of Human Resource and Development.

Objectives of School Health Program

- To provide age-appropriate information about health and nutrition to the children in schools
- To promote healthy behaviors among the children that they will inculcate for life
- To detect and treat diseases early in children and adolescents including identification of malnourished and anemic children with appropriate referrals to PHCs and hospitals
- To promote use of safe drinking water in schools
- To promote safe menstrual hygiene practices by girls
- To promote yoga and meditation through Health and Wellness Ambassadors
- To encourage research on health, wellness and nutrition for children

Target population: All students of all the government and government aided schools in the country.

11.3 HEALTH PROBLEMS OF SCHOOL CHILDREN

Children are vulnerable to wide spectrum of communicable and chronic disease conditions including nutritional deficiencies, substance abuse, mental health concerns, violence, injury and reproductive and sexual health problems. A number of these issues can be prevented through informed health choices. A focused and comprehensive intervention that targets risk factors and social determinants of health conditions as well as empowers children and adolescents to adopt healthy behaviors can play an important role in reducing the burden of these diseases. More children than ever are attending school, and for longer periods of their lives, therefore, schools can do more than perhaps any other single institution to improve the well-being and competence of children and adolescents.

It is a well-known fact that establishing healthy behaviors during childhood is easier and more effective that trying to change unhealthy behavior during adulthood. Therefore, schools play a critical **role in helping students establish healthy behaviors for their lifetime.**

Health and education are strongly connected—healthy children achieve better results at school, which in turn are associated with improved health later in life. Setting up positive and healthy school environment, then, plays an important role in improving the health, well-being, overall academic achievement.

As more children survive to school age and with increased emphasis on Sarva Shiksha Abhiyan (SSA) and Right to Education Act (2010), the number of children attending school has increased considerably.

For millions of young people including adolescents around the world, the onset of adolescence brings not only changes to their bodies, but also new vulnerabilities due to limited access to quality services, and health information, particularly on sexual and reproductive health, injuries and violence and digital challenges (e.g., cyber-bullying and pornography, Internet addiction).

As per National Mental Health Survey 2015–16, prevalence of mental disorders in age group 13–17 years was 7.3% and nearly equal in both genders. Approximately 59.1% of the girls and 31.1% of boys in the age group of 15–19 years are anemic in India (NFHS-5). A large proportion of girls are coerced into unwanted sex or marriage, putting them at risk of unwanted pregnancies, unsafe abortions, sexually transmitted infections, including HIV. AIDS related deaths have fallen for every other age group except for adolescents where it has increased.

As per NFHS-4, more than one-fourth (26.8%) of the girls in the country are still getting married below the legal age, 8% of girls aged 15–19 years were already mothers or pregnant at the time of survey, 58% girls in the age of 15–24 years use a hygienic method during menstruation and more than one-third married female 15–24 years (37%) have experienced physical, sexual, or emotional violence by their husbands. India has over a billion mobile users but access to toilets is only 66%. World Health Organization (WHO) indicates that India has the highest burden of soil-transmitted helminths (STH) in the world, with 220 million children aged 1–14 years estimated to be at risk of worm infestations. NFHS-4 data also shows that in the age 15–19 years 4.2% girls and 4.8% boys are obese while 42% girls and 44% boys are thin.

11.4 COMPONENTS OF SCHOOL HEALTH SERVICES

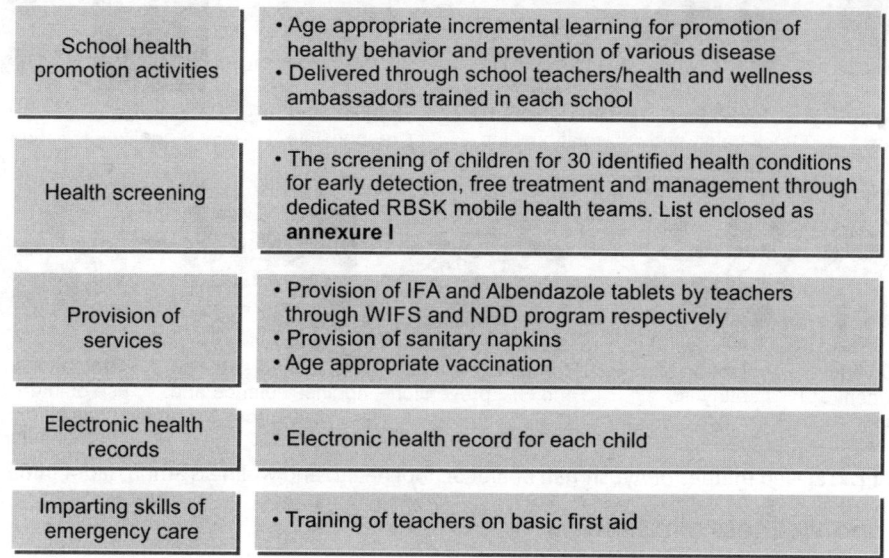

Fig. 11.1: Package of services under school health according to RBSK.

11.5 INITIATION AND PLANNING OF SCHOOL HEALTH SERVICES

Operationalization of the School Health Program According to RBSK

"Health and Wellness Ambassadors"

- One male and one female, in every school will be trained to transact health promotion and disease prevention information in the form of interesting activities for one hour every week.
- Teachers who are proactive, less than 45 years of age and from science/physical education background to be preferred.
- Cascade model of training will be followed for capacity building of school teachers.
- Their training will be based on the Improving Nutrition, Improving Sexual and Reproductive Health, Enhancing Mental Health, Preventing Injuries and Violence (including GBV), Preventing Substance Misuse, Addressing conditions for Non-communicable Diseases.
- Training will be for 5 days.
- The trained teachers/Health and Wellness Ambassadors will conduct weekly sessions and complete the modules in the academic year as per the proposed schedule.
- To address the queries of the students, a question box will be installed in schools where the students can put in their individual queries anonymously to prevent any bias based on question-asking. The Health and Wellness Ambassadors will take up these questions at the start of each new session and use them for discussion **(Fig. 11.2)**.

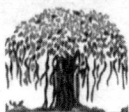 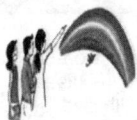 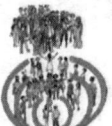 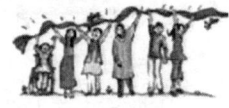 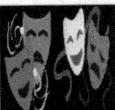 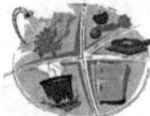

| Growing up healthy | Emotional well-being and mental health | Interpersonal relationships | Values and responsible citizenship | Gender equality | Nutrition, health and sanitation |

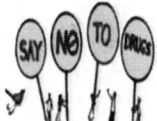 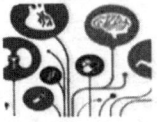 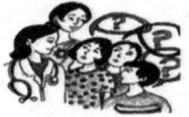 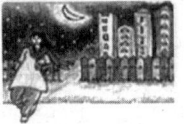 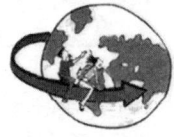

| Prevention and management substance misuse | Promotion of healthy life style | Reproductive health and HIV prevention | Safety and security against violence and injuries | Promotion of safe use of internet and social media behaviors |

Fig. 11.2: Eleven themes of Ayushman Bharat School health and wellness ambassador initiative.

Health and Wellness Messengers

- Students would work as Health and Wellness messengers.
- The Health and Wellness Ambassadors will be supported by two students of each class who would help them facilitate the initiatives and activities under the school health component.
- They will be termed as "Health and Wellness Messengers".
- **Health and Wellness Day:** Every Tuesday to be celebrated as health and wellness day.

Activities in school

Weekly	Fortnightly/monthly	Quarterly	Bi-annual
• Classroom transactions by health and wellness ambassadors • Administration of IFA tablets	• Thematic school assembly • Question box responses	• Thematic AHDs • Parent–Teacher meetings	Administration of albendazole tablet (National deworming day)

School Health Promotion Activities

Age appropriate health promotion		
Primary school	*Middle school*	*High school*
• Health, growth and development • Personal safety • Nutrition and physical activity • Hygiene practices • Prevention of diseases like malaria, dengue, TB, worms infestation, diarrhea and vaccine preventable diseases	• Puberty and related changes • Eye care, oral hygiene • Nutrition • Bullying prevention • Meditation and yoga • Internet safety and media literacy • Prevention of substance abuse • HIV/AIDS • Mental health	• Prevention of substance abuse • Sexual and reproductive health • Violence prevention • Unintentional injury • Road safety • Nutrition • Meditation and yoga

11.6 ROLE OF A SCHOOL HEALTH NURSE

- General examination
- Identify disease or defects or any abnormalities
- First-aid services
- Health education (related to personal hygiene, growth and development, nutrition, etc.)
- School health records
- Immunization records
- Treatment of minor ailments
- Referral services and follow-up visit
- Ensure supplies of drugs
- Health records

11.7 RBSK/SCHOOL HEALTH PROGRAM

- Rashtriya Bal Swasthya Karyakram (RBSK) is an important initiative aiming at early identification and early intervention for children from birth to 18 years to cover 4 'D's viz. Defects at birth, deficiencies, diseases, development delays including disability.
- The 0–6 years' age group will be specifically managed at District Early Intervention Center (DEIC) level while for 6–18 years' age group, management of conditions will be done through existing public health facilities.
- DEIC will act as referral linkage for both the age groups.
- Once the child is screened and referred from school, it would be ensured that the necessary treatment/intervention is delivered at zero cost to the family.
  (*Note:* Objectives and components of RBSK services described in 11.2 and 11.4 division of this chapter.)
- RBSK mobile health team members include medical officer (Ayush 1 male and 1 female), ANM/Nurse, Pharmacist.

Provision of Services

- **Weekly iron folic acid supplementation:**

Age group	Intervention/dose	Regime	Service delivery
6–10 years	45 mg elemental iron and 400 µg of folic acid	Weekly, throughout the period 6–10 years of age	Through teachers
10–19 years	60 mg elemental iron and 500 µg of folic acid	Weekly throughout the period 10–19 years of age	Through teachers

- **Deworming:** To fight against worm infestations, Government of India conducts deworming day twice in year an majority of the times its on 10th August and 10th February as fixed days. Chewable Albendazole tablets 400 mg are administered to children at government, government aided and private schools.
- **Menstrual hygiene:** Sanitary napkins may be provided in the schools for adolescent girls as per MHS guidelines.
- **Health screening:** Under RBSK, identification of 30 diseases including malnutrition and anemia with appropriate referrals. Identification of children with refractive errors may be done and spectacles provided.

Selected health conditions for child health screening and early intervention services	
Defects at birth	**Deficiencies**
• Neural tube defect • Down's syndrome • Cleft lip and palate/cleft palate alone • Talipes (clubfoot) • Developmental dysplasia of the hip • Congenital cataract • Congenital deafness	• Congenital heart diseases • Retinopathy of prematurity • Anemia especially severe anemia • Vitamin A deficiency (Bitot spot) • Vitamin D deficiency (Rickets) • Severe acute malnutrition • Goiter
Diseases of childhood	**Developmental delays and disabilities**
• Skin conditions (scabies, fungal infection and eczema) • Otitis media • Rheumatic heart disease • Reactive airway disease • Dental conditions • Convulsive disorders • Vision impairment	• Hearing impairment • Neuromotor impairment • Motor delay • Cognitive delay • Language delay • Behavior disorder (Autism) • Learning disorder • Attention deficit hyperactivity disorder
• Congenital hypothyroidism, sickle cell anemia, beta thalassemia (Optional)	

- **Physical and mental fitness:** Health and Wellness Ambassadors through classes on yoga and meditation through will inculcate the habits of yoga and meditation among children since their childhood.
- **HEADSSS:** Home, education, employment, eating, activity, drugs, sexuality, safety, suicidal thinking and depression status.
- **Research:** Research and studies on health, wellness and nutrition for children to assess the impact of the program.
- **Other preventive services:** For example, age appropriate vaccination of children through local health staff.

Electronic Health Records

- Student Health Card as electronic health record will include health screening and service access data for each student.
- Under the RBSK, the screening and referral records of all the school children will be digitalized.

Upgrading Skills in Emergency Care

- There should be a first aid box available in each school.
- The teachers and students will be made aware of the various services available to attend to emergencies like the ambulance, fire brigade, police, closest health facility, etc. Sessions on basic first-aid will be taken up and linkages with local disaster response teams will be made, to build the capacity of school teachers and children to respond to emergencies.

Traditional recommendation for school environment
- **Location:** It should be far away from busy roads, factories, market places etc.
- **Classroom:** 40 students per class room. Space per student not less than 10 sq.ft.

- **Desk:** Single desks (minus type) and chairs (with back-rest) should be provided.
- **Color:** Preferably white.
- **Lighting:** Preferably natural light coming from the left.
- **Ventilation:** Combined door and window area should be at least 25 percent of the floor space and window should be placed on different wall to ensure the cross ventilation.
- **Eating area:** Separate mid-day meals eating facilities room
- **Water:** Continuous independent source of safe and portable water
- **Sanitation:** One urinal for 60 students and one latrine for 100 students should be made available separately for boys and girls.

To enhance the quality of education across the country, the Government of India has taken following steps:

- **Samagra Shiksha:** Samagra Shiksha **an integrated scheme covering all classes from pre-primary to senior secondary has been revamped and aligned with the recommendations of NEP 2020.** The scheme aims to ensure that all children have access to quality education with an equitable and inclusive classroom environment which should take care of their diverse background, multilingual needs, different academic abilities and make them active participants in the learning process. The scheme has been extended for a period of five years i.e., from 2021-22 to 2025-26.
- **SARTHAQ:** Implementation Plan for School Education, called 'Students' and Teachers' Holistic Advancement through Quality Education (SARTHAQ)' was released on 8th April 2021. The plan keeps in mind the concurrent nature of education and adheres to the spirit of federalism. States and UTs are given the flexibility to adapt this plan with local contextualization and also modify as per their needs and requirements. This implementation plan delineates the roadmap and way forward for implementation of NEP, 2020 for the next 10 years, which is very important for its smooth and effective implementation.
- **NISHTHA:** An integrated teacher training program 1.0, 2.0, and 3.0 has been introduced for different stages of school education—teachers, head teachers/principals and other stakeholders in educational management and administration.
- **NIPUN Bharat:** National initiative for proficiency in reading with understanding and numeracy (NIPUN Bharat) has been launched under Samagra Shiksha on 5th July 2021, for ensuring that every child in the country necessarily attains foundational literacy and numeracy (FLN) by the end of Grade 3.
- **Padhe Bharat Badhe Bharat: Library grant and promotion of reading:** In order to inculcate reading habit among students of all ages, strengthening of school libraries is being undertaken through provision of books by providing library grant for government schools, under the newly launched centrally sponsored scheme of Samagra Shiksha from 2018-19. The fund for library grant ranges from ₹5,000/- to ₹20,000/- based on the category of the school.
- **Khele India Khile India: Grant for sports and physical education:** Realizing the need for holistic development of children, under the Samagra Shiksha, sports and physical education component has been introduced for the first time for encouragement of Sports, Physical activities, yoga, co-curricular activities, etc. A provision has been made for government schools for sports grant of ₹5,000 for primary schools, ₹10,000 for upper primary schools and up to ₹25,000 for secondary and senior secondary schools for meeting the expenses.
- **PM Poshan:** The Cabinet Committee on Economic Affairs (CCEA) approved the Pradhan Mantri Poshan Shakti Nirman (PM POSHAN), a modified version of the existing National

Scheme for Mid-Day Meal in Schools (MDM) on 29th September, 2021. PM POSHAN Scheme covers all school children studying in I-VIII classes in Government and Government-aided schools.

- **DIKSHA** (one nation, one digital platform) is the nation's digital infrastructure for providing quality e-content for school education in states/UTs and QR coded Energized Textbooks for all grades are available on it. 35 of the 36 states and UTs have on boarded on DIKSHA platform and contextualized the content as per the local need.
- Ministry has undertaken a proactive initiative, named, 'MANODARPAN' covering a wide range of activities to provide psychosocial support to students, teachers and families for Mental Health and Emotional Well-being during the COVID outbreak and beyond.

Global School Health Standards

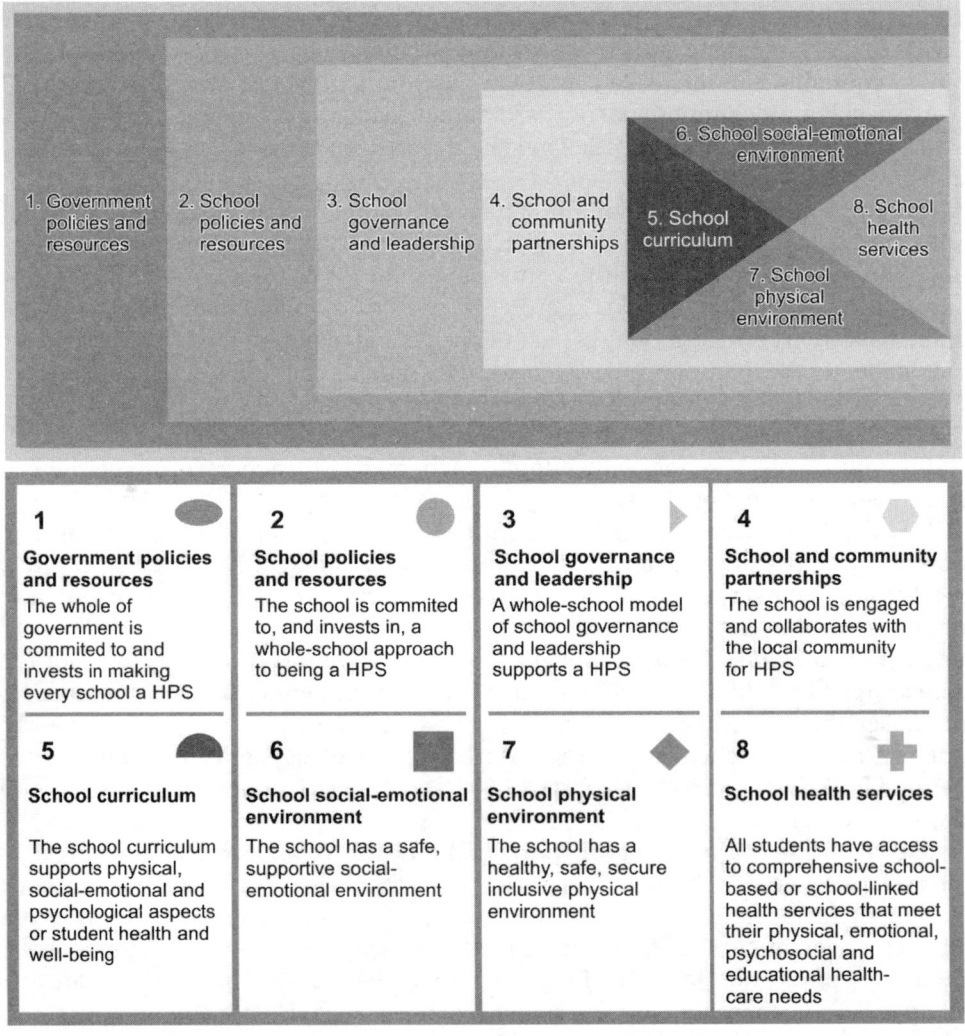

Fig. 11.3: Overview of global school health standards for health promoting schools.

BIBLIOGRAPHY

1. EFA 2000 Assessment - Thematic Study on School Health and Nutrition
2. https://nhm.gov.in/New_Updates_2018/NHM_Components/RMNCHA/AH/guidelines/Operational_guidelines_on_School_Health_Programme_under_Ayushman_Bharat.pdf
3. https://nhm.gov.in/New_Updates_2018/NHM_Components/RMNCHA/AH/Training_Materials/Curriculum-on-Health-and-Wellness-of-School-Going-Children-English.pdf
4. https://pib.gov.in/PressReleasePage.aspx?PRID=1744059
5. https://vikaspedia.in/health/nrhm/national-health-programmes-1/rashtriya-bal-swasthya-karyakram-rbsk

Annexures

CHAPTER OUTLINE

1. List of Important Incubation Period
2. List of Diseases with their Vectors
3. NIN Recommendations (EAR, RDA, Reference Man and Woman, CU)
4. List of Important Public Health Days, Weeks and Fortnights
5. Famous Acronyms

1. LIST OF IMPORTANT INCUBATION PERIOD

Disease causative organism	Incubation period (IP)
Chickenpox	14–16 days
Smallpox	7–17 days
Mumps	14–21 days
Measles	10–14 days
Rubella (German measles)	14–21 days
Poliomyelitis poliovirus	7–14 days
Tuberculosis	Weeks–years
Diphtheria	2–6 days
Pertussis (Whooping cough)	7–14 days
Typhoid fever	10–14 days
Staphylococcal food poisoning	1–6 hours
Salmonella	12–24 hours
Cl. perfringens	6–24 hours

Disease causative organism	Incubation period (IP)
Botulism	12–36 hours
Chikungunya fever	4–7 days
Meningococcal meningitis	3–4 days
Hepatitis A	15–45 days
Hepatitis E	15–60 days
Hepatitis B	45–180 days
Hepatitis C	30–120 days
Hepatitis D	30–90 days
Hepatitis E	21–45 days
L. donovani (Leishmaniasis/Kala-azar)	1–4 months
HIV/AIDS	Months–10 years
Q Fever	2–3 weeks
Trachoma	5–12 days
Tetanus	6–10 days
Rabies	3–8 weeks
Dengue	3–10 days
Malaria plasmodium falciparum	9–14 days
Malaria plasmodium vivax	8–17 days
Malaria plasmodium malariae	18–40 days
Malaria plasmodium ovale	16–18 days
Lymphatic filariasis	8–16 months
KFD (Kyasanur forest disease)	3–8 days
Japanese encephalitis	5–15 days
Bubonic plague	2–7 days
Pneumonic plague	1–3 days
Septicemic plague	2–7 days
Ebola	2–21 days
Swine Flu (H1N1)	1–4 days
Zika	3–12 days
Monkey pox	6–13 days
SARS (Severe Acute Respiratory Syndrome)	3–5 days
Avian Flu (H5N1)	2–5 days
CCHF (Crimean-Congo Hemorrhagic Fever)	1–3 days (tick bite), 5–6 days (infected body fluids like blood)
Yellow fever	2–6 days
Influenza	18–72 hours

Disease causative organism	Incubation period (IP)
Nipah virus	14–16 days
Hantavirus	1–8 weeks
COVID-19	4–14 days
Ascariasis	2 months
Ancylostomiasis (Hookworm)	5 weeks–9 months
Guinea worm	1 year
Taeniasis	8–14 weeks
Scrub typhus	10–12 days
Yaws	3–5 weeks
Anthrax	1–7 days
Brucellosis	5–60 days
Syphilis	9–90 days
Gonorrhea	1–5 days
Lymphogranuloma venereum	3–12 days
Donovanosis	3–21 days
Molluscum contagiosum	14–50 days
Chancroid	3–5 days

BIBLIOGRAPHY

1. http:/www.who.int./topic/infectious_disease/factsheets/en/
2. K Park. Park's Textbook of Preventive and Social Medicine, 23rd ed. Jabalpur: Bhanot Publishers; 2016.

2. LIST OF DISEASES WITH THEIR VECTORS

Vector	Disease transmitted
Anopheles	• Malaria • Filariasis (outside India)
Culex	• Japanese encephalitis (*C. tritaeniorhynchus*) • West nile fever • Viral arthritis • Bancroftian filariasis (*C. quinquefasciatus*)
Aedes	• Dengue • Chikungunya • Filariasis • Zika • Yellow fever • Rift valley fever
Mansonoides	• Malayan (Brugian) filariasis • Chikungunya

Ticks		
Hard tick		• Tick paralysis • Tick encephalitis • Tick hemorrhagic fever • Tularemia • Babesiosis (Human) • Crimean-Congo Hemorrhagic fever • Kyasanur forest disease (KFD) • Lyme disease
Soft tick		• Q Fever • Relapsing fever (Borreliosis)
Flies		
Sandfly (*Phlebotomus argentipes*)		• Sandfly fever • Oroya fever • Oriental sore • Kala-azar (*Visceral leishmaniasis*) • Chandipura virus
Housefly (*Musca domestica*)		• Diarrheal and dysentrical disease • Polio • Anthrax • Yaws • Trachoma • Conjunctivitis
Tse Tse Fly (*Glossina palpalis*)		Sleeping sickness
Black fly (*Simulium*)		Onchocerciasis (River blindness)
Deer fly, Horse fly		LOA LOA (Kind of filariasis)
Flea		• Plague • Endemic typhus • Chiggerosis • Hymenolepis diminuta • Tungiasis (ectoparasite)
Louse		• Epidemic typhus • Trench fever • Relapsing fever • Pediculosis
Mite		• Scrub typhus • Rickettsialpox
Itch mite		Scabies
Cyclops		• Guinea worm disease • *D Latus* (Fish tapeworm)
Aquatics snail		Schistosomiasis (Bilharziasis)
Reduviid bug (Triatomine Bug)		Chagas disease

Annexures

BIBLIOGRAPHY

1. K Park. Park's Textbook of Preventive and Social Medicine, 23rd ed. Jabalpur: Bhanot Publishers; 2016. p 768.
2. Vectorbornediseases;availableat;http://www.who.int/mediacentre/factsheets/fs387/en/, accessed on 15 November 2016.

3. NIN RECOMMENDATIONS (EAR, RDA, REFERENCE MAN AND WOMAN, CU)

Table 1: Summary of EAR (estimated average requirements) for Indians—2020.

Age group	Category of work	Body Wt (kg)	Energy* (Kcal/d)	Fats/Oils (visible) (#) (g/d)	Protein (g/d)	CHO (g/d)
Men	Sedentary	65	2,110	25	42.9	100
	Moderate		2,710	30		
	Heavy		3,470	40		
Women	Sedentary	55	1,660	20	36.3	100
	Moderate		2,130	25		
	Heavy		2,720	30		
	Pregnant woman	55 + 10	+350	30	+7.6 (2nd trimester) +17.6 (3rd trimester)	135
	Lactation 0–6 m		+600	30	+13.6	155
	7–12 m		+520		+10.6	155
Infants	0–6 m	5.8	550	–	6.7	–
	6–12 m	8.5	670	25	8.8	–
Children	1–3 y	11.7	1,010	25	9.2	100
	4–6 y	18.3	1,360	25	12.8	100
	7–9 y	25.3	1,700	30	19.0	100
Boys	10–12 y	34.9	2,220	35	26.2	100
Girls	10–12 y	36.4	2,060	45	26.6	100
Boys	13–15 y	50.5	2,860	50	36.4	100
Girls	13–15 y	49.6	2,400	35	34.7	100
Boys	16–18 y	64.4	3,320	40	45.1	100
Girls	16–18 y	55.7	2,500	35	37.3	100

*Adequate intake: There is no RDA for energy. The EAR is equivalent to the Estimated Energy Requirement (EER).#: Visible fat requirement is in proportion to EER.

Table 2: Summary of RDA (recommended dietary allowances) for Indians—2020.

Age group		Category of work	Body Wt (kg)	Protein (g/d)	CHO (g/d)	Calcium (mg/d)	Magnesium (mg/d)	Iron (mg/d)	Zinc (mg/d)	Iodine (µg/day)	Thiamine (mg/d)	Riboflavin (mg/d)	Niacin (mg/d)	Vit B6 (mg/d)	Folate (µg/d)	Vit B12 (µg/d)	Vit C (mg/d)	Vit A (µg/d)	Vit D (IU/d)
Men		Sedentary	65	54.0	130	1,000	385	19	17	150	1.4	2.0	14	1.9	300	2.5	80	1000	600
		Moderate									1.8	2.5	18	2.4					
		Heavy									2.3	3.2	23	3.1					
		Sedentary	55	45.7	130	1,000	325	29	13.2	150	1.4	1.9	11	1.9	220	2.5	65	840	600
		Moderate									1.7	2.4	14	1.9					
		Heavy									2.2	3.1	18	2.4					
Women		Pregnant woman	55 + 10	+9.5 (2nd trimester) +22.0 (3rd trimester)	175	1,000	385	40	14.5	250	2.0	2.7	+2.5	2.3	570	+0.25	+15	900	600
		Lactation 0–6 m		+16.9	200	1,200	325	23	14	280	2.1	3.0	+5	+0.26	330	+1.0	+50	950	600
		7–12 m		+13.2	200						2.1	2.9	+5	+0.17	330				
Infants		0–6 m*	5.8	8.1	55	300	30	—	—	100	0.2	0.4	2	0.1	25	1.2	20	350	400
		6–12 m	8.5	10.5	95	300	75	3	2.5	130	0.4	0.6	5	0.6	85	1.2	27	350	400
Children		1–3 y	11.7	11.3	130	500	135	8	3.0	90	0.7	0.9	7	0.9	110	1.2	27	390	600
		4–6 y	18.3	15.9	130	550	155	11	4.5	120	0.9	1.3	9	1.2	135	1.2	32	510	
		7–9 y	25.3	23.3	130	650	215	15	5.9	120	1.1	1.6	11	1.5	170	2.5	43	630	
Boys		10–12 y	34.9	31.8	130	850	270	16	8.5	150	1.5	2.1	15	2.0	220	2.5	54	770	600
Girls		10–12 y	36.4	32.8	130	850	255	28	8.5	150	1.4	1.9	14	1.9	225	2.5	52	790	600
Boys		13–15 y	50.5	44.9	130	1000	355	22	14.3	150	1.9	2.7	19	2.6	285	2.5	72	930	600
Girls		13–15 y	49.6	43.2	130	1000	325	30	12.8	150	1.6	2.2	16	2.2	245	2.5	66	890	600
Boys		16–18 y	64.4	55.4	130	1050	405	26	17.6	150	2.2	3.1	22	3.0	340	2.5	82	1,000	600
Girls		16–18 y	55.7	46.2	130	1050	335	32	14.2	150	1.7	2.3	17	2.3	270	2.5	68	860	600

*Adequate intake: There is no RDA for energy. The EAR is equivalent to the Estimated Energy Requirement (EER).

Annexures

Table 3: Reference Indian man and woman.

	Reference Indian man	Reference Indian woman
Age	19–39 years	19–39 years
Weight	65 kg	55 kg
Height	1.77 m	1.62 m
BMI	20.76	20.99
Others	Indian man or woman must be engaged in 8 hours of work, 8 hours for sleep, 4-6 hours for seating and moving around and 2 hours spending for recreation and household activity will be considered as a reference Indian male or female.	

Table 4: Consumption unit (CU) according to gender and type of work.

Lifestyle	Male		Female	
Sedentary	1.0		0.8	
	Teacher, Tailor, Barber, Executives, Shoemaker, Priest, Retired Personnel, Landlord, Peon, Postman, etc.		Teacher, Tailor, Executives, Housewife, Nurse, etc.	
Moderate	1.2		0.9	
	Fisherman, Basket maker, Potter, Goldsmith, Agricultural worker, Carpenter, Mason, Rickshaw puller, Electrician, Fitter, Turner, Welder, Industrial Laborer, Coolie, Weaver, Driver, etc.		Servant maid, Coolie, Basket maker, weaver, Agricultural worker, Bidi-maker, etc.	
Heavy	1.6		1.2	
	Stone cutter, Blacksmith, Mine Worker, Wood cutter, Gang man, etc.		Stone cutter	
For male/female below 21 years of age.				
Age group	CU required		Age group	CU required
1–3 years	0.4		7–9 years	0.7
3–5 years	0.5		9–12 years	0.8
5–7 years	0.6		12–21 years	1.0

*for infants, take zero consumption coefficient.

Important Units of Calorie

- 1 g of carbohydrate gives = 4 kcal
- 1 g of protein gives = 4 kcal
- 1 g of fat gives = 9 kcal
- 1 g of dietary fiber gives = 2 kcal
- 1 g of alcohol gives = 7 kcal
- 1 calorie = 4.184 joules
- 1 kcal = $10^3 * 4.184$
  = 4,184 joules
  = 4.184 kilo joules

Annexures

BIBLIOGRAPHY

1. Recommended Dietary Allowances & Estimated Average Requirements for Indians – 2020, https://www.nin.res.in/nutrition2020/RDA_short_report.pdf

4. LIST OF IMPORTANT PUBLIC HEALTH DAYS, WEEKS AND FORTNIGHTS

Month	Date	Observed as
January	12	National Youth Day
	24	National Girl Child Day
	30	World Leprosy Eradication Day
February	4	World Cancer Day
	10	National Deworming Day
	12	Sexual and Reproductive Health Awareness Day
March	3	World Birth Defects Day
	4	National Safety Day
	6	Glaucoma Day
	8	International Women's Day
	11	No Smoking Day
	2nd Thursday	World Kidney Day
	15	World Disabled Day/World Consumer Rights Day
	16	Measles Immunization Day
	20	World Oral Health Day
	21	World Forestry Day/World Down Syndrome Day
	22	World Day for Water/World Disable Day
	23	World Metrological Day
	24	World TB Day
	26	World Epilepsy Day (Purple Day)
April	2	World Autism Day
	7	World Health Day
	11	World Parkinson Day/National Safe Motherhood Day
	17	World Hemophilia Day
	18	World Heritage Day
	19	World Liver Day
	22	Earth Day
	25	World Malaria Day
	Last Week	World Immunization Week
May	1st Tuesday	World Asthma Day
	1–7th	Anti-Malaria Week

Annexures

Month	Date	Observed as
	8	World Red Cross Day/World Thalassemia Day
	11–18	Retinoblastoma Awareness Week
	12	World Chronic Fatigue Syndrome Awareness Day/International Nurses Day
	15	International Day of Families/International Kangaroo Care Awareness Day
	16	National Dengue Day
	28	International Women's Health Day/World Menstrual Hygiene Day
	31	World Anti-Tobacco Day
June	5	World Environment Day
	8	World Brain Tumor Day
	14	World Blood Donor Day
	17	World Day to Combat Desertification and Drought
	19	World Sickle Cell Day
	21	World Yoga Day
	26	International Day Against Drug Abuse and Illicit Trafficking
	1st to 30th	Anti-Malaria Month
July	1	Doctors Day (In India)
	11	World Population Day
	28	World Hepatitis Day
	29	ORS Day
August	1–8	World Breastfeeding Week
	10	National Deworming Day
	12	International Youth Day
	25th Aug–8th Sept.	Eye Donation Fortnight
September	1 to 7	National Nutrition Week
	8	World Literacy Day
	10	World Suicide Prevention Day
	12	World Oral Health Day
	21	World Alzheimer's Day
	26	World Day of the Deaf
	28	World Rabies Day
	29	World Heart Day
October	1	International Day for the Elderly/National Voluntary Blood Donation Day
	2	National Anti-Drug Addiction Day
	2nd Wednesday	World Disaster Reduction Day

Month	Date	Observed as
	2nd Thursday	World Sight Day
	10	World Mental Health Day
	11	World Obesity Day/International Day of Girl Child
	12	World Arthritis Day
	15–19	World Obesity Awareness Week
	15	World Handwashing Day
	16	World Food Day/World Anesthesia Day
	17	World Trauma Day
	20	World Osteoporosis Day
	21	World Iodine Deficiency Disorder Day
	24	World Polio Day/UN Day
	26	World Obesity Day
	29	World Stroke Day
	30	World Thrift Day
November	3rd Wednesday	World COPD Day
	10	World Immunization Day
	12	World Pneumonia Day
	13	World Alzheimer Day
	14	World Diabetes Day
	17	World Prematurity Day/World Epilepsy Day
	18 to 24	World Antimicrobial Awareness Week
	19	World Toilet Day
	15–21	Newborn Care Week
	25	International Day for Elimination of Violence Against Women
December	1	World AIDS Day
	2	National Pollution Prevention Day
	3	International Day of Persons with Disabilities
	9	World Patient's Safety Day
	10	Human Rights Day
	12	Universal Health Coverage Day

BIBLIOGRAPHY

1. List of important health days; available at; http://www.rajswasthya.nic.in/important%20health%20days.pdf, accessed on 10 September, 2016.
2. Official who health days, who, available at; http://www.who.int/mediacentre/events/official_days/en/, accessed on 14 September, 2016.
3. Program calendar, available at; www.gujhealth.gov.in, accessed on 12 September, 2016.

5. FAMOUS ACRONYMS

- **Bridge: B**oosting **R**outine **I**mmunization **D**emand **G**eneration
  This is an interpersonal communication skill (IPC) training based on SBCC (Social and behavioral change communication) for frontline health workers such as auxiliary nurse midwife (ANM), accredited social health activist (ASHA) and anganwadi worker (AWW) to improve immunization coverage.
- **5 R** for improving coverage and quality of routine immunization. To reach every child with:
  1. Right vaccine
  2. Right condition of the vaccine
  3. Right quantity of the dose of the vaccine
  4. Right timing of the vaccine
  5. Right place for the vaccine administration
- **eVIN : E**lectronic **V**accine **I**ntelligence **N**etwork
  - It is a web-based vaccine management system to improve efficiency of vaccination system.
  - It is a joint initiative of Ministry of Health and Family Welfare (MOHFW) and United Nations Development Programme (UNDP).
  - A unique innovation that brings together technology, people and processes to strengthen the vaccine supply chain by digitizing information on vaccine stocks and storage temperatures.
- **CoWIN:** COVID Vaccine Intelligence Network
- It is an Indian government web portal for COVID 19 vaccination registration. It also provides vaccination certificate. This portal also integrated with arogya setu app.
- **SAANS: S**ocial **A**wareness **a**nd **A**ctions to **N**eutralize **P**neumonia **S**uccessfully
  - It aims to reduce childhood pneumonia related mortality less than three per thousand live births by 2025.
  - It is to increase awareness among caregiver to prevent and early identification of childhood pneumonia.
- **3 DELAY:** Model for maternal mortality (**3 D**)
  1. **Delay** in decision-making for medical help
  2. **Delay** in reaching appropriate health facility
  3. **Delay** in receiving adequate care in health facility
- **ANMOL: A**uxiliary **N**urse **M**idwifery **O**nline
  - It is a tablet-based application developed for collection of reproductive and child health (RCH)-related information which provide readily available services, such as due list, desk board, guidance based on data entered on it.
- **5As:** It is 5As intervention for supporting smoking cessation:
  1. **Ask:** Ask all patients about current smoking status
  2. **Assess:** Assess readiness or willingness to quit
  3. **Advise:** Advise all smokers to quit and provide information on benefits of quitting smoking
  4. **Assist:** Assist all smokers in quitting smoking
  5. **Arrange:** Arrange follow-up
- **5Rs:** It is motivational tool specially used for those smokers who are not ready to quit:
  1. **Relevance:** Show the relevance of smoking
  2. **Risks:** Help the patients to identify the negative consequences of smoking

3. **Rewards:** Help the patient to know the benefits of stopping of smoking
4. **Roadblocks:** Ask the patients to know the barriers to quitting
5. **Repetition:** This motivational interaction should be repeated everytime

☐ **7Cs:** It is tool of effective communication:
1. **Clarity:** It is message with clear ideas and in a language that is easy to understand.
2. **Completeness:** It should convey all the necessary information required by audiences thus it brings the desired response.
3. **Conciseness:** Communicating message with least possible words thus it is time saving.
4. **Concreteness:** Communication which is specific based on facts and figures.
5. **Correctness:** No grammatical error in the communication and accuracy in stating facts.
6. **Consideration:** Before putting any message in front of receiver consider their problems from their points of view.
7. **Courtesy:** Courtesy means the message must have sender's expression as well as must have the respect for the receiver. Courtesy strengthen the relations.

☐ **Frames: Brief intervention for harmful alcohol consumption:**
- **F: Feedback of personal risks or impairment:** Let the people to know that they are drinking at hazardous level and risk associated with this hazardous drinking pattern can be a powerful motivator for change.
- **R: Responsibility:** The decision to change drinking patterns is the responsibility of the person alone.
- **A: Advice:** Advice to change drinking behavior.
- **M: Menu:** Provide **Menu** of strategies for changing drinking behaviors.
- **E: Empathy:** Brief interventions implementation should be in the context of a warm, reflective, empathic, and collaborative form.
- **S: Self-efficacy:** Support the person's self-efficacy for change, and communicate a sense of optimism.

☐ **MPOWER package:** The MPOWER policy package can reverse the tobacco epidemic and prevent millions of tobacco-related deaths.
1. **M**: Monitor tobacco use and prevention policies,
2. **P**: Protect people from tobacco smoke,
3. **O**: Offer help to quit tobacco use,
4. **W**: Warn about the dangers of tobacco,
5. **E**: Enforce bans on tobacco advertising, promotion and sponsorship, and
6. **R**: Raise taxes on tobacco.

☐ **WASH:**
- **W:** Water
- **S:** Sanitation
- **H:** Hygiene
- UNICEF has introduced this WASH strategy since 2006 for improving availability of drinking water at the most remote rural area and also improvement in the sanitation facilities.
- WASH is essential in healthcare facilities, schools and early childhood development centers.

Annexures

- **GATHER approach:** It is the counseling approach commonly used in family planning while dealing with the choice of methods of contraception:
  - **G: Greet** (show respect and trust)
  - **A: Ask** (encourage them to tell the problem)
  - **T: Tell** (provide accurate and specific needed information)
  - **H: Help** (help them to make correct decisions)
  - **E: Explain** (clear the doubts or any misunderstanding)
  - **R: Return** (follow-up visit)
- **25 by 25 initiative:**
  - It is the target set under WHO's NCD global monitoring framework.
  - It means reduction by 25% in premature mortality from non-communicable diseases by 2025.
- **STEPS approach:** It is approach developed by WHO for the surveillance of risk factors related to non-communicable diseases:
  - **STEP 1: Behavioral measurements** (It includes details about tobacco use, alcohol use, diet, physical activity and history of raised BP and history of diabetes).
  - **STEP 2: Physical measurements** (**In the core list** it includes measurement of height, weight and blood pressure. While in the **expanded** form measurement of hip circumference and heart rate is added to core list).
  - **STEP 3: Biochemical measurements** (In the core list measurement of blood glucose and blood lipids included while TG, HDL, and cholesterol measurements are added in the expanded form)
- **DASH: D**ietary **A**pproach for **S**top **H**ypertension:
  - **D**ietary **A**pproaches to **S**top **H**ypertension is a diet plan that is rich in fruits, vegetables, fibers, minerals and low in saturated fat, trans fat and sodium.
  - In this strategy diet plan is decided as per the level of activity and age.
  - It is very important that aerobic exercise should be complementing this DASH plan to have good results in lowering blood pressure.
- **GOBI-FFF:** It is an initiative of UNICEF to reduce child mortality.
  - **G:** Growth monitoring
  - **O:** Oral rehydration
  - **B:** Breastfeeding
  - **I:** Immunization
  - **F:** Female literacy
  - **F:** Family Spacing
  - **F:** Food Supplements for at risk pregnant women
- **SAFE strategy:** This strategy was launched in 1996 by WHO to eliminate trachoma.
  - **S: Surgery** for trichiasis and entropion
  - **A: Antibiotic** (use of Azithromycin as mass treatment)
  - **F: Facial hygiene** (facial cleanliness)
  - **E: Environmental** (environmental improvement)
- **5 S strategy for management in health:** Adopted from Japanese methods of management.

Indian word	Japanese word	Description
Sort	Seiri	Segregate things as wanted and unwanted
Set in order	Seiton	Arrange all necessary items in order so easily can be retrieved
Shine	Seiso	Cleanliness of the workplace should be maintained on daily basis
Standardize	Seiketsu	Standardize level of each activities to compare
Sustain	Shitsuke	Adequate training and motivation should be given to sustain the achieved results

BIBLIOGRAPHY

1. https://nhm.gov.in/New_Updates_2018/NHM_Components/Immunization/Guildelines_ for_immunization/BRIDGE_Operational_Guidelines.pdf
2. https://www.in.undp.org/content/india/en/ home/projects/gavi1.html
3. https://nhm.gov.in/index1.php?lang=1&level=4&sublinkid=1336&lid=716
4. https://imi2.nhp.gov.in/
5. https://www.maternity world wide.org/what-we-do/three-delays-model/
6. https://www.cowin.gov.in/

Index

Page numbers followed by *f* refer to figure and *t* refer to table.

A

Abdomen inspection, assessment of 225
Abdominal cramps 173
Abiotic components 83
Abscess 309
Absolute insulin deficiency 400
Accredited Social Health Activist 43, 384
    components of 43
    incentives 166, 356
    role of 356
Acquired immunodeficiency syndrome 335, 452
Activated health education model 184
Active life expectancy 21
Acute encephalitis syndrome 374
Acute respiratory syndrome, severe 452
Admission and discharge criteria 164
Adolescent girls, scheme for 232
Adoption 238
Aedes 453
    mosquito 258
Aflatoxicosis 171
Aflatoxins 170
Age appropriate health promotion 444
Age specific death rate 20
Aged person, care of 211
AGMARK 178
Agricultural Products (Grading and Marketing) Act 178
Agriculture 82
Air 3, 85
    change, standards of 95
    quality, monitoring of 119
Air pollutants
    primary 99
    secondary 99
Air pollution 99
    control measures for 100
    reducing
        indoor 64
        outdoor 64
Air quality index
    and health impact, level of 120
    classification of 119
    objectives of 119
Air-borne 258
    infection 326

Airway disease, reactive 446
Albendazole 155
Albumin 220
Alcohol 395
All health-related information, repository of 72
Alphavirus 302
Amebiasis 304
    life cycle 305
Amicrofilaraemia, asymptomatic 316
Amino acids 124
Amphixenoses 320
Analytic epidemiology, second method of 281
Ancylostomiasis 305, 453
Anemia
    prevalence 24, 153*t*
    testing of 155
    treatment of 155
Anemia Control Program 154
Anemia Mukt Bharat 152
    strategy of 154*f*
Anganwadi
    population norms for 149
    services scheme 232
Anhydrous 175
Anicteric leptospirosis 325
Animal birth control 389
Animal bite wound, management of 322
Animal health component 389
    strategies for 389
Animal population, increased density of 320
Animal products, increased trade in 320
Annual mass drug administration 316, 386
Anopheles 453
Antenatal care 217
Anthrax 319, 320, 324, 374, 453
Anthropometric measurements 129, 224
Anthropometry 220
    blood pressure recording 221
    breast self-examination 221
    electronic BP apparatus 221
    height recording 220
    temperature recording 221
    urine testing 223
    weight recording 220
Anthroponotic cutaneous leishmaniasis 317
Anthropozoonoses 319

Antibody, synthesis of 123
Antigenemia 385
Antigenic shift 262
Anti-rabies
   serum 389
   vaccine 389
      regime of 322
Anus inspection, assessment of 225
Aquatic ecosystem 84
Aquatics snail 454
Arbovirus infections 319
Arterial disease, peripheral 405
Arthritis 309
Arthropod infections 309
Ascariasis 307, 453
Ascorbic acid 125, 127
Asexual cycle 310
Atal Mission for Rejuvenation and Urban Transformation 103
Atal Vayo Abhyuday Yojana 237
Attack rate, secondary 287, 288, 292
Audiovisual aids 203
Auditory effects 100
Auto disable syringe 227
Autoimmune 416
Auxiliary Nurse Midwife 69
   responsibilities of 353
   role of 432
Avian flu 452
Ayurveda 1
AYUSH services 64
Ayushman Bharat 71, 74
   Digital Mission 71
   Health Account number (health ID) 72
   School Health and Wellness Ambassador initiative 444f

B

Back pain 227
Backwashing 91
Bacteria 252
Bacterial food poisoning 172t
Bag technique 212
   basics of 214
Balanced and healthy diets 64
Bancroftian filariasis, chronic 316
Bang's disease 326
Bar-code system 115
Basic health worker committee 33
Basic home 213
Basic needs indicators 23
Bathrooms and toilets 237

Battered child syndrome 233
Bed turnover ratio 22
Bedaquiline 367
Bed-occupancy rate 22
Behavior change 183, 195
   models of 184
   stages of 188f
   techniques of 184
Behavior, steps of change in 184
Behavioral health 17
Beta blockers 417
Beta thalassemia 446
Beti Bachao Beti Padhao Scheme 232
Bio-chemical estimations 130
Biodiversity 82, 84
   loss of 84
Biological oxygen demand 111
Biological transmission 258
Biomedical waste management 114
   Rules 114, 115
Bio-medical wastes
   disposal of 116
   treatment of 116
Bio-security preparedness 71
Biotic components 83
Birth and Death Registration Act 5
Black death 323
Black fly 454
Bleaching powder 93
Blinding 272
   double 272
   single 272
   trachoma 338
   triple 272
   type of 272
Blindness 290, 411, 412
   causes of 412
   prevalence of 411
Block public health units 71
Blood
   lipids, abnormal 405
   tests 417
Blood pressure
   high 417
   measurement of 403
   tracking of 404
Blumberg antigen 302
Boiling 93
   advantages of 93
Bradycardia 416
Break point chlorination 93
Breast and axillae inspection, assessment of 225

Index

Breast cancer 418, 423
    management algorithm for 419*f*
    risk factors for 418
    warning signs of 419
Breastfeeding
    benefits of 152*f*
    continued 151
    exclusive 150
    initiating 150
Breteau index 282, 313
Brickmaker's anemia 305
Bronchitis
    acute 100
    chronic 100
Brucellosis 257, 319, 320, 326, 374, 453
Bubonic plague 323, 452
Bull necked 293
Bureau of Indian Standards 178
    certification 177
Burial 108

C

Calcivirus 302
Calorie, important units of 457
Cancer 399
    breast 409, 418
    cervical 418
    development, phases of 418*f*
    oral 418
    statistics 25, 428
    warning signals for 418
Canicola fever 325
Capacity building 433
Carbohydrate 123
    complex 123
Carbon monoxide 99
Cardiovascular diseases 394, 405, 435
Cardiovascular system inspection, assessment of 225
Care
    after 238
    continuity of 68, 430
    primary 64
Caregiver after vaccination 354
Carpal tunnel syndrome 416
Case control study 267
    advantages of 268
    disadvantages of 268
Case fatality rate 20
Catarrhal stage 294
Catastrophic health expenditures 63
Causation theory, web of 250
Causative agent 287, 292
Cellulitis 309
Central Consumer Protection Authority 181
Central Council of Health 47
Central sector components 71
Central surveillance unit 375
Centrally sponsored scheme components 71
Cerebrovascular disease 405
Certificate Program in Community Health 54
Certification 261
Cervical cancer 419, 423
    management algorithm for 420*f*
    prevention of 421
    risk factors for 419
    signs of 420
    symptoms of 420
Cervix 409
Chadah committee 33
Chaga's disease 257
Chancroid 453
Chandipura virus disease 374
Chemical control 311
Chemical disinfection 93
Chemical oxygen demand 111
Chickenpox 258, 288, 374, 451
Chief District Health Officer 359
Chikungunya 314, 374
    fever 320
    prevention and control of 385
Child abuse 232
    risk factors for 233
    types of 233
Child health screening 446
Child Marriage Restraint Act 5
Child Protection Services Scheme 232
Childhood vaccine preventable disease 23
Children's home 238
Chinese medicine 2
Chlorination, desirable level of 93
Chlorinator 93
Chlorine
    demand 92
    solution 93
    tablet 94
Chlorofluorocarbons 101
Chloronome 93
Chloroquine 44
Cholera 169, 227, 257, 275, 298, 374
Chronic disease 400
Chronic obstructive
    lesion, stage of 316
    pulmonary disease 425

Cigarettes and other Tobacco Products Act 398
Clean India Mission 103
Climate Change 101
   and National Program 101
   on health, indirect impacts of 102
   positive impacts of 102
   threat of 102
Clofazimine 356, 367
Clostridium perfringens 451
Codex alimentarius commission 177
Cohort study
   advantages of 270
   analysis of 270
   design overview 269
   disadvantages of 270
   steps of 272
   synonyms of 269
Cold chain, managing 226
Colon 409
Combined cohort study 270
Commercial sex workers 232, 235
Commissioner of Food Safety 179
Committee to review 33
Common cancer 418
   cases of 25
Common health problems, management of 227
Common nutritional
   challenges 129
   disorders 139
Communicability, period of 260, 287
Communicable disease 260, 287, 389, 393
Communication 193, 195
   barriers to effective 192
   basic methods of 189
   behavior change 197
   channels of 190
   common channel of 190
   face-to-face 190
   formal 192
   improving factors 193*f*
   in health education, concepts of 183
   informal 192
   message 190
   non-verbal 192
   one-way 192
   overcoming barriers to 193
   process 190
   receiver 190
   sender 190
   skills 189
   social and behavior change 194
   social behavior change 197*f*
   theory 185
   two-way 192
   types of 192
   with caregivers 227
Community assessment 206
Community based approach 138
Community diagnosis 246
Community health 1, 3
   center 49, 427
Community health nurse 11, 208, 220
   competencies for 11
   function of 209
   in family health services, role and responsibilities of 208
   in supportive supervision and training, role and responsibilities of 218
   major roles of 12
   qualities of 12, 12*f*
   role and responsibilities of 206, 212
Community health nursing 1, 4
   approaches 206
   areas of concern for 10
   characteristics of 4
   objectives of 10
   Practice 5
   principles of 10
   scope of 10
Community health officer 75
   role of 432
   roles and responsibilities of 370
Community healthcare services 207
Community level, management at 227
Community mobilization 423
Community nursing diagnosis 206
Community Nutrition Education Program 138
Community participation
   advantages of 42
   and citizen engagement 80
   in health planning 41
   initiatives for 42
Community volunteers 384
Compact fluorescent lamp 117
Complementary feeding to baby, benefits of 152*f*
Compliment fixation test 318
Condoms 44
Condyloma acuminate 337
Conjunctiva 255, 338
Conservancy system 108

Index

Constipation 135
Construction and Demolition Waste Management Rules 114
Consumer Protection Act 181
Contact infection 326
Contact with soil 256
Contagion theory 249
Container index 313
Contractual manpower 425
Controlled tripping 108
Convalescent stage 294
Convulsive disorders 446
Cook thoroughly 176
Cooked food 176
Cooking competitions 169
COP-26 Glasgow 103
Cornea 338
Coronary heart disease 394, 405
Corrective actions 84
Cost benefit analysis 29
Cost effectiveness analysis 28
Cost minimization analysis 28
Cost utility analysis 28
Counseling 215
    basics of 215
    benefits of 215
    key components of 215
    tasks involved in 215
Counselor characteristics 216
Counselor skills 216
Country's fuel-efficiency standards 102
COVID-19 296, 448, 453
C-planning process 195f
Crimean-Congo hemorrhagic fever 334, 374, 452
Critical care hospital blocks 71
Cross ventilation 95
Cross-sectional study, type of 266
Crude death rate 19
Cryptic filariasis 316
Culex 453
    gelidus 318
    tritaeniorhynchus 318
    vishnui groups 318
Culicine mosquitoes 318
Cultural anthropological norms 320
Cushing's syndrome 403
Cutaneous leishmaniasis 317
Cyclical trend 280
Cyclops 454
Cycloserine 367
Cyclozoonoses 319
Cytomegalovirus infection 257
Cytotoxin 172

D

Dapsone 356
Daylight factor 97
Deaf 414
Deafness 413
    causes of 414
Death rate, specific 19
Decentralized Non-governmental Organization Scheme 429
Deer fly 454
Defects at birth 446
Demonic theory 248
Dengue 275, 312, 374, 452
    fever 313, 320
    hemorrhagic fever 313
    prevention and control of 385
    virus 258
Dental conditions 446
Dermatitis 399
Dermatophytosis 320
Dever's epidemiological model 250
Deworming 155, 445
Diabetes mellitus 135, 400, 423
    complications of 399
    etiological classification of 400
    insulin-dependent 400
    management of 401
    type 1 400
    type 2 400
Diabetic coma 402
Diabetic ketoacidosis 402
Diagnose anemia 153t
Diarrhea 135, 173, 227, 290, 374
    management of 161
    prevention and control of 160
    treatment of 162
Diarrheal disease, acute 374
Diet consistency, modifications in 134
Diet planning
    concept of 133
    principles of 134
Diet surveys, types of 130
Dietary fiber 123
Dietary intake methods 130
Digi doctor 72, 73
Digital health ecosystem 72

Digital infrastructure for knowledge sharing (DIKSHA) 448
Dihydrate 175
Diphtheria 293, 319, 374, 451
Directorate General of Health Services 47
Disability
    years lived with 432
    years lost to 21
Disability rates 21
    types 21
Disability-adjusted life years 21, 414
Disability-free life expectancy 21
Disaster, strengthening 71
Disease
    causation, postulates of 252
    control 261
    determinants of 244
    development of 241
    distribution of 244
    frequency 244
    important 335
    infectious 71, 260
    natural history of 247, 262, 263*f*
    specific profile 24*t*
    supernatural theory of 1
    types of 88, 374
    under eradication 374
    with vectors, list of 453
    with water, classification of 88
    X status 286
Disease causation
    factors of 248
    theories of 247
    wheel of 251*f*
Disease causative organism 451
    incubation period 451
Disease transmission
    different modes of 255
    modes of 254
Disinfection 92
    types of 92
Disposable delivery kits 44
District Cancer Control Program 429
District Consumer Disputes Redressal Forum 181
District Health Knowledge Institute 80
District Surveillance Unit 375
District Tuberculosis Center 359
District Viral Hepatitis Management Unit 392
Diversity and quantity of family food supplies 136
Donovanosis 453
Dose-response relationship 253
Dracunculiasis 308
Droplet nuclei 258
Drug 214
Drug-resistant tuberculosis 363, 365, 366
    pre-extensively 366
Drug-sensitive tuberculosis, regimen for 365
Duplicate samples 131
Dysentery 227, 374

E

Early visual impairment 411
Ears inspection 224
Earth and water 3
Eating area 447
Eating patterns 273
Ebola 452
    river 334
    virus disease 334
Echinococcosis 319
Economic evaluation, types of 28
Economic growth 55
Economic status 17
Ecosystem 82, 83
    structure of 83*f*
Eczema 446
Edema, malignant 324
Edible oils packaging order 179
Education 17
Effective gatekeeping 68
Effluent, disposal of 111
Egyptian chlorosis 305
Egyptian medicine 2
Elders abuse 232, 234
Electronic health records 446
Electronic medical record 72, 73
Elimination of tuberculosis, joint effort for 371
Emergency care, upgrading skills in 446
Emissions strategies, reducing 103
Emotional abuse 233
Emotional dimension 16
Encephalitic stage, acute 318
End tuberculosis strategy 369
Endemic ascites 171
Endemic treponematoses 340
Endocrine disorders 403
Enteric fever 299, 374
Enteritis 227
Enterobacteriaceae 319
Enterotoxin 172
Environment 250
    and health, concept of 85
    factor 287
    health 82

Index

indicators 22
laws and rules 112
modification 205
preparation of 224
science 82
Enzymes 123
E-pharmacy and telemedicine services 72
Epidemic Disease Act 5
Epidemic dropsy 170
Epidemic jaundice 302
Epidemic preparedness 71
Epidemiological study designs, classification of 265
Epidemiological triad 249
Epidemiological triangle 250
Epidemiology
    basic tools of 245
    components of 244
    concepts of 259
    made easy 241
    objectives of 244
    uses of 246
Equipment 214
    preparation of 224
Ergotism 171
Essential newborn care 217
Essential primary health services 68
Estimated average requirements 455t
Ethambutol 367
Ethionamide 367
Evidence, level of 284
Evidence-based
    approach 207
    medicine, hierarchy of 284
Evidence-based public health 283
    characteristics of 283
    steps of 284
E-waste management rules 117
Excreta disposal, methods of 108
Exophthalmos 417
Extrapulmonary tuberculosis 364
Eye
    health 431
    inspection 224
    prominent 417

F

Face and skull inspection 224
Family composition 209
Family coping 210
Family diet survey 130
Family environment 210
Family function 210
Family health
    assessment 209
    nursing plan 209
    services 208, 209
        principles of 209
    status 210
Family life education 211
Family meal requires, modification of 133
Family planning 210
Family process 210
Family record 230
Family resources 210
Fat 124
    invisible 124
    soluble vitamins 124, 125
    sources of 124
    trans 124
    visible 124
Fatty acids, types of 124t
F-diagram 108, 109f
Feeding
    complementary 150
    interval and frequency of 134
Feticide, female 232, 235
Fever 135
Field work, preparation for 277
Filariasis 314
Filtration process 91f
Fingers 256
Fire 3
First census 5
Fisheries 82
Flavivirus 302
    genus 318
Flea 454
Flies 256, 454
Floor 85
    space 86
Fluid 256
Fluorosis 399
Folic acid 125
    fortified 156
    supplementation 155
Folk media 191, 202
Fomite-borne 258
Fomites 256
Food 256
    adulteration 170
    analyst 179
    balance sheets 131
    behavior 136

function of 122
preparation and handling 171
production and processing 171
pyramid 128, 128f
related diseases 169
specimens 174
storage 172
Food Adulteration Act, prevention of 179
Food poisoning 257, 300
mechanisms of 172t
Food safety 169, 175
officer 179
regulation 176
standards 177
Food Safety and Standards Act 177-179
Food Safety Commissioners 177
Food-borne
diseases 102, 169, 171
hazards, major 173t
illness 171
infection 174, 326
Food-poisoning, treatment of 174
Foot and mouth disease 320
Forestry 82
Formulated plan, write-up of 31
Foster care 238
Fruit products order 179
Fumonisins 170
Fungal infection 446

G

Gallbladder 409
Gastric aspirate 174
Gastroenteritis 374
acute 257
Genital warts 337
Genitalia inspection, assessment of
female 225
male 225
Geriatric clinic 427
Geriatric field 426
Geriatric medicine 427
Geriatric unit 427
Germ theory 249
German measles 291, 451
Gestational diabetes mellitus 401
Global School Health Standards 448
overview of 448f
Glucose 175
Glycemic index 123

Goiter 434
Gonorrhea 453
Good documentation, characteristic of 229
Good human relations 201
Good listener, listening ladder for 193
Graves' disease 416
Greek medicine 2
Green co-rating system 103
Green highways 102
Green House Gas Program 103
Gross Domestic Product 27
Gross National Product 27
Group approach 201
Group discussion 202
Group on medical education and support
manpower 34
Guinea worm 308, 453

H

Handicapped person, care of 211
Handling animal byproducts and wastes 320
Handwashing
and sanitation 160
demonstration 162
Hansen's disease 340
Hanta virus 332, 453
Hard tick 454
Hardness, level of 87
Hashim committee 67
Hashimoto's thyroiditis 416
Hazards 98, 100
of inadequate lighting 97, 97f
of overcrowding 86
of poor sanitation 110
Head and neck, assessment of 224
Health 13
and disease, determinants of 13
and education 440
biological determinants of 17
care delivery indicators 21
communication, methods in 201, 201f
concept of 13
major 205f
consequences of child abuse 234, 234f
data consent manager 73
determinants of 16, 16f, 17
dimensions of 14
environmental determinants of 17
financing and financial protection 79
human resources for 80

Index

indicators of 18
institution, peripheral 360
museums and exhibitions 202
nursing approaches, types of 206
persons 396
policy indicators 22
positive 13
promoting schools 448*f*
screening 445
situation, analysis of 30
sociocultural determinants of 17
spectrum of 264
status, assessment of 220
system 46
Health and wellness
   ambassadors 443
   center 71, 75
      key elements of 51*f*
      level, management at 228
      sub-health centers, care at 399
   day 444
   messengers 444
Health behavior 185
   categories of 183
   preventive 183
Health belief model 184, 185
   limitations of 185
Health education 198, 205
   and health promotion, basics of 198
   approach 199
   emphasis of 198
   models of 200
   planning of 203, 203*f*
   principles of 200
   tools of 201*t*
Health facility 360
   registry 72, 73
   status of 23*t*
   type 23
Health planning 29, 32
   basics of 26
   cycle 29
   stages of 29, 29*f*
Health problem 23, 23*t*, 198
   of school children 442
Health promotion 203
   components of 204*f*
   intervention in 205
   principles of 204
Health services 17

integration of 33
norms 80
Health survey
   and development committee 32
   and planning committee 32
Health-adjusted life expectancy 21
Healthcare 38, 45
   planning and organization 26
   professionals registry 73
   services 64
   system, levels of 231*f*
Healthcare Delivery System 230*t*
   institutional framework of 46
   overview of 45
   rural area 48
   urban area 49
Healthcare providers 72
   role of 198
Healthy diet 133
Healthy environment 211
Healthy worker effect 270
Hearing loss 414
   and deafness 413
   causes of 414
Hearing, hard of 414
Heart attack 405
   preventing 405
   warning signs of 405
Heart disease, congenital 405
Hemagglutination inhibition test 318
Hemoglobin
   estimation 222
   levels 153*t*
Hemorrhagic fever 374
Hemorrhagic jaundice 325
Hepacivirus 302
Hepatitis 227, 389
   A 257, 302, 374, 389
   acute 374
   B 147, 257, 302, 389, 391
      immunization of 390
      vaccination 391
   B-0 346
   C 389, 391
      virus 302
   D 389
   E 302, 374, 389
      virus 302
   infectious 302
   post-transfusion 302

Hill's criteria 253, 270
Historical cohort study 270
Home based care for young child 166
　home visits 167f
　schedule of visits under 167f
Home based newborn care 166
Home care, types of 213
Home visit
　activities of 213
　advantages of 212
　assessed during 213
　limitations of 213
　objectives of 212
　purpose of 212
Homeopathic medicine 3
Hookworm 305, 453
Hormones 123
Horrock's apparatus 93
Horse fly 454
Horticulture waste 114
Hospice 240
　care centers 236
Hospital Management Society, objectives of 44
Hospital-acquired infection 258
Hospitals and doctors, voluntary for 73
House 85
　and health 85
　index 282, 313
Housefly 454
Housing criteria 86
Human cycle 310
Human development index 14
Human health component 388
　strategies of 389
Human immunodeficiency virus 25, 452
　transmission, risk of 379t
Human papillomavirus 419
Human rabies 374
Human resource 163
　development 373
Human tuberculosis 319
Humoral theory 248
Humors theory 2
Hydatid disease 331
Hydrocarbon 99
Hyperaldosteronism 403
Hypercholesterolemia 251
Hyperglycemia 402
Hyperlipidemia 405
Hyperparathyroidism 403

Hypertension 135, 251, 273, 394, 402, 423
　classification of 403
　complications of 399
　risk factors for 403
　stop 404
　symptoms of 404
Hyperthyroidism 403, 415, 416
　diagnosed 417
　signs of 417
　symptoms of 417
Hypnozoites 312
Hypochlorite, high test 93
Hypoglycemia 402
Hypotheses
　evaluation 280
　generation 280
Hypothyroidism 415
　congenital 446
　signs of 416
　symptoms of 416

I

Iceberg phenomenon 263
Icteric leptospirosis 325
Illness behavior 183
Immunization 223, 226, 353, 415
　complete 353
　planning for 226
　services 211
　session
　　preparing and conducting 227
　　routine 353
　　site 226
Impounding reservoirs 88
Inadequate cooking temperature 171
India's contribution globally 23
Indian Factories Act 5
Indirect policy instruments 143
Indoor air pollution 100
Infant and child mortality rate 24
Infant and young child feeding 150, 217
　benefits of 152
　practices 141
Infant mortality rate 20
Infections 170
　chain of 255f
　concept of chain of 254
　initial 336
　intestinal 298
　latent 260

nosocomial 258
reservoir of 316
source of 287, 292, 300
subclinical 253
Infectious disease, chronic 338
Infective organism, lifecycle of 319
Influenza 258, 292, 374, 452
Infrastructure and human resource development 64
Initiation and planning of school health services 443
Innovation theory
   diffusion of 185, 186
   limitations of diffusion of 187
Insects 85
In-service training 219
Institutional level diet survey 131
Instrument 214
   utility 93
Insulin deficiency, relative 400
Integrated Child Development Services Scheme 147
Integrated Disease Surveillance Program 372
Integrated District Public Health Laboratories 71
Integrated Solid Waste Management System Hierarchy 107
Integrated vector control 385
Integumentary system, assessment of 224
Intensified Diarrhea Control Fortnight 141, 160
Intermittent system, disadvantages of 89
International Organization for Standardization 177
Internet 202
Intestinal parasites 257
Intoxications 170
Intrathoracic tuberculosis, pediatric 364
Invasion 172
Inventory method 131
Iodine 94
   deficiency disorders 140
Ionizing radiation, effects of 101f
Iron 156
   deficiency anemia 140
      treatment of 156
   folic acid 445
   tablet 44, 217
Irritability 417
Isoniazid, high dose 367
Isoniazid-resistant tuberculosis 366
Itch mite 454

J

Janata Government Plan 36
Japanese encephalitis 318, 349, 374, 452
   prevention and control of 386
Jaundice 135, 374
   infectious 325
Joint pain 227
Jungalwala committee 33
Juvenile Justice (Care and Protection of Children) Act 239
Juvenile mass treatment 341

K

Kala-azar 316, 317
   strategies for elimination of 385
Kartar Singh committee 34
Kasturba Poshan Sahay Yojna 147
Keep food at safe temperatures 176
Key vital statistics, status of 23t
Khele India Khile India 447
Kidney 409
   diseases 403
Koch's postulate, limitations of 253
Koch's postulates 252
Krishnan committee 35
Kyasanur-forest disease 327, 374, 452,

L

Latrines, service type 108
Lead poisoning 399
Learning and adaptive system 63
Leishmania 316
   donovani 316
Leishmaniasis 316, 319
Leprosy 25, 340
   classification of 355
   treatment of 356
   type of 356
Leptospira, spread of 320
Leptospirosis 319, 325, 374
Levofloxacin 362, 367
Life index, physical quality of 14
Lifestyle and behavioral changes 205
Light 85
   measurement units 97
Lighting
   criteria 96
   types of 96f
Lignans 124

Linezolid 367
Liver 409
Lost life, years of 21
Louse 454
Low vision, functional 411
Lower gastrointestinal tract symptoms 173
Lung
   disease 435
   disorders 409
Lyme disease 258
Lymphatic filariasis 316, 452
   elimination of 316
      strategies for 385
Lymphedema, management of 316
Lymphogranuloma venereum 453

M

Macrominerals 127
Mahamari 323
Mahila Arogya Samiti 69
Malaria 24, 257, 309, 374
   control
      administrative framework, hierarchy of 381
      strategies 311
   diagnosis 382
   eliminate 383
      global technical strategy for 381
   epidemiology of 381
   free status, elimination and attainment of 382
   prevention 382
   treatment 382
   vaccine 312
Malaria plasmodium
   falciparum 452
   malariae 452
   ovale 452
   vivax 452
Malnutrition, double burden of 409
Malta fever 326
Man's environment, ecological changes in 320
Management and institutional reforms 80
Manodarpan 448
Manpower 82
   training and development 433
Mansonoides 453
Manure pits 108
Mass approach 201, 202
Mass blood survey 316
Mass media 191
Maternal and child health 210
Maternal mortality ratio 20

Meal and diet planning, concept of 132
Meal planning 132
   factors affecting 132
   steps of 132
Measles 258, 263, 275, 289, 348, 349, 374, 451
Meat food products order 179
Mechanical filters 90
Mechanical transmission 257
Medical education, significant changes in 32
Medical model 200
Medicine
   indigenous systems of 46
   vaccines and technology, access to 80
Mediterranean fever 326
Meningitis 295, 374
Meningococcal
   meningitis 374
   septicemia 295
Meningoencephalitis 374
Menstrual cycle, irregular 417
Menstrual hygiene 445
Mental dimension 15
Mental fitness 446
Mental status 224
Mentally healthy 15
Mesopotamian medicine 2
Metabolism 121
Metazoonoses 319
Metformin 401
Methylene blue reduction test 176
Miasmatic theory 248
Microfilaremia, asymptomatic 316
Microminerals 127
Micronutrient deficiencies 140
Mid-level health provider 53
   role of 53
Milk, pasteurization of 176
Miner's disease 305
Minerals 82, 124
   types of 127
Ministry of Women and Child Development,
      major schemes of 149
Mission 27
   POSHAN 2.0 144
Mission Indradhanush 141
   intensified 141, 158
Mite 454
Mitigation strategies 103
Modern era, theories of 249
Modern society, part of 189
Molluscum contagiosum 337, 453

Index

Monkey disease 327
Monkey pox 297, 452
Mononucleosis, infectious 257
Mono-resistant tuberculosis 366
Morbidity management and disability prevention 386
Mortality data, analysis of 241
Mortality indicators 19
Mortality rate, proportional 20
Mosquito cycle 310
Mother and Child Protection Card 141
Motivation 196, 200
Motivational model 200
Mouth and throat inspection 224
MPOWER strategy 437
Mucocutaneous leishmaniasis 317
Mucosa 256
Mud fever 325
Mudaliar committee 32
Multi-disciplinary teams 234
Multidrug-resistant tuberculosis 366
Multifactorial theory 250
Multiple organ dysfunction syndromes 325
Multipurpose health worker, role of 356
Multi-sectoral involvement 162
Mumps 290, 374, 451
Muscle
    cramps 416
    weak 417
Musculoskeletal disorders 227, 409
Musculoskeletal system inspection, assessment of 225
Mycobacterium
    indicus pranii vaccine 357
    leprae 253
Mycotoxins 170
Myocardial infarction, causation for 251f

N

Namami Gange 103
Narcotic Drugs and Psychotropic Substances Act 236
Nasha Mukt Bharat Abhiyaan 236
Nasha Mukti Abhiyan 64
National Action Plan for Dog Mediated Rabies Elimination 386
National Action Plan for Drug Demand Reduction 236
National Action Plan for Rabies Elimination, core components of 388
National AIDS Control Program 376, 430
National Air Quality Index 103, 118
National Bio-Diesel Mission 102
National Cancer Control Program 428
National Center for Disease Control 391
National Clean Air Program 118
National Consumer Disputes Redressal Forum 181
National Council for Human Resources 80
National Deworming Day 141, 153
National Digital Health Mission 71, 72
National Framework for Malaria Elimination 383
National Goiter Control Program 434
National Health Authority 72
National Health Mission 66
National Health Package 78
National Health Policy 61, 62, 64, 153
National Health Programs 46, 64, 287, 393
    related to Nutrition 144
National Heritage City Development and Augmentation Yojana 103
National Immunization Schedule 345t
National Iodine Deficiency Disorders Control Program 141, 434
National Leprosy Eradication Program 354, 357
    domains of 355
    objectives 355
    strategies 355
National Mental Health Survey 442
National Mission for Clean Ganga 103
National Nutrition Mission 141
National Nutritional Policy 142
National Program on Climate Change and Human Health 104
National Program for Control of Blindness and Visual Impairment 431
National Program for Healthcare of Elderly 424, 427
    specific objectives of 425
    vision of 425
National Program for Palliative Care 429
National Program for Prevention and Control of Cancer, Diabetes, Cardiovascular Diseases and Stroke 424
    Deafness 432, 433
National Rabies Control Program 387, 387f
National Rural Health Mission 66, 430
    major initiatives under 67
National Smart Grid Mission 103
National Solar Mission 103
National Strategic Plan 360

for Acquired Immunodeficiency Syndrome 378
for Human Immunodeficiency Virus 378
for Tuberculosis 360
National Tobacco Control Cell 436
National Tobacco Control Program 435, 436
structure of 436f
National Tuberculosis Elimination Program 358, 359
chronology of 358
Organogram 359
Structure comprises 359
National Urban Health Mission 67, 69
institutional framework of 69
National Vector Borne Disease Control Program 153, 380
evolution of 380
National Viral Hepatitis Control Management Unit 391
National Viral Hepatitis Control Program 389
Natural resources 82
Nausea 173
Neck inspection 225
Negative predictive value 286
Negri bodies 322
Neisseria meningitidis 295
Neonatal morbidity 166
Neonatal mortality 166
Nerve involvement, peripheral 355
Net domestic product 28
Net national product 28
Neurolathyrism 170
Neurological system, assessment of 226
Neuromuscular weakness 434
Newcastle disease 320
Nicotinic acid 125
NIKSHAY Mitra 371
NIKSHAY Poshan Yojana 367
NIKSHAY Patrika 372
NIKSHAY Sampark 372
NIPAH virus 332, 453
NIPUN Bharat 447
Nirbhaya Nari 64
NISHTHA 447
NITI Ayog 40
Nitrogen dioxide 99, 119
Noise 85, 98
pollution 100
Non-auditory effects 100
Non-communicable disease 393, 394, 400, 408, 409, 423

basics of 393
chronic 408
management of 399
prevention of 396
risk factors for 394, 396f, 397f, 398
screening for 423
Non-degradable pollutants 99
Non-governmental organizations 138
Non-institutional care 238
Nonketotic hyperosmolar diabetic coma 402
Non-persistent pollutants 98
Non-service type latrines 108
Non-typhoidal salmonellosis 374
Non-verbal cues
negative 194
positive 194
Normal diet, types of modification of 134
Nose inspection 224
Nurse
responsibilities of 214
role of 407
Nursing chart 230
Nursing diagnosis 210
Nursing process 206
Nutrient
content, modifications in 134
types of 122
Nutrition
basics of 121
counseling 217
of family 211
policy instruments 143
problems, major 142
rehabilitation center 163
supplementary 169
Nutrition education 136, 138
approaches 137
beneficiary groups for 139
methods of 136
program 138
Nutritional assessment
and nutrition education 121
methods 129
rationale for 129
Nutritional blindness, basic of 157
Nutritional intervention 205
Nutritional norms
per child 169
revised 148
Nutritional practices 136
Nutritional status

indicators 21
  of children 24
Nutrition-tuberculosis 372

O

O'byrne's distinction 205
Obese, causes of 409
Obesity 273, 408
  methods to diagnosis of 409
  prevention of 411
Observation homes 238
Occult filariasis 316
Occupation 17
Occupational hazards 320
Ochratoxin A 170
Odd's ratio, interpretation of 268
Old age homes 236
Oncology wing, development of 429
One stop center 232
Open shelters 238
Operational standards 237
Opioid substitution therapy 376
Oral cancer 421, 423, 435
  management algorithm for 422f
  risk factors for 421
  signs of 421
  symptoms of 421
Oral pills 44
Oral rehydration
  solution distribution 161
  therapy 174
    establishment of 162
Oral visual examination 423
Oriental sore 316
Orphanages 236, 239
Oryzanol 124
Osmolarity ORS formulation 175t
Osteoarthritis 409
Otitis media 290, 446
Ottawa charter for health promotion 204, 204f
Outbreak investigation, objectives of 276
Outreach 68
Ovary 409
Overcrowding 86
Overweight, causes of 409

P

Padhe Bharat Badhe Bharat 447
Palliative care 239, 429
  centers 236
    continuum 430f

Palpitations 417
Panchayati Raj 48
  Institutions 39, 44, 437
Panel discussion 202
Pantothenic acid 125
Paramedical health staff 373
Paramparagat Krishi Vikas Yojana 103
Paris Agreement 103
Paroxysmal stage 294
Partnerships, inclusive 63
Pea pickers disease 325
Pediculosis 342
Pelvic inflammatory disease 336
People empowerment 207
Periodic fluctuation 280
Peripheral vascular system inspection,
  assessment of 226
Permanent hardness 87
Persistent pollutants 98
Personal health records 72, 73
  module 73
Personal protective measures 311
Persons per room 86
Pertussis 294, 374, 451
Pheochromocytoma 403
Phlebotomus
  argentipes 317
  papatasi 317
Phosphatase test 176
Physical abuse 233
Physical activity 395, 398
Physical dimension 14
Physical exercise 273
Physical fitness 446
Pituitary gland 415
  dysfunction 416
Place distribution 280
Plague 275, 319, 323, 374
Planned behavior
  limitations of theory of 186
  theory of 184, 186
Planning Nutrition Education Programs 138f
Plasma glucose level 401
Pluralism 63
Pneumococcal conjugate vaccine 348
Pneumoconiosis 399
Pneumonia 325
Pneumonic plague 323,
Policies 27
Polio 257, 374
  vaccine, fractional inactivated 347

Poliomyelitis 301
    poliovirus 451
Political system 17
Pollutants
    primary 99
    secondary 99
Pollution
    kinds of 98
    types of 99
Poly-drug resistant tuberculosis 366
Poor ventilation, drawbacks of 96
Population
    aging of 17
    attributable risk 271
    strategy 274
    target 68
Poshan 2.0, objectives of 145
Poshan Abhiyaan 232
    and Mission Poshan 144
Poshan Maah 145
Poshan Vatika 145
Positive predictive value 286
Post-exposure prophylaxis 357
Post-kala-azar dermal leishmaniasis 317
Postnatal care 217
Postpasteurization tests 176
Post-vedic period 5
Post-visit phase 213
Potassium
    chloride 175
    permanganate 94
Potential life lost, years of 20
Poverty-malnutrition, vicious cycle of 142f
Pradhan Mantri Ayushman Bharat Health Infrastructure Mission 70
Pradhan Mantri Jan Arogya Yojana 74-77
Pradhan Mantri Krishi Sinchayee Yojana 103
Pradhan Mantri Matru Vandana Yojana 146, 147, 232
Pradhan Mantri Poshan Shakti Nirman 168, 447
Prediabetes, diagnosis of 401
Premodern era, theories of 248
Pre-pasteurization test 176
Pre-visit phase 213
Primary Health Center 49, 408f, 427
Primary healthcare 50
    approach 200
    comprehensive 50, 75
    elements of 50
    principles of 50
    provision of 223
Primitive medicine 1

Program execution and expansion 433
Propaganda and health education 200t
Prophylactic iron 155
Protein-energy malnutrition 139
Proteins 123
    types 123
Protozoa diseases 316
Public education, system of 439
Public health 1, 5, 243, 284
    days, list of important 458
    development of 5, 6
    important environmental legislation, list of 112
Public hospitals 64
Pulmonary tuberculosis 363
Punitive theory 248
Pupae index 313
Purification of water on
    large scale 90
    small scale 93
Pustule, malignant 324
Pyrazinamide 367
Pyridoxine 125

Q

Q fever 258, 452
Quality of life 14
    indicators of 22
Quality-adjusted life years 21
Quarantine Act 5

R

Rabies 263, 319, 321, 452
    immunoglobin 322
    virus 253
Radiation pollution 101
Radioactive iodine 417
Randomized controlled trial
    advantages of 273
    disadvantages of 273
Rapid diagnostic tests 311
Rapid sand filter 90, 91
Rashtriya Bal Swasthya Karyakram 141, 441, 443f, 445
Rashtriya Kishor Swasthya Karyakram 441
Record
    admission 229
    clinical 229
    importance of 229
    keeping 228
    nurses 229
    principles of 229

Index

purposes of 228
types of 229
Rectum 409
  inspection, assessment of 225
Referral services complex 34
Referral site
  care at 399
  management at 228
Refresher training 219
Refuse 106
Regular periodic surveys 375
Rehabilitation
  phase 165
  services 427
Reinforcement 201
Relapse 312
Renal disease, chronic 403
Renovascular disease 403
Reproductive tract infections 217
Resources, assessment of 30
Respiratory disease 374
  chronic 394
Respiratory disorders 399
Respiratory distress 374
Respiratory infections 287, 402
Respiratory system, assessment of 225
Retrospective cohort studies 270, 281
Rheumatic heart disease 405, 425, 446
Riboflavin 125
Rice bran oil 124
Rickettsial diseases 329
Rifampicin 356, 362, 367
  resistant tuberculosis 366
Right to Education Act 442
Rights of Consumer 181
Road traffic accidents 374
Rogi Kalyan Samiti 42, 44
  composition of 45
  objectives of 44
Rota vaccine 160
Rota virus 347, 348
Roundworm 307
Routine health check-up 223
Routine immunization session, types of 354
Rubella 263, 291, 349, 374, 451
Rule of Halves 404
Rural Primary Healthcare Institutions 38

S

Safe water and raw materials, use of 176
Safer food, keys to 175
Saline intrusion 89
Salmonella 169, 451
Salmonellosis 320
Samagra shiksha 447
Samuel hahneman 3
Sand fly 85, 454
Sanitary latrine 108
  criteria for 109
Sanitary ventilation 95
Sanitation 82, 447
Saprozoonoses 319
SARTHAQ 447
Sarva Shiksha Abhiyan 442
Scabies 341, 446
Schistosomiasis 319
School health
  history of 439
  nurse, role of 445
  objectives of 441
  promotion activities 444
School Health Committee 440
School Health Program 439, 445
  objectives of 441
School health services
  components of 443
  objectives of 441
School nutrition gardens 169
Screening test, example of 286
Scrub typhus 374, 453
Secular trend 280
Selected health conditions 446
Selective mass treatment 341
Separate raw 176
Sepsis 309
Septicemic plague 323, 452
Serum hepatitis 302
Services, expanded range of 52
Sesame oil 124
Set back 85
Sewage 106
  aerobic oxidation of 111
  treatment
    modern 110
    plant, process flow 110*f*
Sex separation 86
Sexual abuse 234
Sexual cycle 310
Sexually transmitted diseases 336
Shaken infant 233
Shigellosis 374
Sick
  care of 211
  person 240

Sickle cell anemia 446
Sick-role behavior 183
Siddha system of medicine 3
Similia Similbus Curentur 3
Single remedy 3
Skilled home 213
Skin 256
    conditions 446
    fold thickness 410
    lesions 355
    smear 355
Sleeping, problems 417
Slim disease 335
Slow sand filter 91
Smallpox 287, 451
Smart cities mission 103
Smog 99
Smoking 251, 273
Social behavior change communication,
    principles of 197
Social change 195
Social cognitive theory 185
Social dimension 15
Social inclusion and environmental sustainability 55
Social indicators 22
Social intervention model 200
Social marketing approach 137
Social mobilization 197
Socio-ecological model 196, 196*f*
Socio-economic
    conditions 17
    indicators 22
Sodium chloride 175
Soft tick 454
Soil health card scheme 103
Soil pollution 100
Soil-transmitted helminths 305, 442
Solar powered toll plazas 103
Solid waste
    disposal, methods of 107
    health hazard of 107
    management
        rules 112
        system 107*f*
Special homes 238
Specific diseases, diet in 135
Spiritual dimension 15
Staphylococcal food poisoning 451
Staphylococcus aureus 169
Starches 123

State Consumer Disputes Redressal Forum 181
State surveillance unit 375
State viral hepatitis management unit 392
Steroids 417
Stool specimens 174
Strategic information management systems 377
Strengthening institutional capacities 377
Stress 395
    reduce 64
Stroke 394, 406, 408*f*
    presenting features of 406
    risk factors for 406
Study design 267
Study population, selection of 269
Sub-national disease certification 370
Subnormal intelligence 434
Subsidiarity 63
Substance abuse 232, 235
Sulfonylureas 401
Sullage 106
Sulphur dioxide 99, 119
Sungai NIPAH 332
Superchlorination 93
Supervision
    approach, types of 218
    importance of 218
Supplementary nutrition, postnatal check-up 44
Supplementary strategies 426
Supportive supervision 218, 219*f*
    steps of 219
Sustainable cities and communities 68
Sustainable development goals 56*f*
Swachh Bharat Abhiyan 64
Swachh Bharat Mission 103
Swadhar Greh Scheme 232
Swamp fever 325
Swasth Nagrik Abhiyan 64
Swine flu 452
Swineherd's disease 325
Syndrome identification 247
Syndromic surveillance 373
Syphilis 257, 453
    primary 337

T

Taeniasis 319, 330, 453
Tanks 88
Telecommunication 192
Television 202
Temporary hardness 87
Terrestrial ecosystem 83

Index

Tetanus 263, 339, 452
Thiamine 125
Thyroid
  diseases 415
  gland 415
  hormone
    regulation of 415f
    synthesis of 434
  scan 417
  ultrasound 417
Thyroiditis 416
Thyroxine 434
Tick 258, 454
Tithi Bhojan 168
Tobacco
  control 398
    cells 437
  dangerous impact of 395, 395f
  use, levels of prevention of 435
Tones formula 205
Total mass treatment 341
Toxic elements 99
Toxic nodular goiter 416
Toxoplasmosis 319
Trace mineral 127
Trachoma 338, 452
Transform malaria surveillance 382
Transient ischemic attack 406
  presenting features of 407
Transition phase 165
Transovarial transmission 258
Transstadial transmission 258
Transtheoretical model 184, 187
  limitations of 188
Tremor 417
Treponema pallidum 336
Triatomine bug 454
Trichothecenes 170
Tridosha theory 2
Triiodothyronine 434
Trisodium citrate 175
Trypanasomes 257
Tse tse fly 454
Tuberculin skin test 362
Tuberculosis 25, 258, 295, 320, 358, 374, 451
  Arogya Sathi 372
  cascade of 362
  infection 361
    diagnosis of 362
    overview of 361
  medications 368
  preventive treatment 361
  symptoms of 370
  treatment of 366
  type of 358
  unit level 360
Tunnel disease 305
Twin pillar strategy 316
Typhoid 227, 299, 374
  fever 257, 451
Typical water purification, components of 90

U

Ujjawala scheme 232
Ultraviolet irradiation 94
Unani medicine 2
Unclean hands and fingers 259
Undulant fever 326
Unique health ID 72
Universal access 68
Universal health coverage 77, 78f
  areas of 79
  expected outcomes of 79
  guiding principles of 79
  vision of 75, 78, 79f
Universal Immunization Program 343
  objectives of 344
Unsafe food, punishment for 180
Unusual syndromes 374
Upper gastrointestinal tract symptoms 173
Urban accredited social health activist 69
Urban beneficiaries 76
Urban health 64
  care facilities 69f
Urban issues 68
Urban primary healthcare 38
  principles of 68
Urban Social Health Activist 69
Urine sugar 220
Utilization rates 22

V

Vaccination 262
  Act 5
Vaccine
  administration of 352f
  contraindication of 353
  preventable disease 282, 374
  reaction, common 353
Vector control 311
Vector-borne disease 102, 257, 282, 374
  classification of 257

Index

Vectors transmit agent 257
Vegetable oil products order 179
Vehicle-borne 257
Ventilation 95, 447
   assessment of 96
Verbal communication 192
   skills 194
Village Health and Nutrition Days 42, 44, 141
Village Health Sanitation and Nutrition Committee 42
Viral hepatitis 302
Virus infected mosquitoes, transportation of 320
Visceral leishmaniasis 317
Vision 26
   impairment 446
Vision 2020 412
   structure of 413f
Visual impairment 411
   moderate 411
      severe 411
   prevalence of severe 411
   severe 411
Vital signs 224
Vitamin 124
   A 125, 350
      basic of 157
      prophylactic 158, 412
   A deficiency 140, 412
      signs of 157f
      treatment of 158
   B1 125
   B12 125, 126
   B2 125, 126
   B3 125, 126
   B5 125, 126
   B6 125, 126
   B7 126
   B9 125, 126
   C 125, 127, 153
   D 125
   E 125
   K 125
   types of 126
Vocal for local 169
Vocational dimension 16
Voluntary health agencies 46
Vomiting 173
Vomitus 174

W

Wage compensation 166
Waist circumference 410
Waist height ratio 411
Waist hip ratio 410
Waste 106
   management 106
   types of 106f
Water 85, 87, 447
   based diseases 88
   breeding diseases 88
   chlorination of 92, 92f
   ground 88
   hardness of 87
   household purification of 93
   pollution 99
   related diseases 88
   removal of hardness of 87f
   remove hardness of 87
   requirement 87
   safe and wholesome 87
   sanitation and hygiene 217
   seal performs 109
   soluble vitamins 125
   source of 88
   surface 88
   uses of 87
   washed diseases 88
Water distribution 89
   systems of 89
Water purification 90
   method 95
Water-borne disease 88, 102, 227, 374, 389
   outbreak 282
Weighment diet survey 130
Weight loss 417
Weight status, classification of 410t
Weil's disease 325
Well
   artesian 89
   chlorination of 94
   deep 89
   kutcha 89
   masonry 89
   pucca 89
   sanitary 89
   shallow 89
   steps 89
   tube 89
Wheel theory 251
Whooping cough 294, 451
Wilson and Jungner criteria 285
Women empowerment 232
Women helpline, universalization of 232
Wool sorter's disease 324

Index

Work, type of 457*t*
Working women hostel 232
Workmen Compensation Act 5
World Trade Organization 177

X

Xerophthalmia, classification of 157, 412

Y

Yang and Yin principle 2
Yatri suraksha 64
Yaws 340, 453
Yellow fever 320, 374, 452
Yersinia enteroclitica 169

Z

Zero human rabies death 387
Zika 452
Zooanthroponoses 319
Zoonoses
    classification of 319
    direct 319
    influencing prevalence of 320
Zoonotic cutaneous leishmaniasis 317
Zoonotic disease 319
    outbreaks 282
Zoonotic infection 319